Diabetic Nephropathy: Pathophysiology and Clinical Management

Diabetic Nephropathy: Pathophysiology and Clinical Management

Editor: Robin Wayne

AMERICAN
MEDICAL PUBLISHERS
www.americanmedicalpublishers.com

AMERICAN
MEDICAL PUBLISHERS
www.americanmedicalpublishers.com

Cataloging-in-Publication Data

Diabetic nephropathy : pathophysiology and clinical management / edited by Robin Wayne.
p. cm.
Includes bibliographical references and index.
ISBN 978-1-63927-114-6
1. Diabetic nephropathies. 2. Diabetic nephropathies--Pathophysiology. 3. Diabetic nephropathies--Treatment.
4. Diabetes--Complications. 5. Kidneys--Diseases. I. Wayne, Robin.
RC918.D53 D53 2022
616.462--dc23

American Medical Publishers,
41 Flatbush Avenue,
1st Floor, New York,
NY 11217, USA

ISBN 978-1-63927-114-6 (Hardback)

Contents

Preface

The purpose of the book is to provide a glimpse into the dynamics and to present opinions and studies of some of the scientists engaged in the development of new ideas in the field from very different standpoints. This book will prove useful to students and researchers owing to its high content quality.

Diabetic nephropathy is a chronic loss of kidney function. It occurs in people suffering from diabetes mellitus. Due to the damage of glomeruli, it causes protein loss in the urine. It also causes low serum albumin that eventually results in nephrotic syndrome. The initial symptoms of diabetic nephropathy appear after five to ten years of its beginning. The first symptom includes nocturia, which is frequent urination at night. Other general symptoms include tiredness, nausea, vomiting, headaches, lack of appetite, itchy skin and swelling in legs. People previously suffering from diabetes have higher possibilities of acquiring diabetic nephropathy. Its risk factors include poor control of blood glucose, uncontrolled high blood pressure, smoking, and a family history of diabetic nephropathy. ACE inhibitor medications are used to reduce the levels of proteinuria and to slow down the progression of diabetic nephropathy. This book presents researches and studies performed by experts across the globe. From theories to research to practical applications, case studies related to all contemporary topics of relevance to this disease have been included herein. This book will serve as a reference to a broad spectrum of readers.

At the end, I would like to appreciate all the efforts made by the authors in completing their chapters professionally. I express my deepest gratitude to all of them for contributing to this book by sharing their valuable works. A special thanks to my family and friends for their constant support in this journey.

Editor

1

Artificially Cultivated *Ophiocordyceps sinensis* Alleviates Diabetic Nephropathy and Its Podocyte Injury via Inhibiting P2X7R Expression and NLRP3 Inflammasome Activation

Chao Wang, Xiao-xia Hou, Hong-liang Rui, Li-jing Li, Jing Zhao, Min Yang, Li-jun Sun, Hong-rui Dong, Hong Cheng, and Yi-Pu Chen

Division of Nephrology, Beijing Anzhen Hospital, Capital Medical University, Beijing 100029, China

Correspondence should be addressed to Hong Cheng; Drchengh@163.com and Yi-Pu Chen; chen_yipu@163.com

Academic Editor: Claudia Rodrigues

Background/Aims. It is known that chronic low-grade inflammation contributes to the initiation and development of both diabetes and diabetic nephropathy (DN), so we designed this study to investigate the role of P2X7R and NLRP3 inflammasome in DN pathogenesis and the antagonistic effects of artificially cultivated *Ophiocordyceps sinensis* (ACOS). *Methods.* A rat model of DN caused by high-fat-diet feeding and low-dose streptozotocin injection and a mouse podocyte injury model induced by high-glucose (HG) stimulation were established, and the intervention effects of ACOS on them were observed. The biological parameters of serum and urine and the pathological manifestations of kidney tissue were examined. The expression of mRNA and protein of P2X7R and NLRP3 inflammasome (NLRP3, ASC, and caspase-1) and downstream effectors (IL-1β and IL-18), as well as podocyte-associated molecules, was determined by real-time quantitative PCR and Western blot assay, respectively. *Results.* The DN rats showed to have developed insulin resistance, elevated fasting blood glucose, increased urinary protein excretion, and serum creatinine level as well as corresponding glomerular pathological alterations including podocyte damages. ACOS significantly antagonized the above changes. The experiments *in vivo* and *in vitro* both displayed that the mRNA and protein expression of P2X7R, NLRP3, ASC, caspasel (procaspase-1 mRNA in the gene level and active caspase-1 subunit P10 in the protein level), IL-1β, and IL-18 was significantly upregulated and the mRNA and protein expression of podocyte-associated molecules was significantly changed (downregulation of nephrin, podocin, and WT-1 expression and upregulation of desmin expression) indicating podocyte injury in the kidney tissue of DN rats and in the HG-stressed mouse podocytes, respectively. ACOS also significantly antagonized all the above changes. *Conclusion.* Our research work suggests that P2X7R and NLRP3 inflammasome are involved in the pathogenesis of DN, and ACOS can effectively inhibit the high expression of P2X7R and the activation of NLRP3 inflammasome, which may contribute to the therapeutic effects of *Ophiocordyceps sinensis*.

1. Introduction

The global prevalence of diabetes has dramatically increased over the recent decades. The International Diabetes Federation reported that the overall prevalence of diabetes was estimated to be 8.8% in people aged 20~79 years worldwide in 2015, which was predicted to rise to 10.4% in 2040 [1]. The China Noncommunicable Disease Surveillance Group reported that the overall prevalence of diabetes was estimated to be 11.6% and the prevalence of prediabetes in Chinese adult population aged 18 years or older was estimated to be 50.1% in 2010 [2]. Diabetic nephropathy (DN), also known as diabetic kidney disease (DKD), is one of the most common chronic microvascular complications of diabetes, which is the leading cause of end-stage renal disease (ESRD) in developed countries and the second cause of ESRD in China [3]. So, diabetes with its kidney complication, DN, has become a worldwide public health problem that seriously threatens human health.

DN is a glomerular disease. Now, it has been recognized that podocyte injury is a pivotal event in the pathogenesis of DN [4]. However, the underlying mechanism of podocyte injury in DN has not been fully clarified. A growing number of studies show that diabetes is characterized by chronic low-grade inflammation, referred to as "metaflammation," which is a relevant factor contributing to the initiation and development of both diabetes and its complications including DN [5–7]. In the past years, it was discovered that the expression of purinergic 2X7 receptor (P2X7R) was significantly upregulated in glomerular cells, mainly in podocytes, in diabetic rat models [8]. It was also observed that the nucleotide-binding oligomerization domain-like receptor protein 3 (NLRP3) inflammasome activation in glomerular cells including podocytes was associated with the onset of DN, while NLRP3 inflammasome deficiency or inhibition could ameliorate DN in mouse models [7, 9]. The above studies have drawn our attention to the pathogenic role of P2X7R and NLRP3 inflammasome in DN.

P2X7R is a member of the P2XR family. It is characterized by the response to extracellular ATP (eATP), with a rapid opening of a ligand-gated cation channel, resulting in potassium ion (K^+) efflux and intracellular potassium depletion. When the level of intracellular potassium reduces below the threshold of 90 mM, the assembly and activation of NLRP3 inflammasome are initiated [10–12]. The NLRP3 inflammasome is an intracellular multiprotein complex consisting of NLRP3, apoptosis-associated speck-like protein containing a caspase recruitment domain (ASC, adaptor protein), and cysteinyl aspartate specific protease-1 (caspase-1, effect protein). Caspase-1 usually exists as an inactive precursor procaspase-1, which can be self-enzymatically hydrolyzed to its active forms, P10 and P20 subunits, during the assembly and activation of NLRP3 inflammasome. The active P10/P20 subunits can turn the inactive precursors of interleukin 1 beta (IL-1β) and IL-18 into the mature forms to induce inflammation [13–15]. In this study, we investigated the relationship between P2X7R with its downstream NLRP3 inflammasome and DN and inspected the effects of *Ophiocordyceps sinensis* on them.

Ophiocordyceps sinensis (once called *Cordyceps sinensis*), a fungus-caterpillar complex formed after the fungus infects the larva of the moth that belongs to Hepialidae, is a well-known traditional Chinese medicine and has been used for centuries in China and Asian countries. Clinical practice and experimental studies have shown that it is effective in the treatment of many kinds of kidney diseases including DN [16–18]. However, so far, there have been no reports of the effects of *Ophiocordyceps sinensis* on P2X7R and NLRP3 inflammasome, as we did in this study. Wild *Ophiocordyceps sinensis* is now too scarce to meet the medical needs in China. So, artificially cultivated *Ophiocordyceps sinensis* (ACOS) has been highly expected for a long time. Fortunately, it has finally succeeded in recent years (Figure 1) [19–21]. In this study, we utilized the ACOS instead of wild *Ophiocordyceps sinensis* for the experiments *in vivo* and *in vitro*, which is the first experimental study of ACOS in the treatment of diseases.

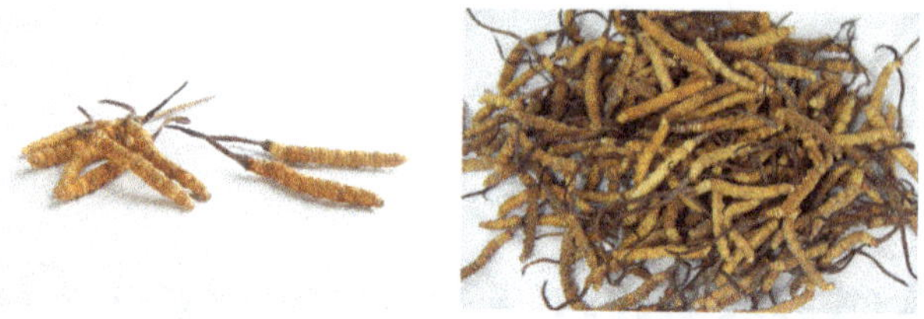

FIGURE 1: Artificially cultivated *Ophiocordyceps sinensis* (ACOS). *Ophiocordyceps sinensis* is a fungus-caterpillar complex formed after the fungus infects the larva of the moth that belongs to Hepialidae. The black part of the complex is the fungal part that is called the fruiting body and consists of stromatophore and stroma; the yellowish-brown part is the dead larva body that is filled with mycelia, called the sclerotium. The *Ophiocordyceps sinensis* in this photo is the ACOS, which has been produced through industrialized artificial cultivation in China now.

In this study, we established a rat model of DN caused by type 2 DM and a mouse podocyte injury model induced by high-glucose (HG) stress and then studied the role of P2X7R and NLRP3 inflammasome in the pathogenesis of DN and the antagonistic effects of ACOS by using these models.

2. Materials and Methods

2.1. Animals and Grouping. Thirty-two male Sprague-Dawley rats weighing 180–200 g at the age of 6 weeks were purchased from Vital River Laboratory Animal Technology Co. (Beijing, China) and were housed in an animal room of specific-pathogen-free cleanliness grade with 50–60% humidity at temperature 20–26°C. Rats were randomly and equally divided into the following 4 groups: control group, DN model group, intervention group with a low dose of ACOS, and intervention group with a high dose of ACOS (HEC Pharm Co., China). The rats in the control group were fed with ordinary chow (energy ratio: fat—12.11%, protein—22.47%, and carbohydrates—65.42%), while the rats in the other three groups were fed with high-fat chow (energy ratio: fat—45.65%, protein—16.46%, and carbohydrates—37.89%). At the end of the 4th week, the insulin resistance index (IRI) was measured with the HOMA-IR formula in the rats fed with high-fat chow. After insulin resistance was confirmed, the rats in the DN model group and two intervention groups were intraperitoneally injected with streptozotocin (Sigma, USA) in a single dose of 35 mg/kg, while the rats in the control group were only injected with an equivalent volume of buffer. 72 h after the injection, the fasting blood glucose (FBG) of each rat was tested and rats are considered to have type 2 DM when their FBG level is >11.1 mmol/L. From the 5th week, the rats in the low- and high-dose intervention groups were given ACOS by gavage in a dose of 2.5 g/kg (LD-ACOS group) and 5.0 g/kg (HD-ACOS group), respectively, every day for 8 weeks, while the rats in the control and model groups were given the equal volume of tap water by gavage every day for 8 weeks.

2.2. Biological Parameters. Body weight was measured at baseline and at the 4th and 13th week. Kidney weight was measured after the rat was sacrificed, and then the ratio of kidney weight/body weight (KW/BW) of each rat was calculated. Urinary protein excretion of 24 h urine sample was tested at baseline and the 13th week. Serum creatinine (SCr) was detected at the 13th week. FBG was detected at the 4th and 13th week and also at 72 h after streptozotocin injection. Glycated hemoglobin (HbA1c) was measured at the 13th week. Fasting insulin was detected at the 4th and 13th week, and then IRI was calculated using the HOMA-IR formula: IRI = fasting blood glucose (mmol/L) × fasting insulin (mIU/L)/22.5 [22, 23].

2.3. Pathological Examination. After the renal tissue was conventionally processed, the 3 μm thick sections were stained with a periodic acid-Schiff reagent for light microscopy. Twenty images of glomerular maximal profiles with a vascular pole and/or urinary pole were taken under a high-power microscope (×400, Olympus, Japan) and were analyzed by Nikon NIS-Elements BR image analysis software (Nikon, Japan). The length (μm) of the two longest perpendicular diameters in every glomerular capillary tuft without Bowman's space was measured, and then the mean value was calculated. The areas of the glomerular mesangial region and capillary tuft were also measured, and then the relative area of the mesangial region (%) was calculated according to the formula: area of the mesangial region/area of the capillary tuft × 100%.

After the renal tissue was processed according to standard techniques. The ultrathin sections were stained with uranium acetate-lead citrate for electron microscopy. For each specimen, ten photographs (×20,000 magnification) covering different regions in the glomerular cross section were taken separately. The length (μm) of the peripheral GBM was measured, and the number of slit pores overlying this GBM length was counted by Nikon NIS-Elements BR image analysis software (Nikon, Japan). The mean of the foot process width ($\bar{W}_{FP}$) was calculated as follows [24]:

$$\bar{W}_{FP} = \frac{\pi}{4} \cdot \frac{\sum \text{GBM length}}{\sum \text{slits}}, \quad (1)$$

where $\sum$slits is the total number of slits counted and $\sum$GBM length is the total GBM length measured in one glomerulus.

2.4. Double Immunofluorescence Staining. For the double staining of an indirect immunofluorescence assay of P2X7R/NLRP3 and podocyte marker synaptopodin, frozen renal tissues of rats were cut into 5 μm thick sections. A rabbit anti-P2X7R polyclonal antibody (1 : 100 dilution, Alomone) or rabbit anti-NLRP3 polyclonal antibody (1 : 100 dilution, Novus) and mouse anti-synaptopodin monoclonal antibody (1 : 50 dilution, Santa Cruz) were used as primary antibodies. Rhodamine-labeled goat anti-rabbit immunoglobulins (Beijing Zhongshan) and FITC-labeled goat anti-mouse immunoglobulins (Beijing Zhongshan) were used as secondary antibodies, respectively. After staining, the tissue sections were observed with a fluorescent microscope (Nikon, Japan).

2.5. Podocyte Culture and Grouping. The conditionally immortalized mouse podocyte cell line was kindly provided by Professor Maria Pia Rastaldi (S. Carlo Hospital, University of Milan). Podocytes were incubated in RPMI-1640 medium (Thermo Fisher Scientific) containing 10% inactivated fetal bovine serum (FBS, Thermo Fisher Scientific) and 10 μ/mL interferon-γ (IFN-γ, Cell Signaling Technology) at 33°C in a humidified air with 5% CO_2. When the cells reached 80–90% confluence, they were transferred to RPMI-1640 medium containing 10% inactivated FBS without IFN-γ and incubated at 37°C in a humidified air with 5% CO_2 for 10–14 days to allow differentiation.

Well-differentiated podocytes were used for experiments. The podocytes were incubated in the RPMI-1640 medium with 5% inactivated FBS and grouped as follows: medium alone (control group), medium containing 30 mM glucose (Sigma) (HG group), medium containing 50 μg/mL ACOS extract (HEC Pharm Co., China) (ACOS control group), and medium containing both 30 mM glucose and 50 μg/mL ACOS extract (HG + ACOS group). According to the LDH release test, 30 mM glucose had no cytotoxic effects on cellular viability (Table 1S, see Supplementary Materials).

2.6. Reverse Transcription and Real-Time Quantitative PCR. Total RNA was extracted from rat renal cortex tissue or cultured podocytes using TRIzol reagent (Invitrogen) following the manufacturer's instructions. 2 μg total RNA from each sample was reverse-transcribed to cDNA with Easy-Script First-Strand cDNA Synthesis SuperMix (TransGen Biotech). The gene-specific primers (SBS Genetech) are listed in Tables 1 and 2. RT-PCR was performed using SYBR Green RT-PCR Master Mix (TransGen Biotech) according to the manufacturer's instruction. The GAPDH was set as the internal control gene in the animal and cellular experiments. The relative quantity of mRNA expression was calculated according to the formula: $2^{-(\text{targetgeneCt} - \text{GAPDHCt})} \times 10^3$, in which Ct was the threshold cycle number. All assays were repeated at least in triplicate independently.

2.7. Western Blot Assay. Total protein lysates were extracted from rat renal cortex tissue or cultured podocytes using RIPA lysis buffer (ComWin Biotech). Protein samples were sonicated five times for 1 s each, centrifuged at 12000 rpm for 10 min at 4°C, and then boiled for 5 min. Protein samples were separated by 10–12% sodium dodecyl sulphate-polyacrylamide gel electrophoresis (SDS-PAGE) and transferred to nitrocellulose membranes (General Electric Co.). After being blocked with 5% skim milk in phosphate-buffered saline with 0.1% Tween 20 for 1 h, the membranes were incubated with a primary antibody at 4°C overnight and then incubated with a secondary antibody at room temperature for 1 h. Details regarding primary and secondary antibodies are listed in Table 3. The blotted proteins were quantified using the Odyssey Infrared Imaging System (LI-COR Biosciences). β-Actin was set as an internal control. The relative expression level of each target protein was displayed as a ratio of target protein/β-actin protein. All the assays were performed at least in triplicate independently.

Table 1: Primer sequences for PCR analysis in animal experiments.

Target	Primer sequence (5′–3′)	Length (bp)
Nephrin	Forward CTGGGGGACAGTGGATTGAC Reverse CCACCAACTGCAAAGAGCAC	158
Podocin	Forward GCTGTCTGCTACTACCGCAT Reverse GTGAGGGATCGATGTGCCAA	125
WT-1	Forward TGCGTCCTATCAGGTTTGCC Reverse CCCAGCGAAATGAGCACAAG	188
Desmin	Forward CTGAGCAAAGGGGTTCCGA Reverse GTGTGACATCCGAGAGTGGA	185
P2X7R	Forward TAACCACTGAGCCGTCCCTA Reverse AGGTCCTCATGCTTGTGCTC	127
NLRP3	Forward TAGCTTCTGCCGAGGTCTCT Reverse ATTGATGGGTCAGTCCGCAG	176
ASC	Forward ACAGTACCAGGCAGTTCGTG Reverse GGTCTGTCACCAAGTAGGGC	143
Procaspase-1	Forward CCGGGGATCCCTCTTCATTG Reverse ACCCTTTCAGTGGTTGGCAT	144
IL-1β	Forward AGGCTGACAGACCCCAAAAG Reverse CTCCACGGGCAAGACATAGG	178
IL-18	Forward ACCGCAGTAATACGGAGCAT Reverse GTCTGGGATTCGTTGGCTGT	110
GAPDH	Forward TGGGTGTGAACCACGAGAA Reverse GGCATGGACTGTGGTCATGA	143

Table 2: Primer sequences for PCR analysis in cellular experiments.

Target	Primer sequence (5′–3′)	Length (bp)
Nephrin	Forward GTCTGGGGACCCCTCTATGA Reverse CAGGTCTTCTCCAAGGCTGT	209
Podocin	Forward CAGAAGGGGAAAAGGCTGCT Reverse GATGCTCCCTTGTGCTCTGT	200
WT-1	Forward TCCGGTCAGCATCTGAAACC Reverse GAGCTGGTCTGAGCGAGAAA	179
Desmin	Forward GTTTCAGACTTGACTCAGGCAG Reverse TCTCGCAGGTGTAGGACTGG	106
P2X7R	Forward CACCGTGCTTACAGGTGCTA Reverse CGGTCTTGGGGAACTCCTTC	115
NLRP3	Forward TCTGCACCCGGACTGTAAAC Reverse CATTGTTGCCCAGGTTCAGC	131
ASC	Forward GACAGTGCAACTGCGAGAAG Reverse CGACTCCAGATAGTAGCTGACAA	106
Procaspase-1	Forward ACAAGGCACGGGACCTATG Reverse TCCCAGTCAGTCCTGGAAATG	237
IL-1β	Forward CGCAGCAGCACATCAACAAG Reverse GTGCTCATGTCCTCATCCTG	118
IL-18	Forward ACTTTGGCCGACTTCACTGT Reverse GTCTGGTCTGGGGTTCACTG	135
GAPDH	Forward TGTGAACGGATTTGGCCGTA Reverse GATGGGCTTCCCGTTGATGA	202

Table 3: Primary and secondary antibodies for Western blot assays.

Primary antibody	Secondary antibody
Rabbit anti-nephrin pAb (Abcam)	IRDye 800-conjugated goat anti-rabbit IgG antibody (LI-COR)
Rabbit anti-podocin pAb (Sigma)	Ditto
Rabbit anti-WT-1 pAb (Abcam)	Ditto
Rabbit anti-desmin pAb (Abcam)	Ditto
Rabbit anti-P2X7R pAb (Alomone)	Ditto
Rabbit anti-NLRP3 pAb (Novus)	Ditto
Rabbit anti-ASC pAb (Santa Cruz)	Ditto
Rabbit anti-caspase-P10 pAb (Santa Cruz)	Ditto
Rabbit anti-IL-1β pAb (Abcam)	Ditto
Mouse anti-IL-18 mAb (Santa Cruz)	IRDye 680-conjugated goat anti-mouse IgG antibody (LI-COR)
Mouse anti-β-actin mAb (Sigma)	Ditto

Table 4: Biological parameters in the different groups at the 13th week ($\bar{x} \pm s$).

Group	BW (g)	KW/BW (mg/g)	FBG (mmol/L)	HbA1c (%)	SCr (μmol/L)	Upro (mg/d)
Control	526.9 ± 51.5	6.1 ± 0.3	6.95 ± 0.53	11.8 ± 0.7	24.9 ± 2.6	6.0 ± 1.5
Model	$452.9 \pm 41.1^{*}$	$8.8 \pm 1.5^{*}$	$32.58 \pm 1.31^{**}$	$20.3 \pm 0.9^{**}$	$34.8 \pm 4.9^{*}$	$33.8 \pm 9.7^{*}$
LD-ACOS	$438.7 \pm 50.1^{*}$	$8.5 \pm 1.1^{*}$	$30.96 \pm 4.03^{**}$	$20.0 \pm 1.1^{**}$	$32.8 \pm 4.2^{*}$	$24.6 \pm 8.1^{*\#}$
HD-ACOS	466.1 ± 105.3	$7.4 \pm 1.1^{*\#}$	$20.25 \pm 7.86^{**\#\#}$	$18.4 \pm 3.2^{**}$	$28.9 \pm 2.5^{*\#}$	$18.4 \pm 4.6^{*\#}$

$^{*}P < 0.05$ and $^{**}P < 0.01$ vs. control group; $^{\#}P < 0.05$ and $^{\#\#}P < 0.01$ vs. model group. BW: body weight; KW: kidney weight; FBG: fasting blood glucose; HbA1c: glycosylated hemoglobin A1c; SCr: serum creatinine; Upro: urinary protein.

2.8. Statistical Analysis. All the data of continuous variables were represented as the mean ± SD and analyzed by using SPSS 21.0 statistical software. One-way ANOVA was used to test the differences among groups. Statistical significance was defined as $P < 0.05$.

3. Results

In the course of the experiment, each one rat died in the model group, LD-ACOS group, and HD-ACOS group. Therefore, at the end of the experiment, only the data of the remaining seven rats in the 3 groups were statistically analyzed.

3.1. Effects of ACOS on the Body Weight and the Ratio of KW/BW of the Rat DN Model. Body weight at baseline among the four animal groups had no statistical difference (247.4 ± 5.9 g, 254.6 ± 9.3 g, 277.8 ± 9.8 g, and 252.6 ± 8.4 g in the DN, LD-ACOS, HD-ACOS, and control groups, respectively, $P > 0.05$). At the 4th week, the body weight of rats in the three groups fed with high-fat chow (412.7 ± 30.7 g, 422.3 ± 27.3 g, and 409.7 ± 31.6 g in the DN, LD-ACOS, and HD-ACOS groups, respectively) was significantly higher than that in the control group (374.4 ± 25.0 g) ($P < 0.05$). At the 13th week, the body weight in the DN group and LD-ACOS group was significantly lower than that in the control group ($P < 0.05$), and the body weight in the HD-ACOS group was higher than that in the DN group, but the difference between them was not yet statistically significant ($P > 0.05$) (Table 4).

At the 13th week, the ratio of KW/BW in the DN group and two intervention groups was significantly higher than that in the control group ($P < 0.05$), while in the HD-ACOS group, the ratio was significantly lower than that in the DN group ($P < 0.05$) (Table 4).

3.2. Effects of ACOS on the Blood Glucose and Insulin Resistance of the Rat DN Model. At the 4th week, the FBG levels among the four groups had no statistical difference (6.11 ± 0.65 mmol/L, 6.03 ± 1.11 mmol/L, 5.91 ± 1.08 mmol/L, and 6.14 ± 0.79 mmol/L in the DN, LD-ACOS, HD-ACOS, and control groups, respectively, $P > 0.05$). The FBG levels of rats in the DN group and two intervention groups were all beyond 11.1 mmol/L at 72 h after streptozotocin injection. At the 13th week, the FBG levels in the DN group and two intervention groups were significantly higher than those in the control group ($P < 0.01$), while in the HD-ACOS group, the level was significantly lower than that in the DN group ($P < 0.01$) (Table 4).

In addition, at the 13th week, the HbA1c levels in the DN group and two intervention groups were significantly higher than those in the control group ($P < 0.01$), and the HbA1c level in the HD-ACOS group was lower than that in the DN group, but the difference between them was not yet statistically significant ($P > 0.05$) (Table 4).

At the 4th week, the levels of blood insulin and IRI in the three groups fed with high-fat chow were significantly higher than those in the control group ($P < 0.05$). At the 13th week, the blood insulin level in the DN group was significantly lower than that in the control group ($P < 0.05$) and the level

TABLE 5: Serum insulin and insulin resistance index in different groups ($\bar{x} \pm s$).

Group	4th week		13th week	
	Serum insulin (mIU/L)	IRI	Serum insulin (mIU/L)	IRI
Control	18.6 ± 1.5	5.03 ± 0.56	20.7 ± 2.2	6.43 ± 1.99
Model	$23.9 \pm 2.6^{*}$	$6.52 \pm 1.29^{*}$	$17.2 \pm 1.4^{*}$	$24.89 \pm 2.81^{**}$
LD-ACOS	$24.5 \pm 4.2^{*}$	$6.49 \pm 0.85^{*}$	19.4 ± 2.2	$24.47 \pm 2.55^{**}$
HD-ACOS	$24.3 \pm 3.0^{*}$	$6.48 \pm 2.11^{*}$	$20.6 \pm 2.3^{\#}$	$18.49 \pm 7.33^{**\#\#}$

$^{*}P < 0.05$ and $^{**}P < 0.01$ vs. control group; $^{\#}P < 0.05$ and $^{\#\#}P < 0.01$ vs. model group. IRI: insulin resistance index.

in the HD-ACOS group was significantly higher than that in the model group ($P < 0.05$). The IRI levels in the DN group and two intervention groups were significantly higher than those in the control group ($P < 0.01$), while the level in the HD-ACOS group was significantly lower than that in the model group ($P < 0.01$) (Table 5).

3.3. Effects of ACOS on the Proteinuria and Renal Function of the Rat DN Model. Urinary protein excretion among the four groups was not statistically different at baseline (5.4 ± 1.6 mg/d, 4.3 ± 0.9 mg/d, 4.4 ± 1.0 mg/d, and 4.9 ± 1.2 mg/d in the DN, LD-ACOS, HD-ACOS, and control groups, respectively, $P > 0.05$). At the 13th week, the urinary protein excretion in the DN group and two intervention groups was significantly higher than that in the control group ($P < 0.05$), while the excretion in the two intervention groups was significantly lower than that in the DN model group ($P < 0.05$) (Table 4).

At the 13th week, the SCr levels in the DN group and two intervention groups were significantly higher than those in the control group ($P < 0.05$), while the level in the HD-ACOS group was significantly lower than that in the DN group ($P < 0.05$) (Table 4).

3.4. Effects of ACOS on the Renal Pathological Parameters of the Rat DN Model. Light microscopy of kidney tissue showed that the average glomerular size, which was represented as an average glomerular diameter, in the DN group and LD-ACOS group was significantly larger than that in the control group ($P < 0.05$), while the size in the two intervention groups was significantly smaller than that in the DN group ($P < 0.05$). The relative area of the mesangial region in the DN group was significantly larger than that in the control group ($P < 0.05$), while the area in the two intervention groups was significantly smaller than that in the DN group ($P < 0.05$) (Figure 2).

Electron microscopy of kidney tissue indicated that the foot processes of podocytes appeared to experience segmental effacement and the average width of foot processes in the DN group and two intervention groups was significantly larger than that in the control group ($P < 0.05$), while the width in the two intervention groups was significantly smaller than that in the DN group ($P < 0.05$) (Figure 2).

3.5. Effects of ACOS on the Expression of Podocyte-Associated Molecules in the Renal Cortex of the Rat DN Model. The results showed that the mRNA and protein expression of nephrin, podocin, and WT-1 was significantly downregulated in the DN group compared with the control group ($P < 0.01$) and was significantly upregulated in the two intervention groups compared with the DN group ($P < 0.01$ or 0.05) (Figure 3).

In contrast, the mRNA and protein expression of desmin was significantly upregulated in the DN group compared with the control group ($P < 0.01$) and was significantly downregulated in the two intervention groups compared with the DN group ($P < 0.01$) (Figure 3).

The above results suggest that podocyte injury occurs in the DN model and ACOS can alleviate the podocyte injury.

3.6. Effects of ACOS on the Expression of P2X7R/NLRP3 Inflammasome and IL-1β/IL-18 in the Renal Cortex of the Rat DN Model. The results showed that the mRNA and protein expression of P2X7R, NLRP3, ASC, and caspase-1 (procaspase-1 mRNA in the gene level and active caspase-1 subunit P10 in the protein level) was significantly upregulated in the DN group compared with the control group ($P < 0.01$), and the above expression was significantly downregulated in the HD-ACOS group compared with the DN group ($P < 0.01$) (Figure 4).

The mRNA and protein expression of downstream effectors of NLRP3 inflammasome, IL-1β and IL-18, was also significantly upregulated in the DN group compared with the control group ($P < 0.01$), and the above expression was significantly downregulated in the HD-ACOS group compared with the DN group ($P < 0.01$) (Figure 5).

The above results suggest that there are enhanced expression and activation of P2X7R/NLRP3 inflammasome and IL-1β/IL-18 in the DN model and ACOS can attenuate the changes.

3.7. The Localization of P2X7R/NLRP3 in Podocytes of the Rat Kidney in the DN Model. As shown in Figure 6, double immunofluorescence staining analysis revealed that the P2X7R (Figure 6(a), red spots) and NLRP3 (Figure 6(b), red spots) both were colocalized with synaptopodin (a podocyte marker; green spots indicate alone localization and yellow spots indicate colocalization) in glomeruli of DN rats. Outside of glomeruli, there was hardly any expression of P2X7R and NLRP3. Furthermore, the expression levels of P2X7R/NLRP3 in podocytes were obviously decreased in the HD-ACOS and LD-ACOS groups compared with the DN group.

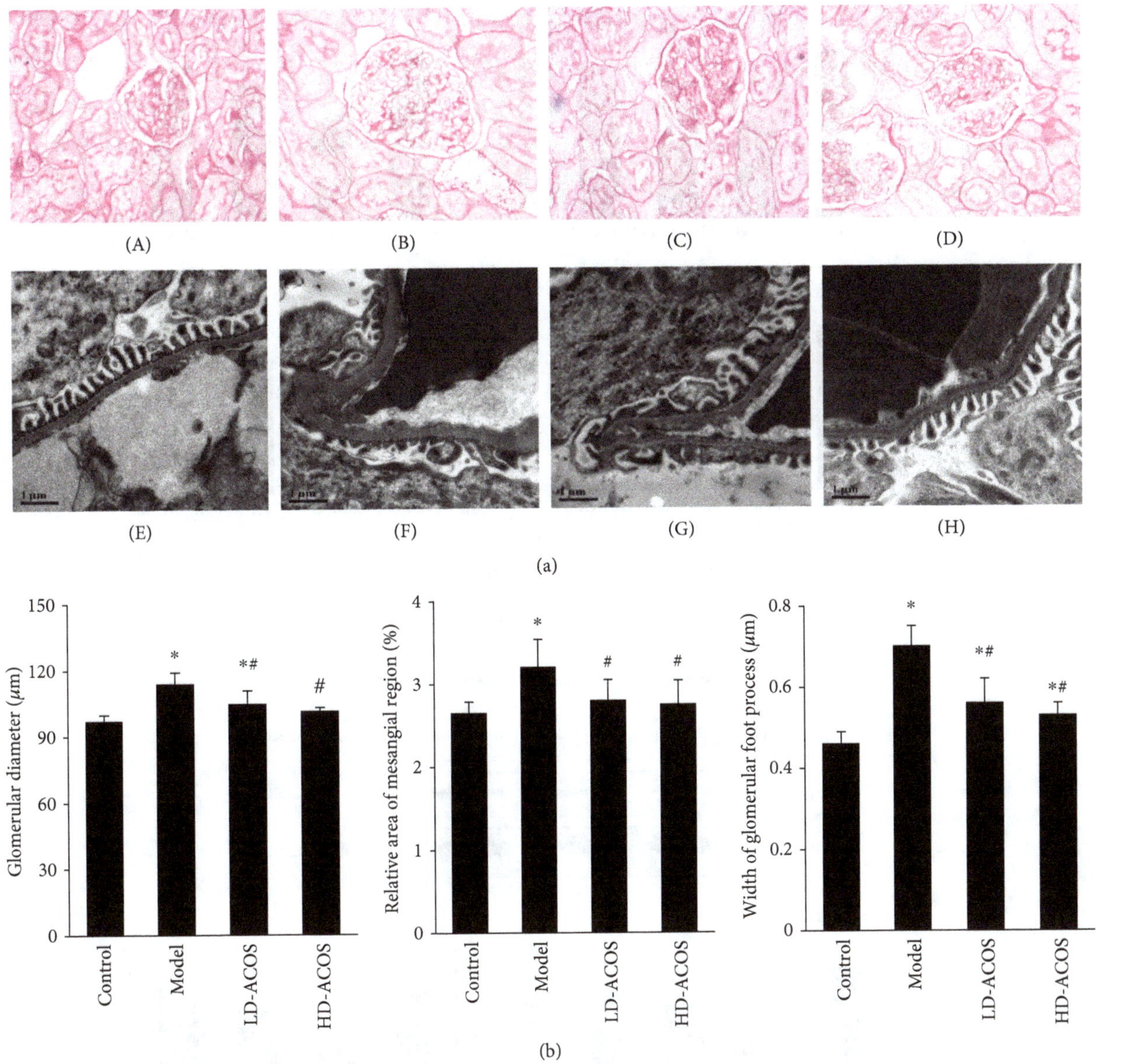

FIGURE 2: Effects of ACOS on the pathological parameters of the rat DN model. (a) Light microscopic images of glomerular size (PAS staining ×400) and electron microscopic images of foot processes of podocytes (×20,000). (A, E) Control group. (B, F) DN model group. (C, G) LD-ACOS group. (D, H) HD-ACOS group. (b) Histograms of the glomerular diameter, relative area of the mesangial region, and foot process width. Values are represented as mean ± SD. $^{*}P < 0.05$ vs. control group, $^{\#}P < 0.05$ vs. DN model group.

The above results suggest that P2X7R and NLRP3 both are expressed on podocytes and ACOS can weaken their expression.

3.8. Effects of ACOS on the HG-Induced Expression of Podocyte-Associated Molecules in Cultured Podocytes. The results showed that the mRNA and protein expression of nephrin, podocin, and WT-1 was significantly downregulated in the HG group compared with the control group ($P < 0.01$) and was significantly upregulated in the HG + ACOS group compared with the HG group ($P < 0.01$ or 0.05) (Figure 7).

On the contrary, the mRNA and protein expression of desmin was significantly upregulated in the HG group compared with the control group ($P < 0.01$) and was significantly downregulated in the HG + ACOS group compared with the HG group ($P < 0.01$ or 0.05) (Figure 7).

We performed an experiment of parallel controls with mannitol and did not find podocyte injury being caused by HG-related high osmotic pressure (Figure 1S, see Supplementary Materials). The results of the cell experiment are consistent with the results of the animal experiment, and both suggest that ACOS can alleviate the HG-induced podocyte injury.

3.9. Effects of ACOS on the HG-Induced Expression of P2X7R/NLRP3 Inflammasome and IL-1β/IL-18 in Cultured Podocytes. The results showed that the mRNA and protein expression of P2X7R, NLRP3, ASC, and caspase-1 (procaspase-1 mRNA in the gene level and active caspase-1

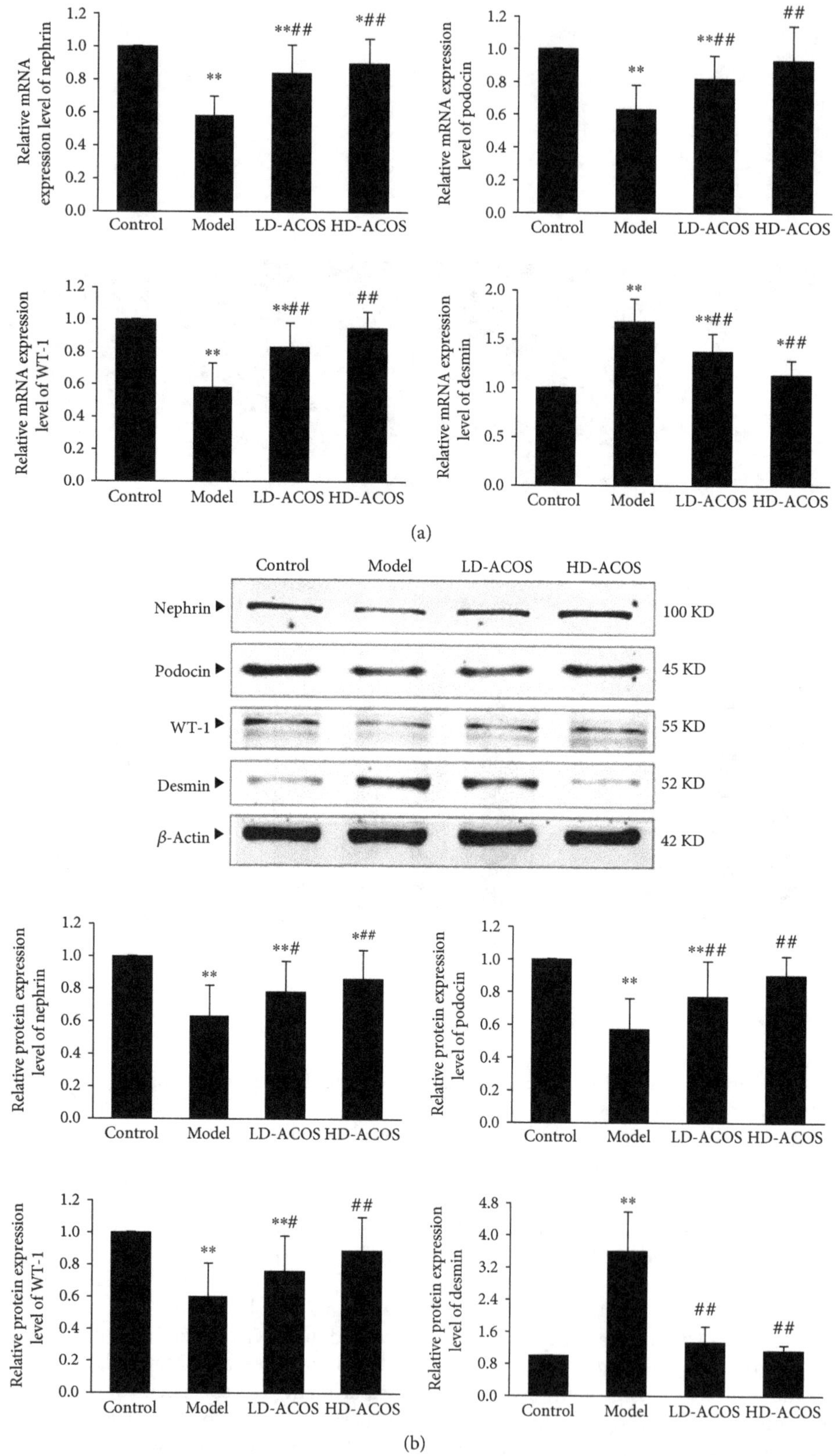

FIGURE 3: Effects of ACOS on the expression of podocyte-associated molecules in the rat DN model. (a) Total RNA was extracted from renal cortex tissue, and the relative mRNA expression levels of nephrin, podocin, WT-1, and desmin were measured by real-time quantitative PCR. (b) Renal cortex tissue was lysed, and total lysates were analyzed by the Western blot assay with antibodies against nephrin, podocin, WT-1, desmin, and β-actin, respectively. The relative protein expression level was expressed as the target protein/β-actin ratio. Values are represented as mean ± SD. $^{*}P < 0.05$ and $^{**}P < 0.01$ vs. control group, $^{\#}P < 0.05$ and $^{\#\#}P < 0.01$ vs. DN model group.

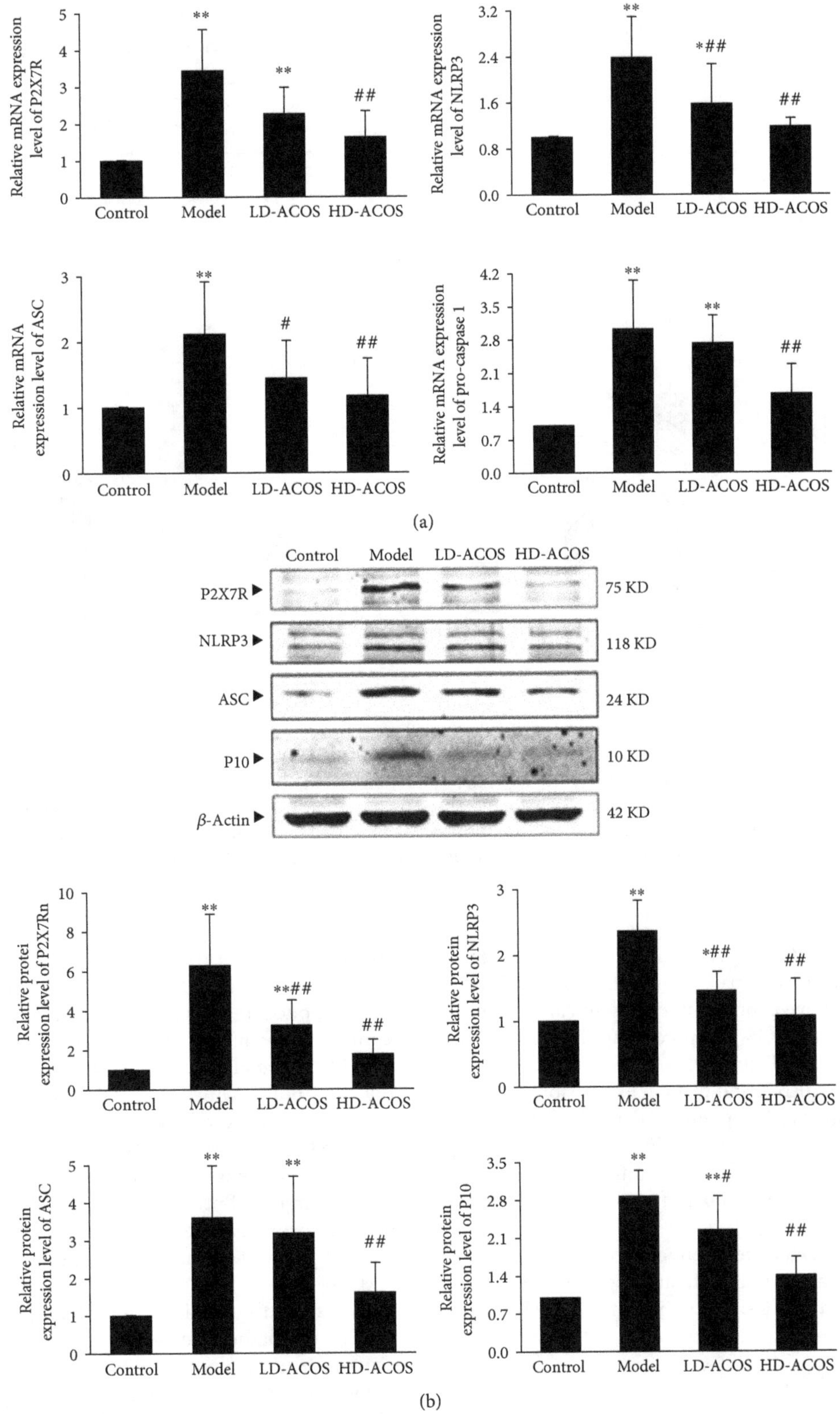

Figure 4: Effects of ACOS on the expression of P2X7R/NLRP3 inflammasome in the rat DN model. (a) Total RNA was extracted from renal cortex tissue, and the relative mRNA expression levels of P2X7R, NLRP3, ASC, and procaspase-1 were measured by real-time quantitative PCR. (b) Renal cortex tissue was lysed, and total lysates were analyzed by the Western blot assay with antibodies against P2X7R, NLRP3, ASC, active caspase-1 subunit P10, and β-actin, respectively. The relative protein expression level was expressed as the target protein/ β-actin ratio. Values are represented as mean ± SD. $^{*}P < 0.05$ and $^{**}P < 0.01$ vs. control group, $^{\#}P < 0.05$ and $^{\#\#}P < 0.01$ vs. DN model group.

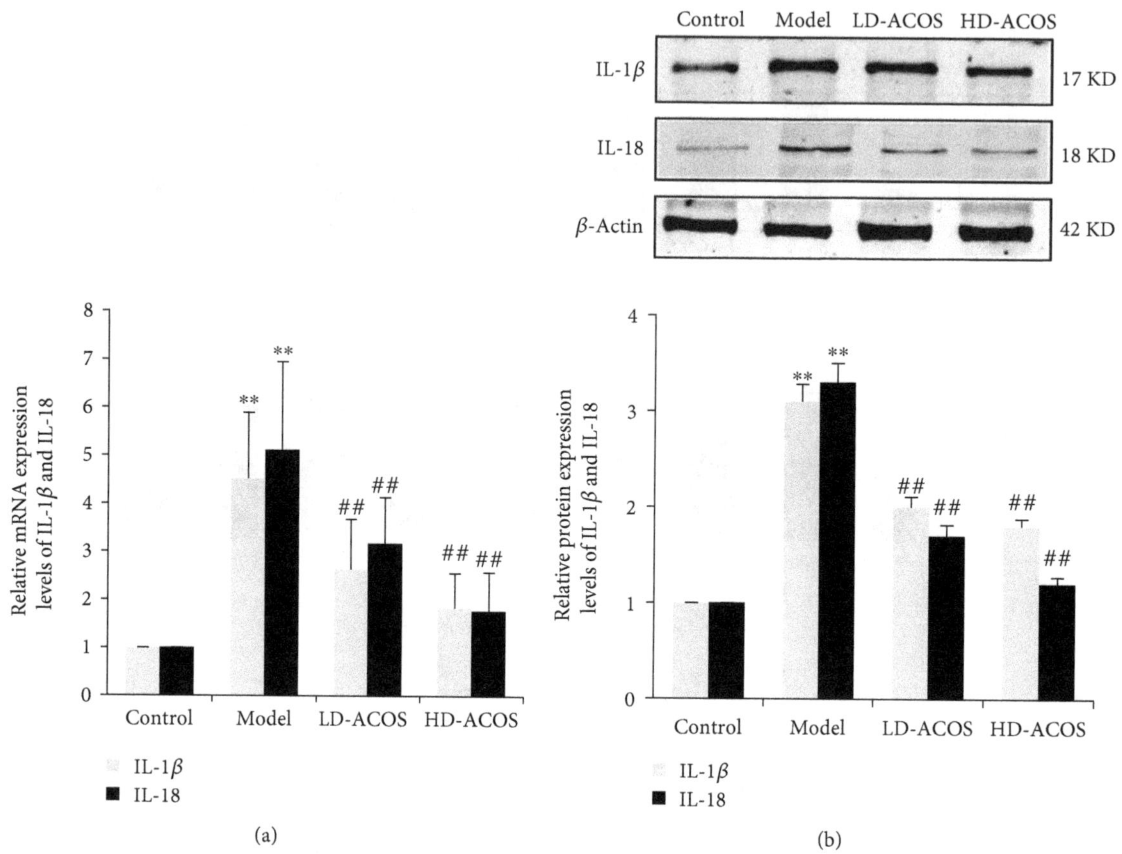

FIGURE 5: Effects of ACOS on the expression of IL-1β/IL-18 in the rat DN model. (a) Total RNA was extracted from renal cortex tissue, and the relative mRNA expression levels of IL-1β and IL-18 were measured by real-time quantitative PCR. (b) Renal cortex tissue was lysed, and total lysates were analyzed by the Western blot assay with antibodies against IL-1β, IL-18, and β-actin, respectively. The relative protein expression level was expressed as the target protein/β-actin ratio. Values are represented as mean ± SD. $^{**}P < 0.01$ vs. control group, $^{\#\#}P < 0.01$ vs. DN model group.

subunit P10 in the protein level) was significantly upregulated in the HG group compared with the control group ($P < 0.01$), and the above expression was significantly downregulated in the HG + ACOS group compared with the HG group ($P < 0.01$ or 0.05) (Figure 8).

Accordingly, the mRNA and protein expression of IL-1β and IL-18 was significantly upregulated in the HG group compared with the control group ($P < 0.01$ or $P < 0.05$), and the above expression was significantly downregulated in the HG + ACOS group compared with the HG group ($P < 0.01$ or 0.05) (Figure 9).

The results of the cell experiment are consistent with the results of the animal experiment, and both suggest that ACOS can attenuate the HG-induced inflammatory reaction in podocytes.

4. Discussion

In this study, we successfully established a rat model of DN caused by type 2 DM, which was induced by high-fat-diet feeding and low-dose streptozotocin injection and characterized by insulin resistance and hyperglycemia [25, 26]. In the model, the rats of DN developed obvious proteinuria, elevated serum creatinine, and podocyte injury showing as foot process segmental effacement with an increased width and significant alteration of the expression of podocyte-associated molecules (downregulation of nephrin, podocin, and WT-1 and upregulation of desmin). In addition, we also successfully established a cell model of podocyte injury, which was produced with the stimulation of HG [27]. In the cell model, the expression of podocyte-associated molecules was also significantly changed, which was similar to what is seen in the rat DN model, suggesting podocyte injury. Both the animal and cell models provide good platforms for us to study *in vivo* and *in vitro* the mechanism of podocyte injury of DN and the intervention effects of ACOS.

It has been recognized that podocyte injury is a pivotal event in the pathogenesis of DN, which contributes to the occurrence and progression of DN [4]. The podocyte injury in DN includes decreased podocyte density and number, foot process effacement, detachment and disruption of the slit diaphragm, podocyte loss and its resulting hypertrophy and/or dedifferentiation, and podocyte death [4]. The above changes of podocytes will cause proteinuria, while the proteinuria itself can further aggravate the podocyte injury to form a vicious cycle, eventually leading to glomerulosclerosis and renal dysfunction [4]. Therefore, in this study,

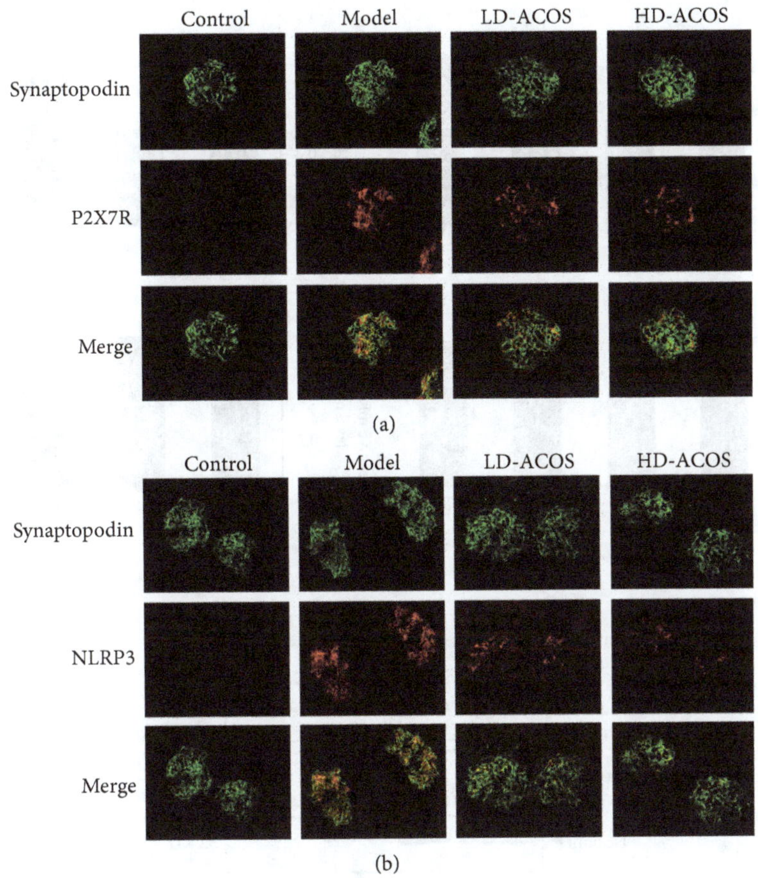

FIGURE 6: Double immunofluorescence staining of the podocyte marker and P2X7R/NLRP3 in renal tissues of the rat DN model. The colocalization of P2X7R (a, red spots) or NLRP3 (b, red spots) and synaptopodin (a podocyte marker; green spots indicate alone localization and yellow spots indicate colocalization) in the frozen renal tissue section of the rat DN model (immunofluorescence microscopy ×400).

we focused on watching the changes of podocytes in the rat DN model and in the HG-stressed cell model.

In the past years, the pathogenic role of P2X7R and NLRP3 inflammasome in kidney diseases was highly noticed [28, 29], and the expression of P2X7R and all the components of NLRP3 inflammasome in podocytes was also affirmed [8, 30, 31]. In 2004, Vonend et al. [8] first reported that the expression of P2X7R in glomeruli, mainly in podocytes, was significantly upregulated in a diabetic rat model. In 2014, Shahzad et al. [7] observed that the NLRP3 inflammasome was activated in the podocytes of the patients with DN and the mouse models of DN and in the glucose-stressed podocytes in culture. Our studies *in vivo* and *in vitro* further confirm their previous findings. Furthermore, because P2X7R is a potent activator of the NLRP3 inflammasome [32], we put them together to watch their changes in the studies *in vivo* and *in vitro* and found that the upregulation of P2X7R expression was always synchronized with the activation of NLRP3 inflammasome and its downstream effectors IL-1β and IL-18. So, our study extends, to a certain extent, the previous observations.

Ophiocordyceps sinensis and its anamorph *Hirsutella sinensis* are widely used in the treatment of kidney diseases in China and have been proven to be effective in the treatment of DN both in clinical practice and in animal experiments [16]. In this study, our experiments with ACOS also affirmed its effectiveness. Moreover, through the experiments *in vivo* and *in vitro*, we found that *Ophiocordyceps sinensis* could significantly inhibit the high expression of P2X7R and the activation of NLRP3 inflammasome in podocytes, which may be one of the important mechanisms for the therapeutic effects of *Ophiocordyceps sinensis* on DN. To our knowledge, no similar research results have been published so far. Our study also showed that ACOS could improve insulin resistance and reduce blood glucose level in a diabetic rat model, which is consistent with previous studies [16, 18, 33]. Undoubtedly, the effects can also contribute to the prevention and treatment of DN.

Wild *Ophiocordyceps sinensis* only grows in China's Qinghai-Tibet Plateau, and its resource is quite limited. The predatory digging and collecting every year not only exhaust the resources but also destroy the fragile ecological environment on the local plateau. Now, wild *Ophiocordyceps sinensis* has been listed by the Chinese government as "National Grade II Protected Species" and has been restricted from picking [19, 20]. So, artificial cultivation of *Ophiocordyceps*

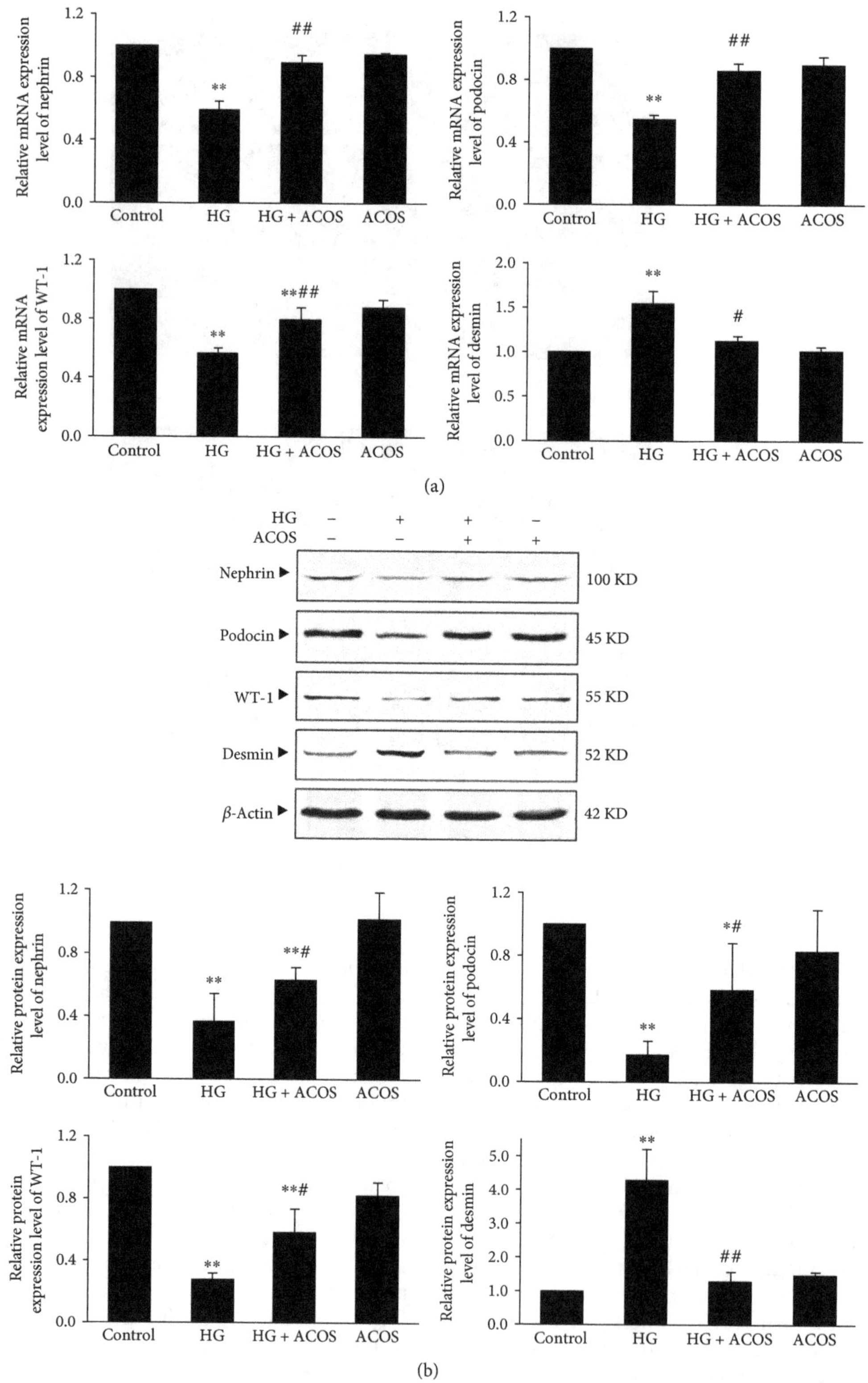

FIGURE 7: Effects of ACOS on the high-glucose-induced expression of podocyte-associated molecules in cultured podocytes. Podocytes were incubated in medium and medium containing 30 mM glucose and/or 50 μg/mL ACOS, respectively. (a) After 6 h of incubation, cells were harvested. Then, the total RNA was extracted, and the relative mRNA expression levels of nephrin, podocin, WT-1, and desmin of podocytes were measured by real-time quantitative PCR. (b) After 24 h of incubation, cells were lysed and the total lysates were used to determine the protein expression levels of nephrin, podocin, WT-1, desmin, and β-actin by the Western blot assay. The relative protein expression level was expressed as the target protein/β-actin protein ratio. Values are represented as mean ± SD ($n = 3$). $^{*}P < 0.05$ and $^{**}P < 0.01$ vs. control group, $^{\#}P < 0.05$ and $^{\#\#}P < 0.01$ vs. HG group.

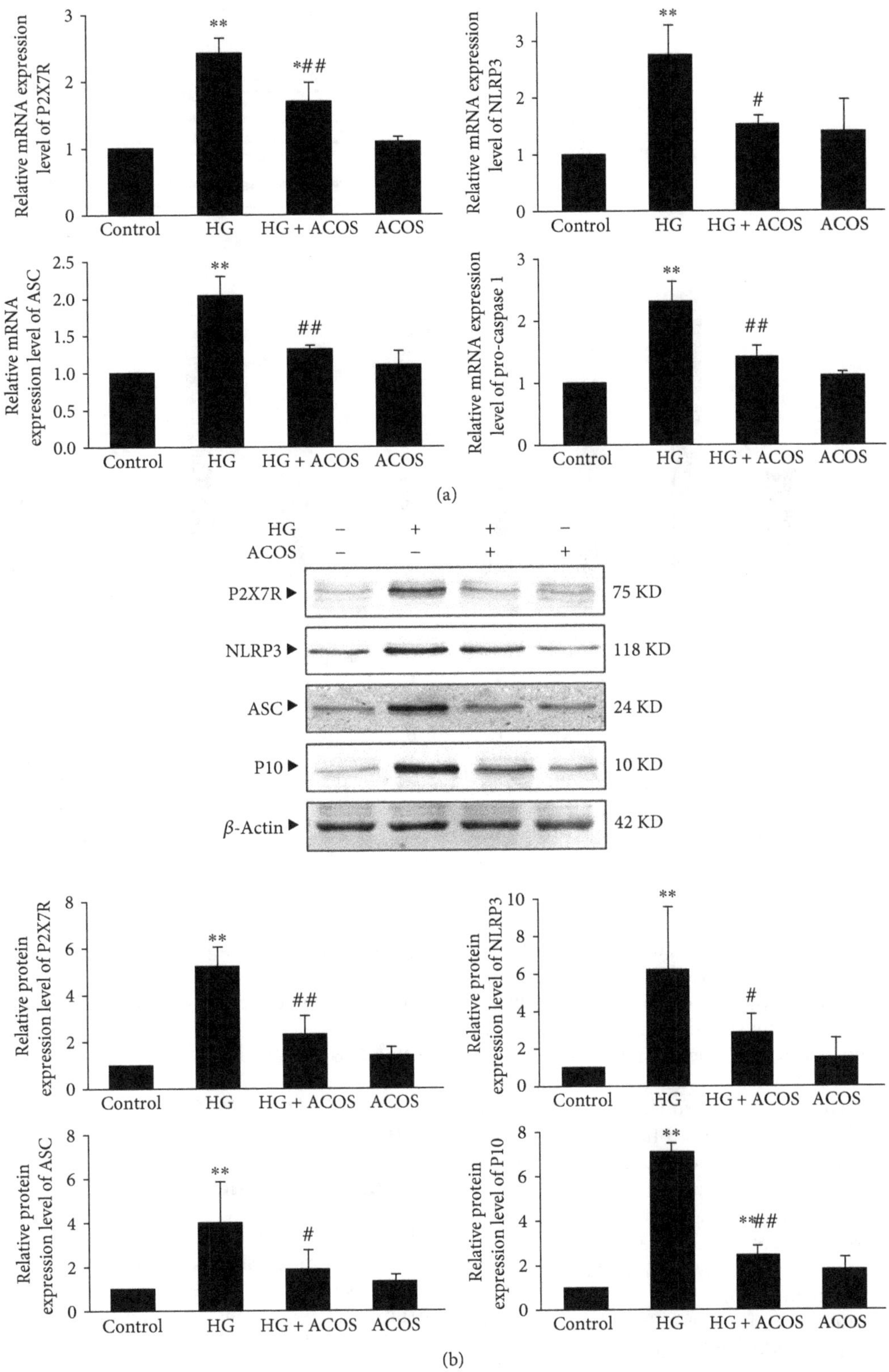

FIGURE 8: Effects of ACOS on the high-glucose-induced expression of P2X7R/NLRP3 inflammasome in cultured podocytes. Podocytes were incubated in medium and medium containing 30 mM glucose and/or 50 μg/mL ACOS, respectively. (a) After 6 h of incubation, cells were harvested. Then, the total RNA was extracted, and the relative mRNA expression levels of P2X7R, NLRP3, ASC, and procaspase-1 were measured by real-time quantitative PCR. (b) After 24 h of incubation, cells were lysed and the total lysates were used to determine the protein expression levels of P2X7R, NLRP3, ASC, active caspase-1 subunit P10, and β-actin by the Western blot assay. The relative protein expression level was expressed as the target protein/β-actin protein ratio. Values are represented as mean ± SD (n = 3). $^{*}P < 0.05$ and $^{**}P < 0.01$ vs. control group, $^{\#}P < 0.05$ and $^{\#\#}P < 0.01$ vs. HG group.

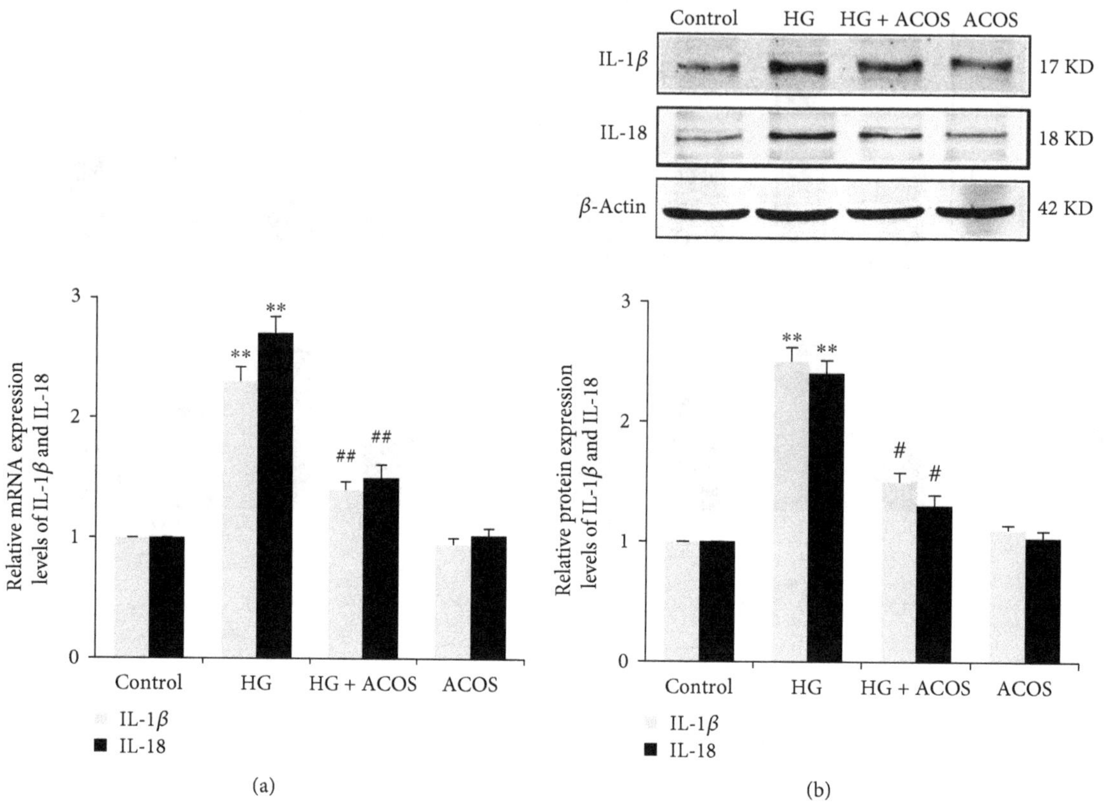

FIGURE 9: Effects of ACOS on the high-glucose-induced expression of IL-1β/IL-18 in cultured podocytes. Podocytes were incubated in medium and medium containing 30 mM glucose and/or 50 μg/mL ACOS, respectively. (a) After 6 h of incubation, cells were harvested. Then, the total RNA was extracted, and the relative mRNA expression levels of IL-1β and IL-18 were measured by real-time quantitative PCR. (b) After 24 h of incubation, cells were lysed and the total lysates were used to determine the protein expression levels of IL-1β, IL-18, and β-actin by the Western blot assay. The relative protein expression level was expressed as the target protein/β-actin protein ratio. Values are represented as mean ± SD ($n = 3$). $^{**}P < 0.01$ vs. control group, $^{\#}P < 0.05$ and $^{\#\#}P < 0.01$ vs. HG group.

sinensis is urgently needed. After more than 30 years of hard work to explore and overcome a lot of technical difficulties, artificial cultivation and industrialized production of *Ophiocordyceps sinensis* were finally successful in 2015 [20], and the ACOS has been verified by the Chinese Academy of Sciences [21]. After molecular systematic analysis [21], nuclear magnetic resonance fingerprint analysis [34], and chemical compound analysis [35, 36], it has been confirmed that the ACOS has no significant difference with wild *Ophiocordyceps sinensis* and its quality fully complies with the standard of Chinese pharmacopoeia. Our study is the first experimental research to treat the disease with ACOS and has gained good results, which clearly displays that the ACOS is effective for the treatment of DN.

In conclusion, our experiments *in vivo* and *in vitro* conducted in the DN rat model and HG-stressed podocyte model suggest that P2X7R and NLRP3 inflammasome are involved in the pathogenesis of DN including its podocyte injury and *Ophiocordyceps sinensis* including ACOS can effectively alleviate the podocyte injury of DN. The therapeutic efficacy may be related to its antagonistic effects on the P2X7R/NLRP3 inflammasome axis. The above research results provide a valuable experimental basis for the clinical application of ACOS in the prevention and treatment of DN.

Conflicts of Interest

The authors declare that they have no conflict of interests.

Authors' Contributions

Chao Wang and Xiao-xia Hou contributed equally to this work.

Acknowledgments

This research was supported by the 3 following Grants: National Natural Science Fund Project (81573745), Beijing Municipal Natural Science Foundation (7172066), and Beijing Development Foundation of Traditional Chinese Medicine (QN2016-23).

References

[1] K. Ogurtsova, J. D. da Rocha Fernandes, Y. Huang et al., "IDF diabetes atlas: global estimates for the prevalence of diabetes for 2015 and 2040," *Diabetes Research and Clinical Practice*, vol. 128, pp. 40–50, 2017.

[2] Y. Xu, L. Wang, J. He et al., "Prevalence and control of diabetes

in Chinese adults," *The Journal of the American Medical Association*, vol. 310, no. 9, pp. 948–959, 2013.

[3] Z. H. Liu, "Nephrology in China," *Nature Reviews Nephrology*, vol. 9, no. 9, pp. 523–528, 2013.

[4] J. S. Lin and K. Susztak, "Podocytes: the weakest link in diabetic kidney disease?," *Current Diabetes Reports*, vol. 16, no. 5, p. 45, 2016.

[5] F. Prattichizzo, V. De Nigris, R. Spiga et al., "Inflammageing and metaflammation: the yin and yang of type 2 diabetes," *Ageing Research Reviews*, vol. 41, pp. 1–17, 2018.

[6] J. Wada and H. Makino, "Inflammation and the pathogenesis of diabetic nephropathy," *Clinical Science*, vol. 124, no. 3, pp. 139–152, 2013.

[7] K. Shahzad, F. Bock, W. Dong et al., "Nlrp3-inflammasome activation in non-myeloid-derived cells aggravates diabetic nephropathy," *Kidney International*, vol. 87, no. 1, pp. 74–84, 2015.

[8] O. Vonend, C. M. Turner, C. M. Chan et al., "Glomerular expression of the ATP-sensitive P2X receptor in diabetic and hypertensive rat models," *Kidney International*, vol. 66, no. 1, pp. 157–166, 2004.

[9] K. Shahzad, F. Bock, M. M. Al-Dabet et al., "Caspase-1, but not caspase-3, promotes diabetic nephropathy," *Journal of the American Society of Nephrology*, vol. 27, no. 8, pp. 2270–2275, 2016.

[10] A. Solini, S. Menini, C. Rossi et al., "The purinergic 2X7 receptor participates in renal inflammation and injury induced by high-fat diet: possible role of NLRP3 inflammasome activation," *Journal of Pathology*, vol. 231, no. 3, pp. 342–353, 2013.

[11] N. Riteau, P. Gasse, L. Fauconnier et al., "Extracellular ATP is a danger signal activating P2X7 receptor in lung inflammation and fibrosis," *American Journal of Respiratory and Critical Care Medicine*, vol. 182, no. 6, pp. 774–783, 2010.

[12] C. Schorn, B. Frey, K. Lauber et al., "Sodium overload and water influx activate the NALP3 inflammasome," *Journal of Biological Chemistry*, vol. 286, no. 1, pp. 35–41, 2011.

[13] K. Schroder and J. Tschopp, "The inflammasomes," *Cell*, vol. 140, no. 6, pp. 821–832, 2010.

[14] F. S. Sutterwala, Y. Ogura, D. S. Zamboni, C. R. Roy, and R. A. Flavell, "NALP3: a key player in caspase-1 activation," *Journal of Endotoxin Research*, vol. 12, no. 4, pp. 251–256, 2006.

[15] S. L. Cassel, S. Joly, and F. S. Sutterwala, "The NLRP3 inflammasome: a sensor of immune danger signals," *Seminars in Immunology*, vol. 21, no. 4, pp. 194–198, 2009.

[16] R. Q. Lin, H. Cheng, and Y. P. Chen, "The application and mechanism research of Ophiocordyceps sinensis and its preparation in treatment of kidney diseases," *Chinese Journal of Integrated Traditional and Western Nephrology*, vol. 10, pp. 914–926–1016–1018, 2009.

[17] X. Y. Xu, J. J. Chai, Y. P. Chen et al., "Hirsutella sinensis attenuates aristolochic acid-induced renal tubular epithelial-mesenchymal transition by inhibiting TGF-β1 and snail expression," *PLoS One*, vol. 11, no. 2, article e0149242, 2016.

[18] H. C. Lo, S. T. Tu, K. C. Lin, and S. C. Lin, "The anti-hyperglycemic activity of the fruiting body of Cordyceps in diabetic rats induced by nicotinamide and streptozotocin," *Life Sciences*, vol. 74, no. 23, pp. 2897–2908, 2004.

[19] X. W. Zhou, L. J. Li, and E. W. Tian, "Advances in research of the artificial cultivation of Ophiocordyceps sinensis in China," *Critical Reviews in Biotechnology*, vol. 34, no. 3, pp. 233–243, 2013.

[20] W. J. Li, C. H. Dong, X. Z. Liu, Q. M. Li, J. M. Xia, and L. Liang, "Research advances in artificial cultivation of Chinese Cordyceps," *Mycosystema*, vol. 35, no. 4, pp. 375–387, 2016.

[21] J. C. Wei, X. L. Wei, W. F. Zheng, W. Guo, and R. D. Liu, "Species identification and component detection of Ophiocordyceps sinensis cultivated by modern industry," *Mycosystema*, vol. 35, no. 4, pp. 404–410, 2016.

[22] M. Gutch, S. Kumar, S. M. Razi, K. K. Gupta, and A. Gupta, "Assessment of insulin sensitivity/resistance," *Indian Journal of Endocrinology and Metabolism*, vol. 19, no. 1, pp. 160–164, 2015.

[23] Y. Si, Y. Zhao, H. Hao et al., "Infusion of mesenchymal stem cells ameliorates hyperglycemia in type 2 diabetic rats: identification of a novel role in improving insulin sensitivity," *Diabetes*, vol. 61, no. 6, pp. 1616–1625, 2012.

[24] K. Koop, M. Eikmans, H. J. Baelde et al., "Expression of podocyte-associated molecules in acquired human kidney diseases," *Journal of the American Society of Nephrology*, vol. 14, no. 8, pp. 2063–2071, 2003.

[25] M. J. Reed, K. Meszaros, L. J. Entes et al., "A new rat model of type 2 diabetes: the fat-fed, streptozotocin-treated rat," *Metabolism*, vol. 49, no. 11, pp. 1390–1394, 2000.

[26] K. Srinivasan, B. Viswanad, L. Asrat, C. L. Kaul, and P. Ramarao, "Combination of high-fat diet-fed and low-dose streptozotocin-treated rat: a model for type 2 diabetes and pharmacological screening," *Pharmacological Research*, vol. 52, no. 4, pp. 313–320, 2005.

[27] M. C. Iglesias-de la Cruz, F. N. Ziyadeh, M. Isono et al., "Effects of high glucose and TGF-beta1 on the expression of collagen IV and vascular endothelial growth factor in mouse podocytes," *Kidney International*, vol. 62, no. 3, pp. 901–913, 2002.

[28] J. W. R. Booth, F. W. K. Tam, and R. J. Unwin, "P2 purinoceptors: renal pathophysiology and therapeutic potential," *Clinical Nephrology*, vol. 78, no. 8, pp. 154–163, 2012.

[29] A. Chang, K. Ko, and M. R. Clark, "The emerging role of the inflammasome in kidney diseases," *Current Opinion in Nephrology and Hypertension*, vol. 23, no. 3, pp. 204–210, 2014.

[30] C. Zhang, K. M. Boini, M. Xia et al., "Activation of Nod-like receptor protein 3 inflammasomes turns on podocyte injury and glomerular sclerosis in hyperhomocysteinemia," *Hypertension*, vol. 60, no. 1, pp. 154–162, 2012.

[31] K. G. Fischer, U. Saueressig, C. Jacobshagen, A. Wichelmann, and H. Pavenstadt, "Extracellular nucleotides regulate cellular functions of podocytes in culture," *American Journal of Physiology-Renal Physiology*, vol. 281, no. 6, pp. F1075–F1081, 2001.

[32] J. Zhao, H. Wang, C. Dai et al., "P2X7 blockade attenuates murine lupus nephritis by inhibiting activation of the NLRP3/ASC/caspase 1 pathway," *Arthritis & Rheumatology*, vol. 65, no. 12, pp. 3176–3185, 2013.

[33] H. C. Lo, T. H. Hsu, S. T. Tu, and K. C. Lin, "Anti-hyperglycemic activity of natural and fermented Cordyceps sinensis in

rats with diabetes induced by nicotinamide and streptozotocin," *American Journal of Chinese Medicine*, vol. 34, no. 5, pp. 819–832, 2006.

[34] G. Chen, L. Huang, W. J. Li et al., "The establishment of NMR characteristic fingerprint of Cordyceps sinensis and its identification study," *World Science and Technology-Modernization of Traditional Chinese Medicine*, vol. 16, no. 11, pp. 2371–2379, 2014.

[35] Z. M. Qian, W. Q. Li, M. T. Sun, X. Z. Liu, E. W. Li, and W. J. Li, "Analysis of chemical compounds in Chinese Cordyceps," *Mycosystema*, vol. 354, no. 4, pp. 476–490, 2016.

[36] K. Zan, R. Su, J. Liu et al., "Comparative study on content of adenosine between cultivated and wild Cordyceps sinensis," *Chinese Pharmaceutical Affairs*, vol. 30, no. 6, pp. 598–603, 2016.

2

Sweet Taste Receptors Mediated ROS-NLRP3 Inflammasome Signaling Activation: Implications for Diabetic Nephropathy

Luping Zhou,[1,2] Wei Huang,[1,3,4] Youhua Xu,[3,4] Chenlin Gao,[1,3,4] Ting Zhang,[1,2] Man Guo,[1,2] Yan Liu,[3,4] Jingya Ding,[1,2] Ludan Qin,[1,2] Zihao Xu,[2] Yang Long,[1] and Yong Xu[1,5]

[1]*Department of Endocrinology, Affiliated Hospital of Southwest Medical University, Luzhou, Sichuan 646000, China*
[2]*The Graduate School of Southwest Medical University, Luzhou, Sichuan 646000, China*
[3]*Faculty of Chinese Medicine, Macau University of Science and Technology, Avenida Wai Long, Taipa, Macau, China*
[4]*State Key Laboratory of Quality Research in Chinese Medicine, Macau University of Science and Technology, Avenida Wai Long, Taipa, Macau, China*
[5]*Key Laboratory of Medical Electrophysiology of Ministry of Education, Collaborative Innovation Center for Prevention and Treatment of Cardiovascular Disease of Sichuan Province, Southwest Medical University, Luzhou, Sichuan 646000, China*

Correspondence should be addressed to Yang Long; xiaolong0325ly@163.com and Yong Xu; xywyll@aliyun.com

Academic Editor: Jan M. Williams

Previous studies demonstrated that ROS-NLRP3 inflammasome signaling activation was involved in the pathogenesis of diabetic nephropathy (DN). Recent research has shown that sweet taste receptors (STRs) are important sentinels of innate immunity. Whether high glucose primes ROS-NLRP3 inflammasome signaling via STRs is unclear. In this study, diabetic mouse model was induced by streptozotocin (STZ) in vivo; mouse glomerular mesangial cells (GMCs) and human proximal tubular cells were stimulated by high glucose (10, 20, and 30 mmol/L) in vitro; STR inhibitor lactisole was used as an intervention reagent to evaluate the role and mechanism of the STRs in the pathogenesis of DN. Our results showed that the expression of STRs and associated signaling components (Gα-gustducin, PLCβ2, and TRPM5) was obviously downregulated under the condition of diabetes in vivo and in vitro. Furthermore, lactisole significantly mitigated the production of intracellular ROS and reversed the high glucose-induced decrease of Ca^{2+} and the activation of NLRP3 inflammasome signaling in vitro ($p < 0.05$). These combined results support the hypothesis that STRs could be involved in the activation of ROS-NLRP3 inflammasome signaling in the pathogenesis of DN, suggesting that STRs may act as new therapeutic targets of DN.

1. Introduction

Oxidative stress and persistent microinflammatory state in circulatory and renal tissues play a key role in the development and progression of diabetic nephropathy (DN) [1, 2]. The NOD-like receptor pyrin 3 (NLRP3) inflammasome is an intracellular platform that recruits the adaptor molecule-apoptosis-associated speck-like protein (ASC) by pyrin domain, and then ASC hydrolyzes procaspase-1, and finally, active caspase-1 cleaves pro-IL-1β into its mature form in response to "danger" signals [3]. Therefore, the pharmacological targeting of the oxygen species- (ROS-) NLRP3-mediated inflammatory response may help with the design of a new approach to develop therapeutic strategies for preventing the deterioration of kidney injury in the pathogenesis of DN. However, the mechanism mediating NLRP3 inflammasome activation in DN has not been completely clarified yet [4].

Among five basic taste qualities, sweet taste permits the identification of energy-rich nutrients, which are very attractive for animals and influence food intake [5, 6]. Studies have revealed two classes of GPCRs that have been identified, including taste 1 receptor family (T1R) and the taste 2 receptor family (T2R), and two subtypes of the T1R family, including T1R member 2 (T1R2) and T1R member 3 (T1R3), form heterodimers to act as sweet taste receptors (STRs), which are expressed in taste buds and in the gastrointestinal tract and respond to various chemically distinct compounds, such as natural sugars, noncaloric artificial and natural sweeteners, some D-amino acids, and sweet-tasting proteins [7]. As a natural ligand for STRs, glucose binding to STRs leads to activation of the heteromeric Gα-gustducin. Phospholipase C β2 (PLCβ2) is subsequently stimulated, leading to release of intracellular Ca^{2+} and activation of the transient receptor potential channel M5 (TRPM5). Finally, taste cells are depolarized, generate action potentials, and release transmitters (ATP) via pannexin-1 hemichannels [8].

Accumulating evidence shows that STRs are ubiquitous throughout the body, including the stomach, pancreas, gut, liver, and brain. These STRs are heavily involved in nutrient sensing, monitoring changes in energy stores, and triggering metabolic and behavioral responses to maintain energy balance and immune response [9–11]. Recent study indicated that sweet taste disorder in patients with abnormal glucose tolerance was associated with increased sugar intake and vascular complications, including DN and diabetic retinopathy [12]. However, whether STRs are also expressed in renal tissue and take part in the activation of ROS-NLRP3 inflammasome signaling under high-glucose stress is unclear. In this study, we detected the expression of T1R2, T1R3, Gα-gustducin, PLCβ2, TRPM5, NLRP3, procaspase-1, and IL-1β in renal tissue of DN model mouse and renal innate cells (mouse GMCs and human proximal tubular cells (HK-2)) under high-glucose stress and then observed the changes of these players using lactisole-blocked STRs, aiming to elucidate the role of STRs in the activation of ROS-NLRP3 inflammasome signaling in the pathogenesis of DN.

2. Materials and Methods

2.1. Establishing the Animal Model and Sample Collection. Male C57BL/6 mouse weighing 20 g was purchased from the Biotechnology Corporation of Dashuo (Chengdu, China). The mouse was randomly allocated into two groups: a control group (NC group, $n = 10$) and a diabetes mellitus group (DM group, $n = 10$). Mouse in the DM group was rendered diabetic by intraperitoneal injection of Streptozocin (STZ, Sigma, USA), which was dissolved in 0.1 M citrate buffer at pH 4.5, at a dose of 40 mg/kg for 4 days. Meanwhile, a mouse in the NC group received an intraperitoneal injection of the same volume of citrate buffer. After 4 days following the STZ injection, fasting blood glucose (FBG) measurements were performed in blood samples from tail veins, and FBG levels of ≥16.7 mmol/L lasting 3 days were confirmed as being "diabetic."

All mice were weighed and 24-hour urinary microalbumin (mAlb) was collected in metabolic cages (Hattera, USA) every two weeks. Urinary protein and urinary creatinine concentrations were measured according to the manufacturers' procedures described in the kits (AfinionTM ACR, Axis-Shield PoC AS, Norway), and urine albumin-creatinine ratios (ACR) were calculated. After 12 weeks, all mice were sacrificed and heart blood was collected to measure blood urea nitrogen (BUN) levels by automatic biochemistry analyzer. Both kidneys were cut along the coronal plane; the right kidneys were used for pathology, and the left renal tissues were preserved in RNA later solution (Thermo Fisher Scientific, USA) until required for qRT-PCR.

2.2. Cell Culture, Stimulation, and Viability Assay. Mouse GMCs (SV40 MES 13) and human proximal tubular cells (HK-2) were purchased from the China Center for Type Culture Collection (CCTCC) and were cultured in Dulbecco's modified Eagle's medium (DMEM, Glbco) containing 5.6 mmol/L glucose and 10% fetal bovine serum (FBS, Glbco) at 37°C and 5% CO_2.

Initially, to determine proper concentrations of high glucose and lactisole, cells were randomly divided into the following groups: (1) normal control group (NC group, 5.6 mmol/L glucose); (2) high-glucose treatment group (HG group; cells were treated with culture medium containing 10 mmol/L, 20 mmol/L, and 30 mmol/L glucose); (3) osmotic pressure group (OP group, with medium that contained 5.6 mmol/L glucose + 24.4 mmol/L mannitol); (4) lactisole (Sigma-Aldrich, MO, USA) at 3, 5, and 10 mmol/L as an inhibitor of STR intervention group.

The cells in each group were induced for 6, 12, or 24 h before the culture supernatant was collected, and the protein and mRNA were extracted for further study. Viability of GMCs was determined by 3-(4,5-dimethylthiazol-2-yl)-2,5-diphenyltetrazolium bromide (MTT). For MTT analysis, absorbance at 570 nm was measured for the experimental groups using a microplate reader according to the manufacturer's instruction. Each experiment was performed in duplicate and repeated thrice.

2.3. Immunohistochemistry and Immunofluorescence Staining. Sections were incubated with the following primary antibodies: anti-T1R2 (goat polyclonal antibody; 1 : 100 dilution; Santa Cruz, USA), anti-T1R3 (goat polyclonal antibody; 1 : 100 dilution; Santa Cruz, USA), anti-NLRP3 (rabbit monoclonal antibody; 1 : 100 dilution; CST, USA), and anti-IL-1β (rabbit monoclonal antibody; 1 : 100 dilution; CST, USA) overnight at 4°C. After sections were washed with PBS, they were incubated with horseradish peroxidase (HRP) or fluorescein isothiocyanate fluorescent dye-conjugated secondary antibodies (1 : 200 dilution, Biosynthesis Biotech, China) for 2 h at room temperature. For visualizing the signals, sections were treated with peroxidase substrate DAB (3,3-diaminobenzidine) and counterstained with hematoxylin.

GMCs were grown on coverslips in 6-well plates. After overnight adherence, cells were incubated with different compounds for 24 h as described above and then were fixed in 4% paraformaldehyde and then blocked with 5% rabbit serum. The cells were incubated overnight with the anti-NLRP3, caspase-1, and IL-1β antibody (1 : 100 dilution). Images were taken with a fluorescence microscope (Leica, Germany), and the values of semiquantitative analysis for average intensity were assessed by Image-Pro Plus 6.0 software.

2.4. Protein Extraction and Western Blotting. Total protein was extracted from kidney, mouse GMCs, and human proximal tubular cells using a protein extraction kit (Kaiji, Shanghai, China). Proteins were separated by sodium dodecyl sulfate-polyacrylamide gel electrophoresis and transferred to a polyvinylidene difluoride (PVDF) membrane (Millipore). Immunoblotting was performed using anti-T1R2 antibody (1 : 800 dilution), anti-T1R3 antibody (1 : 1000 dilution), anti-NLRP3 antibody (1 : 800 dilution), anti-procaspase-1 antibody (rabbit monoclonal antibody; 1 : 800 dilution; CST, USA), anti-IL-1β antibody (1 : 800 dilution), and anti-GAPDH antibody (mouse; 1 : 800 dilution; Beyotime, China).

2.5. RNA Extraction and Quantitative Real-Time PCR (qRT-PCR) Analysis. Total RNA was isolated from kidney and GMCs using an RNA extraction kit (ComWin Biotech, Beijing, China). The isolated RNA was subjected to reverse transcription using the PrimeScript RT Reagent Kit (TaKaRa). The synthesized cDNA was used as a template for the quantitative PCR analysis. The house-keeping gene β-actin was quantified as an internal control. The primer sequences for all studied genes are listed in Table 1. qRT-PCR was performed on 7900HT Fast Real-Time PCR system (Thermo Fisher Scientific, USA). The thermal cycling program used was as follows: an initial step at 95°C for 10 minutes, followed by 40 cycles of denaturation at 95°C for 15 seconds, annealing at 60°C for 34 seconds, and extension at 72°C for 15 seconds. The melting curve of each PCR product was obtained by continuous fluorescence monitoring at a temperature gradient ramp from 60 to 95°C. The quantitative PCR reactions were performed in triplicate to remove any outliers. The relative changes of target genes were analyzed by the $2^{-\Delta\Delta CT}$ method.

2.6. Detection of Intracellular ROS Level. Intracellular production of ROS was measured using the ROS assay kit (Beyotime Institute of Biotechnology, China) with oxidation of 2′,7′-dichlorofluorescin diacetate (DCFH-DA) to fluorescent 2′,7′-dichlorofluorescin (DCF). The fluorescence images were taken with a fluorescence microscope (Leica, Germany) and measured in a plate reader with excitation at 488 nm and emission at 525 nm according to the manufacturer's instructions. The values were expressed as the mean absorbance normalized to the percentage of the normal control.

2.7. Enzyme-Linked Immunosorbent Assay (ELISA). IL-1β protein level in the cells culture supernatant was determined using commercially available ELISA IL-1β kits (Neo-Bioscience, China) according to the manufacturer's protocols. IL-1β protein levels were determined by comparing the samples to the standard curve generated by the kit.

2.8. Ca^{2+} Measurement. GMCs were treated with 30 mmol/L glucose alone or were intervened by 5 mmol/L lactisole following 30 mmol/L glucose for 24 h, respectively. For Ca^{2+} imaging experiments, GMCs on coverslips were incubated with Fura-PE3 AM (1 μM) for 30 min at 37°C in Ca^{2+}-free standard bath solution. The ratio (F_{340}/F_{380}) of Ca^{2+} dye fluorescence was measured by a Nikon Ti-E system with NIS-Elements software. All the experiments were performed at room temperature (23–26°C).

2.9. Data Analysis. All data obtained from at least three independent experiments were expressed as the means ± standard deviation (SD), and between-group comparisons were analyzed using one-way analysis of variance (ANOVA), followed by the LSD post hoc test for multiple comparisons (SPSS 17 software). $p < 0.05$ was considered significant.

3. Results

3.1. STZ-Induced Changes in ACR and Renal Function of Diabetic Mouse. As shown in Figure 1, compared with the NC group, FBG (Figure 1(a)) levels were increased in the DM group ($p < 0.05$), but the body weight (Figure 1(b)) was significantly decreased ($p < 0.05$). More importantly, urinary ACR (Figure 1(c)) and serum BUN (Figure 1(d)) levels, as important features of DN, were increased in the DM groups ($p < 0.05$). The immunohistochemical stainings showed that there were increased NLRP3 and IL-1β expressions in renal tissue of DM group (Figure 1(e)). These data suggest that DN mouse models were successfully achieved by using STZ.

3.2. The Expression of STRs and Associated Signaling Components Was Downregulated in Renal Tissue of DM Mouse Models. The expression of T1R2 and T1R3 in renal tissue was detected by immunohistochemistry (Figure 2(a)), immunofluorescence (Figure 2(b)), and Western blotting (Figure 2(c)). Compared with the NC group, these receptor molecular expression was downregulated in DM group ($p < 0.05$). Consistent with the expression of T1R2 and T1R3, the mRNA expression of STR signaling molecules, Gα-gustducin, PLCβ2, and TRPM5 was also inhibited in DM group ($p < 0.05$) (Figure 2(d)). Combined with the above results, we confirm that the expression of STRs and associated signaling components was downregulated in renal tissue of DM mouse models.

3.3. High Glucose Inhibited the Expression of STRs and Primed NLRP3 Inflammasome Signaling. To determine whether STRs are regulated by glucose in renal innate cells, we first detected T1R2 and T1R3 expression in GMCs (SV-40 MES 13) and human proximal tubular cells (HK-2). Compared with the NC group, both the protein and mRNA levels of T1R2 and T1R3 in SV-40 MES 13 cells were also significantly inhibited following 6, 12, and 24 h of exposure to 30 mmol/L high glucose in a time-dependent manner ($p < 0.05$); the same trend is found in HK-2 cells ($p < 0.05$) (Figure 3(a)). Similarly, the expression of T1R2 and T1R3 in SV-40 MES 13 cells and HK-2 cells was also significantly decreased by different concentrations of high glucose in a dose-dependent manner ($p < 0.05$) (Figure 3(b)). However, both the protein and mRNA levels of NLRP3, cleaved caspase-1, and cleaved IL-1β were also significantly induced by high glucose in a dose-dependent manner ($p < 0.05$) (Figure 3(c)). Meanwhile, high glucose induced inflammatory cytokine IL-1β release from SV-40 MES 13 cells in a dose-dependent

Table 1: Primer sequences for qRT-PCR.

Gene	Forward sequence	Reverse sequence
T1R2	5′-GTCCGCTGCACCAAGCA-3′	5′-GTTCGTCGAAGAAGAGCTGGTT-3′
T1R3	5′-AGCTTCTTCCTCATGCCACA-3′	5′-GCCATAGTCATCATCACTCCCT-3′
Gα-gustducin	5′-TGCATTATATTTTGCGCAGC-3′	5′-AGAACAATGGAGGTGGTTGC-3′
PLCβ2	5′-TGGTAGCCACCACCCTTTCCATTA-3′	5′-AGTTCCACTTCCACATAGGTGCGT-3′
TRPM5	5′-CCAGCATAAGCGACAACATCT-3′	5′-GAGCATACAGTAGTTGGCCTG-3′
NLRP3	5′-AGAAGAGACCACGGCAGAAAG-3′	5′-CTTGGAACCAGGTTGAGTGT-3′
Caspase-1	5′-TGGAAGGTAGGCAAGACT-3′	5′-ATAGTGGGCATCTGGGTC-3′
IL-1β	5′-GTCTTTCCCGTGACCTTC-3′	5′-ATCTCGGAGCCTGTTAGTGC-3′
β-Actin	5′-ACCTCTATGCCAACACAGTG-3′	5′-GGACTCATCGTACTCCTGCT-3′

manner ($p < 0.05$) (Figure 3(d)). These results suggested that high glucose inhibited the expression of STRs and activated NLRP3 inflammasome in *vitro*.

3.4. Lactisole Reversed High-Glucose-Induced Downregulation of STRs. Lactisole, a STR inhibitor, was used to stimulate GMCs. The effect of different concentrations of lactisole on GMCs' viability was assessed by MTT. We observed that 3–5 mM concentration range of lactisole has no effect on the cell viability ($p > 0.05$) and reversed 30 mM high-glucose-induced proliferation in a dose-dependent manner ($p < 0.05$). However, higher concentrations of lactisole (≥10 mM) may inhibit cell viability (Figure 4(a)). Considering the cytotoxicity detected by MTT and the pharmacological concentrations of lactisole reported in the literature [13], we chose the 3 mM and 5 mM lactisole as the intervention reagent. As expected, high-glucose-inhibited T1R2 and T1R3 expression in SV-40 MES 13 cells (Figure 4(b)) and HK-2 cells (Figure 4(c)) was obviously reversed by lactisole in a dose-dependent manner ($p < 0.05$). qRT-PCR showed that high-glucose-inhibited Gα-gustducin, PLCβ2, and TRPM5 were obviously reversed by lactisole in a dose-dependent manner ($p < 0.05$) (Figure 4(d)). Moreover, the intracellular calcium level was measured by using a fluorescent Ca^{2+} indicator Fura-PE3 AM. The results showed that 30 mmol/L glucose stimulation for 24 h induced the decrease of Ca^{2+} after a certain lag period ($p < 0.05$). The intracellular calcium level inhibited by high glucose was significantly reversed by lactisole ($p < 0.05$) (Figure 4(e)). These results suggested that high-glucose-induced downregulation of STRs was reversed by lactisole.

3.5. Lactisole Reversed High-Glucose-Induced Activation of ROS-NLRP3 Inflammasome Signaling. Next, we assessed whether STRs were involved in the high-glucose-induced ROS-NLRP3 inflammasome signaling in SV-40 MES 13 cells. The results showed that high-glucose-induced intracellular ROS production (Figure 5(a)) and the expression of NLRP3, cleaved caspase-1, and cleaved IL-1β (Figure 5(b)) were also abrogated after lactisole treatment in a dose-dependent manner ($p < 0.05$). Meanwhile, high-glucose-induced inflammatory cytokine IL-1β release from SV-40 MES 13 cells was blunted by lactisole ($p < 0.05$) (Figure 4(c)). Consistent with this finding, we used immunofluorescence to detect the expression level of NLRP3, caspase-1, and IL-1β, and we observed the same changes ($p < 0.05$) (Figure 5(d)). These results suggested that STRs signaling is required for high-glucose-induced ROS-NLRP3 inflammasome signaling activation.

4. Discussion

Although inflammatory responses are a critical component in defense against pathogens and damage-associated molecular patterns, too much inflammation is harmful. The molecular underpinnings of this inflammation include nutrient excess-mediated activation of the innate immune NLRP3 inflammasome. How NLRP3 inflammasome formation is triggered remains debatable because several models have been proposed, all of which explain some but not all observations [14, 15]. We reported previously that high glucose and lipopolysaccharide activate ROS-TXNIP-NLRP3 inflammasome signaling in GMCs, but ROS inhibitor N-acetylcysteine (NAC) could not completely inhibit the activation of NLRP3 inflammasome induced by high glucose, suggesting that there may be other pathways by which high glucose primes ROS-NLRP3 inflammasome signaling [16].

A recent paradigm in sensory physiology suggests that several classes of understudied receptors (olfactory receptors (ORs), taste receptors, and orphan GPRs) play key roles in nonsensory tissues, where they serve as selective and sensitive chemoreceptors [17, 18]. Previous research showed that the intestinal STRs, T1R2 and T1R3, were expressed in distinct epithelial cells in the human proximal intestine and that their transcript levels varied with glycemic status in patients with type 2 diabetes [11, 19]. Recent research found that STRs were also expressed in extragustatory organs regulating carbohydrate metabolism. T1R2 and T1R3 are expressed in pancreatic β-cells; inhibition of this receptor by gurmarin or deletion of the T1R3 gene attenuates glucose-induced insulin secretion from β-cells [9, 13]. However, few reports exist on the regulation of taste receptors in renal tissues under the condition of diabetes. Just as ORs were found in a variety of additional tissues including the kidney and considered as a

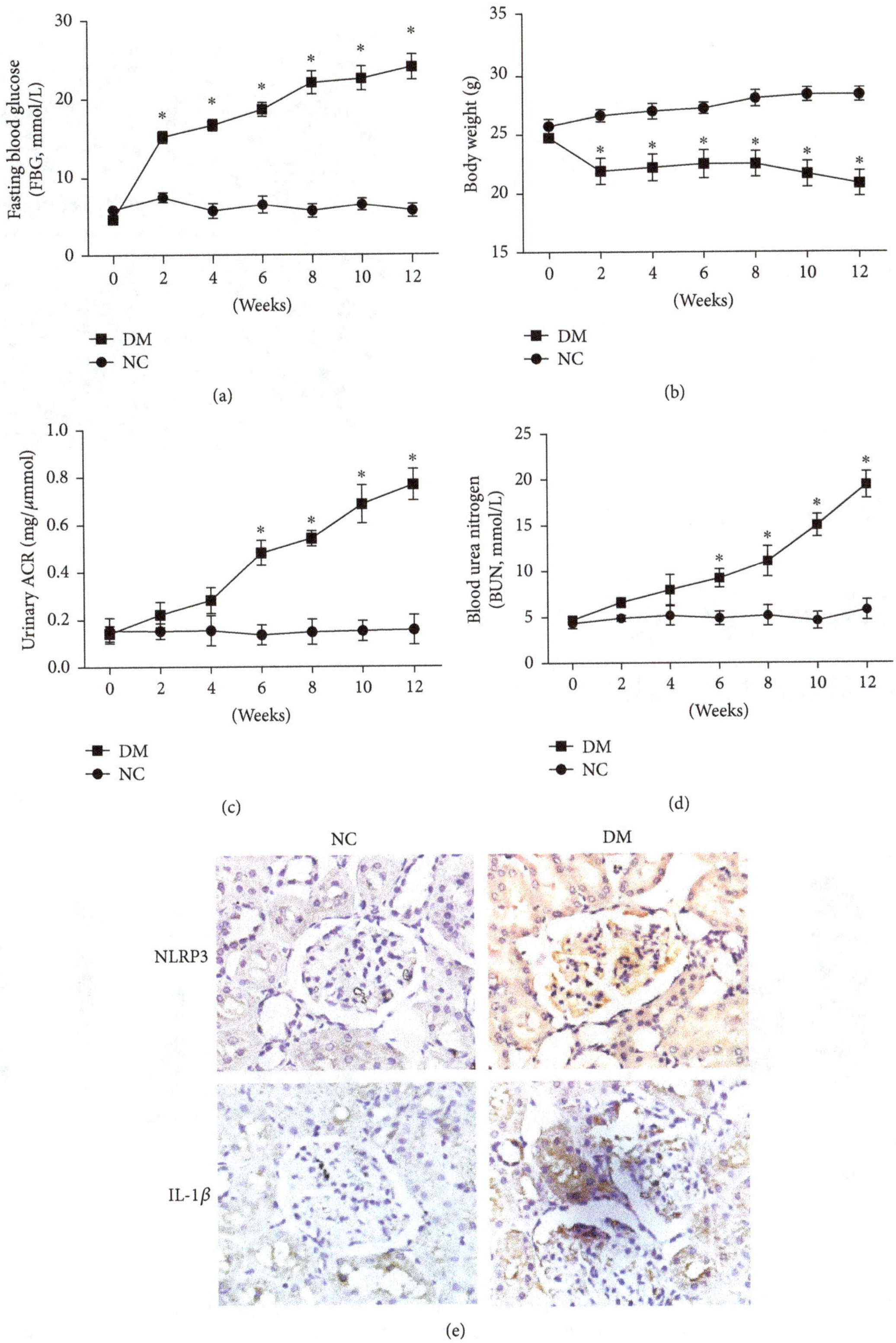

Figure 1: STZ-induced changes in FBG, body weight, ACR, and renal function of diabetic mouse. Male C57BL/6 mice were divided into diabetes mellitus group (DM group, $n = 10$) and normal control group (NC group, $n = 10$). Every two weeks, fasting blood glucose (a), body weight (b), ACR (c), and BUN (d) levels were examined. (e) STZ-induced expression of NLRP3 and IL-1β in renal tissue was observed by immunohistochemistry and light microscopy (200×). Data are presented as means ± SD. $^*p < 0.05$ versus NC group at the same treatment time.

novel mechanism of blood pressure regulation and kidney glucose handling [20], here, our research indicated that STRs and associated signaling components were also expressed in kidney in vivo and in vitro; furthermore, we characterize for the first time that compared with the NC group, these signaling molecule expressions were downregulated in

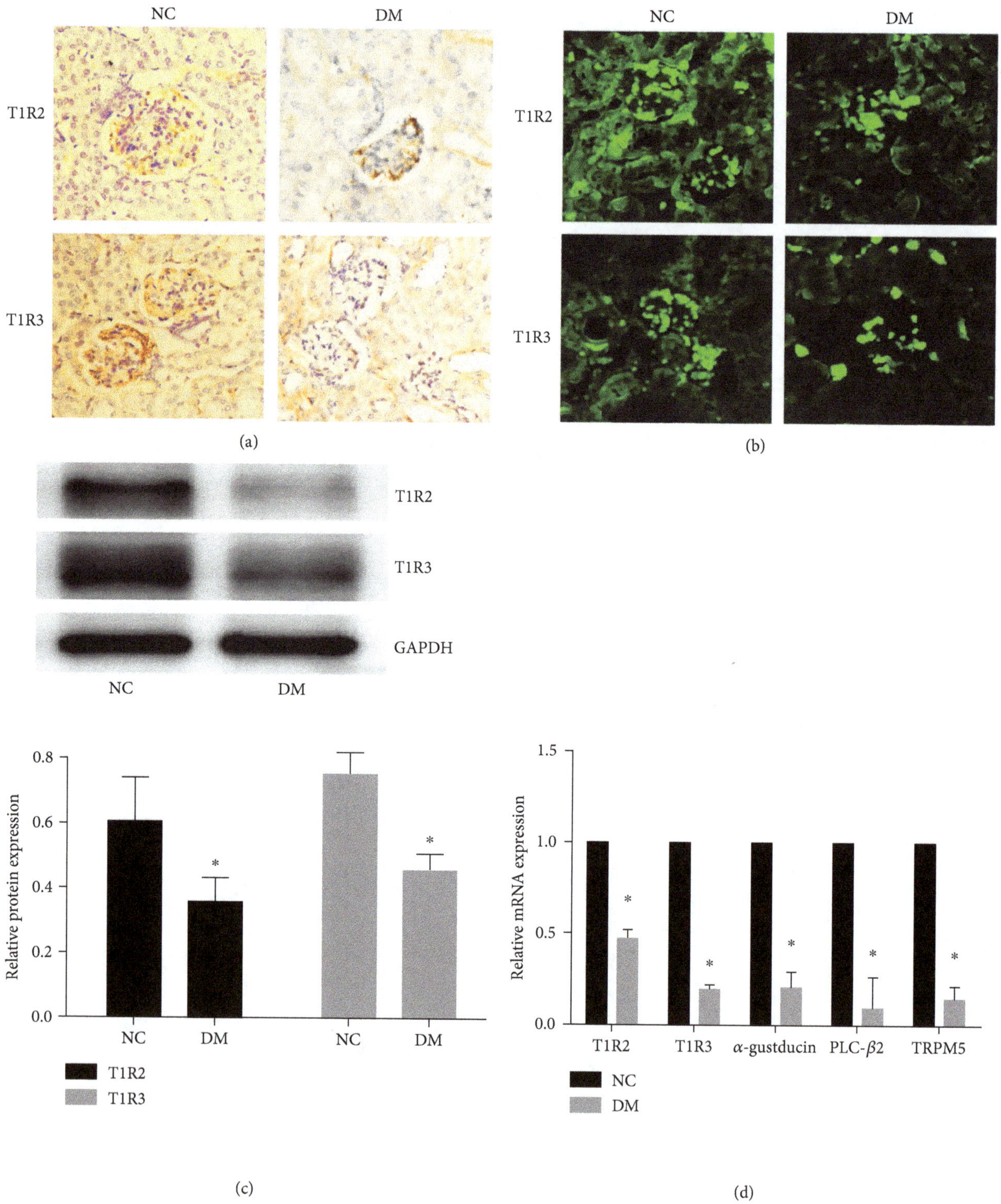

FIGURE 2: The expression of STRs and associated signaling components was downregulated in renal tissue of DM mouse models. Representative images of immunohistochemistry (a) and immunofluorescence (b) staining showed that T1R2 and T1R3 expression was downregulated in renal tissue of DM mouse models. T1R2 and T1R3 expression was represented as the positive yellow-brown stained area (immunohistochemistry, 200×) or green fluorescence area (immunofluorescence, 200×). (c) STR-associated signaling component (α-gustducin, PLCβ2, and TRPM5) mRNA expression in renal tissues was detected by qRT-PCR. Data are presented as means ± SD; the gray graph confirmed these trends. $^*p < 0.05$ versus NC group.

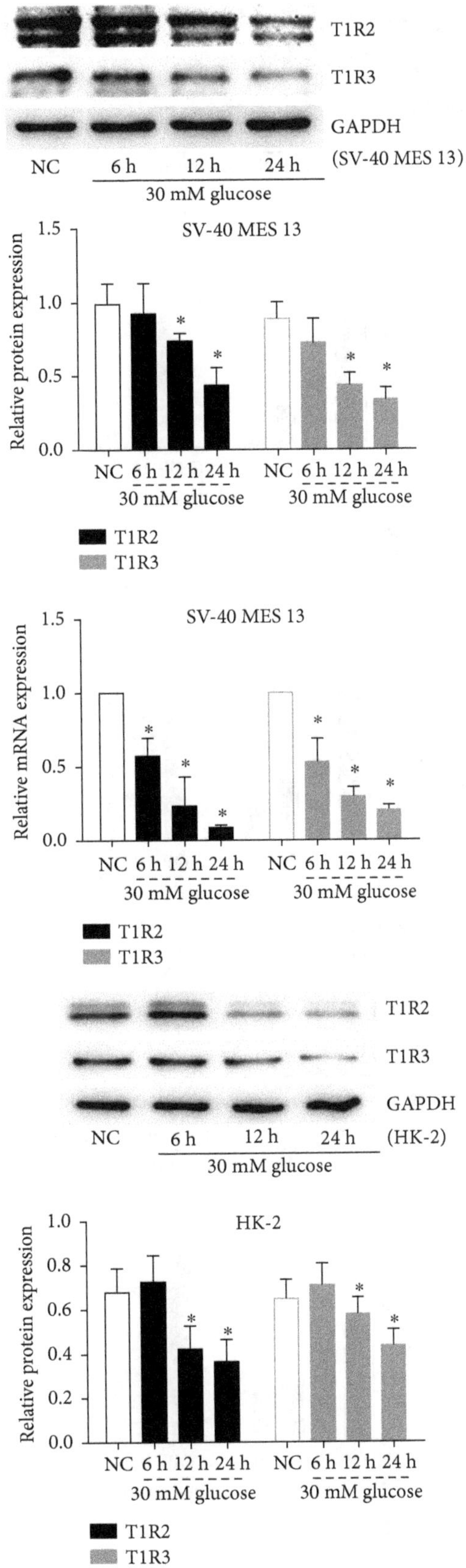

(a)

FIGURE 3: Continued.

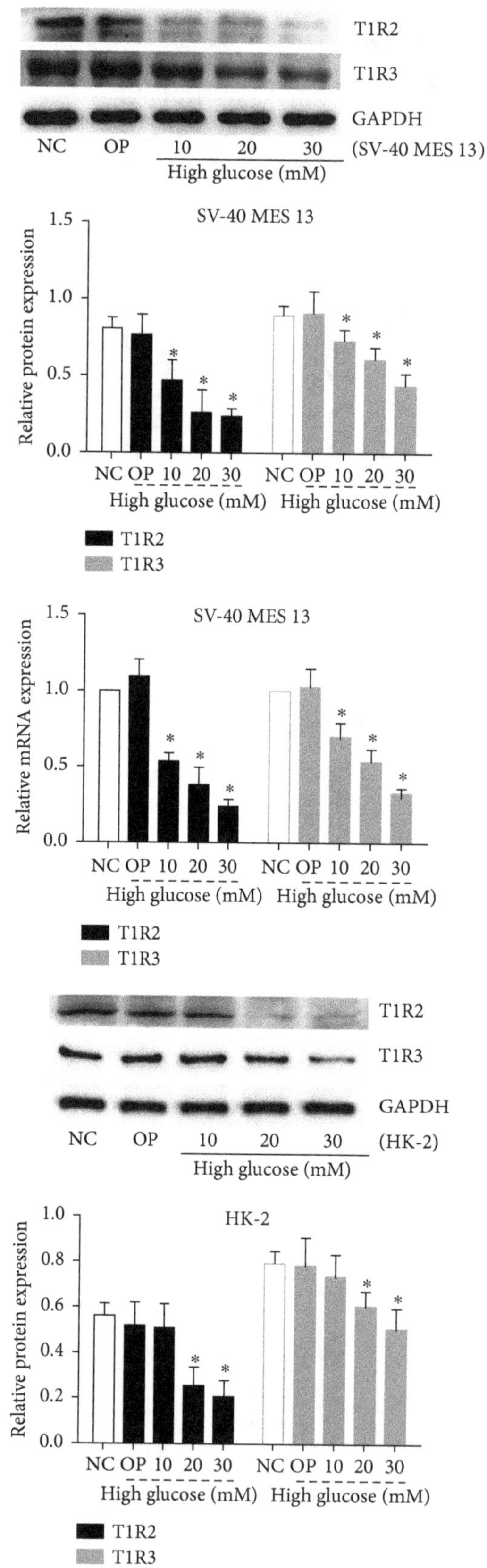

(b)

Figure 3: Continued.

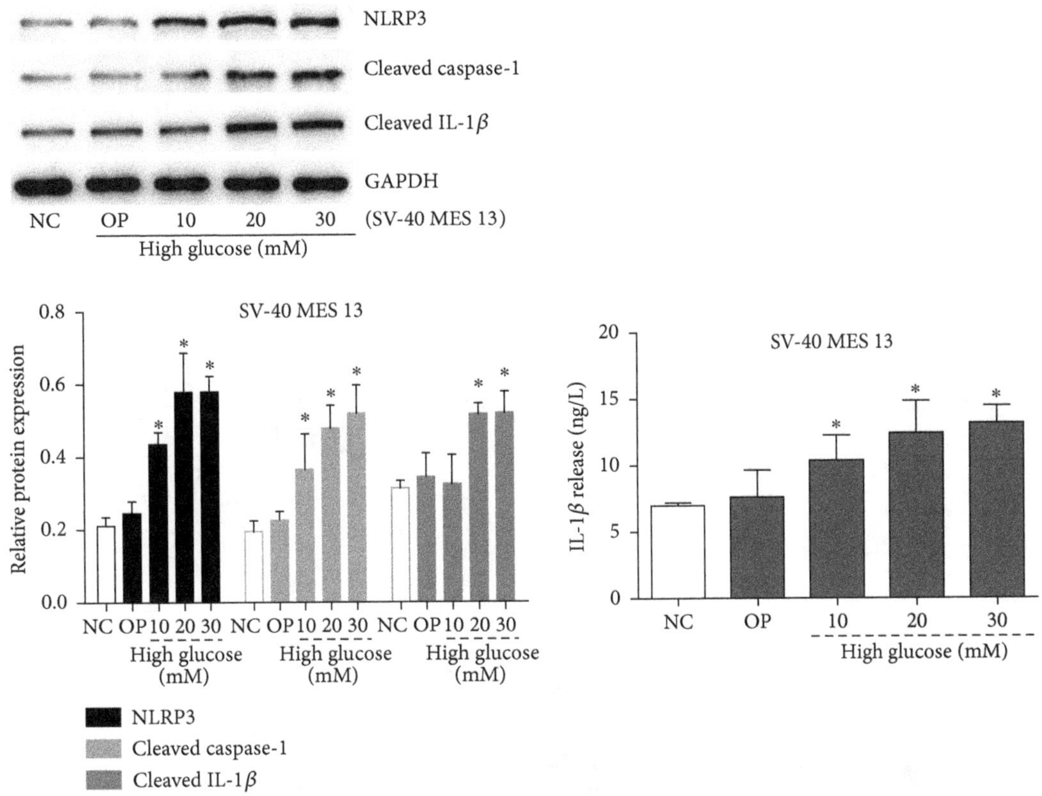

(c) (d)

FIGURE 3: High glucose inhibited the expression of STRs and activated NLRP3 inflammasome. (a) GMCs (SV-40 MES 13) and human proximal tubular cells (HK-2) were treated with 30 mmol/L high glucose for 6, 12, and 24 h, and Western blot or qRT-PCR was performed to detect T1R2 and T1R3 protein or mRNA expression levels. (b) Cells were treated with the indicated concentrations of glucose or mannitol for 24 h. Western blot or qRT-PCR was performed to detect T1R2 and T1R3 protein or mRNA expression levels. (c) Western blotting analysis of NLRP3, cleaved caspase-1, and cleaved IL-1β in GMCs treated with an indicated concentration of glucose or mannitol for 24 h. (d) IL-1β protein level in the GMC culture supernatant was determined by ELISA. Data are expressed as mean ± SD. $^*p < 0.05$ versus NC group.

DM group, suggesting their modulation under the condition of diabetes.

It is becoming increasingly clearer that taste receptors have important roles beyond simply that of gustation. Studies have shown that taste buds express various molecules involved in innate immune responses, including the proinflammatory cytokine tumor necrosis factor (TNF), suggesting that TNF signaling preferentially modulates bitter taste responses [21]. Recently, it is thought that the taste receptors have emerged as key players in the regulation of innate immune defenses in the mammalian respiratory tract [22]. These responses are quick in onset and are complementary to traditional antimicrobial pathways, such as those involving TLRs [23]. Dysfunction or genetic variation of bitter or sweet taste receptors appears to play a key role in respiratory disease and associated with some chronic inflammatory diseases. The chemosensory functions of taste receptors as sentinels of innate immunity may partly explain why these receptors are so widely expressed throughout the body [24]. Although the role of STRs in respiratory tract involved in innate immune defenses has been widely studied and information on the presence and possible role of STRs in kidney is relatively scarce, it remains unclear whether they are known to be modulated by glucose level, let alone whether any taste reception is involved in the regulation of inflammatory cytokines.

Our current aims were, therefore, to investigate whether STRs and associated signaling component expression will be changed after long-term treatment with high glucose in renal innate cells (mouse GMCs and human proximal tubular cells (HK-2)). The present study has also shown that the expression of STRs and associated signaling components (Gα-gustducin, PLCβ2, and TRPM5) was rapidly downregulated upon exposure to glucose in a time- and dose-dependent manner in vitro. GMC proliferation and hypertrophy, ECM accumulation, as well as consequent renal fibrosis induced by high glucose, AGEs, or LPS, have been recognized as major pathogenic events in the progression of renal failure in DN [25]. Accordingly, our study found 30 mmol/L glucose stimulation for 24 h induced decrease of Ca^{2+} after a certain lag period; meanwhile, NLRP3 inflammasome signaling molecules and inflammatory cytokine IL-1β release from GMCs were induced by high glucose, suggesting that STRs could be involved in the activation of NLRP3 inflammasome under high-glucose stress.

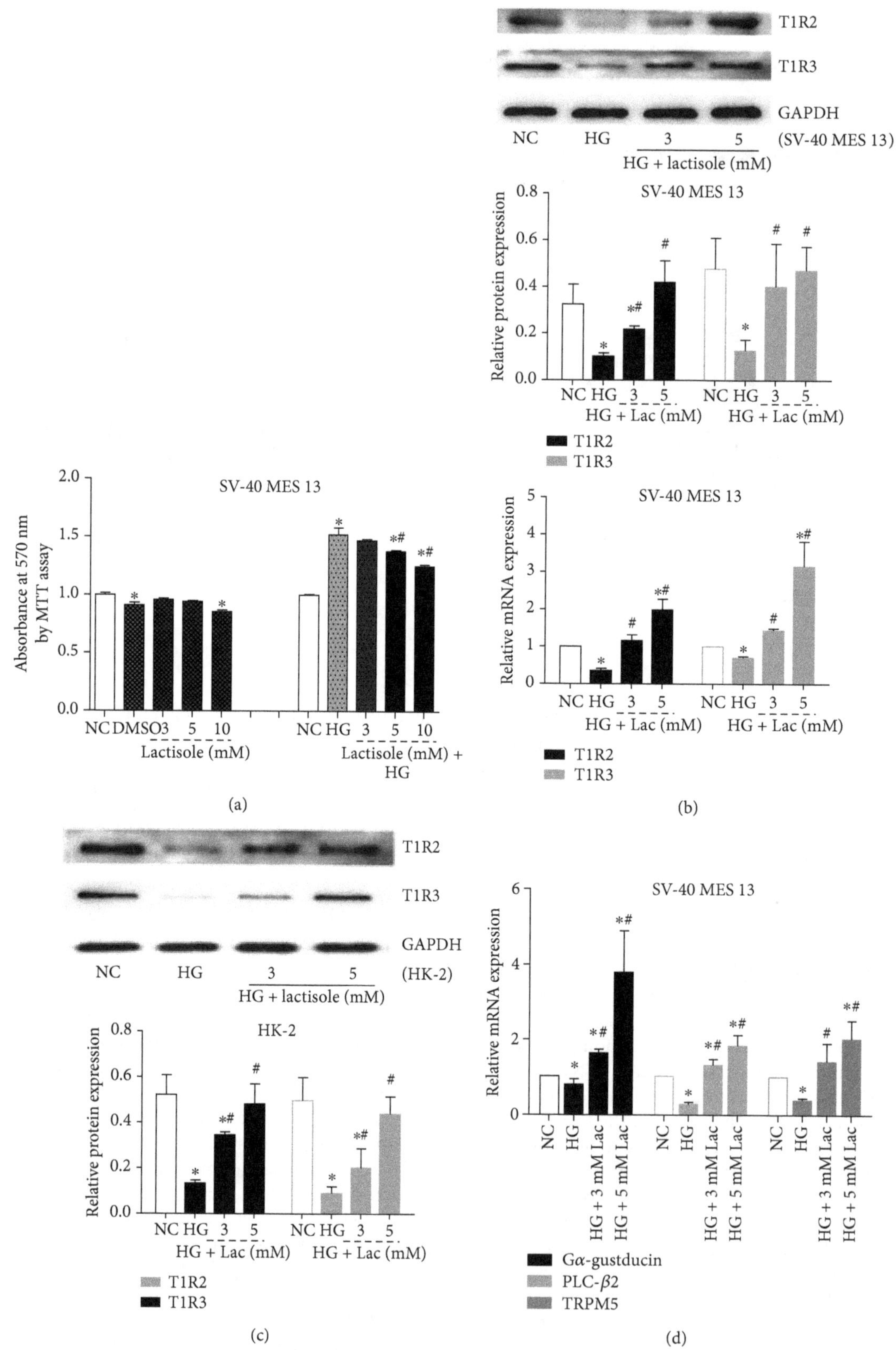

Figure 4: Continued.

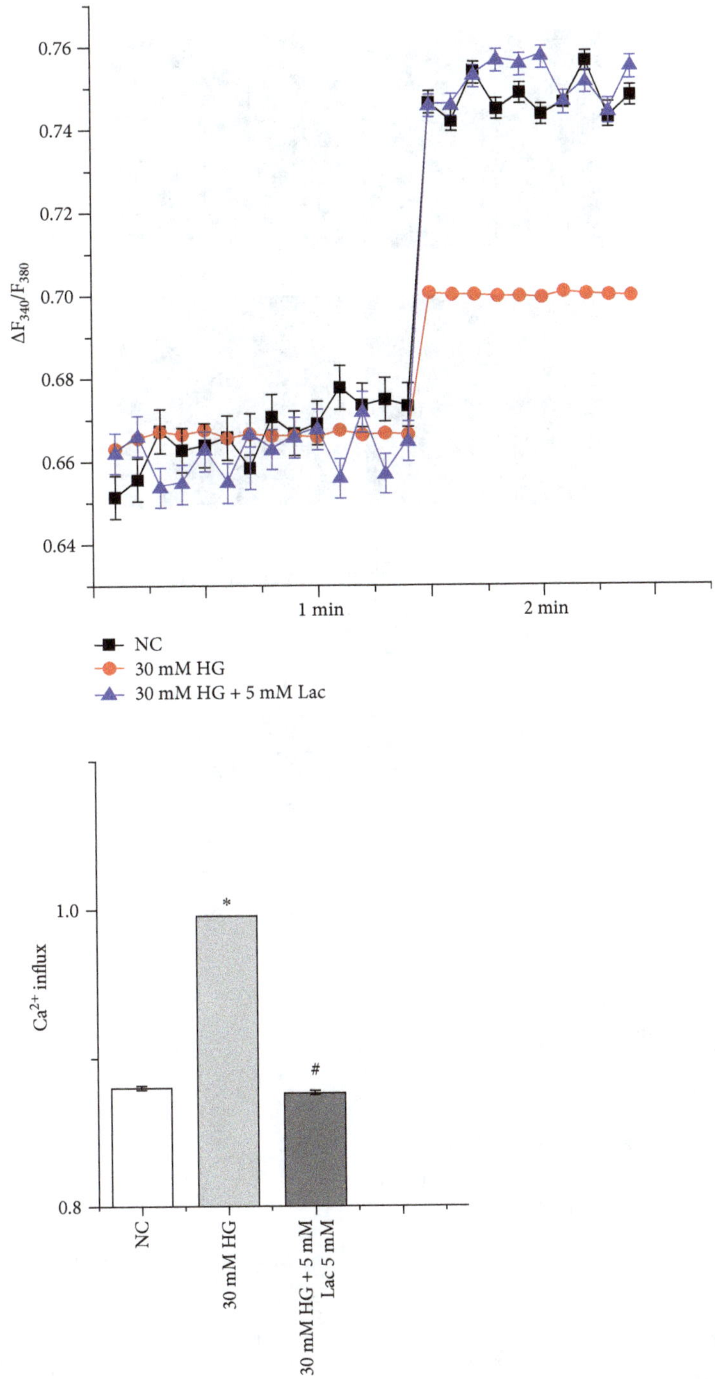

(e)

FIGURE 4: High glucose-induced downregulation of STRs and associated signaling components was reversed by lactisole. Mouse GMCs (SV-40 MES 13) was firstly incubated with 3, 5, and 10 mM lactisole; then 30 mM high glucose (HG) alone was intervened by the indicated concentrations of lactisole following 30 mM high glucose for 24 h. (a) Cell viability was determined by MTT analysis. (b) The protein and mRNA expression of T1R2 and T1R3 in GMCs were detected by Western blotting and qRT-PCR. (c) The protein expression of T1R2 and T1R3 in human proximal tubular cells (HK-2) was detected by Western blot. (d) STR-associated signaling components (α-gustducin, PLCβ2, and TRPM5) were detected by qRT-PCR. (e) GMCs were stimulated with 30 mmol/L glucose in the presence (blue), and absence (red) of 5 mmol/L lactisole, and the Ca^{2+} influx changes in Ca^{2+} dye fluorescence was monitored. Data are expressed as mean ± SD. $^*p < 0.05$ versus NC group. $^\#p < 0.05$ versus 30 mM glucose (HG) stimulation group.

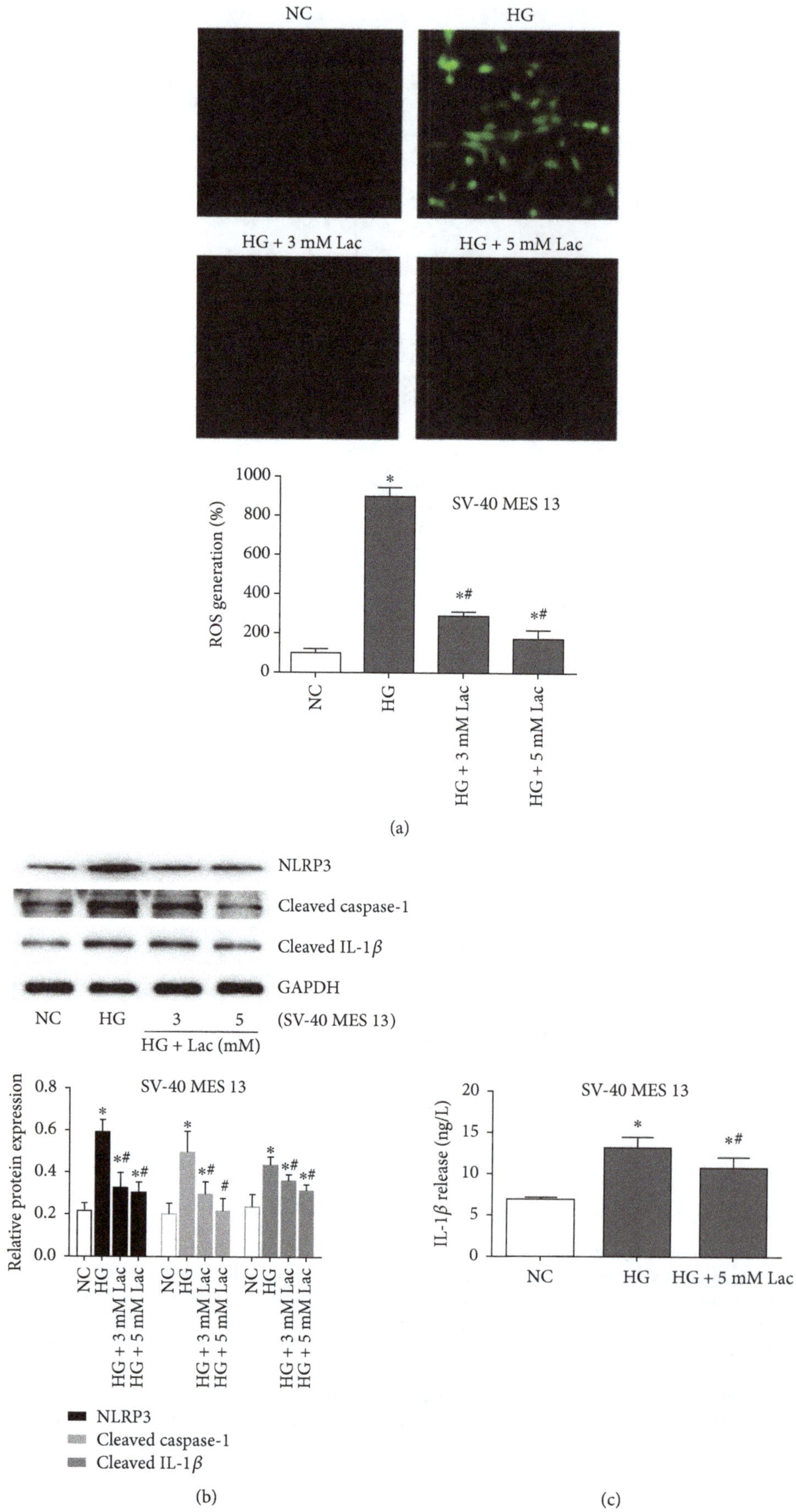

Figure 5: Continued.

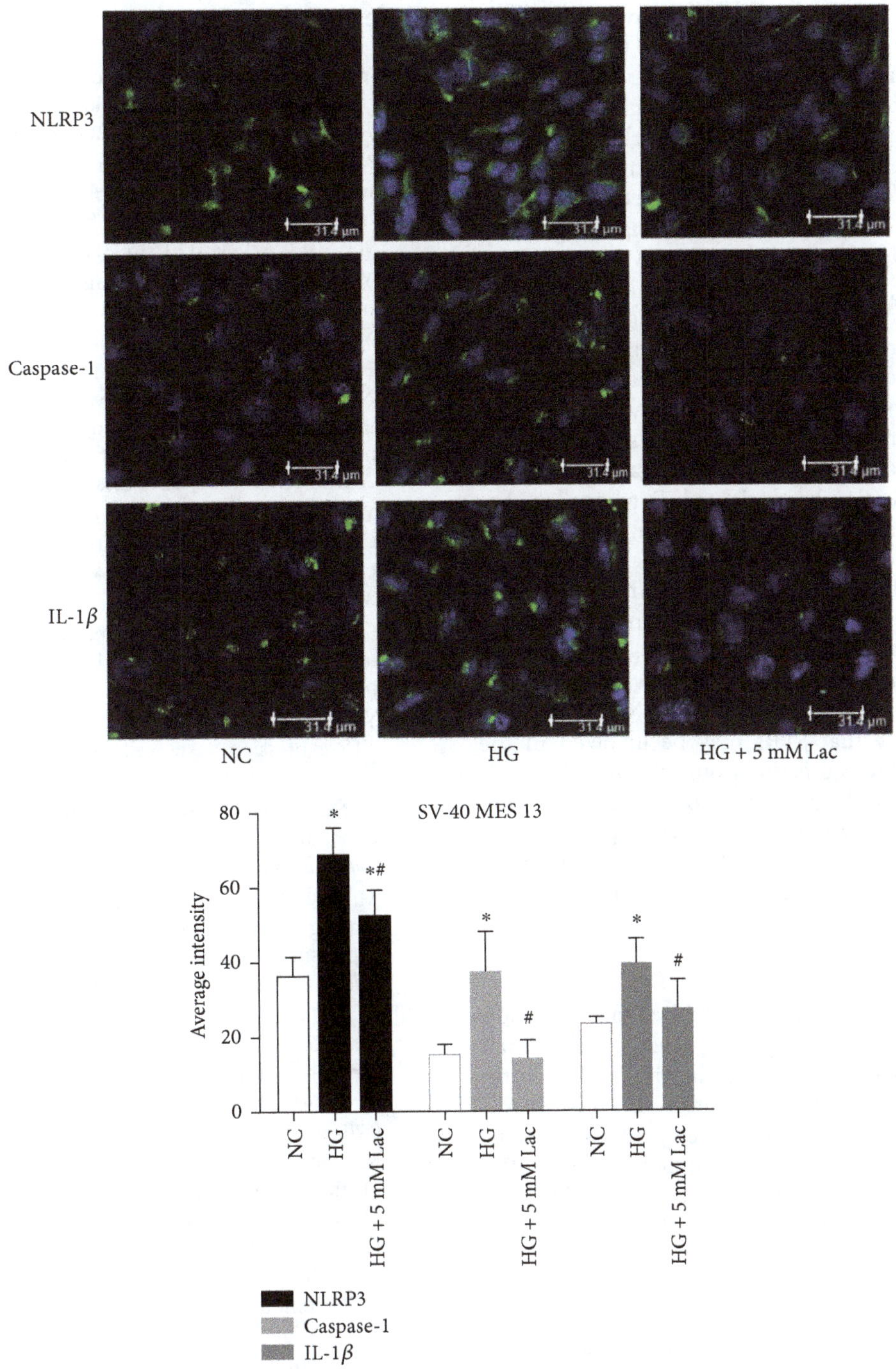

(d)

FIGURE 5: High glucose-induced activation of ROS-NLRP3 inflammasome signaling was reversed by lactisole. (a) The fluorescence images (100×) and quantitative assay for intracellular ROS was determined by detection kits. (b) The protein and mRNA expression of NLRP3, cleaved caspase-1, and cleaved IL-1β were detected by Western blotting. (c) IL-1β protein level in the cell culture supernatant was assayed after lactisole treatment. (d) Immunofluorescence and a laser scanning confocal microscope (400×) detected the expressions of NLRP3, caspase-1, and IL-1β in GMCs as green fluorescence that overlapped with blue fluorescence emitted by the nuclear stain DAPI. The values of semiquantitative analysis for average intensity were assessed and the gray graphs confirmed these trends. Data are expressed as mean ± SD. $^{*}p < 0.05$ versus NC group. $^{\#}p < 0.05$ versus 30 mmol/L glucose (HG) stimulation group.

It is quite likely that a major component of the STRs may be a homodimer of T1R3 [26]. To block the sweet-sensing receptor, the putative compound should inhibit the homodimer of T1R3. Among various inhibitors of sweet taste perception, lactisole, a broad-acting sweet antagonist, suppresses the sweet taste of sugars, protein sweeteners, and artificial sweeteners and is the most interesting candidate since it acts on the specific region of T1R3 [27].

Lactisole is commercially available and may be useful to assess the function and physiological role of the STRs [28]. The present study was conducted to examine whether or not lactisole can be used as an inhibitor of the glucose-sensing receptor. Our data revealed that 5 mM lactisole reversed the high glucose-inhibited STR expression and intracellular calcium level but blocked high glucose-induced intracellular ROS production and NLRP3 inflammasome signaling activation in a dose-dependent manner in mouse GMCs, suggesting that STR-induced signaling pathway may be involved in the regulation of innate immune, and 5 mM lactisole may be useful in assessing the role of the glucose-sensing receptor in mouse GMCs. However, it must be pointed out that the mechanism by which STRs regulate the activation of ROS-NLRP3 inflammasome is not clear, and the specific impact that this modulation of sweet taste signaling has on the development of DN still has to be elucidated. Furthermore, our studies by no means rule out other potential mechanisms by which STRs may mediate oxidative stress and inflammation. Recent research has already showed that the T1R1/T1R3, as a direct sensor of the fed state and amino acid availability, which was found in most tissues, could activate mTOR and inhibit autophagy [29, 30]. In view of mTOR and autophagy involved in the regulation of NLRP3 inflammasome, we speculate that STRs may be involved in the regulation of ROS-NLRP3 inflammasome signaling by modulating mTOR and autophagy. Even so, our study shows that a direct role of the kidney in sweet taste sensing and subsequent regulation of ROS-NLRP3 inflammasome signaling should not be excluded and deserves further research.

5. Conclusion

Our study confirms that high glucose inhibited the expression of STRs and associated signaling components and primed ROS-NLRP3 inflammasome signaling in vivo and in vitro. STR inhibitor lactisole reversed high-glucose-induced activation of ROS-NLRP3 inflammasome signaling. Our study supports the hypothesis that high glucose induced ROS-NLRP3 inflammasome signaling activation in part via STRs, suggesting that STRs may act as new therapeutic targets of DN.

Disclosure

Wei Huang is the co-first author. Yang Long is the cocorresponding author.

Conflicts of Interest

The authors declare that they have no competing interests regarding the publication of this paper.

Acknowledgments

This work was supported by the Program of Collaborative Innovation Center for Prevention and Treatment of Cardiovascular Disease of Sichuan Province and Southwest Medical University. The authors gratefully acknowledge Clinical Center Laboratory for technical assistance.

References

[1] Y.-y. Qiu and L.-q. Tang, "Roles of the NLRP3 inflammasome in the pathogenesis of diabetic nephropathy," *Pharmacological Research*, vol. 114, pp. 251–264, 2016.

[2] M. Lu, N. Yin, W. Liu, X. Cui, S. Chen, and E. Wang, "Curcumin ameliorates diabetic nephropathy by suppressing NLRP3 inflammasome signaling," *BioMed Research International*, vol. 2017, Article ID 1516985, 10 pages, 2017.

[3] Y. He, H. Hara, and G. Núñez, "Mechanism and regulation of NLRP3 inflammasome activation," *Trends in Biochemical Sciences*, vol. 41, no. 12, pp. 1012–1021, 2016.

[4] P. Gao, F.-F. He, H. Tang et al., "NADPH oxidase-induced NALP3 inflammasome activation is driven by thioredoxin-interacting protein which contributes to podocyte injury in hyperglycemia," *Journal of Diabetes Research*, vol. 2015, Article ID 504761, 12 pages, 2015.

[5] Y. Peng, S. Gillis-Smith, H. Jin, D. Tränkner, N. J. P. Ryba, and C. S. Zuker, "Sweet and bitter taste in the brain of awake behaving animals," *Nature*, vol. 527, no. 7579, pp. 512–515, 2015.

[6] G. Miller, "Neuroscience. Sweet here, salty there: evidence for a taste map in the mammalian brain," *Science*, vol. 333, no. 6047, p. 1213, 2011.

[7] Y. Ryusuke and N. Yuzo, "Taste information derived from T1R-expressing taste cells in mice," *Biochemical Journal*, vol. 473, no. 5, pp. 525–536, 2016.

[8] G. Nelson, M. A. Hoon, J. Chandrashekar, Y. Zhang, N. J. P. Ryba, and C. S. Zuker, "Mammalian sweet taste receptors," *Cell*, vol. 106, no. 3, pp. 381–390, 2001.

[9] M. Anya, N. Yuko, M. Jinhui et al., "Expression of the glucose-sensing receptor T1R3 in pancreatic islet: changes in the expression levels in various nutritional and metabolic states," *Endocrine Journal*, vol. 61, no. 8, pp. 797–805, 2014.

[10] A. C. Gerspach, R. E. Steinert, L. Schonenberger, A. Graber-Maier, and C. Beglinger, "The role of the gut sweet taste receptor in regulating GLP-1, PYY, and CCK release in humans," *American Journal of Physiology-Endocrinology and Metabolism*, vol. 301, no. 2, pp. E317–E325, 2011.

[11] K. R. Smith, T. Hussain, E. Karimian Azari et al., "Disruption of the sugar-sensing receptor T1R2 attenuates metabolic derangements associated with diet-induced obesity," *American Journal of Physiology-Endocrinology and Metabolism*, vol. 310, no. 8, pp. E688–E698, 2016.

[12] T. Tsujimoto, K. Imai, S. Kanda, M. Kakei, H. Kajio, and T. Sugiyama, "Sweet taste disorder and vascular complications in patients with abnormal glucose tolerance," *International Journal of Cardiology*, vol. 221, pp. 637–641, 2016.

[13] K. Hamano, Y. Nakagawa, Y. Ohtsu et al., "Lactisole inhibits the glucose-sensing receptor T1R3 expressed in mouse pancreatic β-cells," *Journal of Endocrinology*, vol. 226, no. 1, pp. 57–66, 2015.

[14] M. N. Patel, R. G. Carroll, S. Galván-Peña et al., "Inflammasome priming in sterile inflammatory disease," *Trends in Molecular Medicine*, vol. 23, no. 2, pp. 165–180, 2017.

[15] D. Veltman, T. Laeremans, E. Passante, and H. J. Huber, "Signal transduction analysis of the NLRP3-inflammasome pathway after cellular damage and its paracrine regulation," *Journal of Theoretical Biology*, vol. 415, pp. 125–136, 2017.

[16] H. Feng, J. Gu, F. Gou et al., "High glucose and lipopolysaccharide prime NLRP3 inflammasome via ROS/TXNIP pathway in

mesangial cells: implications for diabetic nephropathy," *Journal of Diabetes Research*, vol. 2016, Article ID 6973175, 11 pages, 2016.

[17] J. Miyamoto, M. Kasubuchi, A. Nakajima, J. Irie, H. Itoh, and I. Kimura, "The role of short-chain fatty acid on blood pressure regulation," *Current Opinion in Nephrology and Hypertension*, vol. 25, no. 5, pp. 379–383, 2016.

[18] B. Kalbe, M. Schlimm, S. Wojcik et al., "Olfactory signaling components and olfactory receptors are expressed in tubule cells of the human kidney," *Archives of Biochemistry and Biophysics*, vol. 610, pp. 8–15, 2016.

[19] P. O'Brien and C. P. Corpe, "Acute effects of sugars and artificial sweeteners on small intestinal sugar transport: a study using CaCo-2 cells as an *in vitro* model of the human enterocyte," *PLoS One*, vol. 11, no. 12, article e0167785, 2016.

[20] B. D. Shepard, L. Cheval, Z. Peterlin et al., "A renal olfactory receptor aids in kidney glucose handling," *Scientific Reports*, vol. 6, no. 1, article 35215, 2016.

[21] P. Feng, M. Jyotaki, A. Kim et al., "Regulation of bitter taste responses by tumor necrosis factor," *Brain, Behavior, and Immunity*, vol. 49, pp. 32–42, 2015.

[22] A. D. Workman, J. N. Palmer, N. D. Adappa, and N. A. Cohen, "The role of bitter and sweet taste receptors in upper airway immunity," *Current Allergy and Asthma Reports*, vol. 15, no. 12, p. 72, 2015.

[23] R. J. Lee, B. Chen, K. M. Redding, R. F. Margolskee, and N. A. Cohen, "Mouse nasal epithelial innate immune responses to *Pseudomonas aeruginosa* quorum-sensing molecules require taste signaling components," *Innate Immunity*, vol. 20, no. 6, pp. 606–617, 2014.

[24] B. M. Hariri and N. A. Cohen, "New insights into upper airway innate immunity," *American Journal of Rhinology & Allergy*, vol. 30, no. 5, pp. 319–323, 2016.

[25] W. Huang, H. L. Guo, X. Deng et al., "Short-chain fatty acids inhibit oxidative stress and inflammation in mesangial cells induced by high glucose and lipopolysaccharide," *Experimental and Clinical Endocrinology & Diabetes*, vol. 125, no. 02, pp. 98–105, 2017.

[26] Y. Nakagawa, M. Nagasawa, H. Mogami, M. Lohse, Y. Ninomiya, and I. Kojima, "Multimodal function of the sweet taste receptor expressed in pancreatic β-cells: generation of diverse patterns of intracellular signals by sweet agonists," *Endocrine Journal*, vol. 60, no. 10, pp. 1191–1206, 2013.

[27] P. Jiang, M. Cui, B. Zhao et al., "Lactisole interacts with the transmembrane domains of human T1R3 to inhibit sweet taste," *The Journal of Biological Chemistry*, vol. 280, no. 15, pp. 15238–15246, 2005.

[28] E. K. Azari, K. R. Smith, F. Yi et al., "Inhibition of sweet chemosensory receptors alters insulin responses during glucose ingestion in healthy adults: a randomized crossover interventional study," *The American Journal of Clinical Nutrition*, vol. 105, no. 4, pp. 1001–1009, 2017.

[29] E. M. Wauson, M. L. Guerra, J. Dyachok et al., "Differential regulation of ERK1/2 and mTORC1 through T1R1/T1R3 in MIN6 cells," *Molecular Endocrinology*, vol. 29, no. 8, pp. 1114–1122, 2015.

[30] E. M. Wauson, E. Zaganjor, A. Y. Lee et al., "The G protein-coupled taste receptor T1R1/T1R3 regulates mTORC1 and autophagy," *Molecular Cell*, vol. 47, no. 6, pp. 851–862, 2012.

3

Role of Nuclear Factor Erythroid 2-Related Factor 2 in Diabetic Nephropathy

Wenpeng Cui,[1] Xu Min,[1] Xiaohong Xu,[2] Bing Du,[3] and Ping Luo[1]

[1]*Department of Nephrology, The Second Hospital of Jilin University, Changchun, Jilin 130041, China*
[2]*Department of Gynaecology and Obstetrics, The Second Hospital of Jilin University, Changchun, Jilin 130041, China*
[3]*Department of Cardiology, The First Hospital of Jilin University, Changchun, Jilin 130031, China*

Correspondence should be addressed to Bing Du; dbdavina@126.com and Ping Luo; luopingjen@163.com

Academic Editor: Wei J. Liu

Diabetic nephropathy (DN) is manifested as increased urinary protein level, decreased glomerular filtration rate, and final renal dysfunction. DN is the leading cause of end-stage renal disease worldwide and causes a huge societal healthcare burden. Since satisfied treatments are still limited, exploring new strategies for the treatment of this disease is urgently needed. Oxidative stress takes part in the initiation and development of DN. In addition, nuclear factor erythroid 2-related factor 2 (Nrf2) plays a key role in the cellular response to oxidative stress. Thus, activation of Nrf2 seems to be a new choice for the treatment of DN. In current review, we discussed and summarized the therapeutic effects of Nrf2 activation on DN from both basic and clinical studies.

1. Introduction

According to the data from the International Diabetes Federation, the number of individuals who suffered from diabetic mellitus was 285 million in 2010, and this number will increase to 439 million in 2030. Diabetic nephropathy (DN), a serious complication of diabetic mellitus, is manifested as increased urinary protein level, decreased glomerular filtration rate (GFR), and final renal dysfunction [1]. DN is the leading cause of end-stage renal disease worldwide. Additionally, DN reduces patient's quality of life and increases the societal healthcare burdens. Various therapeutic approaches, such as glucose, lipid, and blood pressure control; renin-angiotensin system inhibitor application; and lifestyle changes, have been tried to slow the progression of DN [2]. However, the curative effect is not satisfactory, and the developing speed of DN is still the fastest among chronic kidney diseases (CKDs). Therefore, novel strategies for fighting against this disease are urgently needed.

The pathogenesis of DN is complicated. It is suggested that hemodynamic changes, genetic susceptibility, hyperglycemia, dyslipidemia, and oxidative stress take part in the progress and development of DN [3]. Among these issues, oxidative stress and its related inflammation and fibrosis have been reported to aggravate DN in recent years [4]. In our body, mechanisms maintaining the balance between oxidation and reduction are complicated. Nuclear factor erythroid 2-related factor 2 (Nrf2)/antioxidant-responsive element (ARE) pathway is proven to be crucial in this process [5, 6]. Therefore, activation of Nrf2/ARE pathway seems to be a potentially effective method for the treatment of DN. Here, we seek to review the contribution of Nrf2/ARE pathway activation to DN.

2. Oxidative Stress and DN

The nature of oxidative stress is the disproportionate generation of reactive oxygen species (ROS) and endogenous antioxidants. Low ROS level in body is crucial for survival and proliferation. High level of ROS leads to cellular apoptosis. Extremely high level of ROS gives rise to the damage of cellular macromolecules, including DNA [7], lipid [8], and protein [9]. It will cause mutations and followed by tissue injury or even necrotic cell death if those damages were not repaired [10].

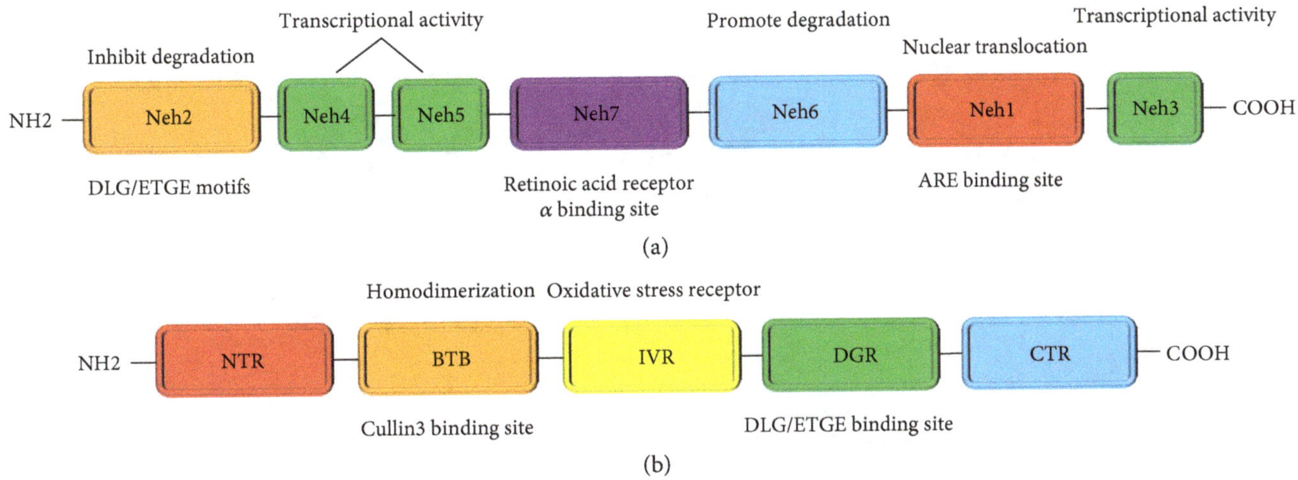

FIGURE 1: Molecular structure of Nrf2 (a) and Keap1 (b) proteins. (a) There are seven domains in the Nrf2 molecule, and a brief explanatory note for the main function of each domain was given. (b) There are five domains in the Keap1 molecule, and a brief explanatory note for the main function of each domain was given.

Under diabetes condition, oxidative stress is triggered through a variety of ways, such as advanced glycation end-product accumulation and activation of polyol pathway, protein kinase C pathway, and renin angiotensin-aldosterone system. It is well accepted that oxidative stress takes part in the pathogenesis of DN. A large number of excellent reviews have shown that oxidative stress accelerates the progress of experimental DN [4, 11, 12]. For example, in type 1 diabetes rats, kidney expression of superoxide dismutase together with glutathione was obviously decreased, while restoring these two enzymes inhibited the progression of DN [13]. For type 2 diabetes rats, similarly, upregulation of malondialdehyde and downregulation of antioxidant enzymes, such as superoxide dismutase and glutathione, were observed in diabetes rat kidney. And, restoration of these enzymes halted hyperglycemia-induced oxidative stress and maintained renal function [14]. Moreover, it is not difficult to obtain similar evidence from clinical studies [15–17]. For example, in new published clinical trials, individuals who suffered from DN were enrolled. Kidney injury was attenuated accompanied by improving oxidative stress biomarkers (nitric oxide, glutathione, and malondialdehyde) after short-term supplementation of selenium or vitamin E [15, 16]. Taken together, antioxidative stress therapy might bring favorable outcomes to patients with DN.

3. Oxidative Stress and Nrf2/ARE Pathway

3.1. Components of Nrf2/ARE Pathway. Nrf2 is a smart transcription factor with a basic leucine zipper motif [18]. It has seven highly conserved Nrf2-ECH homology domains, Neh1 to Neh7 [19, 20]. Neh1 domain includes a basic leucine zipper structure, which facilitates dimerization with small musculoaponeurotic fibrosarcoma (sMaf) protein and binding to ARE [21]. Besides, Neh1 also promotes the cytoplasmic-to-nuclear translocation of Nrf2 [22]. Neh2 domain is highly conserved between species [23] and enables Nrf2 to combine with Kelch-like ECH-associated protein 1 (Keap1) [24, 25]. Additionally, the presences of lysine residues and a serine residue in Neh2 domain are involved in the suppression of proteasome-mediated Nrf2 degradation [26] and Nrf2-Keap1 complex structure modulation, respectively. The functions of Neh3–Neh6 domains are relatively simple. Briefly, Neh3–Neh5 domains are essential for Nrf2 transcriptional activity [27], and Neh6 domain is associated with Nrf2 degradation [28]. Neh7 domain, which has been identified recently, suppresses Nrf2 downstream gene expression through binding to the retinoic acid receptor α [29]. Nrf2 molecular structure is given in Figure 1(a).

Keap1 was first recognized in 1999 with the application of the Neh2 domain of Nrf2 [25]. The Keap1 molecules from different species are slightly different. The number of cysteine residues in the Keap1 molecule from mouse and human beings is 25 and 27, respectively. To be noticed, cysteine residues are sensors for Nrf2 activation [30]. Five domains have been discovered in the Keap1 molecule. They are NTR, BTB, IVR, DGR, and CTR [23]. The BTB domain is required for the homodimerization of Keap1 [31] and the interaction between Keap1 and Cullin3-Rbx1E3 ubiquitin ligase (Cul3-E3-ligase) [32]. The cysteine-rich IVR domain is sensitive to oxidation [33]. Three important cysteine residues (Cys151, Cys273, and Cys288) were identified to be crucial for maintaining the structural integrity of Keap1 [34–36]. The DGR domain is where Keap1 binds to the Neh2 domain of Nrf2 [37]. The Keap1 molecular structure is given in Figure 1(b).

3.2. Working Model of Nrf2/ARE Pathway. Nrf2/ARE pathway plays a crucial role in cellular resistance to oxidative stress [5]. Under rest conditions, Keap1 interacts with Nrf2 to form a complex [38, 39]. At this situation, Keap1 acts as an inhibitor of Nrf2. Moreover, this Nrf2 inhibitor can also interact with Cul3-E3-ligase, which mediates Nrf2 degradation in ubiquitin-proteasome system. After that, the transcription function of Nrf2 is repressed [40] (Figure 2(a)). During oxidative stress, Nrf2 is activated. By modifying the

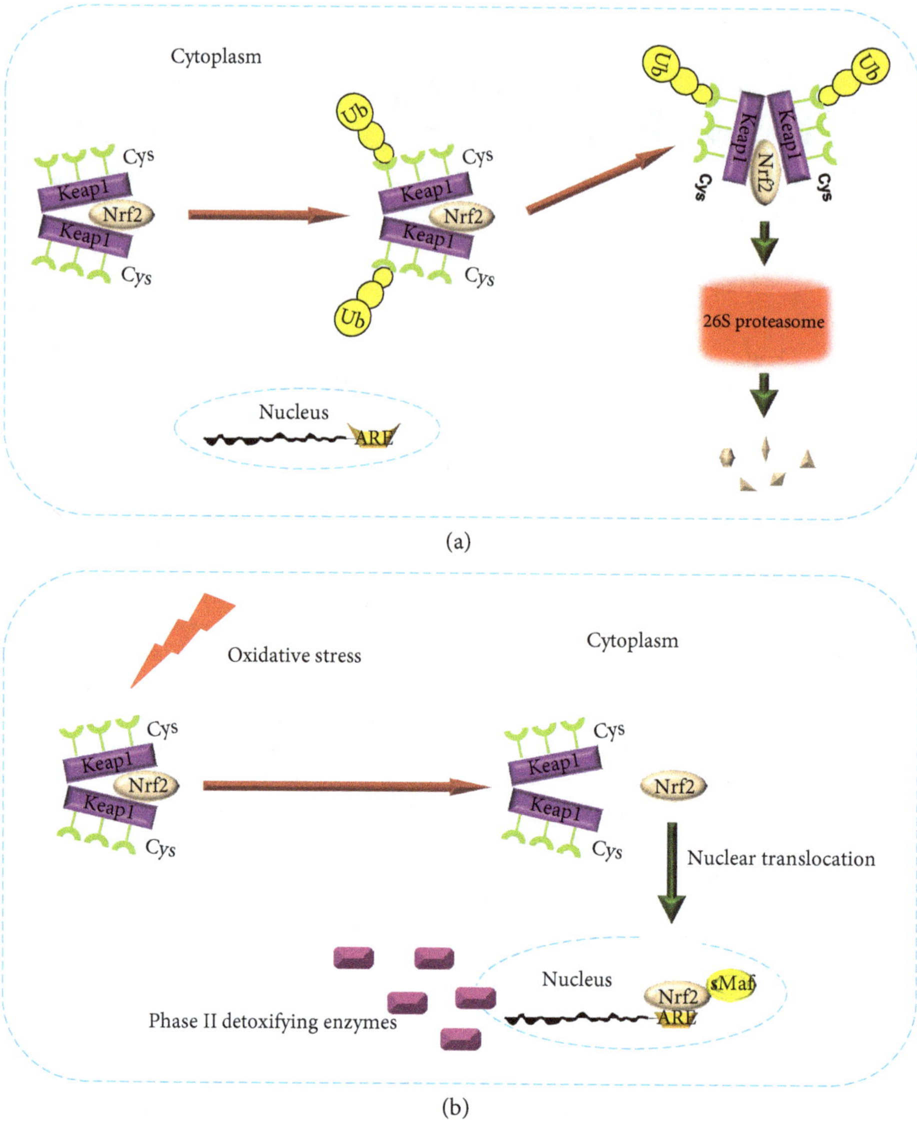

FIGURE 2: Working model of Nrf2/ARE pathway. (a) Working model of Nrf2/ARE pathway under rest conditions. (b) Working model of Nrf2/ARE pathway during oxidative stress.

three important cysteine residues of Keap1, conformational changes occur in the Nrf2/Keap1 complex [30, 35], leading to Nrf2 liberalization, followed by Nrf2 translocation. In the nucleus, Nrf2 binds to ARE with the help of sMaf protein [21]. Then, Nrf2 triggers the transcription of phase II detoxification enzymes and antioxidants, such as heme oxygenase-1 and superoxide dismutase 1 [41–43] (Figure 2(b)).

3.3. Nrf2/ARE Pathway Regulation. As an executor, Nrf2/ARE signaling pathway is regulated by complex mechanisms [44]. The regulation models include transcriptional level, translational level, and posttranslational level. To examine the mechanisms of Nrf2 transcriptional activation, Kwak et al. found that Nrf2 could autoregulate itself via a specific element of its own promoter [45]. Nowadays, microRNAs are thought to take part in the regulation of oxidative stress [46]. It was suggested that Nrf2 gene could be directly down-regulated by miR-28 [47], miR-34a [48], and miR-144 [49]. Additionally, Nrf2 gene could be indirectly regulated by miR-200a-driven Keap1 gene downregulation [50]. Moreover, it is suggested that both DNA methylation [51, 52] and histone modification [53, 54] can regulate Nrf2/ARE pathway. Such information about the epigenetic regulation of Nrf2 and Keap1 was well summarized in a review article [55].

As we talked above, Nrf2 is degraded in ubiquitin-proteasome system. This process keeps Nrf2 protein at a low level and maintains cellular redox homoeostasis by preventing transcription of undesired genes. Therefore, protein level of Nrf2 can be controlled by both regulation of ubiquitin ligases [56] and proteasome activity [57]. In addition to ubiquitin-proteasome system, other proteins can regulate Nrf2 by interacting with the Nrf2-Keap1 complex. For example, autophagy pathway inhibition leads to excessive p62 accumulation. By directly interacting with Keap1, p62 blots Keap1-mediated Nrf2 degradation [58].

Besides regulating transcription and translation, Nrf2 pathway can also be regulated after translation. For example, protein kinase C catalyzes Nrf2 phosphorylation at serine 40 residue, which is critical for promoting Nrf2 separation from Keap1 [59]. Interestingly, p66Shc which takes part in cellular stress response is transcriptionally regulated by Nrf2. However, p66Shc also controls the expression of several Nrf2 downstream genes, like NAD(P)H:quinone oxidoreductase 1 [60]. Taken together, all these signaling pathway regulation methods have the potential to be used for antioxidative stress strategies.

4. Role of Nrf2/ARE Pathway in DN: Evidences in Basic Research

The effects of Nrf2/ARE pathway activation on DN in different experimental models were well documented in the past ten years [61]. Sun et al. revealed proper time nodes of Nrf2 signaling pathway in different processes of DN in rats [62]. In addition, hyperglycemia-induced oxidative stress and accelerated renal injury were more serious in streptozotocin-treated Nrf2 knockout mice than those in wild-type controls [63–65], indicating a beneficial effect of Nrf2 on DN. With the expectation that Nrf2-targeted genes would be increased, Keap1 knockout and knockdown mice were generated. However, Keap1 knockout mice died early because of severe defects [66], and Keap1 knockdown mice show different impact effects on metabolic homeostasis [67–69]. The possible reasons for the discrepancy could be the component and content of the diet and the length of high-fat feeding. To be noticed, genetic and pharmacological activation of Nrf2 is constitutive and intermittent, respectively, and the levels of Nrf2 downstream genes in the genetically modified mice were higher than those induced by pharmacological Nrf2 inducers [70]. Moreover, aberrant Nrf2 activation causes unexpected side effects, which will be discussed at the end of this review. Therefore, either pharmacologically activating Nrf2 pathway or inhibiting Nrf2 degradation intermittently might be considered as potential strategies for treating DN.

Recently, a mount of Nrf2 activators have been applied to explore the therapeutic potential of Nrf2 in experimental DN models. In these studies, Nrf2 activators acted upon a series of targets via different mechanisms. The information of these articles was summarized and listed in Table 1 [57, 71–106].

4.1. Nrf2-Keap1 Complex Modulation. As a novel Nrf2 activation strategy, directly destroying Nrf2-Keap1 complex has been proved to be effective. For example, under diabetes condition, miR-29 was downregulated. Because miR-29 directly targeted to Keap1 mRNA, Nrf2 content was indirectly reduced [81]. Our previous study demonstrated that C66 (a novel curcumin analogue) ameliorated DN by miR-200a-mediated Nrf2 activation [93]. This method of Nrf2 regulation by miR-200a was confirmed by another study from Wei et al. [107]. Taken together, miR-29 activator and miR-200a activator have the potential to be used in the treatment of DN.

Huang et al. claimed that, in HepG2 cells, PKC promoted Nrf2 phosphorylation at Ser-40. This modulation broke the Nrf2-Keap1 complex and promoted the division between Nrf2 and Keap1 [59]. Therefore, developing medicines inhibiting the interaction between Nrf2 and Keap1-Nrf2 will be a valuable topic.

4.2. Reduction of Nrf2 Degradation. The degradation of Nrf2 occurs in the proteasome system. Thus, suppressing the degradation of Nrf2 via inhibiting proteasome activity seems to be a reasonable strategy for DN. Studies from both other and our groups revealed that low dose of MG132, a proteasome inhibitor, had preventive and therapeutic effects on the development and progression of DN in rodents [57, 106].

In addition, minocycline which has been widely used in clinical research is beneficial to the stabilization of endogenous Nrf2 in the kidneys of *db/db* mice, followed by the reduction of glomerular ROS generation. The underlying mechanism might be minocycline could reduce Nrf2 ubiquitination and then decrease its degradation. However, minocycline-mediated amelioration of DN disappeared in diabetic Nrf2 knockout mice [92].

4.3. Cytoplasm-to-Nuclear Shuttling of Nrf2. Under certain condition, Nrf2 shuttles from cytoplasm to nucleus. Nucleus accumulation of Nrf2 was proven to be effective against diabetes-induced kidney injury [94]. Using human renal tubular cells, our previous study claimed that Zinc increased the Nrf2 protein level in nucleus and upregulated the expression of Nrf2 downstream enzymes through promoting Akt/GSK-3β-mediated inhibition of Fyn, which is a Nrf2 nuclear exporter [98]. Following studies confirmed our viewpoint in type 1 diabetic rodents by using fenofibrate [95] and sulforaphane [96], respectively. Interestingly, it was suggested that sulforaphane mainly induced Nrf2 via modification of Keap1 Cys151 [36]. However, Shang et al. demonstrated that sulforaphane attenuated experimental DN partially through GSK-3β/Fyn/Nrf2 pathway [96]. This study provided another possible mechanism underlying the regulation of Nrf2 by sulforaphane. Additionally, Chen et al. found that connexin43 might hinder the nuclear export of Nrf2 by inhibiting c-Src activity and then attenuate renal fibrosis in high glucose-treated glomerular mesangial cells [91]. All these Nrf2 activators promoted Nrf2 nucleus accumulation by blocking Nrf2 export.

Moreover, beneficial effects of facilitating the nuclear import of Nrf2 by other Nrf2 activators, such as hydrogen sulfide [100], hepatocyte growth factor [103], and tert-butylhydroquinone [105], were proved in many experimental DN models, indicating the importance of the regulation of cytoplasm-to-nuclear shuttling of Nrf2 in the treatment of DN.

4.4. Other Underlying Mechanisms for Nrf2 Activation. In a recent study, streptozotocin-treated Nrf2 knockout mice and wild-type controls were administrated with or without sodium butyrate for twenty weeks. Data showed that Nrf2 played a key role in the process of sodium butyrate protection against DN. Additionally, sodium butyrate might upregulate

Table 1: Beneficial effect of Nrf2 activators on experimental DN.

Nrf2 activator	DN model	Results	Ref.
Sulforaphane	T1DM mice; human renal tubular cells	Sulforaphane alleviates renal inflammation, oxidative stress, fibrosis, and dysfunction in DN mice via activation of Nrf2/ARE pathway (HO-1, SOD1, etc.); beneficial effects disappeared when Nrf2 siRNA was applied	[85]
Sulforaphane	T1DM mice; human renal mesangial cells	Sulforaphane normalizes diabetes-induced kidney oxidative damage, fibrosis, and apoptosis, which is mediated by Nrf2/ARE pathway (NQO1, rGCS, and MRP2) activation; beneficial effects disappeared in Nrf2 knockout mice	[86]
Sulforaphane	T2DM mice	Sulforaphane improves kidney oxidative damage, inflammation, and fibrosis in diabetic mice, accompanied by increasing kidney Nrf2 and its downstream gene metallothionein; beneficial effects disappeared in Nrf2 knockout mice	[89]
Sulforaphane	T1DM rats	Sulforaphane ameliorates DN through GSK3β/Fyn/Nrf2 signaling pathway (prevents nuclear export of Nrf2)	[96]
Resveratrol and rosuvastatin	T1DM mice	Resveratrol combined with rosuvastatin treatment normalizes the TGF-β1, FN, and NF-κB/p65 and restores Nrf2 in renal tissues of diabetic rats	[74]
Resveratrol	T1DM rats; rat mesangial cells	Resveratrol reduces albuminuria and mesangial matrix expansion in DN rats and attenuates mesangial cell proliferation, which is associated with upregulation of Nrf2 and glutathione S-transferases Mu	[84]
Resveratrol	T1DM rats	Resveratrol protects against DN by alleviating oxidative damage and inflammation through Nrf2/ARE pathway (SOD, CAT, etc.)	[87]
Resveratrol	Rat primary glomerular mesangial cells	Resveratrol inhibits AGE-induced FN and TGF-β1 in glomerular mesangial cells through Sirt1/Nrf2 signaling pathway activation	[101]
Polydatin (resveratrol analogue)	T1DM rats; rat glomerular mesangial cells	Polydatin inhibits AGE-induced FN and TGF-β1 in glomerular mesangial cells is associated with activation of Sirt1/Nrf2 pathway	[97]
Curcumin	T2DM rats	Curcumin ameliorates albuminuria, kidney pathophysiologic changes, and urinary MDA, accompanied by increasing Nrf2, HO-1, and urinary SOD	[78]
Curcumin	Rat kidney tubular epithelial cells	Curcumin protects renal tubular cells from high glucose-induced EMT through upregulating Nrf2 and HO-1; beneficial effects disappeared when Nrf2 siRNA was applied	[80]
C66 (curcumin analogue)	T1DM mice	C66 protects against DN by upregulating Nrf2 via both increasing miR-200a and inhibiting miR-21; beneficial effects were partially abolished in Nrf2 knockout mice	[93]
Zinc	Human renal tubular cells	Zn sensitizes Nrf2 by facilitating Akt-associated Fyn inhibition (prevents Nrf2 nuclear export) and thus alleviates kidney oxidative and inflammatory damage and fibrosis	[98]
Zinc	Rat kidney tubular epithelial cells	Zinc ameliorates high glucose-mediated apoptosis in rat kidney tubular cells through Akt/ERK/Nrf2 signaling pathway activation (promotes Nrf2 accumulation in nuclear)	[99]
MG132	T1DM mice; human renal tubular cells	MG132 sensitizes Nrf2 by inhibiting proteasome activity and thus attenuates hyperglycemia-induced kidney oxidative and inflammatory damage, fibrosis, and eventual dysfunction; beneficial effects disappeared when Nrf2 siRNA was applied	[57]
MG132	T1DM rats	Low dose of MG132 prevents diabetes-induced kidney damage by Nrf2/ARE pathway activation	[106]
Rutin	Human renal glomerular endothelial cells	Rutin significantly prevents hyperglycemia-induced glomerular endothelial barrier disruption by decreasing ROS through the activation of Nrf2	[71]
Berberine	T1DM mice; rat renal tubular epithelial cells	Berberine ameliorates high glucose-induced EMT and oxidative stress by Nrf2/ARE pathway (HO-1 and NQO1) activation and TGF-β/EMT pathway inhibition; beneficial effects disappeared when Nrf2 siRNA was applied	[72]
Casein kinase 2 interacting protein-1	Rat glomerular mesangial cells	Casein kinase 2 interacting protein-1 downregulates ICAM-1 and FN by Nrf2/ARE pathway (SOD1 and HO-1) activation	[73]
Salvianolic acid A	T1DM mice	Salvianolic acid A protects DN via Nrf2/ARE pathway (HO-1, NQO1, and GPx-1)	[75]

Table 1: Continued.

Nrf2 activator	DN model	Results	Ref.
Sinomenine	Human renal glomerular endothelial cells	Sinomenine reduces ROS level and exerts renal protective effect by activating Nrf2 in high glucose-treated human renal glomerular endothelial cells	[76]
Momordica charantia polysaccharides	T1DM rats	*Momordica charantia* polysaccharides attenuate type 1 DN in rats by upregulating Nrf2, CAT, GSH, and SOD	[77]
Digitoflavone	T1DM mice	Digitoflavone minimizes pathological changes, decreases oxidative and inflammatory damage as well as fibrosis in DN mice, which is mediated by Nrf2 pathway (GCLC and HO-1) activation; beneficial effects disappeared in Nrf2 knockout mice	[78]
Thrombomodulin domain 1	T2DM mice	Thrombomodulin domain 1 improves DN by suppressing inflammation, activating the Nrf2 pathway, and inhibiting apoptosis in the mouse kidney	[82]
Maxacalcitol	T2DM mice	Maxacalcitol alleviates DN by suppressing kidney oxidative and inflammatory damage as well as fibrosis, which is mediated by Nrf2 pathway (GCLC and HO-1) activation	[83]
4-Phenylbutyric acid	T1DM rats	Treatment with 4-phenylbutyric acid attenuates oxidative damage in DN rats via Nrf2 facilitation	[88]
Sodium butyrate	T1DM mice	Sodium butyrate protects against DN through Nrf2 upregulation, which is mediated by suppressing HDAC function; beneficial effects disappeared in Nrf2 knockout mice	[90]
Connexin43	Primary glomerular mesangial cells; type 2 diabetic mice	Connexin43 activates Nrf2/ARE pathway by means of inhibiting c-Src activity to hinder the nuclear export of Nrf2 and then downregulates FN, ICAM-1, and TGF-β1 expression and ultimately attenuates renal fibrosis in diabetic mice	[91]
Minocycline	T1DM/T2DM mice; human/mouse podocytes	Minocycline stabilizes endogenous Nrf2 by reducing its ubiquitination and reduces markers of oxidative damage, thus alleviated DN; beneficial effects disappeared in Nrf2 knockout mice	[92]
Mycophenolate mofetil	T1DM rats	Mycophenolate mofetil attenuates DN at least in part by upregulating Nrf2 pathway (increases the nuclear accumulation of Nrf2)	[94]
Fenofibrate	T1DM mice	Fenofibrate attenuates DN via increasing FGF21 and activating Akt/GSK-3β/Fyn/Nrf2 pathway (prevents Nrf2 nuclear export)	[95]
Hydrogen sulfide	T1DM rats; rat glomerular mesangial cells	Hydrogen sulfide alleviates DN by suppressing oxidative stress (promotes Nrf2 accumulation in nuclear), inflammation, and renin-angiotensin system activity, as well as by reducing mesangial cell proliferation	[100]
Low-dose radiation	T1DM mice	Prevention of low-dose radiation against DN is associated with Akt phosphorylation and Nrf2 upregulation	[102]
Hepatocyte growth factor	Rat mesangial cells	Hepatocyte growth factor ameliorates high glucose-induced oxidative damage in rat mesangial cells by upregulating 8-nitro-cGMP production, accompanied by nuclear accumulation of Nrf2	[103]
Telmisartan	T2DM mice	Telmisartan inhibits NAD(P)H oxidase and upregulates Nrf2 and SOD, leading to the attenuation of diabetes-induced renal damage	[104]
tert-butylhydroquinone	T1DM mice	tert-butylhydroquinone reduces renal damage through nuclear accumulation of Nrf2 as well as its target genes in type 1 diabetic mice	[105]

Nrf2 at the transcriptional level possibly by inhibiting histone deacetylase activity [90]. As a NAD-dependent histone deacetylase in the nucleus, Sirt1 takes part in many biological processes [108] through working on a battery of transcription factors, including Nrf2 [109–111]. Studies revealed that both resveratrol [101] and its analogue (polydatin) [97] activated Nrf2/ARE pathway through upregulating Sirt1 in glomerular mesangial cells and attenuated high glucose caused fibrosis.

Moreover, Nrf2-dependent beneficial effects on the prevention of DN were observed in low dose of radiation-treated mice [102] and high glucose-treated NRK-52E cells [99], respectively. Activation of Nrf2 in these two studies was reported to be responsible to Akt activation; however, whether Fyn was involved in this process was not mentioned [99, 102].

Oxidative stress aggrieves all kinds of kidney resident cells, including epithelium (podocyte), endothelium, glomerular mesangial cell, and tubular cell. According to Table 1, available evidences support that activation of Nrf2/ARE pathway not only attenuates high glucose-induced podocyte [82, 92, 112, 113], endothelium [71, 76], and mesangial cell [73, 86, 91, 97, 101, 103, 105, 107] injury in glomeruli but also alleviates renal tubular cell [72, 80, 81, 98, 99] damage. In addition, sulforaphane [85, 86, 89, 96] and resveratrol [74, 84, 87, 97, 101] are the most well-studied ones among those Nrf2 activators. Besides, curcumin and its analogues (C66) were also introduced in three studies [78, 80, 93] and have emerged to be a potential therapeutic choice, which will be discussed later in this review.

Taken together, breaking the Nrf2-Keap1 complex, blocking Nrf2 degradation, and promoting Nrf2 cytoplasmic-to-nuclear translocation are valuable strategies to increase antioxidant generation. These basic evidences provide us with new ideas for the treatment of oxidative stress-associated kidney injury under diabetes condition.

5. Role of Nrf2/ARE Pathway in DN: Evidences in Clinical Research

Beneficial effects of Nrf2/ARE pathway activation on DN can be observed in not only basic researches but also clinical researches. Additionally, the relationship of genetic variants of Nrf2 (rs2364723, rs10497511, rs1962142, and rs6726395) and diabetes complications in Han descents of Northeast China has been confirmed recently by our group [114]. Moreover, dysregulation of Nrf2 signaling was also observed in human diabetes kidney [64]. Thus, Nrf2 activators began to be used in patients with DN in clinical trials.

The most well-studied promising candidate Nrf2 activator is bardoxolone methyl (BM), which has been used not only for cancer [115] but also for many other oxidative stress and inflammation-involved chronic diseases [116]. BM was first introduced to clinicians because it possesses anticancer effects. When treating patients who suffered from malignant diseases, the investigators surprisingly found that BM could raise estimated GRF (eGFR), accompanied by increasing NQO1 mRNA in peripheral blood mononuclear cells. Interestingly, these improvements were more likely to be observed in a subset of patients with CKD [117, 118]. Based on these observations, this multifunctional medicine was thought to ameliorate renal damage in type 2 diabetes patients.

With the encouraging idea, BM was further studied in a phase 2a clinical trial to evaluate its renoprotective efficacy and safety [119]. In this multicenter clinical trial, short-term (8 weeks) effects of BM on kidney function was evaluated in type 2 diabetes patients and moderate to severe CKD (baseline serum creatinine level ranged from 1.3 to 3.0 mg/dl). All enrolled patients were administrated with 25 mg BM for 4 weeks and 75 mg BM for next 4 weeks. Data showed that the administration of BM obviously increased eGFR and creatinine clearance while decreased serum creatinine and blood urea nitrogen. These results seemed very optimistic; however, two major limitations in this study should not be ignored. First, this was a self-control study and a placebo control group was needed to obtain a more convincing result. Second, the treatment course was not long enough to observe side effects.

Attempting to further verify the beneficial effects of BM in patients who suffered from diabetes and CKD, the BEAM study with a larger sample size was conducted [120]. To overcome the limitations in the previous phase 2a clinical trial, 227 patients who suffered from diabetes mellitus and CKD were enrolled in the BEAM study. Participants were administrated with either placebo or different doses (25, 75 or 150 mg/day) of BM for 52 weeks. Data showed that BM ameliorated eGFR, which persisted during the 52-week treatment period. Moreover, adverse events reported in the BEAM study were moderate and manageable.

After obtaining these exciting results, the BEACON study was performed in June 2011 [121]. The purpose of this study was further confirming the beneficial effects of BM on safely reducing renal and cardiac morbidity and mortality among patients who suffered from diabetes mellitus and CKD. More than two thousands patients who suffered from type 2 diabetes mellitus and stage 4 CKD were recruited and randomly administrated with either placebo or BM (20 mg/day) for 52 weeks. However, the BEACON study was stopped prematurely in October 2012 due to safety concerns about considerable adverse events as well as high mortality rates. Heart failure events (hospitalization or death) occurred in 96 from 1088 patients and 55 from 1097 patients in the BM group and placebo group, respectively. Moreover, composite outcome events (including nonfatal stroke and myocardial infarction, hospitalization because of heart failure, and death because of cardiovascular diseases) occurred in 139 from 1088 patients and 86 from 1097 patients in the BM group and placebo group, respectively. Compared to the placebo group, although eGFR was improved, urinary protein level and blood pressure were also obviously increased in the BM group during the study period.

The main reason for the termination of the BEACON study was high rates of heart failure, and many occurred early after BM initiation. Analyses aiming to find the reasons for heart failure events in the BEACON study were conducted [122, 123]. Chin et al. claimed that both high B-type natriuretic peptide level and heart failure-caused hospitalization before were risk factors of heart failure [122]. Another mechanism underlying cardiovascular events in the BEACON study was also revealed by Chin et al. It was suggested that BM might pharmacologically lead to acute water-sodium retention and hypertension by modulating the endothelin pathway [123]. Besides heart failure events, hypertension was also more likely to happen in patients from the BM group than from the placebo group. There were two possible reasons to explain this phenomenon. First, endothelin pathway regulation by BM leads to sodium and volume retention as we described above. Second, by binding to the promoter of intrarenal angiotensinogen gene, Nrf2 stimulates its expression and then activates the renin-angiotensin system [124]. Therefore, BM might lead to hypertension by both sodium and volume retention and renin-angiotensin system activation.

In the BEACON study, investigators did observed elevated eGFR in the BM group. This phenomenon was possibly due to a similar structure between BM and cyclopentenone prostaglandins, which can cause renal vasodilatation. To be noticed, eGFR was calculated by serum creatinine in the BEAM study and muscle mass will influence the level of serum creatinine [125, 126]. Compared to those in the placebo group, the degree of weight loss and muscle wasting in the BM group was higher, which might cause an overestimation of eGFR in the BM group [127].

Although some adverse events occurred in BM-treated patients, it cannot stop us from exploring new medicines for the treatment of DN. Different to BM, curcumin was proven to be effective in a DN experiment model [78, 80, 93]. In a recent clinical trial with small sample size, 14 patients with diabetic kidney disease were given curcumin (500 mg/day) for 2–4 weeks. It was claimed that short-term curcumin intervention attenuated kidney damage partially by activating Nrf2 pathway [128], which enhanced our confidence.

6. Other Mechanisms of Nrf2 in the Treatment of DN

6.1. Effects of Nrf2 Activation on Anti-Inflammation. Besides having an antioxidant property, Nrf2 was proven to alleviate inflammation, which is also involved in the progression of DN. Alleviation of kidney damages accompanied by downregulation of inflammatory cytokines (monocyte chemotactic protein-1, intercellular cell adhesion molecule-1) was observed in digitoflavone-treated wild-type diabetic mice instead of Nrf2 knockout diabetic mice [79]. However, the mechanism under which Nrf2 regulated these two proinflammatory mediators was not mentioned. Another study revealed direct evidence of inflammation suppression by Nrf2. Kobayashi et al. demonstrated that Nrf2 interfered with transcriptional upregulation of IL-6 and IL-1b by binding to these two genes and inhibiting RNA polymerase II recruitment [129].

6.2. Effects of Nrf2 Activation on Antifibrosis. Fibrosis is an ultimate pathway in the pathogenesis of DN, and TGF-β1 advances kidney fibrosis. It was suggested that Nrf2 ameliorated DN by transcriptional repression of TGF-β1 directly. Gao et al. found that Nrf2 inhibited TGF-β1 through binding to the specific region in TGF-β1 promoter with the help of c-Jun as well as SP1 [130]. This study provided a novel clue for DN prevention and intervention.

7. Side Effects of Nrf2 Activation

Considerable evidence showed beneficial effects of Nrf2 on DN. However, side effects of this molecule should also be noticed. Zoja et al. treated type 2 diabetic rats with a synthetic triterpenoid analogue of BM (RTA405). They demonstrated that RTA405 elevated mortality, aggravated proteinuria, dyslipidemia, kidney function, and liver function [131]. These findings indicated the toxicity of this molecule. In addition, by using another BM analogue (dh404), the deleterious and salutary actions of Nrf2 activation in the treatment of DN were reported to be dose-dependent. Low dose of dh404 might alleviate kidney damage, while high dose of dh404 might lead to deterioration of the kidney function [132, 133]. Therefore, consideration of the appropriate dose is necessary when applying the BM analogues.

Dural roles of Nrf2 in cancer have also been reported [134, 135]. Some studies suggested that aberrant Nrf2 activation was correlated with cancer progression. For example, one important mechanism of hereditary leiomyomatosis and renal cell carcinoma is fumarate hydratase inactivation-induced fumarate accumulation. Sustained fumarate accumulation leads to aberrant Nrf2 activation and then gives rise to fatal consequences [136]. Nrf2 contributes to cancer cell survival not only by upregulating the expression of Bcl-xl and Bcl-2 to inhibit apoptosis [137] but also by raising the rate of glycolysis to promote cell proliferation [138].

Intrarenal renin-angiotensin system causes blood pressure elevation and kidney damage. Another side effect of Nrf2 activation that should be noticed is that Nrf2 can activate the renin-angiotensin system directly [139]. For example, Abdo et al. found that overexpression of Nrf2 promoted angiotensinogen gene transcription in high glucose-treated renal proximal tubule cells. Moreover, application of Nrf2 siRNA reduced angiotensinogen mRNA and protein expression [124].

8. Conclusions

In summary, oxidative stress is an important pathogenesis of DN. As the center of the body antioxidant system, Nrf2/ARE pathway is of great value in the treatment of DN. Modulating Nrf2/ARE pathway through different mechanisms provides new approaches for future clinical research studying the treatment of DN. It was worth noting that there was no evidence to support the application of BM in animal DN before the BEACON study. Therefore, before designing a new clinical trial, investigators should make sure that preliminary studies have been done and should not ignore any negative outcome. Moreover, in order to avoid the occurrence of a large number of serious adverse events, possible side effects of Nrf2 activation need to be monitored during the period of trial conduction.

Conflicts of Interest

The authors declare that they have no competing interests.

Authors' Contributions

Wenpeng Cui, Bing Du, and Ping Luo designed and wrote this manuscript. Xu Min and Xiaohong Xu revised this manuscript. All of the authors read and approved the final manuscript.

Acknowledgments

This study was supported in part by the National Natural Science Foundation of China (no. 81200525), Jilin Province Science and Technology Development Program (funded Projects no. 20150520034JH and no. 20160414014GH), Jilin Province Scientific Research Program (funded Project no. 2016446), and Norman Bethune Program of Jilin University (no. 2015214). The authors would like to express their gratitude to all the physicians participating in this work.

References

[1] M. Haneda, K. Utsunomiya, D. Koya et al., "A new classification of diabetic nephropathy 2014: a report from Joint Committee on Diabetic Nephropathy," *Clinical and Experimental Nephrology*, vol. 19, no. 1, pp. 1–5, 2015.

[2] H. Gallagher and R. J. Suckling, "Diabetic nephropathy: where are we on the journey from pathophysiology to treatment?" *Diabetes, Obesity & Metabolism*, vol. 18, no. 7, pp. 641–647, 2016.

[3] A. G. Miranda-Diaz, L. Pazarin-Villasenor, F. G. Yanowsky-Escatell, and J. Andrade-Sierra, "Oxidative stress in diabetic nephropathy with early chronic kidney disease," *Journal of Diabetes Research*, vol. 2016 no. 6, p. 7047238, 2016.

[4] M. K. Arora and U. K. Singh, "Oxidative stress: meeting multiple targets in pathogenesis of diabetic nephropathy," *Current Drug Targets*, vol. 15, no. 5, pp. 531–538, 2014.

[5] W. Cui, Y. Bai, P. Luo, L. Miao, and L. Cai, "Preventive and therapeutic effects of MG132 by activating Nrf2-ARE signaling pathway on oxidative stress-induced cardiovascular and renal injury," *Oxidative Medicine and Cellular Longevity*, vol. 2013 no. 3, p. 306073, 2013.

[6] J. A. Johnson, D. A. Johnson, A. D. Kraft et al., "The Nrf2-ARE pathway: an indicator and modulator of oxidative stress in neurodegeneration," *Annals of the new York Academy of Sciences*, vol. 1147 no. 12, pp. 61–69, 2008.

[7] Y. Kaya, A. Cebi, N. Soylemez, H. Demir, H. H. Alp, and E. Bakan, "Correlations between oxidative DNA damage, oxidative stress and coenzyme Q10 in patients with coronary artery disease," *International Journal of Medical Sciences*, vol. 9, no. 8, pp. 621–626, 2012.

[8] N. J. Pillon, M. L. Croze, R. E. Vella, L. Soulere, M. Lagarde, and C. O. Soulage, "The lipid peroxidation by-product 4-hydroxy-2-nonenal (4-HNE) induces insulin resistance in skeletal muscle through both carbonyl and oxidative stress," *Endocrinology*, vol. 153, no. 5, pp. 2099–2111, 2012.

[9] P. Piomboni, A. Stendardi, L. Gambera et al., "Protein modification as oxidative stress marker in normal and pathological human seminal plasma," *Redox Report*, vol. 17, no. 5, pp. 227–232, 2012.

[10] D. A. Abed, M. Goldstein, H. Albanyan, H. Jin, and L. Hu, "Discovery of direct inhibitors of Keap1-Nrf2 protein-protein interaction as potential therapeutic and preventive agents," *Acta Pharmaceutica Sinica B*, vol. 5, no. 4, pp. 285–299, 2015.

[11] N. Kashihara, Y. Haruna, V. K. Kondeti, and Y. S. Kanwar, "Oxidative stress in diabetic nephropathy," *Current Medicinal Chemistry*, vol. 17, no. 34, pp. 4256–4269, 2010.

[12] N. Vasavada and R. Agarwal, "Role of oxidative stress in diabetic nephropathy," *Advances in Chronic Kidney Disease*, vol. 12, no. 2, pp. 146–154, 2005.

[13] L. Kishore, N. Kaur, and R. Singh, "Renoprotective effect of *Bacopa monnieri* via inhibition of advanced glycation end products and oxidative stress in STZ-nicotinamide-induced diabetic nephropathy," *Renal Failure*, vol. 38, no. 9, pp. 1528–1544, 2016.

[14] S. Ahmed, N. Mundhe, M. Borgohain et al., "Diosmin modulates the NF-kB signal transduction pathways and downregulation of various oxidative stress markers in alloxan-induced diabetic nephropathy," *Inflammation*, vol. 39, no. 5, pp. 1783–1797, 2016.

[15] F. Bahmani, M. Kia, A. Soleimani, A. A. Mohammadi, and Z. Asemi, "The effects of selenium supplementation on biomarkers of inflammation and oxidative stress in patients with diabetic nephropathy: a randomised, double-blind, placebo-controlled trial," *The British Journal of Nutrition*, vol. 116, no. 7, pp. 1222–1228, 2016.

[16] P. G. Khatami, A. Soleimani, N. Sharifi, E. Aghadavod, and Z. Asemi, "The effects of high-dose vitamin E supplementation on biomarkers of kidney injury, inflammation, and oxidative stress in patients with diabetic nephropathy: a randomized, double-blind, placebo-controlled trial," *Journal of Clinical Lipidology*, vol. 10, no. 4, pp. 922–929, 2016.

[17] S. Ogawa, T. Mori, K. Nako, T. Kato, K. Takeuchi, and S. Ito, "Angiotensin II type 1 receptor blockers reduce urinary oxidative stress markers in hypertensive diabetic nephropathy," *Hypertension*, vol. 47, no. 4, pp. 699–705, 2006.

[18] P. Moi, K. Chan, I. Asunis, A. Cao, and Y. W. Kan, "Isolation of NF-E2-related factor 2 (Nrf2), a NF-E2-like basic leucine zipper transcriptional activator that binds to the tandem NF-E2/AP1 repeat of the beta-globin locus control region," *Proceedings of the National Academy of Sciences of the United States of America*, vol. 91, no. 21, pp. 9926–9930, 1994.

[19] K. Itoh, J. Mimura, and M. Yamamoto, "Discovery of the negative regulator of Nrf2, Keap1: a historical overview," *Antioxidants & Redox Signaling*, vol. 13, no. 11, pp. 1665–1678, 2010.

[20] Y. S. Keum and B. Y. Choi, "Molecular and chemical regulation of the Keap1-Nrf2 signaling pathway," *Molecules*, vol. 19, no. 7, pp. 10074–10089, 2014.

[21] K. Itoh, T. Chiba, S. Takahashi et al., "An Nrf2/small Maf heterodimer mediates the induction of phase II detoxifying enzyme genes through antioxidant response elements," *Biochemical and Biophysical Research Communications*, vol. 236, no. 2, pp. 313–322, 1997.

[22] A. K. Jain, D. A. Bloom, and A. K. Jaiswal, "Nuclear import and export signals in control of Nrf2," *The Journal of Biological Chemistry*, vol. 280, no. 32, pp. 29158–29168, 2005.

[23] K. Itoh, K. I. Tong, and M. Yamamoto, "Molecular mechanism activating Nrf2-Keap1 pathway in regulation of adaptive response to electrophiles," *Free Radical Biology & Medicine*, vol. 36, no. 10, pp. 1208–1213, 2004.

[24] K. I. Tong, Y. Katoh, H. Kusunoki, K. Itoh, T. Tanaka, and M. Yamamoto, "Keap1 recruits Neh2 through binding to ETGE and DLG motifs: characterization of the two-site molecular recognition model," *Molecular and Cellular Biology*, vol. 26, no. 8, pp. 2887–2900, 2006.

[25] K. Itoh, N. Wakabayashi, Y. Katoh et al., "Keap1 represses nuclear activation of antioxidant responsive elements by Nrf2 through binding to the amino-terminal Neh2 domain," *Genes & Development*, vol. 13, no. 1, pp. 76–86, 1999.

[26] D. D. Zhang, S. C. Lo, J. V. Cross, D. J. Templeton, and M. Hannink, "Keap1 is a redox-regulated substrate adaptor protein for a Cul3-dependent ubiquitin ligase complex," *Molecular and Cellular Biology*, vol. 24, no. 24, pp. 10941–10953, 2004.

[27] Y. Katoh, K. Itoh, E. Yoshida, M. Miyagishi, A. Fukamizu, and M. Yamamoto, "Two domains of Nrf2 cooperatively bind CBP, a CREB binding protein, and synergistically activate transcription," *Genes to Cells : Devoted to Molecular & Cellular Mechanisms*, vol. 6, no. 10, pp. 857–868, 2001.

[28] M. McMahon, N. Thomas, K. Itoh, M. Yamamoto, and J. D. Hayes, "Redox-regulated turnover of Nrf2 is determined by

at least two separate protein domains, the redox-sensitive Neh2 degron and the redox-insensitive Neh6 degron," *The Journal of Biological Chemistry*, vol. 279, no. 30, pp. 31556–31567, 2004.

[29] H. Wang, K. Liu, M. Geng et al., "RXRalpha inhibits the NRF2-ARE signaling pathway through a direct interaction with the Neh7 domain of NRF2," *Cancer Research*, vol. 73, no. 10, pp. 3097–3108, 2013.

[30] N. Wakabayashi, A. T. Dinkova-Kostova, W. D. Holtzclaw et al., "Protection against electrophile and oxidant stress by induction of the phase 2 response: fate of cysteines of the Keap1 sensor modified by inducers," *Proceedings of the National Academy of Sciences of the United States of America*, vol. 101, no. 7, pp. 2040–2045, 2004.

[31] L. M. Zipper and R. T. Mulcahy, "The Keap1 BTB/POZ dimerization function is required to sequester Nrf2 in cytoplasm," *The Journal of Biological Chemistry*, vol. 277, no. 39, pp. 36544–36552, 2002.

[32] N. Chauhan, L. Chaunsali, P. Deshmukh, and B. Padmanabhan, "Analysis of dimerization of BTB-IVR domains of Keap1 and its interaction with Cul3, by molecular modeling," *Bioinformation*, vol. 9, no. 9, pp. 450–455, 2013.

[33] A. T. Dinkova-Kostova, W. D. Holtzclaw, R. N. Cole et al., "Direct evidence that sulfhydryl groups of Keap1 are the sensors regulating induction of phase 2 enzymes that protect against carcinogens and oxidants," *Proceedings of the National Academy of Sciences of the United States of America*, vol. 99, no. 18, pp. 11908–11913, 2002.

[34] W. Hur and N. S. Gray, "Small molecule modulators of antioxidant response pathway," *Current Opinion in Chemical Biology*, vol. 15, no. 1, pp. 162–173, 2011.

[35] R. Saito, T. Suzuki, K. Hiramoto et al., "Characterizations of three major cysteine sensors of Keap1 in stress response," *Molecular and Cellular Biology*, vol. 36, no. 2, pp. 271–284, 2015.

[36] K. Takaya, T. Suzuki, H. Motohashi et al., "Validation of the multiple sensor mechanism of the Keap1-Nrf2 system," *Free Radical Biology & Medicine*, vol. 53, no. 4, pp. 817–827, 2012.

[37] A. Uruno and H. Motohashi, "The Keap1-Nrf2 system as an in vivo sensor for electrophiles," *Nitric Oxide : Biology and Chemistry*, vol. 25, no. 2, pp. 153–160, 2011.

[38] J. D. Hayes and M. McMahon, "NRF2 and KEAP1 mutations: permanent activation of an adaptive response in cancer," *Trends in Biochemical Sciences*, vol. 34, no. 4, pp. 176–188, 2009.

[39] Y. Katoh, K. Iida, M. I. Kang et al., "Evolutionary conserved N-terminal domain of Nrf2 is essential for the Keap1-mediated degradation of the protein by proteasome," *Archives of Biochemistry and Biophysics*, vol. 433, no. 2, pp. 342–350, 2005.

[40] D. Stewart, E. Killeen, R. Naquin, S. Alam, and J. Alam, "Degradation of transcription factor Nrf2 via the ubiquitin-proteasome pathway and stabilization by cadmium," *The Journal of Biological Chemistry*, vol. 278, no. 4, pp. 2396–2402, 2003.

[41] K. J. Min, J. H. Kim, I. Jou, and E. H. Joe, "Adenosine induces hemeoxygenase-1 expression in microglia through the activation of phosphatidylinositol 3-kinase and nuclear factor E2-related factor 2," *Glia*, vol. 56, no. 9, pp. 1028–1037, 2008.

[42] S. Kalayarasan, P. N. Prabhu, N. Sriram, R. Manikandan, M. Arumugam, and G. Sudhandiran, "Diallyl sulfide enhances antioxidants and inhibits inflammation through the activation of Nrf2 against gentamicin-induced nephrotoxicity in Wistar rats," *European Journal of Pharmacology*, vol. 606, no. 1-3, pp. 162–171, 2009.

[43] S. Ruiz, P. E. Pergola, R. A. Zager, and N. D. Vaziri, "Targeting the transcription factor Nrf2 to ameliorate oxidative stress and inflammation in chronic kidney disease," *Kidney International*, vol. 83, no. 6, pp. 1029–1041, 2013.

[44] B. Harder, T. Jiang, T. Wu et al., "Molecular mechanisms of Nrf2 regulation and how these influence chemical modulation for disease intervention," *Biochemical Society Transactions*, vol. 43, no. 4, pp. 680–686, 2015.

[45] M. K. Kwak, K. Itoh, M. Yamamoto, and T. W. Kensler, "Enhanced expression of the transcription factor Nrf2 by cancer chemopreventive agents: role of antioxidant response element-like sequences in the nrf2 promoter," *Molecular and Cellular Biology*, vol. 22, no. 9, pp. 2883–2892, 2002.

[46] X. Cheng, C. H. Ku, and R. C. Siow, "Regulation of the Nrf2 antioxidant pathway by microRNAs: new players in micromanaging redox homeostasis," *Free Radical Biology & Medicine*, vol. 64 no. 9, pp. 4–11, 2013.

[47] M. Yang, Y. Yao, G. Eades, Y. Zhang, and Q. Zhou, "MiR-28 regulates Nrf2 expression through a Keap1-independent mechanism," *Breast Cancer Research and Treatment*, vol. 129, no. 3, pp. 983–991, 2011.

[48] N. Li, S. Muthusamy, R. Liang, H. Sarojini, and E. Wang, "Increased expression of miR-34a and miR-93 in rat liver during aging, and their impact on the expression of Mgst1 and Sirt1," *Mechanisms of Ageing and Development*, vol. 132, no. 3, pp. 75–85, 2011.

[49] A. Stachurska, M. Ciesla, M. Kozakowska et al., "Cross-talk between microRNAs, nuclear factor E2-related factor 2, and heme oxygenase-1 in ochratoxin A-induced toxic effects in renal proximal tubular epithelial cells," *Molecular Nutrition & Food Research*, vol. 57, no. 3, pp. 504–515, 2013.

[50] G. Eades, M. Yang, Y. Yao, Y. Zhang, and Q. Zhou, "miR-200a regulates Nrf2 activation by targeting Keap1 mRNA in breast cancer cells," *The Journal of Biological Chemistry*, vol. 286, no. 47, pp. 40725–40733, 2011.

[51] T. O. Khor, Y. Huang, T. Y. Wu, L. Shu, J. Lee, and A. N. Kong, "Pharmacodynamics of curcumin as DNA hypomethylation agent in restoring the expression of Nrf2 via promoter CpGs demethylation," *Biochemical Pharmacology*, vol. 82, no. 9, pp. 1073–1078, 2011.

[52] C. Zhang, Z. Y. Su, T. O. Khor, L. Shu, and A. N. Kong, "Sulforaphane enhances Nrf2 expression in prostate cancer TRAMP C1 cells through epigenetic regulation," *Biochemical Pharmacology*, vol. 85, no. 9, pp. 1398–1404, 2013.

[53] F. Correa, C. Mallard, M. Nilsson, and M. Sandberg, "Activated microglia decrease histone acetylation and Nrf2-inducible anti-oxidant defence in astrocytes: restoring effects of inhibitors of HDACs, p38 MAPK and GSK3beta," *Neurobiology of Disease*, vol. 44, no. 1, pp. 142–151, 2011.

[54] Z. Li, L. Xu, N. Tang et al., "The polycomb group protein EZH2 inhibits lung cancer cell growth by repressing the transcription factor Nrf2," *FEBS Letters*, vol. 588, no. 17, pp. 3000–3007, 2014.

[55] Y. Guo, S. Yu, C. Zhang, and A. N. Kong, "Epigenetic regulation of Keap1-Nrf2 signaling," *Free Radical Biology & Medicine*, vol. 88, no. Pt B, pp. 337–349, 2015.

[56] N. F. Villeneuve, A. Lau, and D. D. Zhang, "Regulation of the Nrf2-Keap1 antioxidant response by the ubiquitin proteasome system: an insight into cullin-ring ubiquitin ligases," *Antioxidants & Redox Signaling*, vol. 13, no. 11, pp. 1699–1712, 2010.

[57] W. Cui, B. Li, Y. Bai et al., "Potential role for Nrf2 activation in the therapeutic effect of MG132 on diabetic nephropathy in OVE26 diabetic mice," *American Journal of Physiology Endocrinology and Metabolism*, vol. 304, no. 1, pp. E87–E99, 2013.

[58] A. Lau, X. J. Wang, F. Zhao et al., "A noncanonical mechanism of Nrf2 activation by autophagy deficiency: direct interaction between Keap1 and p62," *Molecular and Cellular Biology*, vol. 30, no. 13, pp. 3275–3285, 2010.

[59] H. C. Huang, T. Nguyen, and C. B. Pickett, "Phosphorylation of Nrf2 at Ser-40 by protein kinase C regulates antioxidant response element-mediated transcription," *The Journal of Biological Chemistry*, vol. 277, no. 45, pp. 42769–42774, 2002.

[60] M. Miyazawa and Y. Tsuji, "Evidence for a novel antioxidant function and isoform-specific regulation of the human p66Shc gene," *Molecular Biology of the Cell*, vol. 25, no. 13, pp. 2116–2127, 2014.

[61] T. Miyata, N. Suzuki, and C. van Ypersele de Strihou, "Diabetic nephropathy: are there new and potentially promising therapies targeting oxygen biology?" *Kidney International*, vol. 84, no. 4, pp. 693–702, 2013.

[62] Q. Sun, Z. Y. Shen, Q. T. Meng, H. Z. Liu, W. N. Duan, and Z. Y. Xia, "The role of DJ-1/Nrf2 pathway in the pathogenesis of diabetic nephropathy in rats," *Renal Failure*, vol. 38, no. 2, pp. 294–304, 2016.

[63] K. Yoh, A. Hirayama, K. Ishizaki et al., "Hyperglycemia induces oxidative and nitrosative stress and increases renal functional impairment in Nrf2-deficient mice," *Genes to Cells : Devoted to Molecular & Cellular Mechanisms*, vol. 13, no. 11, pp. 1159–1170, 2008.

[64] T. Jiang, Z. Huang, Y. Lin, Z. Zhang, D. Fang, and D. D. Zhang, "The protective role of Nrf2 in streptozotocin-induced diabetic nephropathy," *Diabetes*, vol. 59, no. 4, pp. 850–860, 2010.

[65] B. H. Choi, K. S. Kang, and M. K. Kwak, "Effect of redox modulating NRF2 activators on chronic kidney disease," *Molecules*, vol. 19, no. 8, pp. 12727–12759, 2014.

[66] N. Wakabayashi, K. Itoh, J. Wakabayashi et al., "Keap1-null mutation leads to postnatal lethality due to constitutive Nrf2 activation," *Nature Genetics*, vol. 35, no. 3, pp. 238–245, 2003.

[67] V. R. More, J. Xu, P. C. Shimpi et al., "Keap1 knockdown increases markers of metabolic syndrome after long-term high fat diet feeding," *Free Radical Biology & Medicine*, vol. 61 no. 8, pp. 85–94, 2013.

[68] Y. K. Zhang, K. C. Wu, J. Liu, and C. D. Klaassen, "Nrf2 deficiency improves glucose tolerance in mice fed a high-fat diet," *Toxicology and Applied Pharmacology*, vol. 264, no. 3, pp. 305–314, 2012.

[69] J. Xu, S. R. Kulkarni, A. C. Donepudi, V. R. More, and A. L. Slitt, "Enhanced Nrf2 activity worsens insulin resistance, impairs lipid accumulation in adipose tissue, and increases hepatic steatosis in leptin-deficient mice," *Diabetes*, vol. 61, no. 12, pp. 3208–3218, 2012.

[70] M. S. Yates, Q. T. Tran, P. M. Dolan et al., "Genetic versus chemoprotective activation of Nrf2 signaling: overlapping yet distinct gene expression profiles between Keap1 knockout and triterpenoid-treated mice," *Carcinogenesis*, vol. 30, no. 6, pp. 1024–1031, 2009.

[71] X. Wang, X. Zhao, T. Feng, G. Jin, and Z. Li, "Rutin prevents high glucose-induced renal glomerular endothelial hyperpermeability by inhibiting the ROS/Rhoa/ROCK signaling pathway," *Planta Medica*, vol. 82, no. 14, pp. 1252–1257, 2016.

[72] X. Zhang, H. He, D. Liang et al., "Protective effects of berberine on renal injury in streptozotocin (STZ)-induced diabetic mice," *International Journal of Molecular Sciences*, vol. 17, no. 8, p. 1327, 2016.

[73] W. Gong, C. Chen, F. Xiong et al., "CKIP-1 ameliorates high glucose-induced expression of fibronectin and intercellular cell adhesion molecule-1 by activating the Nrf2/ARE pathway in glomerular mesangial cells," *Biochemical Pharmacology*, vol. 116 no. 9, pp. 140–152, 2016.

[74] M. M. Hussein and M. K. Mahfouz, "Effect of resveratrol and rosuvastatin on experimental diabetic nephropathy in rats," *Biomedicine & Pharmacotherapy = Biomedecine & Pharmacotherapie*, vol. 82 no. 8, pp. 685–692, 2016.

[75] P. Wu, Y. Yan, L. L. Ma et al., "Effects of the Nrf2 protein modulator salvianolic acid A alone or combined with metformin on diabetes-associated macrovascular and renal injury," *The Journal of Biological Chemistry*, vol. 291, no. 42, pp. 22288–22301, 2016.

[76] Q. Yin, Y. Xia, and G. Wang, "Sinomenine alleviates high glucose-induced renal glomerular endothelial hyperpermeability by inhibiting the activation of RhoA/ROCK signaling pathway," *Biochemical and Biophysical Research Communications*, vol. 477, no. 4, pp. 881–886, 2016.

[77] M. Raish, A. Ahmad, B. L. Jan et al., "*Momordica charantia* polysaccharides mitigate the progression of STZ induced diabetic nephropathy in rats," *International Journal of Biological Macromolecules*, vol. 91 no. 10, pp. 394–399, 2016.

[78] B. H. Kim, E. S. Lee, R. Choi et al., "Protective effects of curcumin on renal oxidative stress and lipid metabolism in a rat model of type 2 diabetic nephropathy," *Yonsei Medical Journal*, vol. 57, no. 3, pp. 664–673, 2016.

[79] Y. Yang, G. Chen, X. Cheng et al., "Therapeutic potential of digitoflavone on diabetic nephropathy: nuclear factor erythroid 2-related factor 2-dependent anti-oxidant and anti-inflammatory effect," *Scientific Reports*, vol. 5 no. 6, p. 12377, 2015.

[80] X. Zhang, D. Liang, L. Guo et al., "Curcumin protects renal tubular epithelial cells from high glucose-induced epithelial-to-mesenchymal transition through Nrf2-mediated upregulation of heme oxygenase-1," *Molecular Medicine Reports*, vol. 12, no. 1, pp. 1347–1355, 2015.

[81] L. Zhou, D. Y. Xu, W. G. Sha et al., "High glucose induces renal tubular epithelial injury via Sirt1/NF-kappaB/microR-29/Keap1 signal pathway," *Journal of Translational Medicine*, vol. 13 no. 11, p. 352, 2015.

[82] S. M. Yang, S. M. Ka, H. L. Wu et al., "Thrombomodulin domain 1 ameliorates diabetic nephropathy in mice via anti-NF-kappaB/NLRP3 inflammasome-mediated inflammation, enhancement of NRF2 antioxidant activity and inhibition of apoptosis," *Diabetologia*, vol. 57, no. 2, pp. 424–434, 2014.

[83] K. Nakai, H. Fujii, K. Kono et al., "Vitamin D activates the Nrf2-Keap1 antioxidant pathway and ameliorates nephropathy in diabetic rats," *American Journal of Hypertension*, vol. 27, no. 4, pp. 586–595, 2014.

[84] B. Jiang, L. Guo, B. Y. Li et al., "Resveratrol attenuates early diabetic nephropathy by down-regulating glutathione s-transferases Mu in diabetic rats," *Journal of Medicinal Food*, vol. 16, no. 6, pp. 481–486, 2013.

[85] W. Cui, Y. Bai, X. Miao et al., "Prevention of diabetic nephropathy by sulforaphane: possible role of Nrf2 upregulation and activation," *Oxidative Medicine and Cellular Longevity*, vol. 2012 no. 9, p. 821936, 2012.

[86] H. Zheng, S. A. Whitman, W. Wu et al., "Therapeutic potential of Nrf2 activators in streptozotocin-induced diabetic nephropathy," *Diabetes*, vol. 60, no. 11, pp. 3055–3066, 2011.

[87] P. Palsamy and S. Subramanian, "Resveratrol protects diabetic kidney by attenuating hyperglycemia-mediated oxidative stress and renal inflammatory cytokines via Nrf2-Keap1 signaling," *Biochimica et Biophysica Acta*, vol. 1812, no. 7, pp. 719–731, 2011.

[88] Z. F. Luo, B. Feng, J. Mu et al., "Effects of 4-phenylbutyric acid on the process and development of diabetic nephropathy induced in rats by streptozotocin: regulation of endoplasmic reticulum stress-oxidative activation," *Toxicology and Applied Pharmacology*, vol. 246, no. 1-2, pp. 49–57, 2010.

[89] H. Wu, L. Kong, Y. Cheng et al., "Metallothionein plays a prominent role in the prevention of diabetic nephropathy by sulforaphane via up-regulation of Nrf2," *Free Radical Biology & Medicine*, vol. 89 no. 12, pp. 431–442, 2015.

[90] W. Dong, Y. Jia, X. Liu et al., "Sodium butyrate activates NRF2 to ameliorate diabetic nephropathy possibly via inhibition of HDAC," *The Journal of Endocrinology*, vol. 232, no. 1, pp. 71–83, 2017.

[91] Z. Chen, X. Xie, J. Huang et al., "Connexin43 regulates high glucose-induced expression of fibronectin, ICAM-1 and TGF-beta1 via Nrf2/ARE pathway in glomerular mesangial cells," *Free Radical Biology & Medicine*, vol. 102 no. 1, pp. 77–86, 2017.

[92] K. Shahzad, F. Bock, M. M. Al-Dabet et al., "Stabilization of endogenous Nrf2 by minocycline protects against Nlrp3-inflammasome induced diabetic nephropathy," *Scientific Reports*, vol. 6 no. 10, p. 34228, 2016.

[93] H. Wu, L. Kong, Y. Tan et al., "C66 ameliorates diabetic nephropathy in mice by both upregulating NRF2 function via increase in miR-200a and inhibiting miR-21," *Diabetologia*, vol. 59, no. 7, pp. 1558–1568, 2016.

[94] A. S. Arellano-Buendia, M. Tostado-Gonzalez, F. E. Garcia-Arroyo et al., "Anti-inflammatory therapy modulates Nrf2-Keap1 in kidney from rats with diabetes," *Oxidative Medicine and Cellular Longevity*, vol. 2016 no. 2, p. 4693801, 2016.

[95] Y. Cheng, J. Zhang, W. Guo et al., "Up-regulation of Nrf2 is involved in FGF21-mediated fenofibrate protection against type 1 diabetic nephropathy," *Free Radical Biology & Medicine*, vol. 93 no. 4, pp. 94–109, 2016.

[96] G. Shang, X. Tang, P. Gao et al., "Sulforaphane attenuation of experimental diabetic nephropathy involves GSK-3 beta/Fyn/Nrf2 signaling pathway," *The Journal of Nutritional Biochemistry*, vol. 26, no. 6, pp. 596–606, 2015.

[97] K. Huang, C. Chen, J. Hao et al., "Polydatin promotes Nrf2-ARE anti-oxidative pathway through activating Sirt1 to resist AGEs-induced upregulation of fibronetin and transforming growth factor-beta1 in rat glomerular messangial cells," *Molecular and Cellular Endocrinology*, vol. 399 no. 1, pp. 178–189, 2015.

[98] B. Li, W. Cui, Y. Tan et al., "Zinc is essential for the transcription function of Nrf2 in human renal tubule cells in vitro and mouse kidney in vivo under the diabetic condition," *Journal of Cellular and Molecular Medicine*, vol. 18, no. 5, pp. 895–906, 2014.

[99] X. Zhang, Y. Zhao, Q. Chu, Z. Y. Wang, H. Li, and Z. H. Chi, "Zinc modulates high glucose-induced apoptosis by suppressing oxidative stress in renal tubular epithelial cells," *Biological Trace Element Research*, vol. 158, no. 2, pp. 259–267, 2014.

[100] X. Zhou, Y. Feng, Z. Zhan, and J. Chen, "Hydrogen sulfide alleviates diabetic nephropathy in a streptozotocin-induced diabetic rat model," *The Journal of Biological Chemistry*, vol. 289, no. 42, pp. 28827–28834, 2014.

[101] K. Huang, J. Huang, X. Xie et al., "Sirt1 resists advanced glycation end products-induced expressions of fibronectin and TGF-beta1 by activating the Nrf2/ARE pathway in glomerular mesangial cells," *Free Radical Biology & Medicine*, vol. 65 no. 12, pp. 528–540, 2013.

[102] X. Xing, C. Zhang, M. Shao et al., "Low-dose radiation activates Akt and Nrf2 in the kidney of diabetic mice: a potential mechanism to prevent diabetic nephropathy," *Oxidative Medicine and Cellular Longevity*, vol. 2012 no. 11, p. 291087, 2012.

[103] S. Guoguo, T. Akaike, J. Tao, C. Qi, Z. Nong, and L. Hui, "HGF-mediated inhibition of oxidative stress by 8-nitro-cGMP in high glucose-treated rat mesangial cells," *Free Radical Research*, vol. 46, no. 10, pp. 1238–1248, 2012.

[104] H. Fujita, H. Fujishima, T. Morii et al., "Modulation of renal superoxide dismutase by telmisartan therapy in C57BL/6-Ins2(Akita) diabetic mice," *Hypertension Research : Official Journal of the Japanese Society of Hypertension*, vol. 35, no. 2, pp. 213–220, 2012.

[105] H. Li, L. Zhang, F. Wang et al., "Attenuation of glomerular injury in diabetic mice with tert-butylhydroquinone through nuclear factor erythroid 2-related factor 2-dependent antioxidant gene activation," *American Journal of Nephrology*, vol. 33, no. 4, pp. 289–297, 2011.

[106] Z. F. Luo, W. Qi, B. Feng et al., "Prevention of diabetic nephropathy in rats through enhanced renal antioxidative capacity by inhibition of the proteasome," *Life Sciences*, vol. 88, no. 11-12, pp. 512–520, 2011.

[107] J. Wei, Y. Zhang, Y. Luo et al., "Aldose reductase regulates miR-200a-3p/141-3p to coordinate Keap1-Nrf2, Tgfbeta1/2, and Zeb1/2 signaling in renal mesangial cells and the renal cortex of diabetic mice," *Free Radical Biology & Medicine*, vol. 67 no. 2, pp. 91–102, 2014.

[108] M. C. Haigis and L. P. Guarente, "Mammalian sirtuins—emerging roles in physiology, aging, and calorie restriction," *Genes & Development*, vol. 20, no. 21, pp. 2913–2921, 2006.

[109] D. Yang, X. Tan, Z. Lv et al., "Regulation of Sirt1/Nrf2/TNF-alpha signaling pathway by luteolin is critical to attenuate acute mercuric chloride exposure induced hepatotoxicity," *Scientific Reports*, vol. 6 no. 11, p. 37157, 2016.

[110] X. Xia, B. Qu, Y. M. Li et al., "NFAT5 protects astrocytes against oxygen-glucose-serum deprivation/restoration damage via the SIRT1/Nrf2 pathway," *Journal of Molecular Neuroscience : MN*, vol. 61, no. 1, pp. 96–104, 2016.

[111] S. A. Shah, M. Khan, M. H. Jo, M. G. Jo, F. U. Amin, and M. O. Kim, "Melatonin stimulates the SIRT1/Nrf2 signaling pathway counteracting lipopolysaccharide (LPS)-induced

oxidative stress to rescue postnatal rat brain," *CNS Neuroscience & Therapeutics*, vol. 23, no. 1, pp. 33–44, 2016.

[112] A. Cao, L. Wang, X. Chen et al., "Ursodeoxycholic acid ameliorated diabetic nephropathy by attenuating hyperglycemia-mediated oxidative stress," *Biological & Pharmaceutical Bulletin*, vol. 39, no. 8, pp. 1300–1308, 2016.

[113] C. Wang, C. Li, H. Peng et al., "Activation of the Nrf2-ARE pathway attenuates hyperglycemia-mediated injuries in mouse podocytes," *Cellular Physiology and Biochemistry : International Journal of Experimental Cellular Physiology, Biochemistry, and Pharmacology*, vol. 34, no. 3, pp. 891–902, 2014.

[114] X. Xu, J. Sun, X. Chang et al., "Genetic variants of nuclear factor erythroid-derived 2-like 2 associated with the complications in Han descents with type 2 diabetes mellitus of Northeast China," *Journal of Cellular and Molecular Medicine*, vol. 20, no. 11, pp. 2078–2088, 2016.

[115] K. T. Liby, M. M. Yore, and M. B. Sporn, "Triterpenoids and rexinoids as multifunctional agents for the prevention and treatment of cancer," *Nature Reviews Cancer*, vol. 7, no. 5, pp. 357–369, 2007.

[116] K. T. Liby and M. B. Sporn, "Synthetic oleanane triterpenoids: multifunctional drugs with a broad range of applications for prevention and treatment of chronic disease," *Pharmacological Reviews*, vol. 64, no. 4, pp. 972–1003, 2012.

[117] S. Nagaraj, J. I. Youn, H. Weber et al., "Anti-inflammatory triterpenoid blocks immune suppressive function of MDSCs and improves immune response in cancer," *Clinical Cancer Research : An Official Journal of the American Association for Cancer Research*, vol. 16, no. 6, pp. 1812–1823, 2010.

[118] D. S. Hong, R. Kurzrock, J. G. Supko et al., "A phase I first-in-human trial of bardoxolone methyl in patients with advanced solid tumors and lymphomas," *Clinical Cancer Research : An Official Journal of the American Association for Cancer Research*, vol. 18, no. 12, pp. 3396–3406, 2012.

[119] P. E. Pergola, M. Krauth, J. W. Huff et al., "Effect of bardoxolone methyl on kidney function in patients with T2D and stage 3b-4 CKD," *American Journal of Nephrology*, vol. 33, no. 5, pp. 469–476, 2011.

[120] P. E. Pergola, P. Raskin, R. D. Toto et al., "Bardoxolone methyl and kidney function in CKD with type 2 diabetes," *The New England Journal of Medicine*, vol. 365, no. 4, pp. 327–336, 2011.

[121] D. de Zeeuw, T. Akizawa, P. Audhya et al., "Bardoxolone methyl in type 2 diabetes and stage 4 chronic kidney disease," *The New England Journal of Medicine*, vol. 369, no. 26, pp. 2492–2503, 2013.

[122] M. P. Chin, D. Wrolstad, G. L. Bakris et al., "Risk factors for heart failure in patients with type 2 diabetes mellitus and stage 4 chronic kidney disease treated with bardoxolone methyl," *Journal of Cardiac Failure*, vol. 20, no. 12, pp. 953–958, 2014.

[123] M. P. Chin, S. A. Reisman, G. L. Bakris et al., "Mechanisms contributing to adverse cardiovascular events in patients with type 2 diabetes mellitus and stage 4 chronic kidney disease treated with bardoxolone methyl," *American Journal of Nephrology*, vol. 39, no. 6, pp. 499–508, 2014.

[124] S. Abdo, Y. Shi, A. Otoukesh et al., "Catalase overexpression prevents nuclear factor erythroid 2-related factor 2 stimulation of renal angiotensinogen gene expression, hypertension, and kidney injury in diabetic mice," *Diabetes*, vol. 63, no. 10, pp. 3483–3496, 2014.

[125] N. Noori, C. P. Kovesdy, R. Bross et al., "Novel equations to estimate lean body mass in maintenance hemodialysis patients," *American Journal of Kidney Diseases : The Official Journal of the National Kidney Foundation*, vol. 57, no. 1, pp. 130–139, 2011.

[126] S. S. Patel, M. Z. Molnar, J. A. Tayek et al., "Serum creatinine as a marker of muscle mass in chronic kidney disease: results of a cross-sectional study and review of literature," *Journal of Cachexia, Sarcopenia and Muscle*, vol. 4, no. 1, pp. 19–29, 2013.

[127] J. A. Tayek and K. Kalantar-Zadeh, "The extinguished BEACON of bardoxolone: not a Monday morning quarterback story," *American Journal of Nephrology*, vol. 37, no. 3, pp. 208–211, 2013.

[128] H. Yang, W. Xu, Z. Zhou et al., "Curcumin attenuates urinary excretion of albumin in type II diabetic patients with enhancing nuclear factor erythroid-derived 2-like 2 (Nrf2) system and repressing inflammatory signaling efficacies," *Experimental and Clinical Endocrinology & Diabetes : Official Journal, German Society of Endocrinology [and] German Diabetes Association*, vol. 123, no. 6, pp. 360–367, 2015.

[129] E. H. Kobayashi, T. Suzuki, R. Funayama et al., "Nrf2 suppresses macrophage inflammatory response by blocking proinflammatory cytokine transcription," *Nature Communications*, vol. 7 no. 5, p. 11624, 2016.

[130] P. Gao, L. Li, L. Ji et al., "Nrf2 ameliorates diabetic nephropathy progression by transcriptional repression of TGFbeta1 through interactions with c-Jun and SP1," *Biochimica et Biophysica Acta*, vol. 1839, no. 11, pp. 1110–1120, 2014.

[131] C. Zoja, D. Corna, V. Nava et al., "Analogs of bardoxolone methyl worsen diabetic nephropathy in rats with additional adverse effects," *American Journal of Physiology Renal Physiology*, vol. 304, no. 6, pp. F808–F819, 2013.

[132] N. D. Vaziri, S. Liu, S. H. Farzaneh, S. Nazertehrani, M. Khazaeli, and Y. Y. Zhao, "Dose-dependent deleterious and salutary actions of the Nrf2 inducer dh404 in chronic kidney disease," *Free Radical Biology & Medicine*, vol. 86 no. 9, pp. 374–381, 2015.

[133] S. M. Tan, A. Sharma, N. Stefanovic et al., "Derivative of bardoxolone methyl, dh404, in an inverse dose-dependent manner lessens diabetes-associated atherosclerosis and improves diabetic kidney disease," *Diabetes*, vol. 63, no. 9, pp. 3091–3103, 2014.

[134] S. Menegon, A. Columbano, and S. Giordano, "The dual roles of NRF2 in cancer," *Trends in Molecular Medicine*, vol. 22, no. 7, pp. 578–593, 2016.

[135] J. Kim and Y. S. Keum, "NRF2, a key regulator of antioxidants with two faces towards cancer," *Oxidative Medicine and Cellular Longevity*, vol. 2016 no. 6, p. 2746457, 2016.

[136] A. Ooi and K. A. Furge, "Fumarate hydratase inactivation in renal tumors: HIF1alpha, NRF2, and "cryptic targets" of transcription factors," *Chinese Journal of Cancer*, vol. 31, no. 9, pp. 413–420, 2012.

[137] S. K. Niture and A. K. Jaiswal, "Nrf2-induced antiapoptotic Bcl-xL protein enhances cell survival and drug resistance," *Free Radical Biology & Medicine*, vol. 57 no. 4, pp. 119–131, 2013.

4

Neutrophils Infiltrate the Spinal Cord Parenchyma of Rats with Experimental Diabetic Neuropathy

Victoria L. Newton,[1] Jonathan D. Guck,[1] Mary A. Cotter,[2] Norman E. Cameron,[2] and Natalie J. Gardiner[1]

[1] *Division of Diabetes, Endocrinology and Gastroenterology, School of Medical Sciences, Faculty of Biology, Medicine and Health, University of Manchester, Oxford Road, Manchester M13 9PT, UK*
[2] *School of Medical Sciences, University of Aberdeen, Aberdeen, UK*

Correspondence should be addressed to Natalie J. Gardiner; natalie.gardiner@manchester.ac.uk

Academic Editor: Dilek Yavuz

Spinal glial cell activation and cytokine secretion have been implicated in the etiology of neuropathic pain in a number of experimental models, including diabetic neuropathy. In this study, streptozotocin- (STZ-) induced diabetic rats were either untreated or treated with gabapentin (50 mg/kg/day by gavage for 2 weeks, from 6 weeks after STZ). At 8 weeks after STZ, hypersensitivity was confirmed in the untreated diabetic rats as a reduced response threshold to touch, whilst mechanical thresholds in gabapentin-treated diabetic rats were no different from controls. Diabetes-associated thermal hypersensitivity was also ameliorated by gabapentin. We performed a cytokine profiling array in lumbar spinal cord samples from control and diabetic rats. This revealed an increase in L-selectin, an adhesion molecule important for neutrophil transmigration, in the spinal cord of diabetic rats but not diabetic rats treated with gabapentin. Furthermore, we found an increase in the number of neutrophils present in the parenchyma of the spinal cord, which was again ameliorated in gabapentin-treated diabetic rats. Therefore, we suggest that dysregulated spinal L-selectin and neutrophil infiltration into the spinal cord could contribute to the pathogenesis of painful diabetic neuropathy.

1. Introduction

The prevalence of diabetes mellitus is increasing worldwide, which has significant health and economic implications. Associated costs include both primary treatment and also treating the associated secondary complications such as retinopathy, nephropathy, and neuropathy [1]. Distal sensory polyneuropathy (DPN) is the most common of the peripheral nerve disorders associated with diabetes [2]. DPN may be accompanied by paresthesia such as tingling and burning sensations, heightened sensitivity to normally innocuous stimuli, and spontaneous pain. Neuropathic pain serves no useful function [3] and is a debilitating condition [4]. There is currently no effective treatment, with single analgesics usually failing to adequately treat the pain, meaning that patients are offered available therapies in a stepwise and often combinatorial fashion [5, 6]. One of the first-line treatments is gabapentin [7], an analogue of the inhibitory neurotransmitter γ-aminobutyric acid (GABA), an anticonvulsant drug which is also antiallodynic in neuropathic and inflammatory pain states [8]. The underlying mechanisms of analgesia provided by this drug are not thoroughly understood. However, gabapentin can interact with several targets, including the $\alpha 2$-δ subunit of voltage-activated calcium channels [9] and the L-amino acid transporters (LAT-1 and LAT-2; [10]) and has been shown to reduce spinal microglial activation and allodynia in rats with experimental diabetes [11, 12].

The pathogenesis of neuropathic pain involves changes in neuronal activity in the peripheral and central nervous systems and also activation of glial and immune cells [13, 14]. Glial cells are rapidly activated in response to peripheral nerve injury [15–17] and are responsible for the release of many inflammatory mediators, including chemokines and cytokines important for the establishment and maintenance of neuropathic pain [13, 18]. In rodent models of diabetes, microglia are activated in the dorsal horn of the lumbar spinal cord [11, 19, 20] and their activation has been associated with neuropathic pain. Whilst the intact blood-brain barrier largely prevents circulating immune cells from crossing into the parenchyma, permeability can be modulated by trauma or inflammation, enabling recruitment and infiltration of immune cells into the central nervous system (CNS). Peripheral injection of carrageenan into the hind paw, for example, causes an increase in ICAM and VCAM expression in spinal epithelium, changes in tight junction proteins, an increase in brain-barrier permeability, and the consequent migration of neutrophils into the CNS [21]. In both diabetic nephropathy and retinopathy, increased leukostasis and infiltration have been observed and are detrimental to symptom severity [22, 23]. However, to our knowledge, no information exists regarding the transmigration of neutrophils in the spinal cord in painful diabetic neuropathy.

In this study, we identify an increase in L-selectin and in the number of neutrophils present in the parenchyma of the spinal cord of untreated diabetic rats, which could represent a novel therapeutic target to explore in future studies.

2. Methods

2.1. Induction of Diabetes and Drug Delivery. All experiments were carried out using mature adult male Sprague-Dawley rats (495–570 g, bred at The Institute of Medical Science, Aberdeen University) in accordance with the UK Animals (Scientific Procedures) Act 1986. Diabetes was induced using streptozotocin (STZ in sterile saline; 40 mg/kg i.p.; $n = 12$). Age- and weight-matched rats were used as nondiabetic controls ($n = 6$). Diabetic rats were either untreated or treated daily for 2 weeks with gabapentin (50 mg/kg/day by gavage; Spectrum Chemical Manufacturing Corp, Gardena) starting 6 weeks following STZ injection.

2.2. Behavioural Testing. After 8 weeks of diabetes and within 2 hours following gabapentin administration, the behavioural response to mechanical and thermal stimulation of the hind paw was assessed using an automatic Von Frey probe and Hargreaves apparatus, respectively (Ugo Basile, Italy). All animals were habituated to the tester and the environment prior to testing. The Von Frey probe was set to deliver an initial 2 g force over 8 seconds. The stimulus was then increased by a 0.2 log unit increment if there was no response or decreased by the same increment if the animal responded. Testing was performed on each foot and a 50% threshold was determined [24, 25]. An average value for the 2 feet was then calculated. For thermal testing, the time taken for the animal to remove its hind paw from the infrared heat stimulus was recorded 3 times for each foot. The first reading from each foot was discarded, and the mean response time was then calculated.

2.3. Tissue Processing. Rats were killed by isoflurane overdose 1 day after their final behavioural assessment and dose of gabapentin. Blood glucose levels were measured using an Ascensia Breeze 2 machine (Bayer, UK) from blood obtained by cardiac puncture. The lumbar (L3–L6) spinal cord region was rapidly dissected and postfixed in ice-cold 4% paraformaldehyde for 4 hours or frozen on dry-ice.

2.4. Immunohistochemistry. Fixed lumbar spinal cord was cryoprotected at 2–8°C in 10% sucrose in 0.1 M phosphate buffer for 18–24 hours followed by 30% sucrose in 0.1 M phosphate buffer for a further 18–24 hours. Tissue was then embedded in OCT embedding matrix media (Thermo Shandon Ltd., UK) and frozen on dry-ice. Transverse sections were cut by cryostat (16 μm) and thaw-mounted onto Superfrost Plus Slides (Fisher Scientific, UK).

For staining of microglia, one group of slides were first incubated twice for 15 minutes each (0.1 M PBS, 20% (v/v) methanol, 1.5% (v/v) hydrogen peroxide) for peroxidase-conjugated studies. After washing (phosphate buffered saline (PBS)), nonspecific binding in all slides was blocked for an hour (5% goat serum in 0.2% triton-X in PBS at room temperature) and sections were incubated overnight with primary antibody for ionized calcium binding adaptor molecule 1 (rabbit anti-Iba1; Wako, Germany; 1/1000 in 5% goat serum in 0.2% triton-X PBS at 2–8°C;). Biotinylated or fluorescein conjugated anti-rabbit secondary antibody (1/500 in 5% goat serum in 0.2% triton-X PBS; Vector, USA) was allowed to bind primary antibody for 1.5 hours at room temperature. Fluorescent sections were washed then either mounted in Vectorshield containing DAPI (Vector, USA) or incubated for 1 hour at room temperature with AvidinBiotin solution as per manufacturer's instructions (VECTASTAIN® ABC system, Vector, USA). Immunoreactivity was then visualised using DAB as per manufacturer's instructions (Vector, USA). Sections were dehydrated through a 50, 70, 90%, and absolute ethanol series followed by xylene washes, before mounting with Pertex mounting media (CellPath, UK).

For staining of neutrophils and blood vessels, sections were washed and nonspecific binding and autofluorescence were reduced (0.1 M glycine, 5% goat serum, 5% donkey serum in 0.3% triton-X in PBS; for 2 hours at room temperature). Primary antibodies for rabbit anti-neutrophil serum (SJC; 1/10,000; gift A. Dénes, (University of Manchester, UK) from D. Anthony and S. Campbell, University of Oxford, UK, produced [26]) and mouse anti-human laminin (1/1000; Millipore, UK) were applied overnight (in 2.5% goat serum, 2.5% donkey serum 0.3% triton-X in PBS, 2–8°C). After washing, primary antibodies were visualised with donkey anti-rabbit secondary Cyanine- 3-(Cy3-) conjugated antibody (1/1000; Jackson ImmunoResearch, USA) and goat anti-mouse conjugated Alexa Fluor™ 488 (1/1000; Invitrogen Life Technologies, UK) for 2 hours at room temperature (5% goat serum, 5% donkey serum in 0.3% triton-X in PBS).

Negative control sections were produced with each batch of immunostaining, with the absence of primary antibody. Staining was visualised on a Leica DMR microscope and images captured using a Hamamatsu digital C4742-95 digital camera (Japan). Higher power fluorescence images were taken using an Olympus BX51 upright microscope and Coolsnap EZ (Photometrics, USA) camera running MetaVue Software (Molecular Devices, USA), or a Delta Vision (Applied Precision, USA) restoration microscope using a

60x objective, captured using a Coolsnap HQ (Photometrics, USA) camera with a Z optical spacing of 0.2 μm. Raw images were then deconvolved using Softworx (Applied Precision, USA). High magnification images of microglia were captured on a Panoramic 250 slide scanner (3DHISTECH Ltd., Hungary), using a 20x objective and visualised using Pannoramic Viewer 1.15 software (3DHISTECH Ltd., Hungary).

2.5. Cytokine Profile Array. Spinal cords were homogenized in ice-cold lysis buffer (25 mM Tris HCl pH 7.4, 15 mM NaCl, 10 mM NaF, 10 mM Na Pyrophosphate, 2 mM EDTA, 0.2 mM Na_4OV_3, 1 mM PMSF, Protease Inhibitor Cocktail (1 : 200; Sigma Aldrich, UK)) using the FastPrep® bead beater system (MP Biomedicals, USA). The protein concentration of each sample was determined using a BCA assay (Pierce Biotechnology, UK) and 350 μg of lysate was loaded per membrane (Rat Cytokine Array Panel A, R&D Systems, UK), as per manufacturer's instructions. Cytokine levels were visualised and quantified using IRDye® 800CW Streptavidin secondary antibody (1/2000 in assay buffer 6; Li-Cor, UK) and captured on an Odyssey® Infrared Imaging System. Results were analysed using Odyssey 2.1 Software (Li-Cor, UK) and all absorbance values were corrected for background.

2.6. L-Selectin ELISA. Spinal cord lysates from control, untreated diabetic and gabapentin-treated rats (75 μg of protein) were loaded in duplicate and analysed for L-selectin content using a commercial ELISA kit (rat L-selectin/CD62L DuoSet, R&D Systems, UK).

2.7. Spinal Cord Neutrophil Analysis. To determine the number of infiltrating neutrophils, dual labelling was used to visualise both blood vessels and neutrophils present within the parenchyma. Only neutrophils outside of blood vessels were measured, that is, not intraluminal neutrophils. Parenchymal cell counts were performed on 4-5 lumbar spinal cord sections per animal ($n = 6$) and expressed as mean number of neutrophils per section.

2.8. Microglia Analysis. Iba1-immunoreactive cell morphology was analysed from DAB-labelled sections using the method described by Calvo et al. [27]. Briefly, SigmaScan Pro software (SPSS) was used to overlay a grid with squares measuring 10000 μm^2 on regions of the dorsal horn. A minimum of 5 randomly selected squares from a minimum of 4 spinal cord sections per animal were analysed. Only cells with a clearly visible cell body were analysed. Microglia whose processes were greater than double the cell-body length were deemed "surveying." Those cells where processes were less than double the cell-body length were categorised as "effector." Results are presented as the percentage of microglia displaying an "effector" morphology. Iba-1-immunoreactive cells present in the superficial dorsal horn were counted from 3–5 sections per animal and expressed as number of cells per 1×10^5 μm^2.

2.9. Statistical Analysis. Data are expressed as mean values ± standard deviation, unless otherwise stated. A Kruskal-Wallis ranking test was carried out on the Von Frey, and L-selectin ELISA data and 1-way ANOVA with Bonferroni post hoc tests were used to analyse all other data using GraphPad Prism 4 software (GraphPad software, USA).

3. Results

3.1. Gabapentin Reduces Hypersensitivity in STZ-Diabetic Rats. Rats with STZ-induced diabetes displayed mechanical allodynia at 8 weeks compared with age-matched controls (control: 37.0 g ± 3.2 versus untreated diabetic: 17.4 g ± 4.1, $p < 0.001$; Figure 1(a)). Gabapentin-treated diabetic rats (50 mg/kg/day for 2 weeks from 6 weeks after STZ) did not demonstrate the same degree of mechanical sensitivity, as no significant difference was observed between control and gabapentin-treated diabetic rats at 8 weeks (30.6 g ± 5.0, Figure 1(a)). In addition, diabetes-associated thermal hyperalgesia was prevented with gabapentin (untreated diabetic: 7.8 s ± 0.6 versus gabapentin-treated diabetic: 10.1 s ± 1.6, $p < 0.05$; Figure 1(b)). Gabapentin therefore protects against diabetes-associated allodynia and thermal hyperalgesia, without affecting terminal blood glucose levels (control: 8.1 ± 0.4 mmol/L; untreated diabetic: 34.1 ± 4.8 mmol/L ($p < 0.001$); diabetic + gabapentin: 39.2 ± 7.1 mmol/L ($p < 0.001$) compared with blood glucose levels in control rats: 1-way ANOVA with Bonferroni post hoc tests).

3.2. Diabetes-Induced Increase in L-Selectin in the Spinal Cord is Prevented by Gabapentin. An increase in the levels of proinflammatory cytokines has previously been reported in the rat spinal cord at early time points of diabetes (4-5 weeks after STZ: [28, 29]). We therefore conducted a cytokine profiling array using lumbar spinal cord samples (Figures 2(a)–2(c); Table 1) to determine which were altered at the 8-week time point of diabetes. The levels of classical "proinflammatory" cytokines such as TNF-α (Figure 2(d)), IL-1α (Figure 2(e)), and IL-1β (Figure 2(f)) were not significantly different in spinal cord samples from diabetic rats. Indeed, the only significant change (the full panel of results of 29 cytokines is shown in Table 1) was in the expression of L-selectin, which was significantly increased by 55% in spinal cords from untreated diabetic rats compared to control rats; this increase was prevented by gabapentin (Figure 2(g)). This observation was validated using ELISA (untreated diabetic: 0.14 ± 0.13 ρg L-selectin/μg spinal cord protein versus gabapentin-treated diabetic: 0.04 ρg ± 0.02 L-selectin/μg spinal cord protein; $p < 0.05$; Figure 2(h)).

3.3. Glial Cell Profiling in the Dorsal Horn of Rats with 8 Weeks of Experimental Diabetes. A change in spinal microglial number and morphology has previously been reported at early time points of diabetes (2–4 weeks after STZ: [11, 20]). Here, we examined Iba-1-immunopositive microglia at a later time point in the lumbar spinal cord of control, untreated diabetic, and diabetic rats treated with gabapentin (Figure 3). At 8 weeks after STZ, there was a small but significant increase in the numbers of Iba-1-positive cells present in the superficial dorsal horn of untreated diabetic rats (Figures 3(a)–3(d);

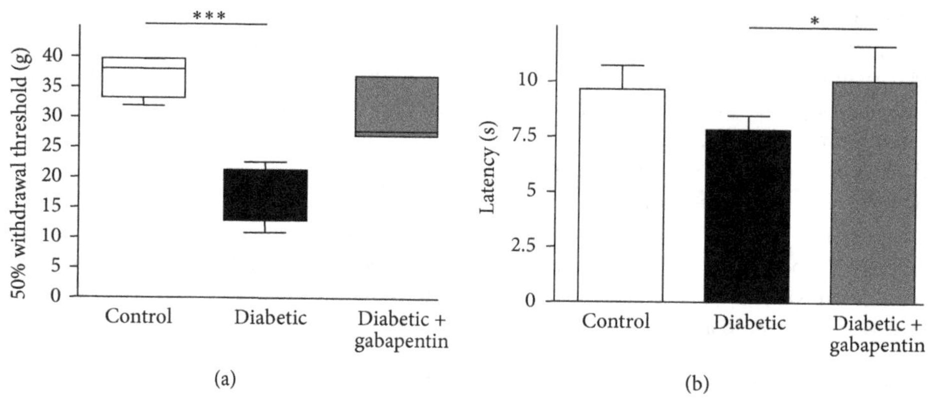

FIGURE 1: Gabapentin corrects diabetes-induced hypersensitivity. (a) Mechanical allodynia was observed in untreated diabetic rats (8 weeks after STZ), whilst diabetic rats treated with gabapentin showed near-control thresholds. Data are displayed as box and whisker plots, $^{***}p < 0.001$, in a Kruskal-Wallis test with Dunn's post hoc tests. (b) Thermal hyperalgesia was determined using a Hargreaves device; again diabetic rats treated with gabapentin showed near-control thresholds $^{*}p < 0.05$, in a 1-way ANOVA with Bonferroni post hoc tests. Data represent mean latency + SD; $n = 6$.

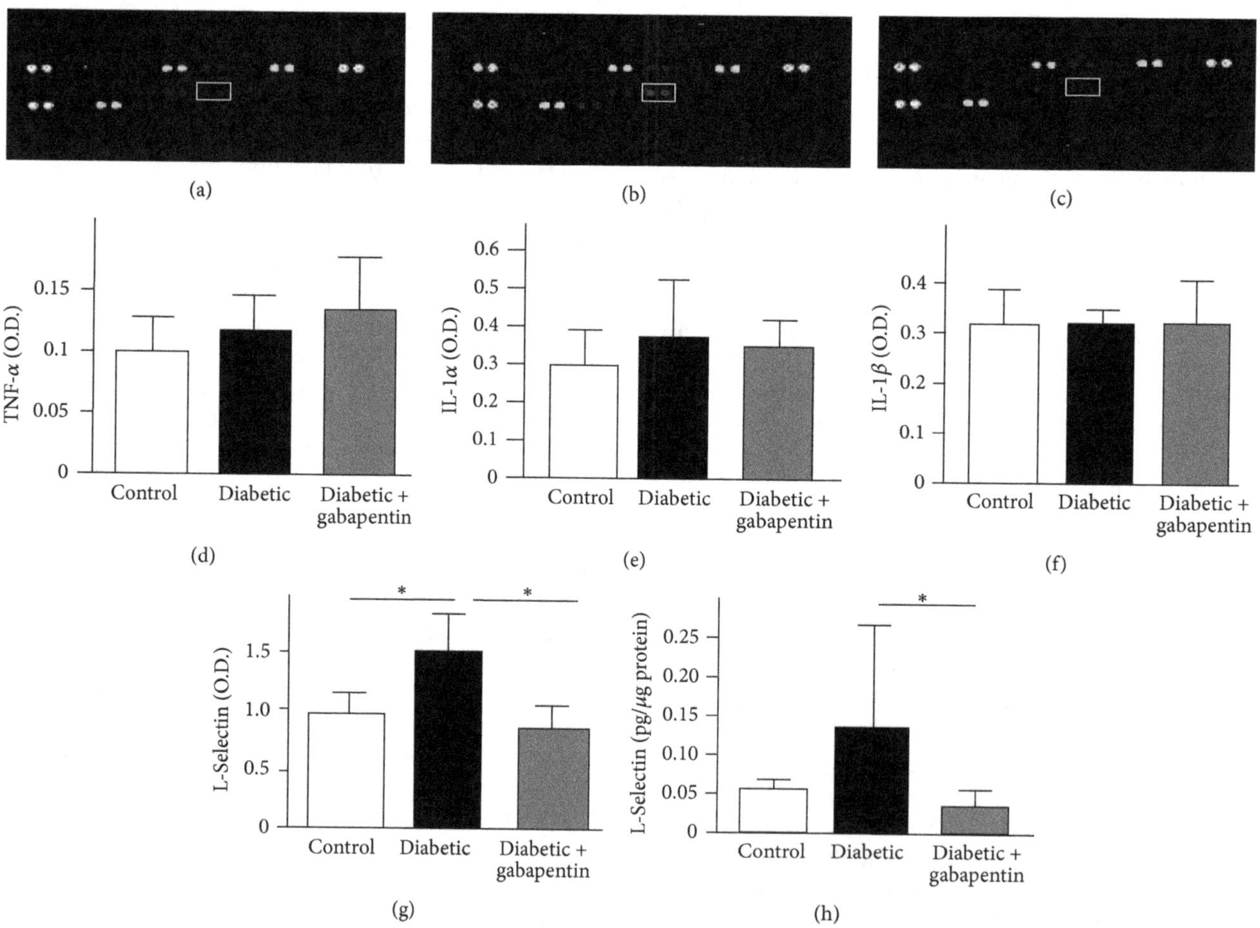

FIGURE 2: L-Selectin is increased in the spinal cord of diabetic rats. Cytokine proteome arrays were used to assay levels of 29 cytokines in (a) control, (b) untreated diabetic, and (c) gabapentin-treated diabetic rats. There was no change in the spinal levels of classically proinflammatory cytokines such as (d) TNF-α, (e) IL-1α, or (f) IL-1β (g). However, L-selectin (highlighted in box in (a)–(c)) was significantly increased in diabetic rat lumbar spinal cord, and this increase was ameliorated by treatment with gabapentin ($^{*}p < 0.05$ in a 1-way ANOVA with Bonferroni post hoc tests. Mean optical densities + SD are displayed; $n = 4$). (h) This was independently confirmed with an ELISA; levels of L-selectin were reduced when diabetic rats were treated with gabapentin ($^{*}p < 0.05$ in a Kruskal-Wallis test with Dunn's multiple comparison test; $n = 5$-6).

Table 1: Rat spinal cord cytokine proteome array. The levels of 29 cytokines in the lumbar spinal cord of control, diabetic, and gabapentin-treated diabetic rats. Mean values ± SD are displayed. $n = 4$. $^{*}p < 0.05$ in a 1-way ANOVA.

Name	Mean OD ± SD						p value
	Control		Diabetic		Diabetic + gabapentin		
IL-1α	**0.30**	0.09	**0.37**	0.15	**0.35**	0.07	*0.60*
IL-1β	**0.32**	0.07	**0.33**	0.03	**0.32**	0.09	*0.96*
IL-1ra	**0.30**	0.03	**0.37**	0.02	**0.33**	0.05	*0.09*
IL-2	**0.25**	0.03	**0.26**	0.06	**0.36**	0.09	*0.10*
CINC-1	**0.39**	0.21	**0.51**	0.34	**0.56**	0.24	*0.68*
CINC-2	**0.10**	0.02	**0.12**	0.02	**0.13**	0.05	*0.40*
CINC-3	**0.31**	0.04	**0.37**	0.04	**0.33**	0.02	*0.12*
IFN-γ	**0.31**	0.05	**0.29**	0.02	**0.27**	0.02	*0.19*
IL-3	**0.26**	0.09	**0.26**	0.05	**0.28**	0.08	*0.91*
IL-4	**0.23**	0.08	**0.25**	0.06	**0.27**	0.08	*0.74*
IL-6	**0.25**	0.04	**0.24**	0.03	**0.20**	0.04	*0.26*
IL-10	**0.25**	0.08	**0.22**	0.03	**0.24**	0.04	*0.82*
CNTF	**6.52**	1.91	**8.68**	2.50	**9.49**	3.47	*0.32*
sICAM-1	**9.18**	3.28	**13.10**	2.74	**12.80**	2.63	*0.15*
Thymus chemokine	**19.90**	0.36	**23.20**	3.03	**17.10**	5.85	*0.13*
Fractalkine	**1.02**	0.24	**1.00**	0.18	**1.02**	0.27	*0.99*
GM-CSF	**0.37**	0.20	**0.34**	0.06	**0.28**	0.04	*0.55*
RANTES	**0.29**	0.06	**0.40**	0.13	**0.40**	0.09	*0.22*
TIMP-1	**0.46**	0.28	**0.75**	0.43	**0.96**	0.94	*0.54*
TNF-α	**0.10**	0.03	**0.12**	0.03	**0.13**	0.04	*0.38*
VEGF	**0.56**	0.17	**0.41**	0.02	**0.49**	0.03	*0.07*
CXCl5	**0.71**	0.1	**1.1**	0.31	**0.72**	0.15	*0.07*
MIG	**0.36**	0.07	**0.35**	0.04	**0.33**	0.07	*0.81*
IL-13	**0.26**	0.17	**0.18**	0.04	**0.22**	0.05	*0.57*
IL-17	**0.22**	0.04	**0.24**	0.06	**0.31**	0.05	*0.10*
MIP-1α	**0.13**	0.02	**0.14**	0.01	**0.13**	0.03	*0.38*
MIP3α	**0.21**	0.04	**0.21**	0.01	**0.19**	0.02	*0.32*
IP-10	**0.27**	0.04	**0.33**	0.01	**0.30**	0.03	*0.06*
L-Selectin	**0.99**	0.18	**1.53**	0.32	**0.87**	0.20	*0.01**

IL-1α: interleukin-1 alpha; IL-1β: interleukin-1 beta; IL-1ra: interleukin-1 receptor antagonist; IL-2: interleukin-2; IL-3: interleukin-3; IL-4: interleukin-4; IL-6: interleukin-6; IL-10: interleukin-10; CNTF: ciliary neurotrophic factor; sICAM: soluble intercellular adhesion molecule; CINC-1: Cytokine-Induced Neutrophil Chemoattractant-1; CINC-2: Cytokine-Induced Neutrophil Chemoattractant-2; CINC-3: Cytokine-Induced Neutrophil Chemoattractant-3; IFN-γ: interferon-gamma; GM-CSF: granulocyte macrophage colony stimulating factor; RANTES: regulated upon activation, normal T-cell expressed and presumably secreted; TIMP-1: tissue inhibitor of metalloproteinases-1; TNF-α: tumour necrosis factor; VEGF: vascular endothelial growth factor; CXCl5: lipopolysaccharide-induced CXC; MIG: monokine induced by gamma interferon; IL-13: interleukin-13; IL-17: interleukin-17; MIP-1α: Macrophage Inflammatory Protein-1 alpha; MIP-3α: Macrophage Inflammatory Protein-3 alpha; IP-10, interferon-gamma-induced protein-10 kDa/CXC motif chemokine 10.

$p < 0.05$ 1-way ANOVA with Bonferroni post hoc tests); however, cell morphology was equivalent in all treatment groups (Figure 3(e); control: 67% ± 4.6: untreated diabetic: 61% ± 8.1; gabapentin-treated diabetic 63% ± 4.8 microglia had "effector" morphology; i.e., processes were less than twice the length of the cell body).

3.4. Increased Numbers of Neutrophils Are Present in the Spinal Cord Parenchyma of Diabetic Rats, Which Is Ameliorated with Gabapentin Treatment. The diabetes-associated upregulation of L-selectin, an adhesion molecule important for neutrophil transmigration [30], suggested possible immune cell recruitment/infiltration into the spinal cord. Therefore, immunohistochemistry was performed to identify whether neutrophils had infiltrated the spinal cord. The spinal cord parenchyma of untreated diabetic rats (arrows, Figures 4(b), 4(e), and 4(h)) contained more neutrophils than control (Figures 4(a), 4(d), and 4(g)) and gabapentin-treated (Figures 4(c), 4(f), and 4(i)) rats. Since rats were not transcardially perfused prior to tissue harvest, only neutrophils present in spinal parenchyma (arrows, Figures 4(k) and 4(l)) were counted and not those contained within blood vessels (asterisks, Figures 4(j) and 4(l)). There was a significant increase in the number of parenchymal neutrophils throughout the spinal cord in untreated diabetic rats compared with control rats (untreated diabetic: 2.60 ± 1.4 versus control: 0.53 ± 0.55; Figure 4(m) $p < 0.01$). Interestingly, this increase was not observed in diabetic animals treated with gabapentin (1.03 ± 0.63, $p < 0.05$ compared with untreated diabetic rats).

4. Discussion

In this study, we demonstrate an increase in the levels of L-selectin, an adhesion molecule important for neutrophil transmigration, in the lumbar spinal cord after 8 weeks of diabetes. In addition, we show an increase in the number of parenchymal neutrophils in the spinal cord of diabetic rats. Together, these data suggest a role for dysregulated L-selectin and spinal vasculature in diabetes that leads to an increase in infiltrating neutrophils in experimental diabetic neuropathy, which is ameliorated by treatment with gabapentin.

The cytokine profiling array did not show diabetes-associated increases in classic proinflammatory cytokines such as IL-1β, TNF-α, fractalkine, and IL-6 cytokines, which are associated with microgliosis and hyperalgesia [11, 20, 28, 29, 31, 32]. Microglial activation has been associated with pain in a number of neuropathy models, notably traumatic nerve-injury models [14] and early time points of STZ-diabetes [11, 31]. However, microgliosis was not associated with viral-induced hypersensitivity [33] and minimal in a nucleoside reverse transcriptase inhibitor- (stavudine-) induced HIV hypersensitivity model [34]. Our finding that there was a small increase in microglial number, but no change in morphology at 8 weeks, perhaps indicates why we did not detect increases in the proinflammatory cytokines in our arrays but does not preclude the possibility that microglial activation may have occurred at an earlier time point. It is also possible that subtle changes in proinflammatory cytokines specifically

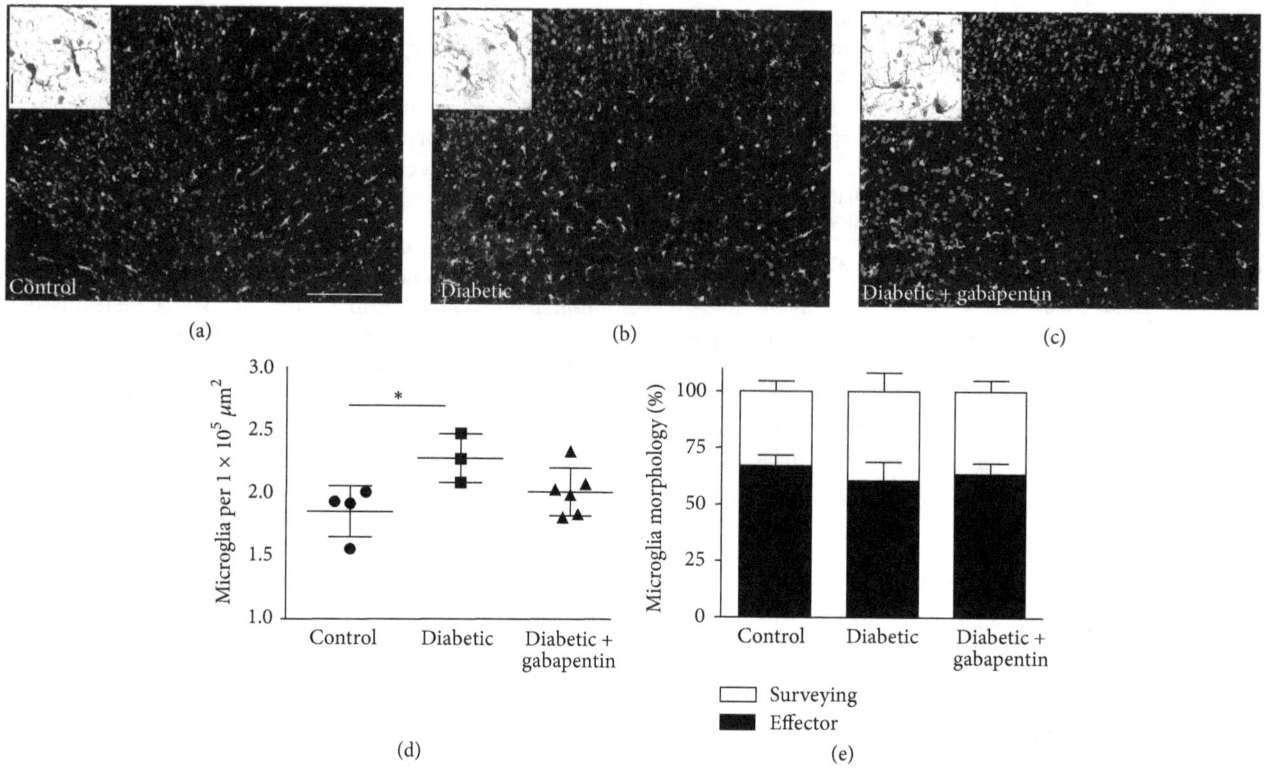

FIGURE 3: Microglial changes in the spinal cord of control, untreated diabetic, and gabapentin-treated diabetic rats. Representative photomicrographs of the L4/5 dorsal horn of the spinal cord of (a) control, (b) untreated diabetic, and (c) diabetic rats treated with gabapentin (a–c), micrographs (and insets) show examples of typical Iba1-immunoreactivity. Scale bars represent 100 μm (main micrograph, (a)–(c)) and 25 μm (insets (a)–(c)). Microglial numbers are increased in the superficial ((d), $^{*}p < 0.05$ 1-way ANOVA Bonferroni post hoc tests) but not deep (e) dorsal horn of diabetic rats; however, morphology of microglia was not significantly different (e).

within the dorsal horn may have not been detected, as whole lumbar spinal cord lysates were used in our assay.

However, interestingly, we found a significant increase in L-selectin (a type I cell adhesion molecule which is constitutively expressed on the cell surface of most circulating leukocytes [30]) in spinal cords from diabetic rats, which was not evident in spinal cords from diabetic rats treated with gabapentin. L-Selectin mediates the initial tethering and rolling of leukocytes along activated endothelial cells and then the transendothelial migration of leukocytes through the vasculature. L-Selectins are cleaved from the cell surface by the action of ADAM17 (disintegrins and metalloproteinase 17) or TACE (TNF-α converting enzyme), a process known as "shedding," which may dramatically regulate migratory cell behaviour [35].

Neutrophils are one of the first types of peripheral immune cell to attend sites of inflammation following injury or infection [36]. They are important in mounting an initial immune response, able to produce both proinflammatory mediators, as well as present antigen to T-cells [37]. In experimental nerve-injury models, the recruitment of immune cells both peripherally and centrally is an important mechanism underlying establishment and maintenance of neuropathic pain [38]. Neutrophil migration into the CNS is well characterised in spinal cord injury models [39], and reductions in leukocyte infiltration in the CNS have been linked to reductions in neuropathic pain [40]. The reactive glycolytic metabolite methylglyoxal is increased in the plasma of both STZ-diabetic mice and diabetic patients [41]. Interestingly, peripheral injection of methylglyoxal induces leukocyte recruitment to the microvasculature of the injection site and approximately 90% of the recruited cells are neutrophils [42], suggesting that recruitment of this cell type may be particularly important in diabetes. In diabetic retinopathy, higher numbers of $CD45^{+}$ immune cells have been recorded in the retina of diabetic mice compared with controls [43]. In diabetic rats too, increased numbers of leukocytes are associated with retinal endothelial cells, when compared with retina from control rats [44]. Similarly, an increase in neutrophils in the kidney has been described in mice with diabetic nephropathy [45]. Increased numbers of neutrophils in the parenchyma of spinal cords from diabetic rats compared with controls indicate commonality between the three major diabetic complications.

This increase in spinal neutrophil recruitment in diabetes could be a consequence of altered afferent activity, spinal sensitisation, structural damage, or altered blood-brain barrier function. Interestingly, the reduction in numbers of neutrophils within the spinal cord parenchyma after gabapentin followed the reduction in allodynia and thermal

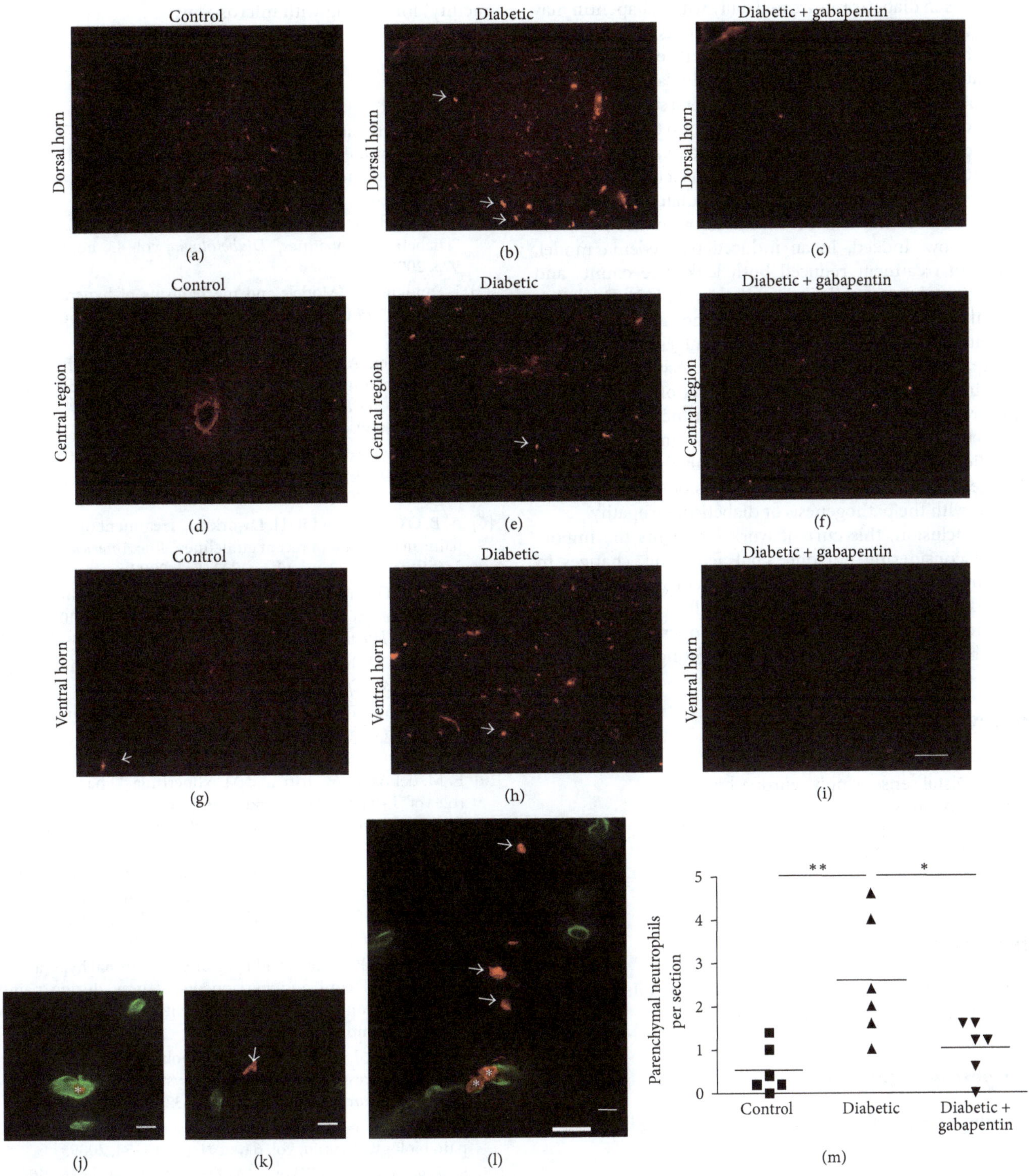

FIGURE 4: Diabetes is associated with an increase in neutrophil numbers within the spinal cord parenchyma, which is ameliorated with gabapentin treatment. (a–i) There is an increase in antineutrophil immunoreactivity within the dorsal horn (a–c), central region (d–f), and ventral horns (g–i) of untreated diabetic rats (arrows, (b), (e), and (h), scale bar represents 100 μm.). Dual immunofluorescence with antilaminin (green) to label blood vessels reveals the presence of intraluminal (asterisks, (j) and (l)) and parenchymal neutrophils (arrows, (k) and (l)). Only parenchymal neutrophils (i.e., those not associated with a vessel) were counted (m) and revealed an increase in neutrophils in the spinal cord of untreated diabetic rats and revealed that gabapentin treatment reduced the numbers to near-control levels ((m), $^{*}p < 0.05$, $^{**}p < 0.01$ in a 1-way ANOVA with Bonferroni post hoc tests. $n = 6$).

hyperalgesia in diabetic rats. The reduced numbers of spinal neutrophils in diabetic rats treated daily with gabapentin may be a downstream consequence of the transitory analgesic effects of gabapentin ([46]). This may be through inhibition of excitatory postsynaptic currents from dorsal horn neurons or a reduction in microgliosis persisting for a sufficient length of time to prevent neutrophil infiltration into the spinal cord. It will be interesting for future studies to examine whether gabapentin has a direct effect on L-selectin expression. This effect may be via the spinal vasculature, neutrophil migration across the endothelium, and/or release from the bone marrow. Indeed, in an induced paw edema model, gabapentin treatment reduced both leukocyte counts and MPO activity (neutrophil marker) in the foot [47]. Depletion of circulating neutrophils has also previously been shown to attenuate the development of hyperalgesia following a peripheral nerve injury [48]. We suggest that future studies will be important to determine the impact of blocking neutrophil recruitment to the spinal cord on neuropathic pain in diabetes. Using intrathecal L-selectin function-blocking antibodies or inhibitors may provide valuable mechanistic evidence linking spinal L-selectin expression and neutrophil invasion with the pathogenesis of diabetic neuropathy.

In conclusion, this current work highlights the importance of considering not only glial activation, changes in ion channel expression, and altered neuronal activity in painful diabetic neuropathy, but also the effect of immune cell infiltration into the spinal cord; this may open more avenues by which to direct future therapeutic targeting.

Abbreviations

CNS: Central nervous system
DPN: Distal sensory polyneuropathy
GABA: γ-Aminobutyric acid
IBA1: Ionized calcium binding adaptor molecule 1
PBS: Phosphate buffered saline
STZ: Streptozotocin.

Disclosure

The funders had no role in study design, data collection, and analysis or preparation of the manuscript.

Competing Interests

The authors declare that they have no competing interests.

Acknowledgments

This work was supported by a GlaxoSmithKline-BBSRC (UK) Ph.D. studentship (VLN; BB/J014478/1) and the authors thank the Centre for Integrated Mammalian Biology, Manchester, for support. Natalie J. Gardiner was supported by the Juvenile Diabetes Research Foundation (Natalie J. Gardiner: JDRF, USA: 2-2009-226). The authors thank Sumia Ali and Sarah Al-Adham for immunocytochemistry advice and Roger Meadows (University of Manchester Bioimaging Facility) for helping with microscopy.

References

[1] N. Hex, C. Bartlett, D. Wright, M. Taylor, and D. Varley, "Estimating the current and future costs of Type1 and Type2 diabetes in the UK, including direct health costs and indirect societal and productivity costs," *Diabetic Medicine*, vol. 29, no. 7, pp. 855–862, 2012.

[2] A. I. Vinik, T. S. Park, K. B. Stansberry, and G. L. Pittenger, "Diabetic neuropathies," *Diabetologia*, vol. 43, no. 8, pp. 957–973, 2000.

[3] J. Sandkühler, "Models and mechanisms of hyperalgesia and allodynia," *Physiological Reviews*, vol. 89, no. 2, pp. 707–758, 2009.

[4] B. S. Galer, A. Gianas, and M. P. Jensen, "Painful diabetic polyneuropathy: epidemiology, pain description, and quality of life," *Diabetes Research and Clinical Practice*, vol. 47, no. 2, pp. 123–128, 2000.

[5] D. Ziegler, "Painful diabetic neuropathy: treatment and future aspects," *Diabetes/Metabolism Research and Reviews*, vol. 24, S1, pp. S52–S57, 2008.

[6] A. B. O'Connor and R. H. Dworkin, "Treatment of neuropathic pain: an overview of recent guidelines," *The American Journal of Medicine*, vol. 122, no. 10, pp. S22–S32, 2009.

[7] N. Attal, G. Cruccu, R. Baron et al., "EFNS guidelines on the pharmacological treatment of neuropathic pain: 2010 revision," *European Journal of Neurology*, vol. 17, no. 9, pp. 1113–1123, 2010.

[8] M. Bialer, "Why are antiepileptic drugs used for nonepileptic conditions?" *Epilepsia*, vol. 53, pp. 26–33, 2012.

[9] J.-K. Cheng and L.-C. Chiou, "Mechanisms of the antinociceptive action of gabapentin," *Journal of Pharmacological Sciences*, vol. 100, no. 5, pp. 471–486, 2006.

[10] E. M. del Amo, A. Urtti, and M. Yliperttula, "Pharmacokinetic role of L-type amino acid transporters LAT1 and LAT2," *European Journal of Pharmaceutical Sciences*, vol. 35, no. 3, pp. 161–174, 2008.

[11] R. Wodarski, A. K. Clark, J. Grist, F. Marchand, and M. Malcangio, "Gabapentin reverses microglial activation in the spinal cord of streptozotocin-induced diabetic rats," *European Journal of Pain*, vol. 13, no. 8, pp. 807–811, 2009.

[12] C. Morgado, P. P. Terra, and I. Tavares, "Neuronal hyperactivity at the spinal cord and periaqueductal grey during painful diabetic neuropathy: effects of gabapentin," *European Journal of Pain*, vol. 14, no. 7, pp. 693–699, 2010.

[13] M. Costigan, J. Scholz, and C. J. Woolf, "Neuropathic pain: a maladaptive response of the nervous system to damage," *Annual Review of Neuroscience*, vol. 32, pp. 1–32, 2009.

[14] S. B. McMahon and M. Malcangio, "Current challenges in glia-pain biology," *Neuron*, vol. 64, no. 1, pp. 46–54, 2009.

[15] S. Jergová and D. Čížková, "Microglial activation in different models of peripheral nerve injury of the rat," *Journal of Molecular Histology*, vol. 38, no. 3, pp. 245–251, 2007.

[16] S.-X. Jin, Z.-Y. Zhuang, C. J. Woolf, and R.-R. Ji, "p38 mitogen-activated protein kinase is activated after a spinal nerve ligation in spinal cord microglia and dorsal root ganglion neurons and contributes to the generation of neuropathic pain," *The Journal of Neuroscience*, vol. 23, no. 10, pp. 4017–4022, 2003.

[17] Z.-Y. Zhuang, Y.-R. Wen, D.-R. Zhang et al., "A peptide c-Jun N-terminal kinase (JNK) inhibitor blocks mechanical allodynia

after spinal nerve ligation: respective roles of JNK activation in primary sensory neurons and spinal astrocytes for neuropathic pain development and maintenance," *Journal of Neuroscience*, vol. 26, no. 13, pp. 3551–3560, 2006.

[18] C. J. Woolf and Q. Ma, "Nociceptors—noxious stimulus detectors," *Neuron*, vol. 55, no. 3, pp. 353–364, 2007.

[19] L. Daulhac, C. Mallet, C. Courteix et al., "Diabetes-induced mechanical hyperalgesia involves spinal mitogen-activated protein kinase activation in neurons and microglia via N-methyl-D-aspartate- dependent mechanisms," *Molecular Pharmacology*, vol. 70, no. 4, pp. 1246–1254, 2006.

[20] M. Tsuda, H. Ueno, A. Kataoka, H. Tozaki-Saitoh, and K. Inoue, "Activation of dorsal horn microglia contributes to diabetes-induced tactile allodynia via extracellular signal-regulated protein kinase signaling," *GLIA*, vol. 56, no. 4, pp. 378–386, 2008.

[21] K. Mitchell, H.-Y. T. Yang, P. A. Tessier et al., "Localization of S100A8 and S100A9 expressing neutrophils to spinal cord during peripheral tissue inflammation," *Pain*, vol. 134, no. 1-2, pp. 216–231, 2008.

[22] F. C. Barouch, K. Miyamoto, J. R. Allport et al., "Integrin-mediated neutrophil adhesion and retinal leukostasis in diabetes," *Investigative Ophthalmology and Visual Science*, vol. 41, no. 5, pp. 1153–1158, 2000.

[23] E. Galkina and K. Ley, "Leukocyte recruitment and vascular injury in diabetic nephropathy," *Journal of the American Society of Nephrology*, vol. 17, no. 2, pp. 368–377, 2006.

[24] S. R. Chaplan, F. W. Bach, J. W. Pogrel, J. M. Chung, and T. L. Yaksh, "Quantitative assessment of tactile allodynia in the rat paw," *Journal of Neuroscience Methods*, vol. 53, no. 1, pp. 55–63, 1994.

[25] W. J. Dixon, "Efficient analysis of experimental observations," *Annual Review of Pharmacology and Toxicology*, vol. 20, pp. 441–462, 1980.

[26] M. A. Trevethick, A. K. Bahl, N. M. Clayton, P. Strong, S. Sanjar, and I. W. Harman, "Neutrophil infiltration does not contribute to the ulcerogenic effects of indomethacin in the rat gastric antrum," *Agents and Actions*, vol. 43, no. 1-2, pp. 39–43, 1994.

[27] M. Calvo, N. Zhu, J. Grist, Z. Ma, J. A. Loeb, and D. L. H. Bennett, "Following nerve injury neuregulin-1 drives microglial proliferation and neuropathic pain via the MEK/ERK pathway," *GLIA*, vol. 59, no. 4, pp. 554–568, 2011.

[28] M. Liu, K. Liao, C. Yu, X. Li, S. Liu, and S. Yang, "Puerarin alleviates neuropathic pain by inhibiting neuroinflammation in spinal cord," *Mediators of Inflammation*, vol. 2014, Article ID 485927, 9 pages, 2014.

[29] M. Bishnoi, C. A. Bosgraaf, M. Abooj, L. Zhong, and L. S. Premkumar, "Streptozotocin-induced early thermal hyperalgesia is independent of glycemic state of rats: role of transient receptor potential vanilloid 1(TRPV1) and inflammatory mediators," *Molecular Pain*, vol. 7, article 52, 2011.

[30] U. Jung and K. Ley, "Mice lacking two or all three selectins demonstrate overlapping and distinct functions for each selectin," *Journal of Immunology*, vol. 162, no. 11, pp. 6755–6762, 1999.

[31] C. Morgado, P. Pereira-Terra, C. D. Cruz, and I. Tavares, "Minocycline completely reverses mechanical hyperalgesia in diabetic rats through microglia-induced changes in the expression of the potassium chloride co-transporter 2 (KCC2) at the spinal cord," *Diabetes, Obesity and Metabolism*, vol. 13, no. 2, pp. 150–159, 2011.

[32] M. Calvo and D. L. H. Bennett, "The mechanisms of microgliosis and pain following peripheral nerve injury," *Experimental Neurology*, vol. 234, no. 2, pp. 271–282, 2012.

[33] J. Blackbeard, V. C. J. Wallace, K. P. O'Dea et al., "The correlation between pain-related behaviour and spinal microgliosis in four distinct models of peripheral neuropathy," *European Journal of Pain*, vol. 16, no. 10, pp. 1357–1367, 2012.

[34] W. Huang, M. Calvo, K. Karu et al., "A clinically relevant rodent model of the HIV antiretroviral drug stavudine induced painful peripheral neuropathy," *Pain*, vol. 154, no. 4, pp. 560–575, 2013.

[35] K. Rzeniewicz, A. Newe, A. Rey Gallardo et al., "L-selectin shedding is activated specifically within transmigrating pseudopods of monocytes to regulate cell polarity in vitro," *Proceedings of the National Academy of Sciences of the United States of America*, vol. 112, no. 12, pp. E1461–E1470, 2015.

[36] J. A. Smith, "Neutrophils, host defense, and inflammation: a double-edged sword," *Journal of Leukocyte Biology*, vol. 56, no. 6, pp. 672–686, 1994.

[37] H. L. Wright, R. J. Moots, R. C. Bucknall, and S. W. Edwards, "Neutrophil function in inflammation and inflammatory diseases," *Rheumatology*, vol. 49, no. 9, pp. 1618–1631, 2010.

[38] L. R. Watkins and S. F. Maier, "Beyond neurons: evidence that immune and glial cells contribute to pathological pain states," *Physiological Reviews*, vol. 82, no. 4, pp. 981–1011, 2002.

[39] E. D. Means and D. K. Anderson, "Neuronophagia by leukocytes in experimental spinalcord injury," *Journal of Neuropathology & Experimental Neurology*, vol. 42, no. 6, pp. 707–719, 1983.

[40] F. Bao, J. C. Fleming, R. Golshani et al., "A selective phosphodiesterase-4 inhibitor reduces leukocyte infiltration, oxidative processes, and tissue damage after spinal cord injury," *Journal of Neurotrauma*, vol. 28, no. 6, pp. 1035–1049, 2011.

[41] A. Bierhaus, T. Fleming, S. Stoyanov et al., "Methylglyoxal modification of Nav1.8 facilitates nociceptive neuron firing and causes hyperalgesia in diabetic neuropathy," *Nature Medicine*, vol. 18, pp. 926–933, 2012.

[42] Y. Su, X. Lei, L. Wu, and L. Liu, "The role of endothelial cell adhesion molecules P-selectin, E-selectin and intercellular adhesion molecule-1 in leucocyte recruitment induced by exogenous methylglyoxal," *Immunology*, vol. 137, no. 1, pp. 65–79, 2012.

[43] J. Yellowlees Douglas, A. D. Bhatwadekar, S. Li Calzi et al., "Bone marrow-CNS connections: implications in the pathogenesis of diabetic retinopathy," *Progress in Retinal and Eye Research*, vol. 31, no. 5, pp. 481–494, 2012.

[44] A. M. Joussen, T. Murata, A. Tsujikawa, B. Kirchhof, S.-E. Bursell, and A. P. Adamis, "Leukocyte-mediated endothelial cell injury and death in the diabetic retina," *The American Journal of Pathology*, vol. 158, no. 1, pp. 147–152, 2001.

[45] R. Mohamed, C. Jayakumar, P. V. Ranganathan, V. Ganapathy, and G. Ramesh, "Kidney proximal tubular epithelial-specific overexpression of netrin-1 suppresses inflammation and albuminuria through suppression of COX-2-mediated PGE2 production in streptozotocin-induced diabetic mice," *The American Journal of Pathology*, vol. 181, no. 6, pp. 1991–2002, 2012.

[46] W. Xiao, A. Boroujerdi, G. J. Bennett, and Z. D. Luo, "Chemotherapy-evoked painful peripheral neuropathy: analgesic effects of gabapentin and effects on expression of the alpha-2-delta type-1 calcium channel subunit," *Neuroscience*, vol. 144, no. 2, pp. 714–720, 2007.

5

Glycopatterns of Urinary Protein as New Potential Diagnosis Indicators for Diabetic Nephropathy

Hanyu Zhu,[1] Moyan Liu,[2] Hanjie Yu,[3] Xiawei Liu,[3] Yaogang Zhong,[3] Jian Shu,[3] Xinle Fu,[3] Guangyan Cai,[1] Xiangmei Chen,[1] Wenjia Geng,[1] Xiaoli Yang,[1] Minghui Wu,[1] Zheng Li,[3] and Dong Zhang[1]

[1]*Department of Nephrology, Chinese PLA General Hospital, Chinese PLA Institute of Nephrology, State Key Laboratory of Kidney Diseases, National Clinical Research Center of Kidney Diseases, Beijing Key Laboratory of Kidney Disease, Beijing, China*
[2]*Department of Nephrology, General Hospital of Jinan Military Command, Jinan, China*
[3]*Laboratory for Functional Glycomics, College of Life Sciences, Northwest University, Xi'an, China*

Correspondence should be addressed to Zheng Li; zhengli@nwu.edu.cn and Dong Zhang; zhangdong1301@126.com

Academic Editor: Wei J. Liu

Diabetic nephropathy is a major cause of chronic kidney disease and end-stage kidney disease. However, so little is known about alterations of the glycopatterns in urine with the development of diabetic nephropathy. Presently, we interrogated glycopatterns in urine specimens using a lectin microarray. The results showed that expression levels of Siaα2-6Gal/GalNAc recognized by SNA exhibited significantly increased tendency with the development of diabetic nephropathy; moreover, SNA blotting indicated glycoproteins (90 kDa, 70 kDa, and 40 kDa) in urine may contribute to this alteration. Furthermore, the glycopatterns of $(GlcNAc)_{2-4}$ recognized by STL exhibited difference between diabetic and nondiabetic nephropathy. The results of urinary protein microarray fabricated by another 48 urine specimens also indicated $(GlcNAc)_{2-4}$ is a potential indictor to differentiate the patients with diabetic nephropathy from nondiabetic nephropathy. Furtherly, STL blotting showed that the 50 kDa glycoproteins were correlated with this alteration. In conclusion, our data provide pivotal information to monitor the development of diabetic nephropathy and distinguish between diabetic nephropathy and nondiabetic renal disease based on precise alterations of glycopatterns in urinary proteins, but further studies are needed in this regard.

1. Introduction

Diabetic nephropathy (DN) is a serious complication of diabetes mellitus and now the major cause of chronic kidney disease (CKD) and end-stage kidney disease (ESRD) throughout the world. However, renal damage associated with diabetes can be classified as either DN or nondiabetic renal disease (NDRD). There are significant differences in the treatment and prognosis of these two types of renal disease. Renal pathological diagnosis is currently the gold standard for distinguishing DN from NDRD, although renal biopsy is invasive.

Urine has some unique advantages (collected noninvasively, a large number of proteins in urinary proteome also belong to plasma proteome); certain proteins in urine not only reflect the status of the entire body, but also correlated with diseases, which is good resource for the analysis of disease processes [1–4]. Valuated urinary proteome analysis is a tool for prediction and monitoring of DN. Transferrin is a glycoprotein with a molecular weight of 76.5 kDa, which was demonstrated that the urinary transferrin could reflect the degree of interstitial fibrosis and tubular atrophy in patients with DN [5]. The low-molecular weight proteome in urine was profiled by capillary electrophoresis-coupled mass spectrometry (CE-MS), and results indicated that the specific collagen fragments in urine could effectively assess DN risk at an early stage [6]. For type 2 diabetic nephropathy, it is reported that urinary cystatin C and NAP (nonalbumin protein) could reflect the progression of type 2 diabetic nephropathy [7]. Liver-type fatty acid-binding protein (L-FABP), an intracellular carrier protein of free fatty acids, is expressed in the liver and kidney, which could serve as a predictive marker for renal and cardiovascular prognosis in type 2 diabetic patients without advanced nephropathy [8]. It is interesting that L-FABP also could be an independent predictor of progression at all stages of type 1 diabetic nephropathy irrespective of stage [9].

Glycosylation is an important posttranscription modification; more than half of known proteins are glycoprotein. It is well known that the glycan attached on glycoproteins has many biological functions, such as maintaining conformation and flexibility of protein, oligosaccharide modification involved in biological processes including cell adhesion, signal transduction, and endocytosis. Abnormal glycosylation had demonstrated correlation with occurrence and development of diseases [10, 11]. Lectin microarray is a powerful technology that uses a panel of lectins immobilized on solid phase substrate for high-throughput analysis of glycans and glycoproteins related to diseases such as cancer and inflammatory diseases [12–14]. Alterations of sialylated MUC1 glycosylation detected by lectin microarray could be indispensable for the development of cholangiocarcinoma [15]. Glycosylated patterns of A1AT (alpha-1-antitrypsin) may serve as potential biomarkers for early detection [16]. For DN, nonenzymatic glycosylation product such as glycated albumin was strongly associated with incident diabetes and its microvascular complications. In addition, the glycated albumin: HbA1c ratio and glycated albumin may be superior to HbA1c associated with the presence of DN [17, 18]. However, there were few reports about enzymatic glycosylation on glycoproteins that altered in development of DN.

In this study, we preformed lectin microarray to investigate altered glycopatterns during the development of DN and evaluate whether glycopattern in urine was a potential biomarker to differentiate DN from NDRD.

2. Materials and Methods

2.1. Study Population. Our study subjects were patients who underwent renal biopsy at the Chinese People's Liberation Army (PLA) General Hospital. The inclusion criteria were as follows: patients aged between 20 and 70 years; patients diagnosed with type 2 diabetes mellitus (type 2) and with persistent overt proteinuria (defined as urinary albumin excretion $\geq$ 300 mg/24 h or urinary protein excretion $\geq$ 500 mg/24 h by at least two tests without evidence of urinary tract infection); patients with serum creatinine less than 442 μmol/L; and patients who were voluntarily admitted to the hospital to undergo renal biopsy. The exclusion criteria were the following: patients who had a confirmed diagnosis of renal diseases before they were diagnosed with type 2 diabetes; with a clinically confirmed diagnosis of NDRD, including lupus nephritis and Henoch-Schönlein purpura nephritis; with familial hereditary nephropathies, such as autosomal dominant polycystic kidney disease; and with an uncertain pathological diagnosis.

The tissue was examined by at least two pathology experts together with another two nephrologists; then the pathological diagnosis was determined. Renal biopsy indications: in clinical practice, the possible diagnosis of NDRD was confirmed by renal biopsy when the following situations occurred: gross/microscopic hematuria; elevated serum creatinine without obvious proteinuria; persistent massive proteinuria with normal renal function and no diabetic retinopathy. The renal biopsy indications for the suspected diagnosis of NDRD at our centre were in accordance with those listed for NDRD in the 2007 Kidney Disease Outcomes Quality Initiative (KDOQI) guidelines. Thus, 19 cases were diagnosed as DN and 18 cases were diagnosed as NDRD which included 10 (membranous nephropathy) MN and 8 IgAN. To evaluate whether glycopattern in urine was a potential biomarker to differentiate DN from NDRD, the presence of other kidney diseases accompanied with DN or NDRD and the patients who had pathological diagnosis of DN combined with NDRD were excluded in this study.

In order to evaluate potential biomarkers for distinguishing DN from NDRD, all the patients were divided into DN and NDRD group. To assess the possibility of urinary glycopatterns as potential biomarkers for monitor the process of DN, we separate the DN group into two subgroups according to the eGFR level. The eGFR level was calculated using the Modification of Diet in Renal Disease (MDRD) Study formula. The DN group I defined as the eGFR > 60 mL/min/1.73 m^2, along with low level 24 h urinary protein (1.41 ± 0.61 g/24 h), means the early stage of kidney disease. The DN group II defined as eGFR < 60 mL/min/1.73 m^2, along with high level 24 h urinary protein (2.64 ± 1.41 g/24 h), means the patients have renal insufficiency, indicating a worse prognosis.

All healthy volunteers (HVs) had no recent illness or medication. All females had no menstrual cycle at the time of collection. The collection of urine samples was done prior to treatment and before the biopsy or at least 1 month after the biopsy. The clinical information was summarized in Table 1.

2.2. Study Approval. The collection and use of all human pathology specimens for research presented here were approved by the Ethical Committee of Northwest University (Xi'an, China), the Department of Nephrology, Chinese PLA General Hospital, Chinese PLA Institute of Nephrology, State Key Laboratory of Kidney Diseases, National Clinical Research Center of Kidney Diseases, Beijing Key Laboratory of Kidney Disease (Beijing, China). Written informed consent was received from participants for the collection of their urine. This study was conducted in accordance with the ethical guidelines of the Declaration of Helsinki.

2.3. Processing of Urine. 15 mL of urine was collected and stored at 4°C immediately. Then, the samples were centrifuged at 3000 rpm for 20 minutes at 4°C to remove cells and debris. The supernatant was frozen at −80°C in 1 mL aliquots. The method of trichloroacetic acid (TCA)/acetone precipitation was utilized to prepare urinary protein; the method of urinary protein precipitation was described elsewhere with

Table 1: Biochemical characteristics of clinical specimens.

	HVs	T2DM	DN (n = 19)		NDRD (n = 18)	
			DN group I	DN group II	MN	IgAN
Number of subjects	10	10	9	10	10	8
Age (years)	59.00 ± 3.05	58.50 ± 6.22	48.00 ± 7.45	52.60 ± 8.33	56.40 ± 6.64	53.63 ± 10.93
Sex (male/female)	4/6	5/5	4/5	8/2	6/4	4/4
BMI (kg/cm^2)	24.2 ± 3.6	25.1 ± 2.9	26.0 ± 3.0	25.7 ± 3.2	27.2 ± 3.8	25.2 ± 3.0
Duration of diabetes (months)	\	63.1 ± 15.5	126.2 ± 63.0	129.6 ± 56.4	69.6 ± 49.8	82.8 ± 50.2
Systolic blood pressure (mmHg)	119.7 ± 19.3	120.4 ± 21.4	152.1 ± 19.0	152.1 ± 19.0	136.4 ± 20.5	136.4 ± 20.5
Urinary protein (g/24 h)	\	\	1.41 ± 0.61	2.64 ±1.41	3.28 ± 1.56	2.84 ± 2.21
Creatinine (μmol/L)	\	63.70 ± 10.93	81.34 ± 14.87	140.83 ± 52.00	82.07 ± 29.88	114.70 ± 46.65
eGFR (ml · min^{-1}· 1.73 m^{-2})	\	\	78.68 ± 23.38	49.37 ± 18.64	83.99 ± 31.77	61.08 ± 30.57
HbAlc (%)	\	6.6 ± 0.9	7.3 ± 1.6	7.2 ± 1.9	6.8 ± 1.0	7.0 ± 1.8
Diabetic retinopathy	\	\	5 (55.6%)	6 (60.0%)	3 (30%)	1 (12.5%)

little modification [19–21]. Briefly, 3 mL mixed urine specimen was mixed with 30 mL TCA 10%-acetone solution 90% (v/v), followed by overnight incubation at −20°C. The mixture was centrifuged at 10,000g for 15 min at 4°C; after that, protein precipitate was resuspended by 2 mL ice-cold acetone; after centrifugation, the protein was left to dry on ice for 1 h. Pellet resuspension was performed with 500 μL 10 mM PBS buffer (pH 7.4) with 1% Tween-20 at ambient temperature for 15 min, sonicated for another 15 min in ultrasound bath. The protein concentration was determined by Bradford assay (Sigma-Aldrich, St. Louis, MO).

2.4. Lectin Microarrays. To reduce the differences between subjects and to tolerate individual variation, urinary protein was pooled equivalently according to sample classification, and each class was divided into three biological replications. The urinary proteins (80 μg) were mixed with equal volume of Na_2CO_3 solution (100 mM, pH 9.3) and then labeled with Cy3 fluorescent dye (GE Healthcare, Biosciences, Piscataway, NJ, USA); the mixture was incubated for 3 h at ambient temperature in darkness. After that, the labeled protein was purified with Sephadex G-25 columns (GE healthcare) according to the manufacturer's instructions to remove uncombined fluorescent dye. The lectin microarray was fabricated by using 37 exogenous plant lectins as purchased from Vector Laboratories (Burlingame, CA), from Sigma-Aldrich (St. Louis, MO), and from Calbiochem Merck (Darmstadt, Germany) with different binding preferences covering N- and O-linked glycans. The lectins were dissolved to a concentration of 1 mg/mL in the manufacturer's recommended buffer, which contained 1 mmol/L appropriate monosaccharide. Lectins were spotted on the homemade epoxysilane-coated slides with Stealth micro spotting pins (SMP-10B) (TeleChem, USA) by a Capital smart microarrayer (CapitalBio, Beijing). Please refer to Qin et al. [22] for the sugar-binding specificities of the lectins, and layout of the lectin microarray was showed in Figure 1(a). Each lectin was spotted in triplicate per slide. After that, the slides were incubated in a humidity-controlled incubator at 50% humidity overnight and then put in vacuum dryer for 2 h at 37°C to immobilize. Then, the slides were blocked with the blocking buffer containing 1% (w/v) BSA in 10 mM PBS (pH 7.4) for 1 h at 25°C and then rinsed twice with 1 × PBST (0.2% Tween-20 in 10 mM PBS, pH 7.4), followed by a final rinse in 10 mM PBS. Previously, we had determined that 4 μg labeled protein was used to ensure that all binding signals were produced in the linear binding range of each lectin for the lectin microarrays [22]. Therefore, 4 μg of Cy3-labeled protein mixed with 0.5 mL of incubation buffer containing 2% (w/v) BSA, 500 mM glycine, and 0.1% Tween-20 in 10 mM PBS was applied to incubate with the lectin microarrays, and an incubation was performed in the chamber at 25°C for 3 h in a rotisserie oven set at 4 rpm. After incubation, the slide was washed with 1 × PBST twice for each for 10 min and washed twice with 10 mM PBS for 5 min and then dried by centrifugation at 600 rpm for 5 min at room temperature. The microarrays were scanned with the 70% photomultiplier tube and 100% laser power settings using a GenePix 4000B Microarray Scanner (Axon Instruments, USA).

2.5. Data Acquisition and Analysis. The fluorescence signal intensity of each spot was extracted by GenePix 3.0 software (Axon Instruments, Inc., USA). To avoid the nonspecific adsorption, if the signal intensity of one lectin spot was less than average background + standard deviation (SD), it is regarded as invalid spot and removed. After data filtered, the median of the effective data points of each sample was counted. To eliminate fluorescence bias between different data sets, the fluorescence signals of each lectin microarray were treated by max-normalization [23–25]. Briefly, the signals of each lectin were normalized to the highest signal intensity among 37 lectins. After normalization, the processed data of the parallel data sets were compared with each other based upon fold changes according to the following criteria: fold changes ≥ 1.5 or ≤0.67 and $p < 0.05$ in the pairs indicated up- or downregulation of certain kind of glycopatterns, respectively. Differences between the arbitrary two data sets or multiple data sets were tested using Student's t-test or Kruskal-Wallis test; the histogram and ROC

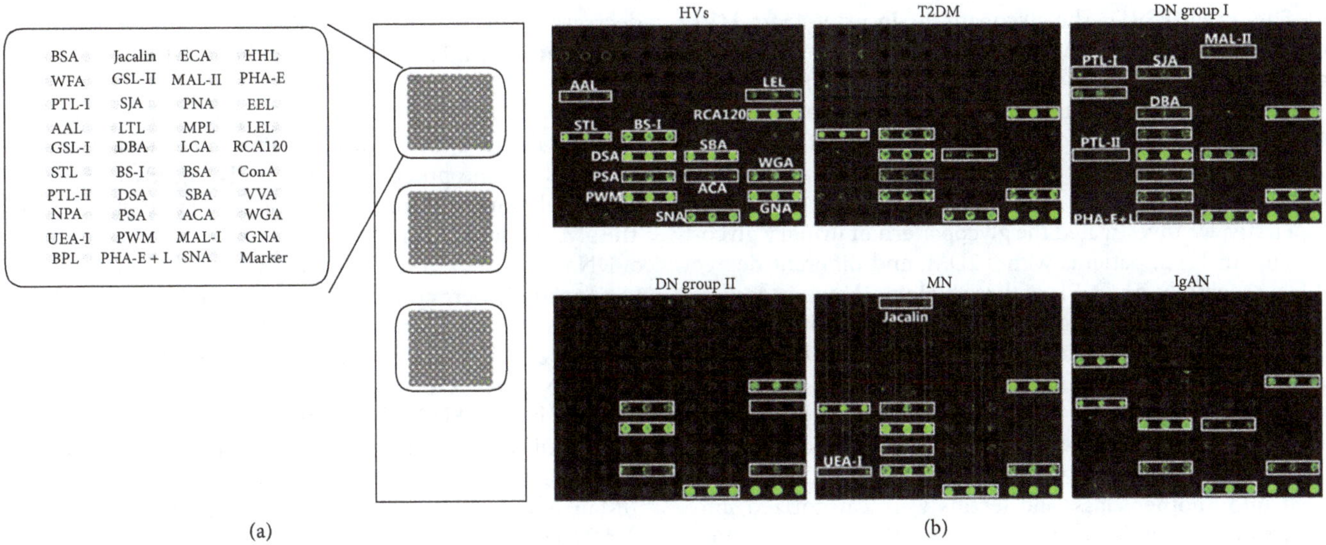

FIGURE 1: Glycopatterns of urine glycoproteins from HVs, patients with T2DM, DN group I, and DN group II by lectin microarrays. (a) The layout of the lectin microarray. Each lectin was spotted in triplicate on one slide. Cy3-labeled BSA was spotted as a location marker and BSA as a negative control. (b) The profile of Cy3-labeled urinary proteins from HVs; patients with T2DM, DN group I, DN group II, MN, and IgAN bound to the lectin microarrays, respectively. The lectins showing the effective data were marked with white frames.

curve analysis were performed by GraphPad Prism 6. The data were further analyzed by Expander 6.4 (version 6.4; http://acgt.cs.tau.ac.il/expander/) in order to perform hierarchical clustering analysis; the unweighted pair group method was constructed with arithmetic-mean tree using Pearson's correlation as the metric of similarity. The Spearman rank-order coefficient (rs) was calculated by Spearman rank correlation analysis.

2.6. Urinary Protein Microarrays. In order to verify the results of the lectin microarrays, a urinary protein microarray was produced by using another 48 individuals urine samples; the detailed sample information was showed in Table S1 (see Supplementary Material available online at https://doi.org/10.1155/2017/5728087). The fabrication and incubation of urinary protein microarrays were similar with lectin microarrays. Briefly, urinary proteins were dissolved in spotting buffer containing 0.5 mg/mL BSA in 10 mM PBS (pH 7.4) to a concentration of 1 mg/mL and spotted on the home-made epoxysilane-coated slides with Stealth micro spotting pins (SMP-10B) by a Capital smart microarrayer. A urinary protein microarray was produced by spotting 48 individual urine samples (7 HVs, 9 T2DM patients, 15 patients with DN (7 DN group I, 8 DN group II), and 17 patients with NDRD (9 MN and 8 IgAN)) on the surface of the epoxy slide. Each urine specimen was spotted in triplicate per slide and incubated in a humidity-controlled incubator at 50% humidity overnight for immobilization. Then, the slides were blocked with the blocking buffer for 1 h; after washing, the blocked slide incubated with 4 μg Cy3 labeled lectin diluted in 0.5 mL of incubation buffer for 3 h at room temperature in the dark. The slide was washed with 1 × PBST twice for each for 10 min and washed once with 10 mM PBS for 5 min and then dried by centrifugation at 600 rpm for 5 min. The slides were scanned with the 70% photomultiplier tube and 100% laser power settings using a GenePix 4000B Microarray Scanner and the signal intensity was extracted by GenePix 3.0 software.

2.7. SDS-PAGE and Lectin Blotting. Urinary glycoproteins were further analyzed using lectin blotting. Firstly, the pooled urinary proteins were analyzed by SDS-PAGE. Briefly, urinary proteins were mixed with 5 × loading buffer and boiled for 5 min at 100°C; after that, the samples were spun down and loaded on a 10% polyacrylamide resolving gel and a 3% stacking gel, and protein molecular weight marker (Thermo Scientific, Waltham, USA) was run in gel simultaneously. After being immobilized, the gel was stained by alkaline silver. For lectin blotting analysis, the proteins in gels were transferred to a PVDF membrane (Millipore, MA, USA) at 100 V for 90 min in wet transfer device (Beijing Liuyi Instrument Factory, China). Subsequently, the membranes were washed twice with TBST buffer (150 mM NaCl, 10 mM Tris-HCl, and 0.05% v/v Tween-20, pH 7.5) and blocked for 1 h with Carbo-Free Blocking Solution (Vector, Burlingame, CA) for 1 h at ambient temperature. The membranes were then incubated with 3 μg/ml Cy5 (GE Healthcare, Biosciences, Piscataway, NJ, USA) labeled lectins in previous blocking solution with gentle shaking overnight at 4°C below protection from light. The membranes were washed twice each for 10 min with TBST and scanned by Storm 840 PhosphorImager (Molecular Dynamics, Sunnyvale, CA) in red fluorescence channel 635 nm excitation/650LP emission.

3. Result

3.1. Alterations of Urinary Glycopatterns with the Development of DN. About 30–40% of patients with type 1 or type 2 diabetes develop evidence of nephropathy, responsible for

40~50% of all ESRD. The glycopatterns in urine from HVs and patients were evaluated by the lectin microarrays. The glycopatterns of Cy3-labeled pooled urinary proteins from HVs and all patients bound to the lectin microarrays were shown in Figure 1(b). The normalized fluorescent intensities (NFIs) for each lectin were summarized as the mean values ± SD in Table S2.

Firstly, we investigated the glycopattern of urinary glycoproteins in HVs, patients with T2DM, and different degree of DN separately. The NFIs of three biological replicates were imported EXPANDER 6.4 for hierarchical clustering analysis (HCA). The NFIs values mapped to the range of 2 to −2 interval were color coded, with red and green indicating an increase and decrease in the abundance of glycopatterns, respectively. The HCA revealed that both DN groups were clustered into one class, whereas the HVs and T2DM clustered into another class, and lectins were categorized into three independent groups according to the NFIs of lectins showing the positive signals in HVs and patients (Figure 2(a)). The results indicated that the abundance of glycan patterns was different between HVs, T2DM, and DN groups. Further, the NFIs of each lectin from HVs and patients were compared based on fold change in pairs, with all p values below 0.05, to evaluate whether the glycopatterns of urinary glycoproteins were altered with the development of DN (Table 2). Compared the alterations of glycopatterns in urine between HVs and T2DM, the results showed that the α-Fuc binder AAL, LacNAc, poly-LacNAc and $(GlcNAc)_n$ binder LEL, Galβ1-3GalNAcα-Ser/Thr (T-antigen) binder ACA, and multivalent Sia and $(GlcNAc)_n$ binder WGA exhibited significantly decreased NFIs in T2DM (all fold change = 0, $p < 0.001$). In addition, the α-Gal/GalNAc binder BS-I, (β-1,4)-linked GlcNAc binder DSA, and α- or β-linked terminal GalNAc binder SBA showed significantly decreased NFIs in T2DM (all fold change ≤ 0.60, $p < 0.05$) (Figure 2(b)).

Evaluating the alterations of urinary glycopatterns with the development of DN, the results showed that there were 6 lectins (e.g., the Siaα2-3Galβ1-4Glc(NAc)/Glc binder MAL-II, GalNAc and GalNAcα-1,3Gal binder PTL-I, and terminal in GalNAc and Gal binder SJA) that exhibited significantly increased NFIs in DN group I compared with HVs and T2DM, and high-Mannose, Manα1-6(Manα1-3)Man binder Con A showed significantly increased NFIs in DN group II compared with HVs and T2DM ($p < 0.01$). However, the α- or β-linked terminal GalNAc binder SBA and Fucα-1,6GlcNAc binder PSA revealed significantly decreased NFIs in DN group II compared with HVs and T2DM (all fold change = 0, $p < 0.001$). The $(GlcNAc)_{2-4}$ binder DSA and Siaα2-6Gal/GalNAc binder SNA exhibited significantly increased NFIs (all fold change ≥ 2.88, $p < 0.05$) in both DN groups compared with HVs and T2DM, and the Manα1-3Man binder GNA, α-Gal/GalNAc binder BS-I, α-Fuc binder AAL, and α- or β-linked terminal GalNAc binder SBA exhibited increased NFIs (all fold change ≥ 1.61, $p < 0.05$) in DN group I compared with T2DM. However, the $(GlcNAc)_{2-4}$ binder STL exhibited significantly decreased NFIs in both DN groups compared with HVs and T2DM (all fold change = 0, $p < 0.001$). And the α-Gal/GalNAc binder BS-I and $(GlcNAc)_n$ and branched $(LacNAc)_n$ binder PWM showed decreased NFIs (fold change = 0.54, $p < 0.05$) in DN group II compared with HVs (showed in Figure 2(b)).

3.2. Alterations of Urinary Glycopatterns Associated with Different Degree of DN. Although the albuminuria and eGFR could reflect the process of DN, it also needs to find new sensitive biomarkers for monitoring the development of DN. The glycopatterns of urinary glycoproteins in different degree of DN were analyzed. The NFIs of each lectin from DN group I and group II were compared based on fold change (Table 2), and the results demonstrated that there were 9 lectins (e.g., the Siaα2-3Galβ1-4Glc(NAc)/Glc binder MAL-II, GalNAc and GalNAcα-1,3Gal binder PTL-I, and terminal in GalNAc and Gal binder SJA) that exhibited significantly decreased NFIs in DN group II compared with group I (all fold change = 0, $p < 0.001$). However, the high-Mannose, Manα1-6(Manα1-3)Man binder Con A showed significantly increased NFIs in DN group II compared with DN group I ($p < 0.001$) (showed in Figure 1(b)). Besides that, the Sia2-6Gal/GalNAc binder SNA showed significantly increased NFIs in DN group II compared with group I (fold change = 2.54, $p < 0.01$). The α-Gal/GalNAc binder BS-I, $(GlcNAc)_n$ and branched $(LacNAc)_n$ binder PWM, and Manα-1,3 man binder GNA exhibited significantly decreased NFIs (all fold change ≤ 0.55, $p < 0.05$) in DN group II compared with DN group I (Figure 2(b)).

3.3. Alteration of Glycopatterns between DN and NDRD. Currently, it is difficult to distinguish DN from NDRD in clinical practice. Renal biopsy is still a reliable clinical detection for diagnosis of DN. Here, the differences of urinary protein glycopatterns were investigated between DN (DN group I and DN group II) and NDRD (MN and IgAN). As a result of HCA, DN groups and NDRD were separated and lectins were categorized into four independent groups according to the NFIs of lectins, which revealed that the glycopatterns in urine showed difference between DN and NDRD (Figure 3(a)). The fold change between DN and NDRD groups was summarized in Table 3.

The results showed that there were 5 lectins (the Siaα2-3Galβ1-4Glc(NAc)/Glc binder MAL-II, GalNAc and GalNAcα-1,3Gal binder PTL-I, terminal in GalNAc and Gal binder SJA, GalNAcα1-3((Fucα1-2))Gal binder DBA, and Gal and T-antigen binder PTL-II) to show high NFIs in DN group I and high-Mannose, Manα1-6(Manα1-3)Man binder ConA to show high NFIs in DN group II compared with NDRD ($p < 0.001$). However, the $(GlcNAc)_{2-4}$ binder STL showed high NFIs in NDRD compared with DN groups, and α-Fuc binder AAL, α- or β-linked terminal GalNAc binder SBA and Fucα-1,6GlcNAc binder PSA showed high NFIs in NDRD compared with DN groups II ($p < 0.001$). In addition, the Galβ1-3GalNAcα-Ser/Thr(T) binder Jacalin and Fucα1-2Galβ1-4Glc(NAc) binder UEA-I exhibited high NFIs in MN compared with both DN groups ($p < 0.001$). Besides that, the β-D-GlcNAc binder DSA showed significantly higher NFIs in both DN groups than that in patients with IgAN (fold change = 3.28, $p < 0.001$), the Siaα2-6Gal/GalNAc binder SNA showed significantly increased NFIs in DN group II compared with NDRD (fold change ≥ 2.56, $p < 0.001$), and

TABLE 2: Fold change of the urinary glycopatterns based upon ratio of the NFIs of each lectin between HVs, T2DM, and DN groups.

Lectin name	Specificity	Fold change[a]					
		T2DM/HVs	DN group I/HVs	DN group I/T2DM	DN group II/HVs	DN group II/T2DM	DN group II/DN group I
MAL-II	Siaα2-3Galβ1-4Glc(NAc)/Glc	—	/***	/***	—	—	0***
PTL-I	GalNAc, GalNAcα-1,3Gal, GalNAcα-1,3Galβ-1,3/4Glc	—	/***	/***	—	—	0***
SJA	Terminal in GalNAc and Gal, anti-A and anti-B human blood group	—	/***	/***	—	—	0***
AAL	α-Fuc, Fucα1-6 GlcNAc (core fucose)	0***	3.30**	/***	0***	—	0***
LEL	LacNAc and poly LacNAc, $(GlcNAc)_n$	0***	0***	—	0***	—	—
DBA	αGalNAc, Tn antigen, GalNAcα1-3((Fucα1-2))Gal (blood group A antigen)	—	/***	/***	—	—	0***
RCA120	β-Gal, Galβ-1,4GlcNAc (type II), Galβ1-3GlcNAc (type I)	0.799	1.05	1.31	1.17	1.46	1.12
STL	$(GlcNAc)_{2-4}$, core (GlcNAc) of N-glycan	1	0***	0***	0***	0***	—
BS-I	α-Gal/GalNAc, Galα-1,3Gal	0.60*	0.97	1.61*	0.54*	0.89	0.55*
ConA	High-Mannose, Manα1-6(Manα1-3)Man, terminal GlcNAc	—	—	—	/***	/***	/***
PTL-II	Gal, blood group H, T-antigen	—	/***	/***	—	—	0***
DSA	(β-1,4)-linked GlcNAc	0.21**	2.88***	13.61***	2.88***	13.61***	1
SBA	α- or β-linked terminal GalNAc, $(GalNAc)_n$, GalNAcα1-3Gal, blood-group A	0.32*	1.16	3.63*	0***	0***	0***
PSA	Fucα-1,6GlcNAc, α-D-Man, α-D-Glc	1.31	1.52	1.16	0***	0***	0***
ACA	Galβ1-3GalNAcα-Ser/Thr (T antigen), sialyl-T(ST)	0***	0***	—	0***	—	—
WGA	Multivalent Sia and $(GlcNAc)_n$	0***	0***	—	0***	—	—
PWM	$(GlcNAc)_n$, branched $(LacNAc)_n$	0.59	1.04	1.76	0.54*	0.92	0.521*
GNA	Manα1-3Man	1.46	2.39**	1.64*	1.17	0.80	0.488*
PHA-E + L	Bisecting GlcNAc, biantennary N-glycans, tri- and tetraantennary complex-type N-glycan	—	/**	/**	—	—	0**
SNA	Sia2-6Gal/GalNAc	1.37	4.34**	3.16*	11.03***	8.05***	2.54**

[a]Fold changes of lectins bound to DN compared to healthy control and diabetic calculated with mean value of normalized florescence intensities of lectins obtained from 3 biological reduplicates. —, no significant difference; /, the denominator of the fold-change was infinite; 0, the numerator of the fold-change was zero. * versus $p < 0.05$; ** versus $p < 0.01$; *** versus $p < 0.001$; p value was calculated by Student's t-test.

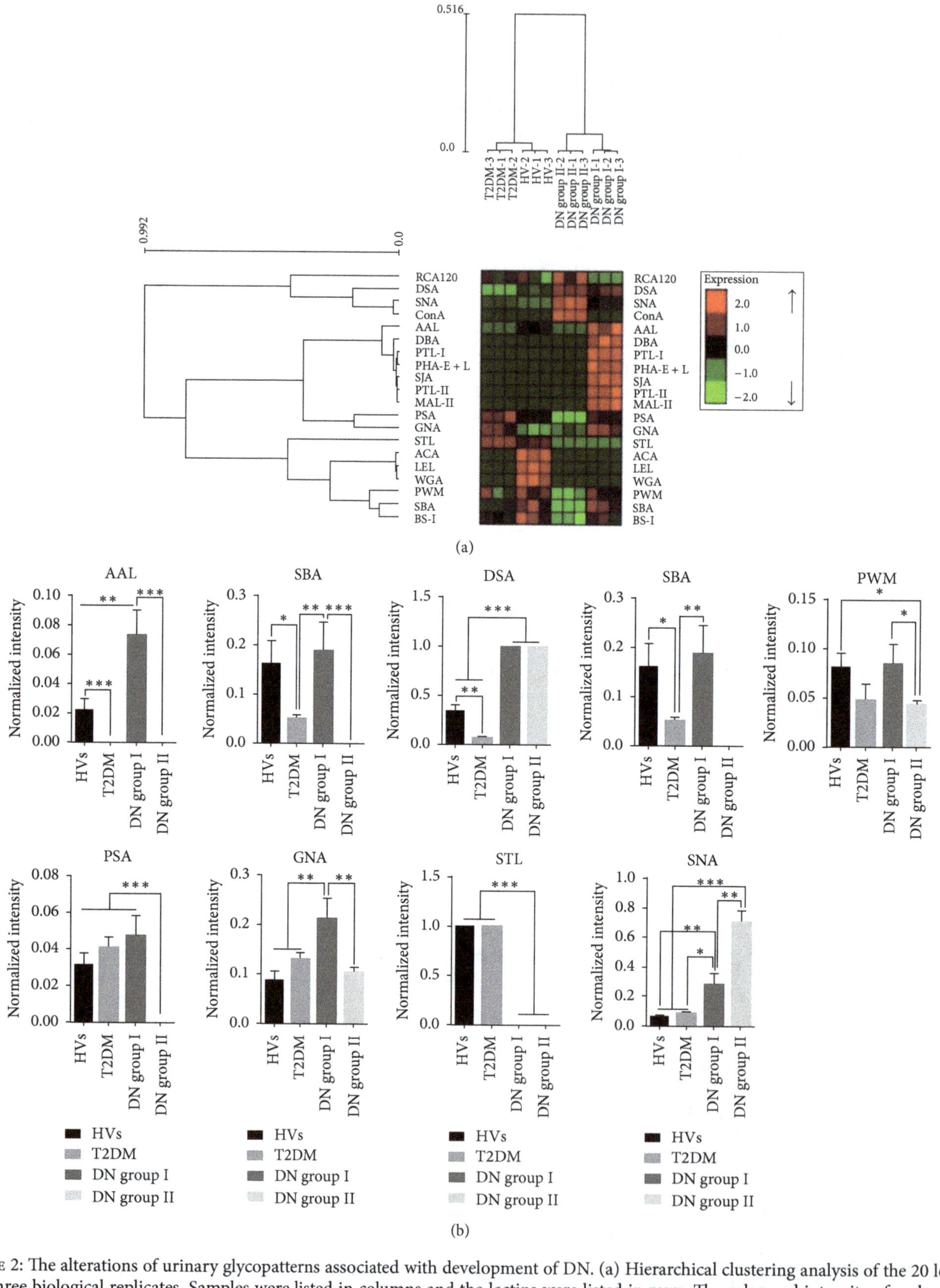

FIGURE 2: The alterations of urinary glycopatterns associated with development of DN. (a) Hierarchical clustering analysis of the 20 lectins with three biological replicates. Samples were listed in columns and the lectins were listed in rows. The color and intensity of each square indicated expression levels relative to other data in the row. Red: high, green: low, and black: medium. (b) Comparing the NFIs of the urinary glycopatterns based upon ratio of each lectin between HVs, T2DM, and DN groups. Significant differences between groups were analyzed according to Student's t-test, respectively ($^{*}p < 0.05$, $^{**}p < 0.01$, and $^{***}p \leq 0.001$). The data were the averaged NFIs ± SD of three biological replicates.

TABLE 3: Fold change of the urinary glycopatterns based upon ratio of the NFIs of each lectin between DN groups and NDRD.

Lectin name	Specificity	Fold change[a]			
		DN group I/MN	DN group I/IgAN	DN group II/MN	DN group II/IgAN
Jacalin	Galβ1-3GalNAcα-Ser/Thr(T), GalNAcα-Ser/Thr(Tn)	0^{***}	—	0^{***}	—
MAL-II	Siaα2-3Galβ1-4Glc(NAc)/Glc,	$/^{***}$	$/^{***}$	—	—
PTL-I	GalNAc, GalNAcα-1,3Gal, GalNAcα-1,3Galβ-1,3/4Glc	$/^{***}$	$/^{***}$	—	—
SJA	Terminal in GalNAc and Gal, anti-A and anti-B human blood group	$/^{***}$	$/^{***}$	—	—
AAL	α-Fuc, Fucα1-6 GlcNAc (core fucose)	$/^{**}$	0.65	—	0^{*}
DBA	αGalNAc, Tn antigen, GalNAcα1-3((Fucα1-2))Gal (blood group A antigen)	$/^{***}$	$/^{***}$	—	—
RCA120	β-Gal, Galβ-1,4GlcNAc (type II), Galβ1-3GlcNAc (type I)	0.22^{***}	1.74^{*}	0.24^{***}	1.95^{**}
STL	$(GlcNAc)_{2-4}$, core (GlcNAc) of N-glycan	0^{***}	0^{***}	0^{***}	0^{***}
BS-I	α-Gal/GalNAc, Galα-1,3Gal	0.41^{**}	$/^{**}$	0.22^{***}	$/^{***}$
ConA	High-Mannose, Manα1-6(Manα1-3)Man, terminal GlcNAc	—	—	$/^{***}$	$/^{***}$
PTL-II	Gal, blood group H, T-antigen	$/^{***}$	$/^{***}$	—	—
DSA	(β-1,4)-linked GlcNAc	—	3.28^{***}	—	3.28^{***}
SBA	α- or β-linked terminal GalNAc, $(GalNAc)_n$, GalNAcα1-3Gal, blood-group A	$/^{**}$	4.64^{*}	—	0^{***}
PSA	Fucα-1,6GlcNAc, α-D-Man, α-D-Glc	0.46^{*}	$/^{**}$	$/^{**}$	—
UEA-I	Fucα1-2Galβ1-4Glc(NAc)	0^{***}	—	0^{***}	—
PWM	$(GlcNAc)_n$, branched $(LacNAc)_n$	0.50^{**}	1.20	0.26^{***}	0.62^{**}
GNA	Manα1-3Man	1.49	3.80^{**}	0.73	1.85^{**}
PHA-E + L	Bisecting GlcNAc, biantennary N-glycans, tri- and tetra-antennary complex-type N-glycan	$/^{**}$	—	—	—
SNA	Sia2-6Gal/GalNAc	1.00	1.80	2.56^{***}	4.57^{***}

[a]Fold changes of lectins bound to DN groups compared to NDRD calculated with mean value of normalized florescence intensities of lectins obtained from 3 biological reduplicates. —, no significant difference; /, the fold-change was infinite; 0, the numerator of the fold-change was zero. $*$ versus $p < 0.05$; $**$ versus $p < 0.01$; $***$ versus $p < 0.001$, p value was calculate by Student's t-test.

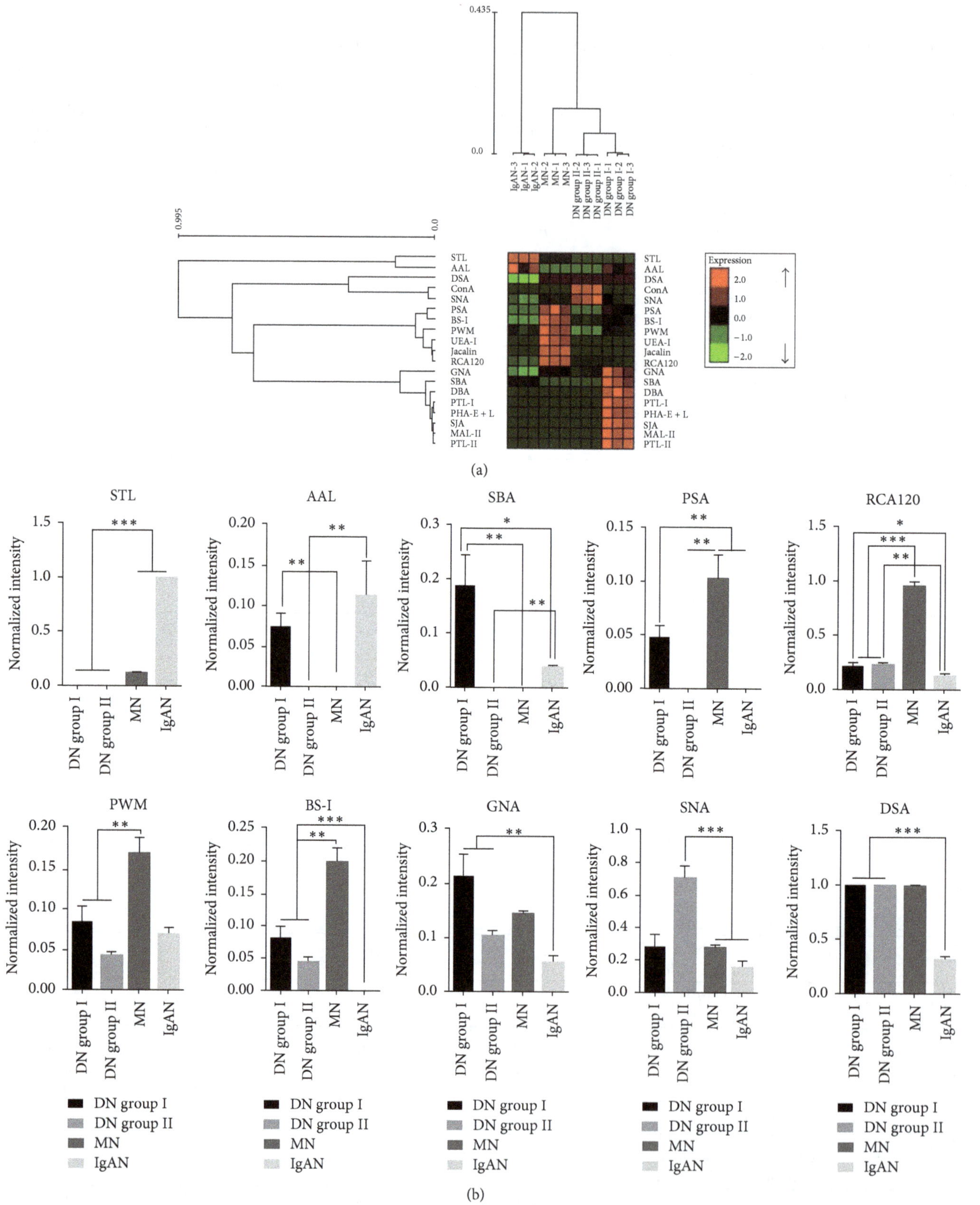

Figure 3: The alterations of glycopatterns between DN and NDRD. (a) Hierarchical clustering analysis of the 19 lectins with three biological replicates. DN groups and NDRD were listed in columns, and the lectins were listed in rows. (b) Ten lectins revealed significant differences between DN and NDRD. Significant differences between groups were analyzed according to Student's t-test, respectively ($^{*}p < 0.05$, $^{**}p < 0.01$, and $^{***}p \leq 0.001$). The data were the averaged NFI ± SD of three biological replicates.

the Manα1-3Man binder GNA associated with increased NFIs in both DN groups compared with IgAN (fold change ≥ 1.85, $p < 0.01$). And the β-Gal/GalNAc binder RCA120 and α-Gal/GalNAc binder BS-I exhibited increased NFIs in both DN groups compared with patients with IgAN (fold change ≥ 1.74, $p < 0.05$) but showed decreased NFIs compared with MN (fold change ≤ 0.41, $p < 0.05$) However, the $(GlcNAc)_n$ and branched $(LacNAc)_n$ binder PWM exhibited significantly decreased NFIs (all fold change ≤ 0.50, $p < 0.01$) in both DN groups compared with MN (Figure 3(b)).

3.4. Assessment of Urinary Glycopatterns as Potential Biomarkers for Diagnosis of DN. The most reliable way of biomarker discovery is to test the candidates with a large cohort of samples that have clear and sufficient clinical records. Here, a urinary protein microarray is produced by spotting 48 individual urine samples (7 HVs, 9 T2DM patients, 15 patients with DN (7 DN group I, 8 DN group II), and 17 patients with NDRD (9 MN and 8 IgAN)) on the surface of the epoxy slide. Each urine sample was spotted in triplicate, and the layout of the urinary protein microarrays was shown in Figure 4(a). SNA and STL that revealed significant differences ($p < 0.05$) in urinary glycopatterns according to the results of the lectin microarrays were selected to validate the alteration of the targeted glycopatterns in individual sample and evaluate the reliability of urinary glycopatterns as potential biomarkers for diagnosis of DN.

As a result, SNA staining showed increased signals in both DN groups compared with HVs and patients with T2DM and significant difference between DN group I and group II ($p < 0.05$). Interestingly, the signals of SNA staining showed an increasing trend with development of DN (Figure 4(b)). The result of correlation analysis indicated that the abundance of Siaα2-6Gal/GalNAc was positive correlation with the progression of DN (rs = 0.888). On the contrary, the signals of STL staining were significantly lower in both DN groups than that in NDRD ($p < 0.001$). ROC analysis showed that the ROC integral was 0.969 and $p < 0.0001$, which indicated the glycopattern of $(GlcNAc)_{2-4}$ recognized by STL in urine glycoprotein could be a potential diagnostic indicator to differentiate DN and NDRD (Figure 4(c)). These results were consistent with lectin microarrays.

3.5. Lectin Blotting Analysis. In order to investigate precisely alterations of glycopatterns associated with DN, SDS-PAGE and lectin blotting analysis were performed with SNA and STL staining (Figure 4(d)). SNA staining showed obvious binding patterns with six distinct protein bands of approximately 120, 90, 70, 50, 40, and 25 kDa marked as b1–b6, respectively. The band of b4 showed strong staining signals in all samples except HVs. There were four bands (b2, b3, b5, and b6) to show increased signals in both DN groups compared with T2DM. Moreover, the glycoprotein bands (b2, b3, and b5) at about 90 kDa, 70 kDa, and 40 kDa exhibited increased staining signals in DN group II compared with group I (Figure 4(e)). Therefore, the abundance of Siaα2-6Gal exhibited general increase in urine with development of DN. Comparing DN and NDRD, the band of b4 (50 kDa) showed strong staining signals in both DN and NDRD groups but did not exhibit significant difference, whereas the bands of b3 (70 kDa) and b5 (40 kDa) revealed stronger staining intensities in DN groups than those in MN and IgAN.

STL staining showed obvious binding patterns with one distinct urinary protein band (b4) in both DN and NDRD at about 50 kDa. The binding signals of this glycoprotein band were significant higher in MN and IgAN than that in DN groups but have no difference between DN groups.

4. Discussion

Glycosylation is an important co- and posttranslational modification of glycoprotein, involved in many biological processes such as embryogenesis and neoplasm metastasis. The altered oligosaccharide moiety of glycoprotein was considered to be associated with the occurrence and development of diseases [26–29]. Abnormal glycosylation of certain glycoprotein in urine could be a more sensitive biomarker for disease diagnosis and monitoring. It is reported that aberrantly excreted urinary *O*-glycosylated proteins (clusterin, leucine-rich alpha-2-glycoprotein, and kininogen) could serve as potential biomarkers for the early detection of early stage ovarian cancer [30]. As a powerful tool, lectin microarray was used to investigate the glycopatterns of protein for decades. With the development of mass spectrometry, the glycan profile could be analysis by MS. However, as a rapid analysis approach, lectin microarray owned some unique advantages. First of all, the proteins do not need to enzymolysis prior to analysis, and the target is simple to prepare. Secondly, the linkage information of glycopatterns could be obtained by lectin microarray; however, mass spectrometry has difficulty in discriminating between the many structural isomers presented by glycans [31]. There is no denying that MS has advantage to acquire precisely information about the component of glycan. Notwithstanding intense efforts by multiple research groups, the use of mass spectrometry as a standalone technique for complete characterization of glycans is still far from complete [32].

In this study, glycopatterns of urine glycoprotein in patients with DN were compared with controls (healthy volunteers and patients with T2DM) and patients with NDRD (MN and IgAN), respectively. As a result, STL showed strong binding signals in HVs and patients with T2DM and IgAN; in addition, DSA exhibited strong binding signals in patients with DN and MN. It indicated that GlcNAc and polymers of GlcNAc were predominant glycopatterns in urine of patients. In urinary glycoprotein, $Hex_5HexNAc_4$-N-Asn was typically N-glycan observed which is similar to our findings [33]. As a result of lectin microarrays, there were 9 and 15 lectins to show binding signals in patients with T2DM and DN group I, which indicated more glycopatterns emerged in urine of patients in middle and advanced stage of DN without renal insufficiency (DN group I) compared with patients with T2DM. However, when compared to patients with overt proteinuria and renal insufficiency (DN group II), the situation was changed, only 7 lectins (e.g., WFA, GSL-II, and PNA) exhibited effective binding signals in DN group II, and 9 lectins (e.g., WFA, GSL-II, and PNA) failed to detect binding

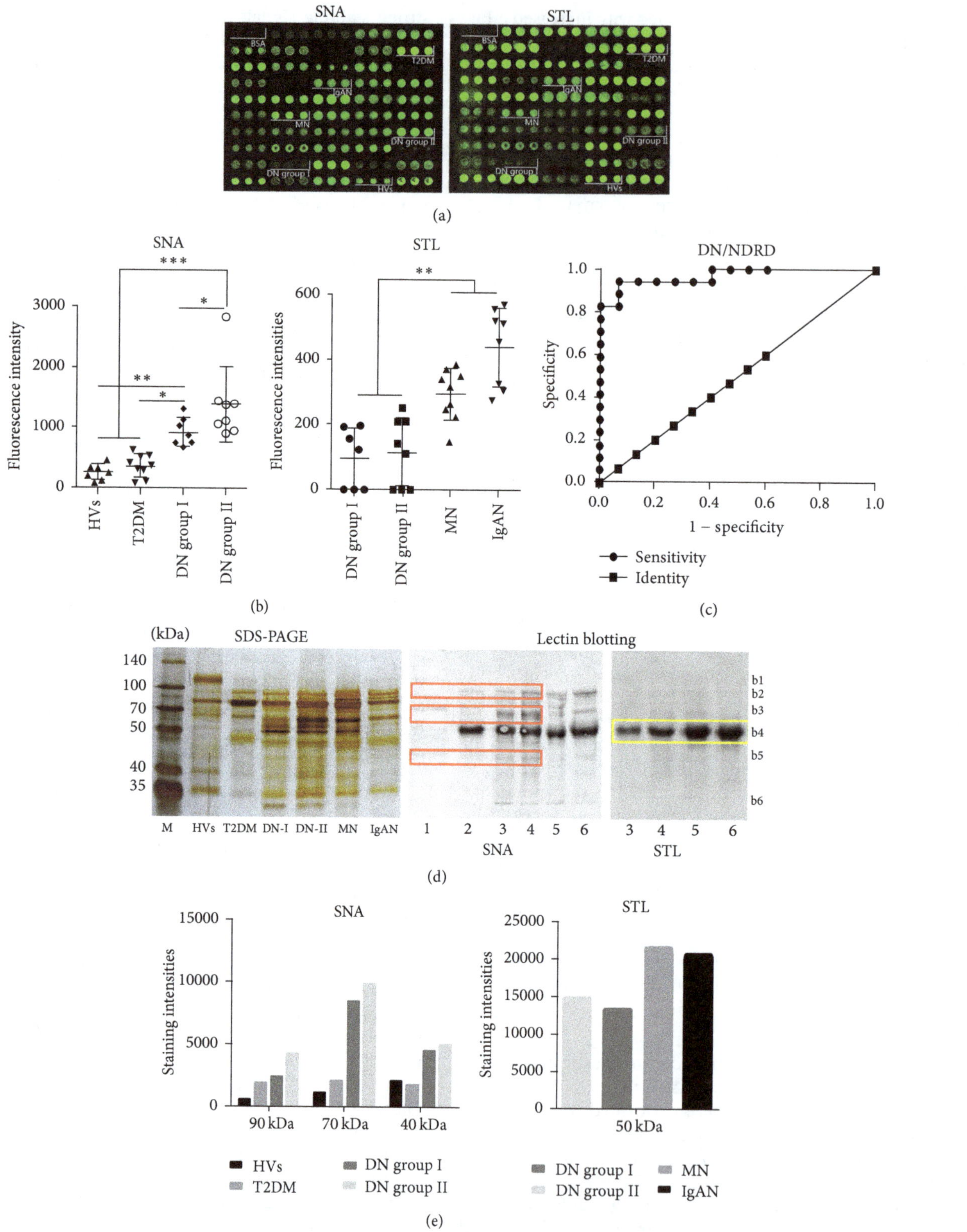

Figure 4: Validation of the differential expressions of the glycopatterns in the urine associated with DN. (a) Scan images of Cy3-labeled SNA and STL incubating to urinary protein microarray, respectively. The incubation images were extracted by GenePix 3.0. (b) Scatter plot analysis of the original data obtained from the urinary protein microarrays. The statistical significance of the differences between groups was calculated by Kruskal-Wallis test. (c) ROC curve analysis of STL to differentiate DN and NDRD, AUC = 0.968, and $p < 0.0001$. (d) SDS-PAGE and lectin blot of pooled urinary protein using SNA and STL, M, marker; lane 1, HVs; lane 2, patients with T2DM; lane 3, DN group I; lane 4, DN group II; lane 5, patients with MN; lane 6, patients with IgAN. (e) The lectin binding strength of selected protein bands is displayed, and the binding strength was counted by image J.

signals compared with DN group I. Furthermore, there were 3 lectins (BS-I, PWM, and GNA) to exhibit decreased NFIs in DN group II compared with DN group I. These findings demonstrated that the glycopatterns, especially the glycopatterns modified by Gal/GalNAc, were decreased as occurred in renal insufficiency. Inoue et al. reported the global reduction of the binding to lectins in urine samples of DN at macroalbuminuria stage [30]. Our finding further clarified that glycopatterns showed global reduction when occurring in renal insufficiency in stage of overt proteinuria. In rat diabetic nephropathy model which was induced by streptozotocin injection, the staining intensities of Gal/GalNAc binders PNA and RCA showed remarkable decrease in model after being induced for 5 weeks [34]. It is known that around 70% of the urinary proteins are estimated to be derived from the kidney and the urinary tract [35]. Therefore, we suspected that the general reduction in signature glycopatterns of Gal/GalNAc in kidney may contribute to the decrease of these glycopatterns in urinary glycoprotein with development of DN; the relationship between glycopatterns in kidney and urine will be clarified in next step.

In present study, we found that the glycopatterns of Siaα2-6Gal/GalNAc showed increased tendency with development of DN, and urinary protein microarray also confirmed this result. Our finding suggested Siaα2-6Gal/GalNAc is potential indicator for monitoring of DN. Furthermore, lectin blotting analysis was employed to investigate the precise alterations of Siaα2-6Gal/GalNAc. Generally, it showed higher staining signals in DN groups than that in HVs and T2DM. The glycoprotein bands at about 90 kDa, 70 kDa, and 40 kDa showed increased staining signals with development of DN. These results indicated the sialylation of these glycoproteins was increased and it may contribute to the upregulation of expression level of Siaα2-6Gal/GalNAc in urinary glycoprotein with development of DN. It is known that the level of serum sialic acid could indicate extensive vascular damage in T2DM and predict microvascular complications occurring in diabetics [36, 37]. As a result of our finding, the expression level of Siaα2-6Gal/GalNAc in urinary glycoprotein correlated with development of DN in stage of overt proteinuria. Similarly, it is reported that a 41 kDa of sialylated glycoprotein orosomucoid which contained Siaα2-6Gal/GalNAc increased excretion in DN, and it could be a potential biomarker for DN [38–40]. In addition, it is reported that the excretion of transferrin (76.5 kDa) and alpha-1-antitrypsin (46 kDa) showed marked increase in urine of patients with DN, which could reflect the development of microalbuminuria; moreover, urinary transferrin is a sensitive indicator of glomerular damage [41, 42]. Therefore, the glycopatterns of Siaα2-6Gal/GalNAc and glycoprotein modified by Siaα2-6Gal/GalNAc (especially the glycoproteins with molecular weight about 90 kDa, 70 kDa; and 40 kDa) in urine could be valuable potential diagnosis indicators for monitoring of DN, and these glycoproteins will be characterized by MS in future.

Although certain clinical manifestations such as shorter duration of diabetes, absence of retinopathy, presence of microscopic hematuria, and active urinary sediment are markers associated with NDRD in type 2 diabetes with clinical renal disease, and the histories of diabetes mellitus, systolic blood pressure, glycated HbA1c, hematuria, diabetic retinopathy, and hemoglobin are independently related to DN, renal biopsy remains indispensable to differentiate between DN and NDRD [43–48]. In this study, we examined the difference between DN and NDRD in urinary glycopatterns; our result showed that the relative abundance of $(GlcNAc)_{2-4}$ in urinary glycoprotein could effectively distinguish between DN and NDRD, and ROC curve analysis also indicated that the glycopatterns recognized by STL have the potential to serve as a clinical predictor to distinguish between DN and NDRD. It demonstrated that the patients with IgAN exhibit circulating IgA1 with reduced Gal (galactose-deficient IgA1) [49–51]. It reported that deficiency of the β1,4GalT1 glycosyltransferase in genetic remodeling mouse could cause IgAN. Because of deficiency of the β1,4GalT1, β4-galactosylation of the *N*-glycans on the serum IgA was completely absent, which led to the exposure of GlcNAc of *N*-linked glycans [52]. In addition, urinary excretion of galactose-deficient IgA1 was elevated in patients with IgAN and the urinary Gd-IgA1 levels correlated with proteinuria [53]. Hiki et al. reported that *O*-glycans attached to serum IgA are truncated to expose GlcNAc, which correlates with antibody glomerular deposition in IgAN [54]. Therefore, we concluded that the exposure of GlcNAc on *N*-/*O*-glycans of IgA correlated with the increasement of $(GlcNAc)_{2-4}$ in urinary glycoprotein from patients with IgAN.

In conclusion, we investigated the correlation of alterations of protein glycopatterns in urine samples from HVs, patients with T2DM, and patients with DN and NDRD. Our finding revealed that the elevated expression level of Siaα2-6Gal/GalNAc in urine was correlated with development of DN in stage of macroalbuminuria, and $(GlcNAc)_{2-4}$ in urine could be a clinical predictor to distinguish between DN and NDRD. It should be pointed out that the sample size in this study is small, and more samples are being recruited to verify our findings and glycoprotein which associated with abnormal glycopatterns will be isolated and identified in next step. This study provided a new method to monitor the development of DN and distinguish between DN and NDRD based on the urinary glycopatterns analysis.

Competing Interests

All the authors declared no competing interests.

Authors' Contributions

Hanyu Zhu and Moyan Liu contributed equally to this work.

Acknowledgments

This study was supported by (1) National Key Research and Development Program (2016YFC1305502); (2) the National Natural Science Foundation of China (no. 61471399; no. 61671479); (3) Innovation Nursery Fund of PLA General Hospital (no. 15KMZ04); (4) National Clinical Research Center for Kidney Disease (no. 2013BAI09B05); (5) the State Key Development Program for Basic Research of China (no. 2013CB530800); (6) Technology Project of Beijing (no. D13110700470000).

References

[1] F. Locatelli, B. Canaud, K.-U. Eckardt, P. Stenvinkel, C. Wanner, and C. Zoccali, "The importance of diabetic nephropathy in current nephrological practice," *Nephrology Dialysis Transplantation*, vol. 18, no. 9, pp. 1716–1725, 2003.

[2] T. Pisitkun, R.-F. Shen, and M. A. Knepper, "Identification and proteomic profiling of exosomes in human urine," *Proceedings of the National Academy of Sciences of the United States of America*, vol. 101, no. 36, pp. 13368–13373, 2004.

[3] W. Sun, F. Li, S. Wu et al., "Human urine proteome analysis by three separation approaches," *Proteomics*, vol. 5, no. 18, pp. 4994–5001, 2005.

[4] C. Shao, M. Li, X. Li et al., "A tool for biomarker discovery in the urinary proteome: a manually curated human and animal urine protein biomarker database," *Molecular & Cellular Proteomics*, vol. 10, no. 11, pp. 1–8, 2011.

[5] M. Kanauchi, Y. Akai, and T. Hashimoto, "Transferrinuria in type 2 diabetic patients with early nephropathy and tubulointerstitial injury," *European Journal of Internal Medicine*, vol. 13, no. 3, pp. 190–193, 2002.

[6] G. Currie and C. Delles, "Urinary proteomics for diagnosis and monitoring of diabetic nephropathy," *Current Diabetes Reports*, vol. 16, no. 11, article no. 104, 2016.

[7] S. S. Kim, S. H. Song, I. J. Kim et al., "Urinary cystatin C and tubular proteinuria predict progression of diabetic nephropathy," *Diabetes Care*, vol. 36, no. 3, pp. 656–661, 2013.

[8] S.-I. Araki, M. Haneda, D. Koya et al., "Predictive effects of urinary liver-type fatty acid-binding protein for deteriorating renal function and incidence of cardiovascular disease in type 2 diabetic patients without advanced nephropathy," *Diabetes Care*, vol. 36, no. 5, pp. 1248–1253, 2013.

[9] N. M. Panduru, C. Forsblom, M. Saraheimo et al., "Urinary liver-type fatty acid-binding protein and progression of diabetic nephropathy in type 1 diabetes," *Diabetes Care*, vol. 36, no. 7, pp. 2077–2083, 2013.

[10] J. W. Dennis, M. Granovsky, and C. E. Warren, "Glycoprotein glycosylation and cancer progression," *Biochimica et Biophysica Acta (BBA)—General Subjects*, vol. 1473, no. 1, pp. 21–34, 1999.

[11] K. Ohtsubo and J. D. Marth, "Glycosylation in cellular mechanisms of health and disease," *Cell*, vol. 126, no. 5, pp. 855–867, 2006.

[12] S. Hu and D. T. Wong, "Lectin microarray," *PROTEOMICS—Clinical Applications*, vol. 3, no. 2, pp. 148–154, 2009.

[13] J. Katrlík, P. Gemeiner, and A. Šedivá, "Lectin microarray and surface plasmon resonance biochips for detection of glycosylation and glyco-biomarkers," *Current Opinion in Biotechnology*, vol. 24, p. S25, 2013.

[14] P. Syed, K. Gidwani, H. Kekki, J. Leivo, K. Pettersson, and U. Lamminmäki, "Role of lectin microarrays in cancer diagnosis," *Proteomics*, vol. 16, no. 8, pp. 1257–1265, 2016.

[15] A. Matsuda, A. Kuno, T. Nakagawa et al., "Lectin microarray-based sero-biomarker verification targeting aberrant O-linked glycosylation on Mucin 1," *Analytical Chemistry*, vol. 87, no. 14, pp. 7274–7281, 2015.

[16] Y. Liang, T. Ma, A. Thakur et al., "Differentially expressed glycosylated patterns of α-1-antitrypsin as serum biomarkers for the diagnosis of lung cancer," *Glycobiology*, vol. 25, no. 3, pp. 331–340, 2015.

[17] E. Selvin, A. M. Rawlings, M. Grams et al., "Fructosamine and glycated albumin for risk stratification and prediction of incident diabetes and microvascular complications: a prospective cohort analysis of the Atherosclerosis Risk in Communities (ARIC) study," *The Lancet Diabetes and Endocrinology*, vol. 2, no. 4, pp. 279–288, 2014.

[18] N. Wang, Z. Xu, P. Han, and T. Li, "Glycated albumin and ratio of glycated albumin to glycated hemoglobin are good indicators of diabetic nephropathy in type 2 diabetes mellitus," *Diabetes/Metabolism Research and Reviews*, 2016.

[19] T. Fujimoto, M. Miya, M. Machida et al., "Improved recovery of human urinary protein for electrophoresis," *Journal of Health Science*, vol. 52, no. 6, pp. 718–723, 2006.

[20] P. Tantipaiboonwong, S. Sinchaikul, S. Sriyam, S. Phutrakul, and S.-T. Chen, "Different techniques for urinary protein analysis of normal and lung cancer patients," *Proteomics*, vol. 5, no. 4, pp. 1140–1149, 2005.

[21] R. Magistroni, G. Ligabue, V. Lupo et al., "Proteomic analysis of urine from proteinuric patients shows a proteolitic activity directed against albumin," *Nephrology Dialysis Transplantation*, vol. 24, no. 5, pp. 1672–1681, 2009.

[22] Y. Qin, Y. Zhong, M. J. Zhu et al., "Age- and sex-associated differences in the glycopatterns of human salivary glycoproteins and their roles against influenza A virus," *Journal of Proteome Research*, vol. 12, no. 6, pp. 2742–2754, 2013.

[23] K. T. Pilobello, L. Krishnamoorthy, D. Slawek, and L. K. Mahal, "Development of a lectin microarray for the rapid analysis of protein glycopatterns," *ChemBioChem*, vol. 6, no. 6, pp. 985–989, 2005.

[24] A. Kuno, Y. Ikehara, Y. Tanaka et al., "Multilectin assay for detecting fibrosis-specific glyco-alteration by means of lectin microarray," *Clinical Chemistry*, vol. 57, no. 1, pp. 48–56, 2011.

[25] H. Tateno, M. Toyota, S. Saito et al., "Glycome diagnosis of human induced pluripotent stem cells using lectin microarray," *Journal of Biological Chemistry*, vol. 286, no. 23, pp. 20345–20353, 2011.

[26] T. M. Block, M. A. Comunale, M. Lowman et al., "Use of targeted glycoproteomics to identify serum glycoproteins that correlate with liver cancer in woodchucks and humans," *Proceedings of the National Academy of Sciences of the United States of America*, vol. 102, no. 3, pp. 779–784, 2005.

[27] P. A. Norton, M. A. Comunale, J. Krakover et al., "N-linked glycosylation of the liver cancer biomarker GP73," *Journal of Cellular Biochemistry*, vol. 104, no. 1, pp. 136–149, 2008.

[28] D. Isailovic, R. T. Kurulugama, M. D. Plasencia et al., "Profiling of human serum glycans associated with liver cancer and cirrhosis by IMS-MS," *Journal of Proteome Research*, vol. 7, no. 3, pp. 1109–1117, 2008.

[29] J. W. Dennis, M. Granovsky, and C. E. Warren, "Glycoprotein glycosylation and cancer progression," *Biochimica et Biophysica Acta—General Subjects*, vol. 1473, no. 1, pp. 21–34, 1999.

[30] A. K.-W. Mu, B.-K. Lim, O. H. Hashim, and A. S. Shuib, "Identification of O-glycosylated proteins that are aberrantly excreted in the urine of patients with early stage ovarian cancer," *International Journal of Molecular Sciences*, vol. 14, no. 4, pp. 7923–7931, 2013.

[31] K. T. Pilobello, D. E. Slawek, and L. K. Mahal, "A ratiometric lectin microarray approach to analysis of the dynamic mammalian glycome," *Proceedings of the National Academy of Sciences of the United States of America*, vol. 104, no. 28, pp. 11534–11539, 2007.

[32] G. Gupta, A. Surolia, and S.-G. Sampathkumar, "Lectin microarrays for glycomic analysis," *OMICS A Journal of Integrative Biology*, vol. 14, no. 4, pp. 419–436, 2010.

[33] A. Halim, J. Nilsson, U. Rüetschi, C. Hesse, and G. Larson, "Human urinary glycoproteomics; attachment site specific analysis of N- and O-linked glycosylations by CID and ECD," *Molecular & Cellular Proteomics*, vol. 11, no. 4, Article ID M111.013649, 2012.

[34] A. Ravidà, L. Musante, M. Kreivi et al., "Glycosylation patterns of kidney proteins differ in rat diabetic nephropathy," *Kidney International*, vol. 87, no. 5, pp. 963–974, 2015.

[35] V. Thongboonkerd and P. Malasit, "Renal and urinary proteomics: current applications and challenges," *Proteomics*, vol. 5, no. 4, pp. 1033–1042, 2005.

[36] K. Prajna, J. Ashok Kumar, S. Rai et al., "Predictive value of serum sialic acid in type-2 diabetes mellitus and its complication (Nephropathy)," *Journal of Clinical and Diagnostic Research*, vol. 7, no. 11, pp. 2435–2437, 2013.

[37] M. A. Crook, J. C. Pickup, P. J. Lumb, F. Georgino, D. J. Webb, and J. H. Fuller, "Relationship between plasma sialic acid concentration and microvascular and macrovascular complications in type 1 diabetes: the EURODIAB complications study," *Diabetes Care*, vol. 24, no. 2, pp. 316–322, 2001.

[38] K. Inoue, J. Wada, J. Eguchi et al., "Urinary fetuin-A is a novel marker for diabetic nephropathy in type 2 diabetes identified by lectin microarray," *PLoS ONE*, vol. 8, no. 10, Article ID e77118, 2013.

[39] M. F. A. Bierhuizen, M. De Wit, C. A. R. L. Govers et al., "Glycosylation of three molecular forms of human α1-acid glycoprotein having different interactions with concanavalin A. Variations in the occurrence of di-, tri-, and tetraantennary glycans and the degree of sialylation," *European Journal of Biochemistry*, vol. 175, no. 2, pp. 387–394, 1988.

[40] H. Jiang, G. Guan, R. Zhang et al., "Increased urinary excretion of orosomucoid is a risk predictor of diabetic nephropathy," *Nephrology*, vol. 14, no. 3, pp. 332–337, 2009.

[41] K. Sharma, S. Lee, S. Han et al., "Two-dimensional fluorescence difference gel electrophoresis analysis of the urine proteome in human diabetic nephropathy," *Proteomics*, vol. 5, no. 10, pp. 2648–2655, 2005.

[42] R. N. Moresco, M. B. Sangoi, J. A. M. De Carvalho, E. Tatsch, and G. V. Bochi, "Diabetic nephropathy: traditional to proteomic markers," *Clinica Chimica Acta*, vol. 421, pp. 17–30, 2013.

[43] A. A. Ghani, S. Al Waheeb, A. Al Sahow, and N. Hussain, "Renal biopsy in patients with type 2 diabetes mellitus: indications and nature of the lesions," *Annals of Saudi Medicine*, vol. 29, no. 6, pp. 450–453, 2009.

[44] D. Wilfred, V. Mysorekar, R. Venkataramana, M. Eshwarappa, and R. Subramanyan, "Nondiabetic renal disease in type 2 diabetes mellitus patients: a clinicopathological study," *Journal of Laboratory Physicians*, vol. 5, no. 2, pp. 94–99, 2013.

[45] S. Liang, X.-G. Zhang, G.-Y. Cai et al., "Identifying parameters to distinguish non-diabetic renal diseases from diabetic nephropathy in patients with type 2 diabetes mellitus: a meta-analysis," *PLoS ONE*, vol. 8, no. 5, Article ID e64184, 2013.

[46] J. Zhou, X. Chen, Y. Xie, J. Li, N. Yamanaka, and X. Tong, "A differential diagnostic model of diabetic nephropathy and non-diabetic renal diseases," *Nephrology Dialysis Transplantation*, vol. 23, no. 6, pp. 1940–1945, 2008.

[47] S. G. Sharma, A. S. Bomback, J. Radhakrishnan et al., "The modern spectrum of renal biopsy findings in patients with diabetes," *Clinical Journal of the American Society of Nephrology*, vol. 8, no. 10, pp. 1718–1724, 2013.

[48] M.-Y. Liu, X.-M. Chen, X.-F. Sun et al., "Validation of a differential diagnostic model of diabetic nephropathy and non-diabetic renal diseases and the establishment of a new diagnostic model," *Journal of Diabetes*, vol. 6, no. 6, pp. 519–526, 2014.

[49] J. D. Marth and P. K. Grewal, "Mammalian glycosylation in immunity," *Nature Reviews Immunology*, vol. 8, no. 11, pp. 874–887, 2008.

[50] H. Suzuki, R. Fan, Z. Zhang et al., "Aberrantly glycosylated IgA1 in IgA nephropathy patients is recognized by IgG antibodies with restricted heterogeneity," *Journal of Clinical Investigation*, vol. 119, no. 6, pp. 1668–1677, 2009.

[51] R. Coppo and A. Amore, "Aberrant glycosylation in IgA nephropathy (IgAN)," *Kidney International*, vol. 65, no. 5, pp. 1544–1547, 2004.

[52] T. Nishie, O. Miyaishi, H. Azuma et al., "Development of immunoglobulin A nephropathy-like disease in β-1,4-galactosyltransferase-I-deficient mice," *American Journal of Pathology*, vol. 170, no. 2, pp. 447–456, 2007.

[53] H. Suzuki, L. Allegri, Y. Suzuki et al., "Galactose-deficient IgA1 as a candidate urinary polypeptide marker of IgA nephropathy?" *Disease Markers*, vol. 2016, Article ID 7806438, 6 pages, 2016.

[54] Y. Hiki, H. Odani, M. Takahashi et al., "Mass spectrometry proves under-O-glycosylation of glomerular IgA1 in IgA nephropathy," *Kidney International*, vol. 59, no. 3, pp. 1077–1085, 2001.

6

Association of *EPHX2* R287Q Polymorphism with Diabetic Nephropathy in Chinese Type 2 Diabetic Patients

Liang Ma,[1] Meihua Yan,[2] Xiaomu Kong,[3] Yongwei Jiang,[1] Tingting Zhao,[2] Hailing Zhao,[2] Qian Liu,[1] Haojun Zhang,[2] Peng Liu,[4] Yongtong Cao,[1] and Ping Li[2]

[1]*Clinical Laboratory, China-Japan Friendship Hospital, Beijing, China*
[2]*Beijing Key Lab Immune-Mediated Inflammatory Diseases, Institute of Clinical Medical Science, China-Japan Friendship Hospital, Beijing, China*
[3]*Department of Endocrinology, China-Japan Friendship Hospital, Beijing, China*
[4]*Graduate School of Peking Union Medical College, Chinese Academy of Medical Sciences and Peking Union Medical College, Beijing, China*

Correspondence should be addressed to Yongtong Cao; caoyongtong92@sina.com and Ping Li; lp8675@163.com

Academic Editor: Janet H. Southerland

The aim of this study was to investigate the relationship between *EPHX2* rs751141 (R287Q polymorphism) and diabetic nephropathy (DN) in Chinese type 2 diabetes (T2D). This case-control study explored the association between *EPHX2* rs751141 and DN in a total of 870 Chinese T2D patients (406 T2D patients with DN and 464 T2D patients without DN). DNA was extracted from peripheral leukocytes of the patients and rs751141 was genotyped. The A allele frequency of rs751141 was significantly lower in DN patients (20.94%) compared with non-DN controls (27.8%) ($P = 0.001$), and the A allele of rs751141 was associated with a significantly lower risk of DN after adjustment for multiple covariates in the additive genetic model (OR = 0.68, 95% CI = 0.52–0.88, $P = 0.004$). Significant association between rs751141 and homocysteine (Hcy) level on the risk of DN was observed, indicating that in patients with the highest Hcy levels, the A allele showed marked association with lower risk of DN in all three genetic models. In conclusion, the A allele of exonic polymorphism in EPHX2 rs751141 is negatively associated with the incidence of DN in the Chinese T2D population, which could be modulated by Hcy level status.

1. Introduction

In China, as of 2010, there were more than 110 million adults with diabetes mellitus and another more than 490 million with prediabetes [1]. Approximately 30–40% of type 2 diabetes (T2D) patients develop diabetic nephropathy (DN), a common microvascular complication of DM that may eventually require renal replacement therapy [2]. This is a warning sign for healthcare systems to be vigilant not only for adequate management but also for identifying risk factors involved in the pathogenesis of DN. In addition to conventional modifiable risk factors (hypertension, smoking, hyperlipidemia, and hemodynamic changes), hereditary components are also considered to be a significant risk factor for DN. Since DN occurs in familial clusters, genetic factors may contribute to DN development although the incidence and severity of DN are affected by the extent of blood glucose status [3, 4]. Therefore, identifying the genetic factors of DN can be of great significance in the prediction and prevention of DN in T2D in the Chinese population.

Epoxyeicosatrienoic acids (EETs) are involved in regulation of renal blood flow and long-term arterial blood pressure. Moreover, renal and cardiovascular diseases are associated with decreased renal and vascular levels of EETs [5]. In different animal models, high levels of EETs have been shown to protect kidney injury through anti-inflammatory, antiplatelet, and antiproliferative activities and endothelial-derived hyperpolarizing role [6–8]. However, EETs are degraded to corresponding diols by a soluble epoxide hydrolase (sEH) that is encoded by the *EPHX2* gene on chromosome 8p21-p12 [9]. Reducing sEH activity by a small molecular inhibitor can increase EET levels and decrease their degradation [10–12]. Gene knockout of *EPHX2* can improve endothelial function and reduce renal injury in streptozotocin-induced diabetic mice [13]. Furthermore, *EPHX2* deletion attenuates renal injury and inflammation in DOCA-salt hypertension [14]. Several single nucleotide polymorphisms (SNPs) of *EPHX2* have been identified, and one of the known SNPs is R287Q polymorphism (rs751141). The presence of an A instead of a G allele results in a lower sEH activity of approximately 25–58% [15].

Although the relationship between rs751141 and risk of IgA nephropathy has been investigated [16], patients carrying the A allele of rs751141 possessed better kidney survival than those with the G allele. However, the association between rs751141 and DN is unknown. Accordingly, we tested the hypothesis that an association exists between *EPHX2* rs751141 and risk of DN in the Chinese with T2D and whether Hcy level affects this association.

2. Materials and Methods

This study was approved by the institutional ethics committee of the China-Japan Friendship Hospital, Beijing, China. Signed informed consent was obtained from all participants. A total of 870 Chinese T2D patients were recruited from the China-Japan Friendship Hospital, between February 2015 and June 2016.

T2D was defined by the World Health Organization (WHO) 1999 criteria. This was a clinic-based case-control study. Cases were persons with type 2 diabetes and DN, and controls were persons with type 2 diabetes who did not have DN. Inclusion criteria for cases were diagnosed with T2D, age between 35 and 85 years old, and 24 h urinary albumin > 500 mg/L or an albumin creatinine ratio (ACR) > 30 mg/g. Inclusion criteria for controls were T2D duration ≥ 7 years, age between 35 and 85 years old, and 24 h urinary albumin < 150 mg/L or an ACR < 30 mg/g. Exclusion criteria for both groups consisted of known proteinuria before the onset of diabetes, other primary or secondary renal diseases (e.g., IgA nephropathy, membranous nephropathy, lupus nephritis, obstructive renal disease, renal stone disease, and acute urinary tract infection), and malignancy.

2.1. Data Collection. Demographic information, smoking habit, history of hypertension, body mass index (BMI), systolic blood pressure (SBP), diastolic blood pressure (DBP), 24 h urinary albumin excretion and ACR, high-density lipoprotein cholesterol (HDL-C), low-density lipoprotein cholesterol (LDL-C), total cholesterol (TC), triglycerides (TG), and homocysteine (Hcy) of each participant were obtained. Body weight and height were measured using standard methods, and BMI was calculated as weight (kg) divided by height squared (m^2). Resting blood pressure was measured twice according to standard protocol and the results were averaged. Serum concentrations of fasting TG, TC, LDL-C, HDL-C, and Hcy were measured using an automated biochemical analyzer (AU5800 Clinical Chemistry System, Beckman Coulter, Brea, CA, USA). A1C was measured using the D-10 Hemoglobin Testing System (Bio-Rad, Hercules, CA, USA).

2.2. DNA Extraction. DNA was extracted from peripheral blood using the QIAamp DNA Blood Mini Kit (Qiagen, Hilden, Germany) following the manufacturer's recommendations and then stored at −20°C or amplified immediately. The concentration of DNA was determined using the NanoDrop 1000 spectrophotometer (Thermo Scientific, Waltham, MA, USA).

2.3. Amplification and Detection of EPHX2 Gene R287Q Polymorphism. Genotyping was confirmed using TaqMan SNP Genotyping Assay (Applied Biosystems, Waltham, MA, USA). In all, 50 ng DNA was amplified in a 25 μl reaction mixture containing 12.5 μl of Premix Ex Taq (Probe qPCR) (Takara, Japan), 5 pmol of each primer (Applied Biosystems) and 3 pmol of each probe (Applied Biosystems) for the amplification of *EPHX2*. The primer and probe sequences were custom designed and synthesized by Applied Biosystems. The primer sequences were F:5′-CGGGAGGAG CAGATGACTCT-3′ and R:5′-TGGAGTGTGCCTGTTTG TTTTC-3′. The probe sequences were FAM-5′-CATAGC TAGGACCCGGTAACCTGCCT-3′-TAMRA and 5′VIC-5′-CCATAGCTAGGACCTGGTAACCTGCCT-3′-TAMRA.

Amplification was performed using a real-time polymerase chain reaction (PCR) detector (LightCycler 480, Roche Diagnostics, Penzberg, Germany) with a PCR temperature profile consisting of denaturation at 95°C for 10 minutes following 40 cycles of denaturation at 95°C for 15 seconds, annealing and elongation at 65°C for 60 seconds.

2.4. Genotyping Using DNA Sequencing. To confirm the genotyping results, 50 samples were randomly selected for DNA sequencing. rs751141 was amplified for DNA sequencing using the following designed primers F:5′-TTACAGGAA GAAGGGGATGG-3′ and R:5′-GGCAGGTAGAAGGCAA GACC-3′. Amplifications followed standard protocol, and the PCR products were purified using the QIAquick PCR Purification Kit (Qiagen) and subsequently analyzed by direct sequencing with an automated DNA sequencer (3500 Genetic Analyzer, Applied Biosystems).

2.5. Statistical Analysis. Quantitative clinical data (age, BMI, blood pressure, duration of diabetes, total cholesterol, HDL-C, LDL-C, TG, and Hcy) were non-Gaussian distribution and presented as median (interquartile range), and Wilcoxon's test was used to compare the difference in clinical characteristics between DN and DM groups. Genotype distribution and allelic frequency were analyzed using the chi-square test. Deviations from Hardy-Weinberg were also tested using the chi-square test. Finally, multiple logistic regression analyses were carried out to examine the association between rs751141 and risk of DN adjusted for age, sex, duration of diabetes, history of hypertension, smoking status, cholesterol, TG, and Hcy levels in additive,

Table 1: Characteristics of DM patients with DN (cases) and without DN (controls).

	DM patients with DN ($n = 406$)[a]	DM patients without DN ($n = 464$)[a]	P
Age (years)	63 (54, 71)	61 (54, 68)	0.001
Sex, male (%)	63.55 (258/406)	58.41 (271/464)	0.121
BMI (kg/m^2)	25.80 (23.89, 28.36)	25.36 (23.20, 27.68)	0.006
Duration of diabetes (years)	15 (9, 21)	13 (10, 18)	0.097
History of hypertension (%)	78.82 (320/406)	49.35 (229/464)	<0.001
Smoking (%)	34.73 (141/406)	28.23 (131/464)	0.039
SBP (mmHg)	138 (125, 150)	127 (120, 140)	<0.001
DBP (mmHg)	80 (74, 84)	80 (70, 80)	0.048
A1C (%)	7.6 (6.5, 9.3)	7.9 (6.7,9.3)	0.148
Hcy (umol/L)	13.63 (11.03, 17.12)	11.48 (9.51, 13.42)	<0.001
TC (mmol/L)	4.25 (3.44, 5.06)	4.14 (3.53, 4.86)	0.36
HDL-C (mmol/L)	0.96 (0.78, 1.18)	1.02 (0.85, 1.24)	0.004
LDL-C (mmol/L)	2.39 (1.85, 2.98)	2.38 (1.94, 2.97)	0.535
TG (mmol/L)	1.71 (1.20, 2.56)	1.42 (0.99, 2.18)	<0.001

BMI: body mass index; DBP: diastolic blood pressure; Hcy: homocysteine; HDL-C: high-density lipoprotein cholesterol; LDL-C: low-density lipoprotein cholesterol SBP: systolic blood pressure; TC: triglyceride. [a]Data are shown as median (interquantile range) or %.

recessive, or dominant models. To define these models, take SNP rs751141 as an example where A is the minor allele. For the dominant model, AA and GA were coded as 1 in the regression model and GG was coded 0. For the recessive model, AA was coded as 1 while GG and GA were coded as 0. For the additive model, AA, GA, and GG were coded as 2, 1, and 0, respectively.

Power calculation was performed by Quanto software (version 1.2.4, University of Southern California, Los Angeles, CA, USA). Data were analyzed with the SPSS software (version 17.0, IBM, Armonk, NY, USA). P values of < 0.05 were considered significant.

Table 2: Genotype distribution and allele frequency of rs751141 in DM patients with DN and without DN participants.

Genotype	Genotype frequencies: DM patients with DN	Genotype frequencies: DM patients without DN	P
GG	250	251	
GA	142	168	0.001
AA	14	45	
A allele	20.94%	27.8%	0.001
G allele	79.06%	72.2%	

DM: diabetes mellitus; DN: diabetic nephropathy.

3. Results

3.1. Baseline Characteristics. A total of 870 participants were included in this study. Cases included 406 DM patients with DN patients (258 males and 148 females), and controls included 464 DM patients without DN (271 males and 191 females) (Table 1). Variables such as smoking, BMI, blood pressure, HDL-C, history of hypertension, TG, and Hcy were found to be elevated in DN patients compared to controls (Table 1).

3.2. Distribution of EPHX2 R287Q Genotype. Distribution of allele frequencies of rs751141 was in accordance with the Hardy-Weinberg equilibrium in both DM with DN and without DN participants ($P = 0.683$ and $P = 0.354$, resp.). Genetic distribution of rs751141 (GG, GA, and AA) was found to be significantly different between DM participants with and without DN ($P = 0.001$) as well as allele frequencies (A and G alleles) ($P = 0.001$) (Table 2).

3.3. Association of R287Q Polymorphism with DN Risk. To confirm the association between the genotyping of rs751141 and the possibility of DN, further multiple logistic regression analysis was performed. Three statistical models were used as unadjusted, adjusted for age and sex, and adjusted for age, sex, Hcy, BMI, duration of diabetes, hypertension, smoking, total cholesterol, and TG levels. Results indicated the risk of DN with rs751141 in these models (Table 3). Additive and recessive models were significantly different in participants with DM patients with DN and DM patients without DN. Furthermore, the dominant model displayed a tendency toward significant difference ($P = 0.059$). AA genotyping was found to significantly decrease the risk of DN compared with GG genotyping in unadjusted and adjusted models ($P < 0.001$).

3.4. R287Q Genotype and Hcy Level Interaction. Participants were randomly divided into three equal groups based on Hcy levels (low level: 4.29–10.78 umol/L; medium level: 10.79–13.93 umol/L; high level: 13.94–55.99 umol/L). The three genetic models of additive, recessive, and dominant showed significant association with DN in the high level of Hcy groups in unadjusted ($P = 0.005$, $P = 0.02$, and $P = 0.02$, resp.) and adjusted models ($P = 0.004$, $P = 0.015$, and $P = 0.019$, resp.), indicating that the A allele carriers in the high Hcy group were at lower risk of DN, while no significant

Table 3: Odds ratios and 95% confidence interval for DN under three genetic models.

Genetic models	Unadjusted OR (95% CI)	P	Adjusted[a] OR (95% CI)	P	Adjusted[b] OR (95% CI)	P
Additive	0.69 (0.55–0.86)	<0.001	0.66 (0.52–0.83)	<0.001	0.68 (0.52–0.88)	0.004
Recessive	0.33 (0.18–0.62)	<0.001	0.33 (0.17–0.65)	0.001	0.28 (0.14–0.60)	0.001
Dominant	0.72 (0.55–0.95)	0.018	0.67 (0.50–0.90)	0.008	0.73 (0.53–1.01)	0.059
GA versus GG	0.83 (0.63–1.10)	0.201	0.77 (0.57–1.05)	0.097	0.87 (0.62–1.23)	0.43
AA versus GG	0.31 (0.17–0.58)	<0.001	0.30 (0.15–0.60)	<0.001	0.27 (0.13–0.58)	<0.001
Allele (A versus G)	0.69 (0.55–0.86)	<0.001				

CI: confidence interval; DN: diabetic nephropathy; OR: odds ratio. [a]Adjusted for age and sex. [b]Adjusted for age, sex, Hcy, BMI, duration of diabetes, hypertension, smoking, total cholesterol, and TG levels.

Table 4: Association of R287Q with risk of DN in different Hcy-level groups.

Hcy level (umol/L)	Genotype	Unadjusted OR (95% CI)	P	Adjusted[a] OR (95% CI)	P
Low: 4.29–10.78 ($n = 290$)	Additive	0.67 (0.44–1.02)	0.063	0.67 (0.41–1.10)	0.113
	Recessive	0.42 (0.14–1.27)	0.12	0.18 (0.03–0.98)	0.05
	Dominant	0.65 (0.38–1.11)	0.12	0.74 (0.40–1.38)	0.35
Medium:10.79–13.93 ($n = 290$)	Additive	0.74 (0.49–1.11)	0.14	0.81 (0.51–1.30)	0.38
	Recessive	0.22 (0.05–0.98)	0.047	0.27 (0.06–1.28)	0.10
	Dominant	0.82 (0.51–1.32)	0.41	0.93 (0.53–1.65)	0.81
High:13.94–55.99 ($n = 290$)	Additive	0.57 (0.38–0.84)	0.005	0.52 (0.33–0.81)	0.004
	Recessive	0.32 (0.13–0.82)	0.02	0.27 (0.09–0.78)	0.015
	Dominant	0.56 (0.34–0.92)	0.02	0.51 (0.29–0.90)	0.019

DN: diabetic nephropathy; Hcy: homocysteine. [a]Adjusted for age, sex, BMI, duration of diabetes, hypertension, smoking, total cholesterol, and TG levels.

association was observed in the medium ($P = 0.38$, $P = 0.10$, and $P = 0.81$, resp.) and low Hcy groups ($P = 0.113$, $P = 0.05$, and $P = 0.35$, resp.) in the adjusted model (Table 4).

4. Discussion

To our knowledge, this study is the first to describe the association between the polymorphism rs751141 of *EPHX2* and DN, as well as the influence of Hcy levels status on their association. A significant difference in the genotypic distribution of rs751141 between DM with DN and without DN participants was observed ($P = 0.001$), and the frequency of the A allele of rs751141 was significantly higher in the DM without the DN group than in the DM with DN group ($P = 0.001$). This suggests that the presence of the A allele of rs751141 was associated with a protective factor for against DN. This finding is consistent with the hypothesis that decreased endogenous sEH metabolic activity increases EET level, such that A allele carriers were associated with a high level of EET and lower risk of DN compared with individuals with GG genotype after adjustment for sex, age, smoking, BMI, history of hypertension, Hcy level, duration of diabetes, TG, and total cholesterol in the current investigation under the additive and recessive genetic models and that a similar trend was observed under the dominant genetic model ($P = 0.059$). Compared with the GG genotype, the AA genotype was found to confer 73% decreased the risk of DN after adjusting for established DN risk factors. The A allele of rs751141 appears to be an independent protective factor against DN in Chinese T2D patients. Moreover, a previous study found that there was no significant difference in genotype distribution and allele frequency between nondiabetic persons and T2D patients [17].

Studies have demonstrated that the A allele of rs751141 exhibits markedly lower sEH metabolic activity and decreased EET hydrolysis in vitro [15, 18]. sEH is an enzyme with multiple biological functions and is involved in the metabolism of xenobiotics. EETs are the endogenous substrates of sEH [19]. The decreased production of 20-hydroxyeicosatetraenoic acid (20-HETE) and EETs in kidney glomeruli is an important factor in glomerular damage in the early stage of DN [20]. In contrast, studies have shown that increase in EETs exerts renal protective effects and 8-9 EET may have a unique and specific protective role in the glomerular filtration barrier [21]. Levels of EETs depend not only on hydrolysis to dihydroxyeicosatrienoic acids (DHETs) by sEH but also on their production by cytochromes P450 (CYPs). Endothelial CYP2J2 overexpression can metabolize arachidonic acid into EETs, which protects the kidney against development and progression of chronic failure [22]. Previous studies have suggested that endothelial dysfunction is a universal risk factor of cardiovascular and renal diseases [23, 24]. Our findings also support the results of a previous study that the A allele of rs751141 is associated with a significantly lower risk of ischemic stroke in a Chinese population [25, 26], suggesting a protective role of the A allele of rs751141 in type 2 DN.

Interactions between genetic and environmental factors play a substantial role in disease risk [27]. A high Hcy level is considered a major risk factor of DN and accelerates disease progression. In the present study, we also observed the effect of high Hcy level on the association between rs751141 and DN in three genetic models. High Hcy level can downregulate CYP2J2 protein expression by inducing matrix metallopeptidase 9 (MMP-9) activation [28] and upregulate sEH protein expression through endoplasmic reticulum stress, activation of activating transcription factor-6 (ATF6), and DNA methylation in vitro and in vivo [29]. Increased sEH protein expression plays an important role in Hcy-induced endothelial activation, which can be prevented by inhibition of enzyme activity [29]. Levels of EETs depend not only on hydrolysis to dihydroxyeicosatrienoic acids (DHETs) by sEH but also on their production by CYPs. Therefore, decreased CYP2J2 expression and increased sEH expression likely attenuate the protective effect by reducing the production of EETs. Hcy level stratification indicated that a high Hcy level has an important genetic effect on rs751141 on the risk of DN. The A allele showed a protective effect in the high Hcy level group but not in the medium and low Hcy groups. This indicates that interactions between genetic and environmental risk factors may be important for the development of DN. Future studies in a larger population are required to better characterize this potential gene-environment interaction and the mechanistic contribution of *EPHX2* and Hcy to DN risk in persons with T2D.

The present study was performed with 406 patients with DN and 464 control participants with DM, which would have good statistical power to detect associations. However, there are still some limitations. First, the sample size of this study was limited when stratified according to Hcy level. Second, this study was conducted in Chinese and whether the results can be generalized to other ethnic groups need further investigation. Thus, a more extensive examination across various ethnic groups may help clarify the role of *EPHX2* rs751141 in the etiology of DN. Finally, the precise biological mechanism of the protective effect of the A allele of rs751141 against DN needs further elucidation.

In conclusion, our findings revealed that the exonic genetic variant in *EPHX2* rs751141 is significantly associated with the development of type 2 DN in the Chinese patients, suggesting the essential role that sEH plays in the pathogenesis of DN. In addition, Hcy level status affected the genetic risk for type 2 DN. Pharmacologic inhibition of sEH is being investigated as a novel therapeutic strategy for CKD [30, 31]. Therefore, based on our observation, sEH inhibitors may be used selectively to decrease DN risk in carriers of individuals with high genetic risk.

Conflicts of Interest

The authors declare no conflicts of interest.

Acknowledgments

This study was supported by the National Natural Science Foundation of China (Grant nos. 81703892, 8162010803, and 81473526) and the China-Japan Friendship Hospital Youth Science and Technology Excellence Project (Grant no. 2015-QNYC-B-09). The authors thank Nissi S. Wang, MSc, for developmental editing of the manuscript.

References

[1] Y. Xu, L. Wang, J. He et al., "Prevalence and control of diabetes in Chinese adults," *Journal of the American Medical Association*, vol. 310, no. 9, pp. 948–959, 2013.

[2] G. Remuzzi, A. Schieppati, and P. Ruggenenti, "Clinical practice. Nephropathy in patients with type 2 diabetes," *New England Journal of Medicine*, vol. 346, no. 15, pp. 1145–1151, 2002.

[3] L. H. Canani, F. Gerchman, and J. L. Gross, "Familial clustering of diabetic nephropathy in Brazilian type 2 diabetic patients," *Diabetes*, vol. 48, no. 4, pp. 909–913, 1999.

[4] R. Skrunes, E. Svarstad, A. V. Reisaeter, and B. E. Vikse, "Familial clustering of ESRD in the Norwegian population," *Clinical Journal of the American Society of Nephrology*, vol. 9, no. 10, pp. 1692–1700, 2014.

[5] J. D. Imig, "Epoxide hydrolase and epoxygenase metabolites as therapeutic targets for renal diseases," *American Journal of Physiology-Renal Physiology*, vol. 289, no. 3, pp. F496–F503, 2005.

[6] J. D. Imig, "Epoxygenase metabolites: epithelial and vascular actions," *Molecular Biotechnology*, vol. 16, no. 3, pp. 233–252, 2000.

[7] R. J. Roman, "P-450 metabolites of arachidonic acid in the control of cardiovascular function," *Physiological Reviews*, vol. 82, no. 1, pp. 131–185, 2002.

[8] A. A. Spector and A. W. Norris, "Action of epoxyeicosatrienoic acids on cellular function," *American Journal of Physiology-Cell Physiology*, vol. 292, no. 3, pp. C996–C1012, 2007.

[9] Z. Yu, F. Xu, L. M. Huse et al., "Soluble epoxide hydrolase regulates hydrolysis of vasoactive epoxyeicosatrienoic acids," *Circulation Research*, vol. 87, no. 11, pp. 992–998, 2000.

[10] J. D. Imig, X. Zhao, C. Z. Zaharis et al., "An orally active epoxide hydrolase inhibitor lowers blood pressure and provides renal protection in salt-sensitive hypertension," *Hypertension*, vol. 46, no. 4, pp. 975–981, 2005.

[11] J. J. Olearczyk, J. E. Quigley, B. C. Mitchell et al., "Administration of a substituted adamantyl urea inhibitor of soluble epoxide hydrolase protects the kidney from damage in hypertensive Goto-Kakizaki rats," *Clinical Science*, vol. 116, no. 1, pp. 61–70, 2009.

[12] D. Xu, N. Li, Y. He et al., "Prevention and reversal of cardiac hypertrophy by soluble epoxide hydrolase inhibitors," *Proceedings of the National Academy of Sciences*, vol. 103, no. 49, pp. 18733–18738, 2006.

[13] A. A. Elmarakby, J. Faulkner, M. Al-Shabrawey, M. H. Wang, K. R. Maddipati, and J. D. Imig, "Deletion of soluble epoxide hydrolase gene improves renal endothelial function and reduces renal inflammation and injury in streptozotocin-induced type 1 diabetes," *American Journal of Physiology-Regulatory, Integrative and Comparative Physiology*, vol. 301, no. 5, pp. R1307–R1317, 2011.

[14] M. Manhiani, J. E. Quigley, S. F. Knight et al., "Soluble epoxide hydrolase gene deletion attenuates renal injury and inflammation with DOCA-salt hypertension," *American Journal of*

Physiology-Renal Physiology, vol. 297, no. 3, pp. F740–F748, 2009.

[15] B. D. Przybyla-Zawislak, P. K. Srivastava, J. Vazquez-Matias et al., "Polymorphisms in human soluble epoxide hydrolase," *Molecular Pharmacology*, vol. 64, no. 2, pp. 482–490, 2003.

[16] J. P. Lee, S. H. Yang, D. K. Kim et al., "In vivo activity of epoxide hydrolase according to sequence variation affects the progression of human IgA nephropathy," *American Journal of Physiology-Renal Physiology*, vol. 300, no. 6, pp. F1283–F1290, 2011.

[17] K. Ohtoshi, H. Kaneto, K. Node et al., "Association of soluble epoxide hydrolase gene polymorphism with insulin resistance in type 2 diabetic patients," *Biochemical and Biophysical Research Communications*, vol. 331, no. 1, pp. 347–350, 2005.

[18] M. J. Merkel, L. Liu, Z. Cao et al., "Inhibition of soluble epoxide hydrolase preserves cardiomyocytes: role of STAT3 signaling," *American Journal of Physiology-Heart and Circulatory Physiology*, vol. 298, no. 2, pp. H679–H687, 2010.

[19] C. Guangzhi, X. Renfan, W. Yinna et al., "Genetic disruption of soluble epoxide hydrolase is protective against streptozotocin-induced diabetic nephropathy," *American Journal of Physiology-Endocrinology and Metabolism*, vol. 303, no. 5, pp. E563–E575, 2012.

[20] P. Luo, Y. Zhou, H. H. Chang et al., "Glomerular 20-HETE, EETs, and TGF-β1 in diabetic nephropathy," *American Journal of Physiology-Renal Physiology*, vol. 296, no. 3, pp. F556–F563, 2009.

[21] M. Sharma, E. T. McCarthy, D. S. Reddy et al., "8,9-Epoxyeicosatrienoic acid protects the glomerular filtration barrier," *Prostaglandins & Other Lipid Mediators*, vol. 89, no. 1-2, pp. 43–51, 2009.

[22] G. Chen, P. Wang, G. Zhao et al., "Cytochrome P450 epoxygenase CYP2J2 attenuates nephropathy in streptozotocin-induced diabetic mice," *Prostaglandins & Other Lipid Mediators*, vol. 96, no. 1–4, pp. 63–71, 2011.

[23] M. J. Landray, D. C. Wheeler, G. Y. Lip et al., "Inflammation, endothelial dysfunction, and platelet activation in patients with chronic kidney disease: the chronic renal impairment in Birmingham (CRIB) study," *American Journal of Kidney Diseases*, vol. 43, no. 2, pp. 244–253, 2004.

[24] J. A. Suwaidi, S. Hamasaki, S. T. Higano, R. A. Nishimura, D. R. Holmes, and A. Lerman, "Long-term follow-up of patients with mild coronary artery disease and endothelial dysfunction," *Circulation*, vol. 101, no. 9, pp. 948–954, 2000.

[25] L. Zhang, H. Ding, J. Yan et al., "Genetic variation in cytochrome P450 2J2 and soluble epoxide hydrolase and risk of ischemic stroke in a Chinese population," *Pharmacogenetics and Genomics*, vol. 18, no. 1, pp. 45–51, 2008.

[26] M. Liang, J. Yongwei, K. Xiaomu et al., "Synergistic effect of the MTHFR C677T and EPHX2 G860A polymorphism on the increased risk of ischemic stroke in Chinese type 2 diabetic patients," *Journal of Diabetes Research*, vol. 2017, Article ID 6216205, 8 pages, 2017.

[27] M. Rutter, T. E. Moffitt, and A. Caspi, "Gene-environment interplay and psychopathology: multiple varieties but real effects," *Journal of Child Psychology and Psychiatry*, vol. 47, no. 3-4, pp. 226–261, 2006.

[28] K. S. Moshal, D. C. Zeldin, S. D. Sithu et al., "Cytochrome P450 (CYP) 2J2 gene transfection attenuates MMP-9 via inhibition of NF-$\kappa\beta$ in hyperhomocysteinemia," *Journal of Cellular Physiology*, vol. 215, no. 3, pp. 771–781, 2008.

[29] D. Zhang, X. Xie, Y. Chen, B. D. Hammock, W. Kong, and Y. Zhu, "Homocysteine upregulates soluble epoxide hydrolase in vascular endothelium in vitro and in vivo," *Circulation Research*, vol. 110, no. 6, pp. 808–817, 2012.

[30] J. Kim, S. P. Yoon, M. L. Toews et al., "Pharmacological inhibition of soluble epoxide hydrolase prevents renal interstitial fibrogenesis in obstructive nephropathy," *American Journal of Physiology-Renal Physiology*, vol. 308, no. 2, pp. F131–F139, 2015.

[31] X. Zhao, T. Yamamoto, J. W. Newman et al., "Soluble epoxide hydrolase inhibition protects the kidney from hypertension-induced damage," *Journal of the American Society of Nephrology*, vol. 15, no. 5, pp. 1244–1253, 2004.

7

The Iron-Klotho-VDR Axis Is a Major Determinant of Proximal Convoluted Tubule Injury in Haptoglobin 2-2 Genotype Diabetic Nephropathy Patients and Mice

Inbal Dahan,[1] Nadia Thawho,[1] Evgeny Farber,[2] Nakhoul Nakhoul,[3] Rabea Asleh,[4] Andrew P. Levy,[4] Yan Chun Li,[5] Ofer Ben-Izhak,[6,7] and Farid Nakhoul[1,2,3]

[1]*Diabetes and Metabolism Lab, The Baruch Padeh Medical Center, Poriya, Lower Galilee, Israel*
[2]*Nephrology and Hypertension Division, The Baruch Padeh Medical Center, Poriya, Lower Galilee, Israel*
[3]*The Azrieli Faculty of Medicine in Zfat in the Galilee, Bar-Ilan University, Ramat-Gan, Israel*
[4]*The Vascular Medicine Lab, Technion, Faculty of Medicine, Rappaport Institute, Haifa, Israel*
[5]*Department of Medicine, The University of Chicago, Chicago, IL 60637, USA*
[6]*Department of Pathology, Rambam Health Care Campus, Haifa, Israel*
[7]*Technion, Haifa, Israel*

Correspondence should be addressed to Farid Nakhoul; fnakhoul@poria.health.gov.il

Academic Editor: Kim Connelly

The haptoglobin (Hp) genotype (1-1 and 2-2) is a major determinant of nephropathy progression in diabetes mellitus patients. Hp 2-2 diabetic mice have impaired Hb clearance and increased iron deposits and oxidative stress in the proximal tubules (PCT), leading to increased renal injury. However, the precise mechanism of the PCT injury in diabetic nephropathy (DN) remains elusive. In the kidney, 1,25$(OH)_2$D3 suppresses the inflammatory response to renal tubular injury and requires normal renal expression of the α-klotho protein. In this study, we set out to test the hypothesis that the increased renal iron deposits in the PCT of Hp 2-2 DN affect the α-klotho-vitamin D receptor (VDR) axis and thereby exacerbates the PCT injury generated by the iron deposits. Immunohistochemical analysis of human and mouse kidney biopsies along with western blot analysis showed that the increased iron deposits in the PCT of the Hp 2-2 genotype were accompanied with significantly decreased α-klotho and VDR renal expression but significantly increased 1-α-hydroxylase renal expression. In conclusion, the iron-klotho-VDR axis is a major player in the mechanism contributing to iron-mediated PCT injury in diabetic Hp 2-2 mice and patients. Targeting this axis may open the way for new ideas regarding the pathogenesis and treatment of DN.

1. Introduction

Haptoglobin (Hp) is an acute phase protein that acts as an antioxidant by virtue of its ability to bind free hemoglobin (Hb) and prevent heme-iron–mediated oxidation accompanied by tissue damage [1, 2]. Two classes of Hp alleles are known (1 and 2). While the Hp 1 allele is found in all animal species, the Hp 2 allele is present only in humans. The Hp genotype is a major determinant of progression of diabetic nephropathy (DN) [3–5]. The Hp 1 protein is superior to the Hp 2 protein in binding to free Hb and neutralizing its oxidative potential [6–8]. Moreover, Hp 2-2 is significantly associated with the development of reduced glomerular filtration rate (GFR) and end-stage renal disease [5] and is associated with greater incidence of cardiovascular disease compared with Hp 1-1 [9–11]. The difference between the Hp types is exaggerated in the diabetic state as extracorpuscular Hb is increased due to increased red cell fragility, and the ability of Hp to block the oxidative activity of Hb is impaired when Hb becomes glycated [1, 7, 8, 12]. Previously, we reported on the ability to recapitulate the interaction between the Hp genotype and DM in DN mice [13]. This mouse model represents DN with the spectrum of micro- and macrovascular complications similar to the human disease [13]. Using this mouse model, we have demonstrated marked differences in renal structure and function between the Hp 1-1 and Hp 2-2 DM mice; Hp 2-2 DM mice had a significant increase of iron deposits in the lysosomes of the kidney proximal convoluted tubule cells (PCT) with lysosomal and renal damage as well as increased features of glomerular disease characteristic of early human DN [7, 13, 14].

Klotho is a novel antiaging gene encoding a protein with multiple pleiotropic effects [15]. The klotho family of proteins consists of three members: α-klotho, β-klotho, and γ-klotho. The α-*klotho* gene is highly expressed in the distal and proximal convoluted tubular epitheliums of normal adult kidneys [16] and is affected by pathophysiological conditions including long-term hypertension, oxidative stress, diabetes, and chronic renal failure [16–21]. α-Klotho protein exists in two forms: a single pass transmembrane protein and a secreted protein [21]. The secreted form is involved in important biological processes including suppression of oxidative stress [15, 21]. The transmembrane α-klotho functions as a coreceptor for FGF-23, a bone-derived hormone that suppresses phosphate reabsorption and $1{,}25(OH)_2D3$ biosynthesis in the kidney via 1-α-hydroxylase [22]. $1{,}25(OH)_2D3$ stimulates both α-klotho and FGF-23, and both FGF-23 and α-klotho inhibit $1{,}25(OH)_2D3$ [23].

The involvement of vitamin D in kidney injury has been extensively studied. Vitamin D is transported to the liver, where it is first hydroxylated in position 25 to yield 25-hydroxyvitamin D. 25-Hydroxyvitamin D is further hydroxylated by 1-α-hydroxylase in the PCT of the kidney, to yield its active form $1{,}25(OH)_2D3$ [24]. The active $1{,}25(OH)_2D3$ binds to the intracellular vitamin D receptor (VDR) to activate vitamin D response elements within target genes [24, 25]. In the kidney, vitamin D is important for maintaining podocyte health, preventing epithelial to mesenchymal transformation, and suppressing renin gene expression and inflammation [26, 27]. Furthermore, in chronic kidney disease (CKD) patients, as renal function declines, serum levels of $1{,}25(OH)_2D3$ progressively decrease due to PCT injury, leading to a vitamin D-deficient state [27]. However, the precise mechanism of the PCT injury in DN with Hp 2-2 genotype remains elusive and needs to be determined. In this study, we set out to test the hypothesis that the increased iron deposits in the PCT of Hp 2-2 DN mice and patients affect the α-klotho-vitamin D receptor axis, leading to more prominent renal damage and a vitamin D-deficient state.

2. Materials and Method

2.1. Study Design. The current study was carried out to explore the involvement of the iron-klotho-VDR axis in the renal PCT injury of DN mice and patients with the Hp 2-2 genotype compared with Hp 1-1 genotype. The study includes experiments with the genetically engineered mouse model of DN with the Hp 2-2 genotype as well as type 2 diabetic (DM) and nondiabetic (nonDM) CKD patients at different stages (1–4) from The Baruch Padeh Medical Center, Poriya.

Kidney biopsies from patients and mice with different Hp genotypes (2-2 and 1-1) were subject to immunohistochemistry (IHC), and the mice kidney lysates were subjected to western blot analysis.

2.2. Animal Studies. All procedures were approved by the Animal Care Committee of the Technion (protocol number IL-112-11-11). We used our Hp mice model that we used in our previous study [13, 14]. The Hp 2-2 DM mice is a good model for DN since it has increased features of glomerular disease characteristic of early human DN including hyperfiltration, glomerular hypertrophy, and albuminuria [13]. All mice were of C57Bl/6 genetic background. The Hp 2 allele is present only in humans. All other species have only an Hp 1 allele, which is highly homologous with the human Hp 1 allele. Thus, wild-type mice carry the Hp 1 allele (referred to herein as Hp 1-1 mice). The construction of the murine Hp 2 allele and the targeting of its insertion by homologous recombination to the murine Hp genetic locus have been previously described [2]. Each group (Hp 2-2 and Hp 1-1 DM and nonDM) included 3 mice. Seven-week-old male mice were made diabetic by intraperitoneal injection of 50 mg/kg of STZ per day freshly prepared in 10 mM citrate buffer (pH 4.2) for 5 consecutive days. Mice were fed normal chow and exposed to a 12 : 12-hour light-dark cycle. Mice were sacrificed after a DM duration of 2 months (nonDM mice and DM mice were sacrificed at the same age). There were no differences in blood spot glucose levels between mice with the different Hp genotypes. After mice were sacrificed, the kidneys were removed, washed in saline, and either fixed in formalin for morphometric and immunohistological analysis [2] or placed in liquid nitrogen for western blot analysis and biochemical studies.

2.3. Patients. All experiments were approved by the Helsinki Committee of Poriya Hospital, and informed consent was obtained from all participants. The study included 42 biopsies from type 2 DM and nonDM CKD patients (males and females), above 18 years old from our nephrology outpatient clinic in Poriya Medical Center. Excluded from the study were oncology patients and pregnant women. The human kidney biopsies were done only for clinical reasons, but after patient consent, we used them for this study as well. For this study, we used only the renal biopsies from Hp 1-1 and 2-2 genotypes. Twenty-two biopsies were from CKD type 2 DM patients, and 20 biopsies from CKD nonDM patients served as controls. All the study participants were screened for the Hp genotype. Demographic and clinical data concerning the patients (age, sex, diabetic status, comorbidities, and medications used) were obtained directly from the patients or from their medical files.

2.4. Haptoglobin Typing. Hp typing of the study participants was performed on plasma samples by polyacrylamide gel electrophoresis as previously described [28]. In brief, 10 μL of Hb-enriched plasma was subjected to electrophoresis in a nondenaturing gel, and the gel was subsequently immersed in a solution containing a congener of benzidine with a precipitate forming in the gel corresponding to the location of

Hb-Hp complexes. The Hp type of the sample was determined by the banding pattern of the Hp-Hb complexes; each of the three Hp types has a characteristic banding fingerprint.

2.5. Western Blot Analysis. Mice renal tissues were homogenized with a protein lysis buffer containing protease and phosphatase inhibitors. The protein content of lysates was determined by the Bradford assay, and equal amounts of protein were boiled in a loading buffer and analyzed by SDS-PAGE. Gels were transferred to Protran membranes (Whatman), blocked with 5% BSA in TBS-T, incubated with a primary antibody in 5% BSA in TBS-T at 4°C overnight, then washed, and incubated with the HRP-conjugated secondary antibody (1:7500, Jackson) in TBS-T for 45 minutes at RT. Bands were visualized using EZ-ECL Chemiluminescence Detection Kit (Biological Industries), and the intensities of the bands were analyzed using Fujifilm ImageGaugeV software. Primary antibodies for klotho (1:2000; LSBio), β-actin (1:5000; Sigma), GAPDH (1:7500; Abcam), VDR (1:750; Novus Biologicals), and 1-α-hydroxylase (CYP27B1 (1:750; Abcam)) were used; secondary antibodies were HRP-linked goat anti-mouse or goat anti-rabbit (1:5000, Jackson).

2.6. Immunohistochemistry (IHC). Renal tissues from mice and human biopsies were fixed in 4% formaldehyde for 24 hours, paraffin embedded, and sectioned at 5 μm for immunostaining. Sections were deparaffinized in xylene and graded alcohols, followed by antigen retrieval and endogenous peroxidase quenched by H_2O_2. Sections were then incubated overnight at 4°C with primary antibodies at the following dilutions in blocking solution (CAS-block, Invitrogen): klotho (1:400; LSBio), VDR (1:200; Novus Biologicals) and 1-α-hydroxylase (CYP27B1 (1:200; Abcam)). HRP-polymer anti-rabbit (Nichirei and Dako) was used as a secondary antibody. Sections were developed with DAB Chromogen (Thermo Scientific). Slides were counterstained with Mayer's Hematoxylin, dehydrated, and mounted with Entellan (Merck). Images were obtained at 20x and 10x using an Axio Lab.A1 microscope with the Axiocam 105 color digital camera and ZEN software. Exposure times were kept constant for all samples. Quantification of the IHC staining was performed by using Panoramic Viewer and Image-Pro software version 7.

2.7. PAS Staining. Slides were deparaffinized, rehydrated, and then incubated in 2% periodic acid for 15 minutes followed by Schiff's reagent (Merck Millipore) for 25 minutes. Counter-staining was performed with filtered hematoxylin.

2.8. Iron Staining by Modified Perls' DAB Staining. After deparaffinization in xylene and rehydration through graded ethanol, sections from mice and human biopsies were washed in PBS and incubated in a peroxidase blocking solution of 3% H_2O_2 for 10 min. Then the slides were treated in Prussian blue solution for 20 min, washed with PBS, and subsequently incubated with 3,3'-DAB and 2 μL of 30% H_2O_2 DAB (Sigma) for 20 min in a dark humidified chamber. Then slides were counterstained with Mayer's Hematoxylin, dehydrated, and mounted with Entellan (Merck).

TABLE 1: Study participants' characteristics stratified by Hp phenotype.

	Hp 1-1 $n = 7$	Hp 2-2 $n = 35$
Mean age (years)	48.88 ± 15.90	50.77 ± 13.55
Range	26–66	21–67
Male/female (n)	4/3	25/10
M/F ratio	1.33	2.5
DM/nonDM (n)	1/6	21/14
% DM	14%	60%
Mean GFR	58.33 ± 21	48.57 ± 24
Range	29–84	15–96
Mean systemic blood pressure	144/74 ± 20/13	141/72 ± 29/16

2.9. Statistics and Quantification. IHC staining was quantified by Panoramic Viewer and Image-Pro (version 7) software according to the Hot-spot method with the most stained fields in each Hp group accompanied with 95% confidence interval analysis. PAS staining was conducted to ensure that the number of tubules in the different renal sections was similar during the IHC quantification. Positively stained tubules were manually counted within the area of the whole field at optical magnification 10x. The quantification was based on at least 10 fields in each group and included the percentage of the total stained area. The total stained area was calculated based on the ratio of the manually selected stained area to the total area of the field. All manual procedures were performed without knowledge of mouse or patient background.

All results are reported as mean ± SEM. Comparison between groups was performed using 2-tailed Student's t-test, ANOVA, Kruskal-Wallis test, and Tukey's LSD method for pairwise comparisons, with a p value < 0.05 considered statistically significant. Data analysis was done using IBM SPSS software version 20.0.

3. Results

The Hp protein products of the Hp 1 and Hp 2 alleles differ in both their biochemical and their functional properties such as antioxidant ability and Hb clearance from the plasmatic compartment, and these differences are exaggerated in diabetes [6–8]. Hence, in the current study, we stratified the study participants according to their Hp genotype and their diabetes status and explored the involvement of the iron-klotho-VDR axis in the renal PCT injury. The study participants' characteristics are presented in Table 1. Most of our CKD patients (83%, $n = 35$) have the Hp 2-2 genotype and had reduced GFR levels compared with Hp 1-1 genotype. Sixty percent ($n = 21$) of these patients are diabetic nephropathy patients (Table 1). This distribution is in agreement with previous studies that have shown that Hp 2-2 genotype is associated with the development of reduced GFR and increased development of diabetic complications [5–8].

3.1. Increased Iron-Rich Deposits in the PCT Cells of DN Mice and Patients with Hp 2-2 Genotype. We previously

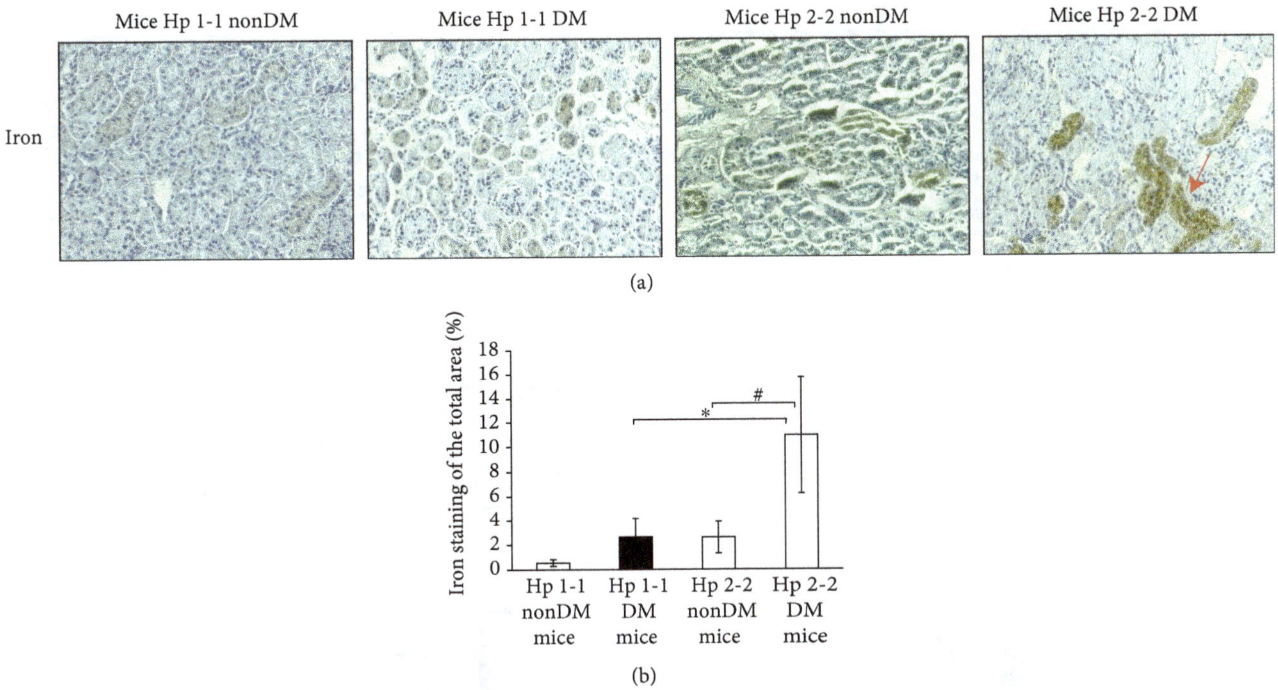

FIGURE 1: Iron staining in Hp 2-2 and Hp 1-1 renal sections of diabetic nephropathy and nondiabetic mice. (a) There was a significant increase of iron deposits represented by the DAB-enhanced Prussian blue staining (brown, indicated by a red arrow) in the proximal convoluted tubule (PCT) of Hp 2-2 diabetic (DM) sections compared with diabetic Hp 1-1 or with Hp 2-2 nondiabetic (nonDM) sections. (b) Quantification of the iron staining shows a significant increase in the percentage of the iron-stained area of Hp 2-2 DM mice compared with DN Hp 1-1 mice ($^*p < 0.001$) or compared with nonDM Hp 2-2 mice ($^\#p < 0.001$).

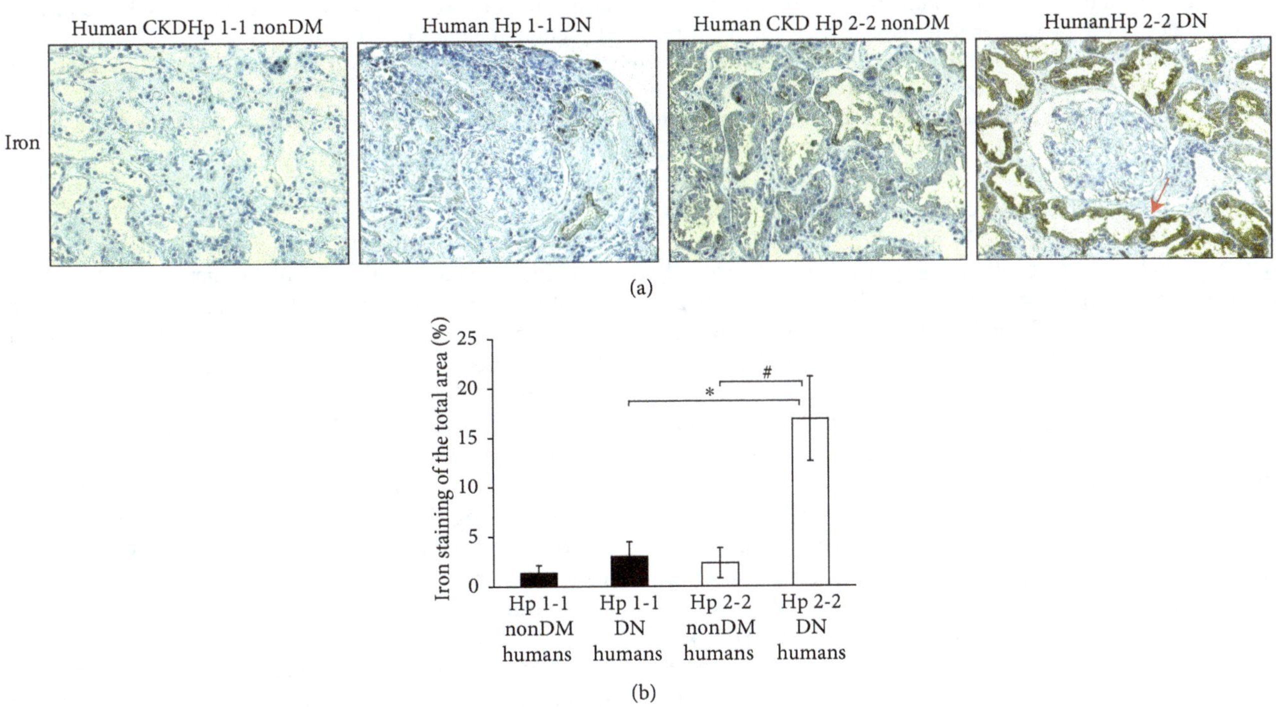

FIGURE 2: Iron staining in Hp 2-2 and Hp 1-1 renal sections of diabetic nephropathy and nondiabetic CKD patients. (a) There was a significant increase of iron deposits represented by the DAB-enhanced Prussian blue staining (brown, indicated by a red arrow) in the PCT of Hp 2-2 diabetic nephropathy (DN) patients compared with DN Hp 1-1 or Hp 2-2 CKD nondiabetic (nonDM) patients. (b) Quantification of the iron staining shows a significant increase in the percentage of the iron-stained area of Hp 2-2 DM patients compared with the DN Hp 1-1 genotype ($^*p < 0.001$) or compared with the nonDM CKD Hp 2-2 genotype ($^\#p < 0.001$).

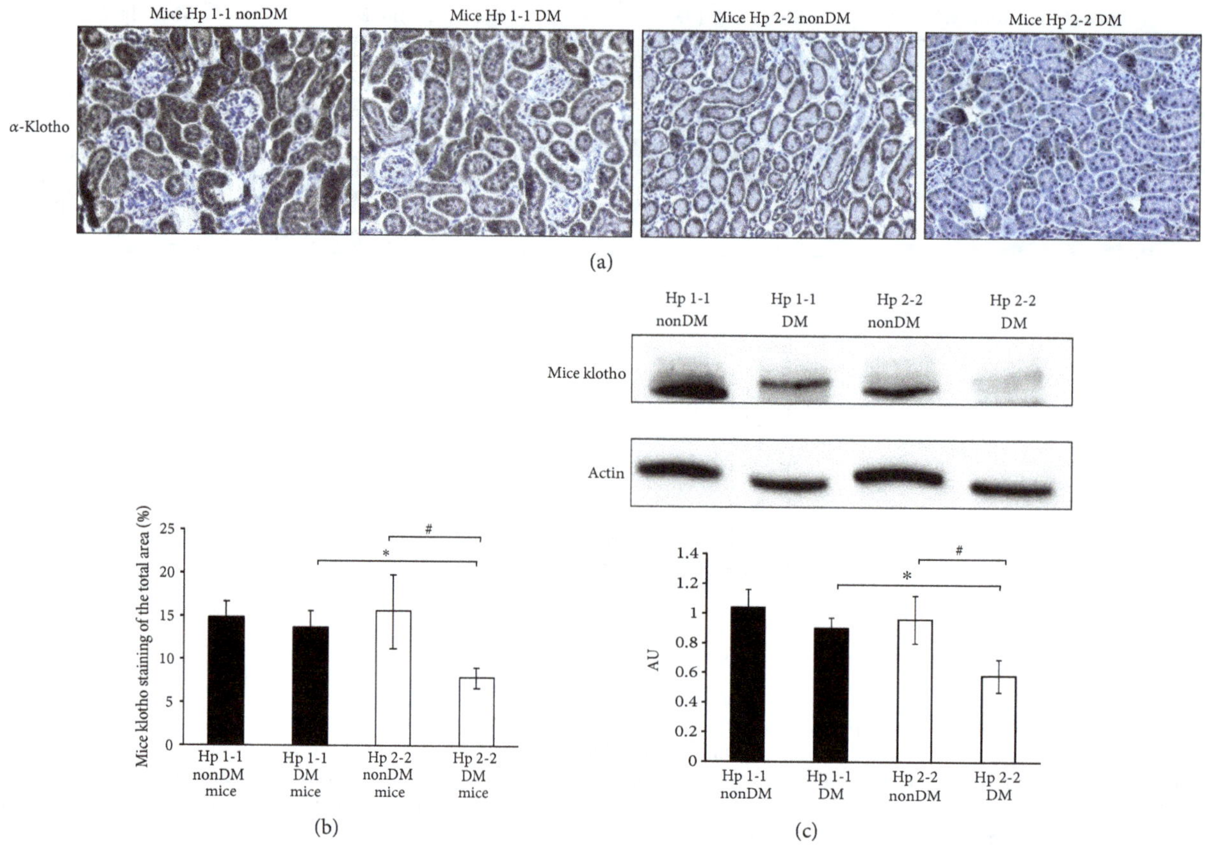

FIGURE 3: (a) α-Klotho renal expression in nondiabetic and diabetic nephropathy mice. (b) The percentage of the α-klotho-stained area is significantly decreased in the renal tubules of Hp 2-2 diabetic (DM) sections compared with Hp 1-1 diabetic ($^{*}p < 0.05$) or with nondiabetic (nonDM) Hp 2-2 sections ($^{\#}p < 0.05$). (c) α-Klotho expression in mice renal lysates from Hp 1-1 and Hp 2-2 nondiabetic (nonDM) and diabetic (DM) mice. Proteins were detected by immunoblotting with antibodies against α-klotho and actin. The values represent the mean ± SEM for 3 independent experiments subjected to 2-tailed, 2-sampled unequal variance Student's *t*-test, with $^{\#}p <$ 0.05 compared with Hp 2-2 nonDM and $^{*}p < 0.05$ compared with Hp 1-1 DM. AU: arbitrary units.

demonstrated an increased accumulation of iron deposits in the renal PCT of Hp 2-2 DN mice [7, 13, 14]. To confirm the prevalence of renal iron deposits in our Hp 2-2 DN mice, renal samples of mice with Hp 1-1 and Hp 2-2 genotypes were stained for iron by using DAB staining. As shown in Figures 1(a) and 1(b), there was a 4-fold increase in the percentage of the iron-stained area in PCT of Hp 2-2 DM mice (11 ± 4.74%) compared with Hp 1-1 DM (2.71 ± 1.45%, $p < 0.001$) or with Hp 2-2 nonDM mice (2.59 ± 1.33%, $p < 0.001$).

To further investigate the prevalence of renal iron deposits also in Hp 2-2 DN patients, renal samples of CKD patients with Hp 1-1 and 2-2 genotypes were stained for iron. There was nearly a 5-fold increase in the iron-stained area in Hp 2-2 DN renal sections (16.86 ± 4.25%) compared with DM Hp 1-1 sections (3.03 ± 1.48%, $p < 0.001$) or compared with nonDM CKD Hp 2-2 sections (2.36 ± 1.51%, $p < 0.001$, Figures 2(a) and 2(b)).

3.2. Decreased Renal α-Klotho Expression in DN Mice and Patients with Hp 2-2 Genotype. Previous studies have indicated that renal *α-klotho* gene expression is regulated by pathophysiological conditions including long-term hypertension, oxidative stress, diabetes, and chronic renal failure in both animal models and humans [16, 17, 20, 29–32]. Hence, we evaluated whether the increased renal iron deposits associated with the Hp 2-2 genotype also affect the α-klotho renal expression both in DN mice and patients. As shown in Figures 3(a) and 3(b), the percentage of the α-klotho-stained area was significantly reduced in the tubules of Hp 2-2 DN mice (7.8 ± 1.22%) compared with DM Hp 1-1 genotype (13.58 ± 2.01%, $p < 0.05$) or with nonDM Hp 2-2 genotype (15.53 ± 4.2%, $p < 0.05$).

In order to strengthen these results, western blot analysis was done using the mice renal lysate (Figure 3(c)). α-Klotho expression was significantly decreased in Hp 2-2 DN mice (0.58 ± 0.11 arbitrary units (AU)) compared with DM Hp 1-1 genotype (0.9 ± 0.07 AU, $p < 0.05$) or with Hp 2-2 nonDM mice (0.96 ± 0.16 AU; $p < 0.05$).

Similar to the results obtained in mice, the percentage of the stained area of renal α-klotho was also reduced by nearly 2-fold in tubules of Hp 2-2 DN patients (7.5 ± 2.36%) compared with DM Hp 1-1 genotype (14.02 ± 5.1%, $p < 0.05$) or with CKD nonDM Hp 2-2 genotype (14.58 ± 5.34%, $p <$ 0.05, Figures 4(a) and 4(b)).

We further investigated whether the decline in renal function among Hp 2-2 CKD patients was associated with an exacerbated decrease in renal α-klotho expression. As

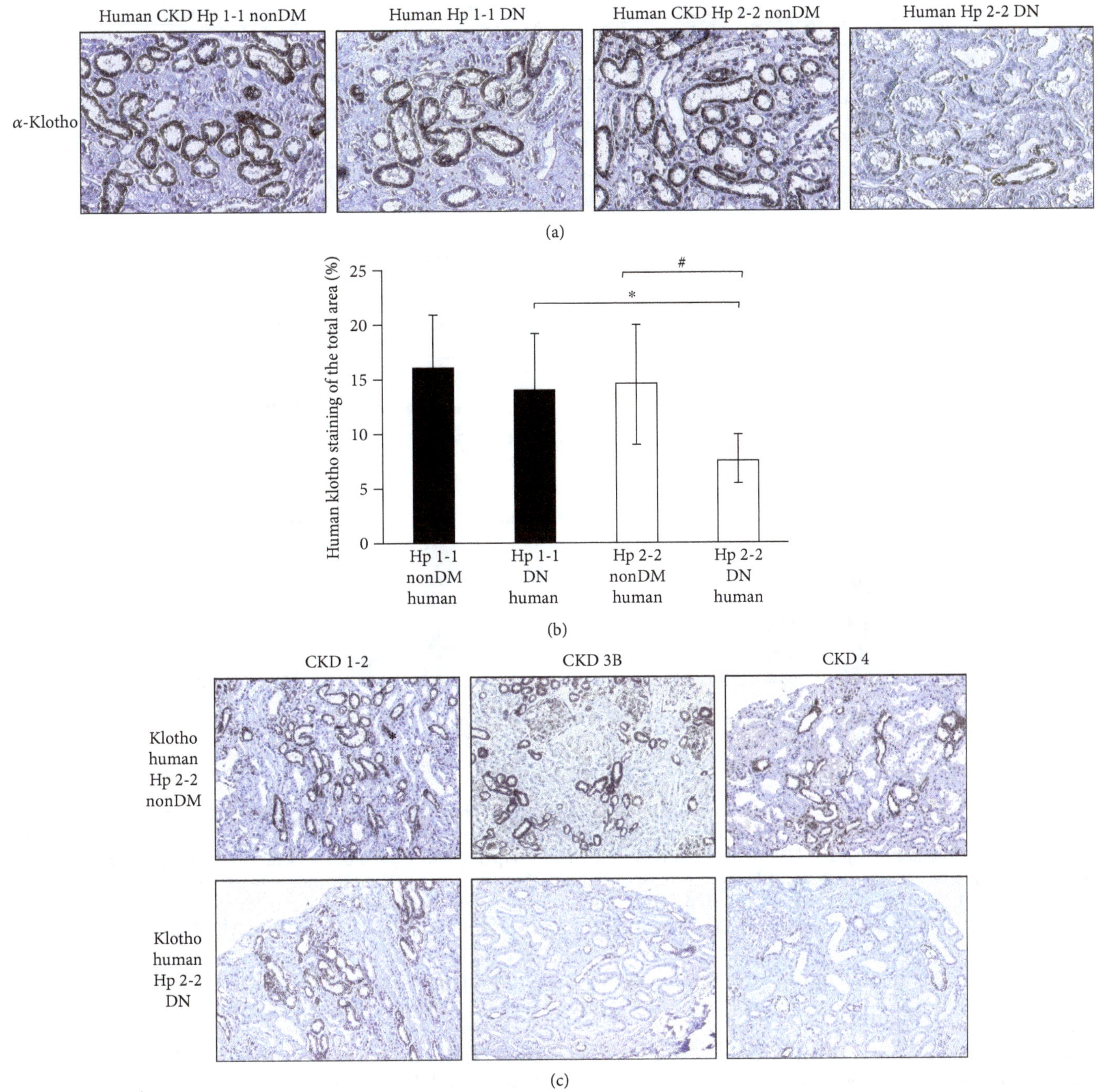

Figure 4: (a) α-Klotho renal expression in nondiabetic and diabetic nephropathy patients. (b) The percentage of the stained area of α-klotho is significantly decreased in the renal tubules of diabetic (DM) biopsies with Hp 2-2 genotype compared with Hp 1-1 diabetic ($^{*}p < 0.05$) or with nondiabetic (nonDM) Hp 2-2 genotype ($^{\#}p < 0.05$). (c) In chronic kidney disease (CKD) patients with the Hp 2-2 genotype, the renal expression of α-klotho declines with the progression in the CKD stage, and it is exacerbated in the diabetic state.

shown in Figure 4(c), the renal α-klotho expression was gradually decreased along with the progression in CKD stages, and this decrease was exacerbated in diabetes.

3.3. Decreased Expression of Renal Vitamin D Receptor (VDR) and Increased Expression of 1-α-Hydroxylase in DN Hp 2-2 Mice and Patients. Normal expression of renal α-klotho is required for normal vitamin D homeostasis via downregulation of 1-α-hydroxylase and upregulation of 24-hydroxylase. Therefore, we tested whether the decrease in α-klotho renal expression shown in the Hp 2-2 DN genotype was accompanied with altered expression of renal VDR and 1-α-hydroxylase. As shown in Figures 5(a) and 5(b), the percentage of the VDR-stained area in mice renal sections was significantly decreased in the PCT of DN Hp 2-2 mice ($8.3 \pm 1.83\%$, $p < 0.05$) compared with DM Hp 1-1 mice ($13.6 \pm 2.9\%$) or with Hp 2-2 nonDM mice ($19.8 \pm 3.4\%$, $p < 0.05$).

Western blot analysis of the mice renal lysates (Figure 5(c)) strengthened these results, as VDR expression was significantly decreased in Hp 2-2 DN mice ($0.47 \pm$

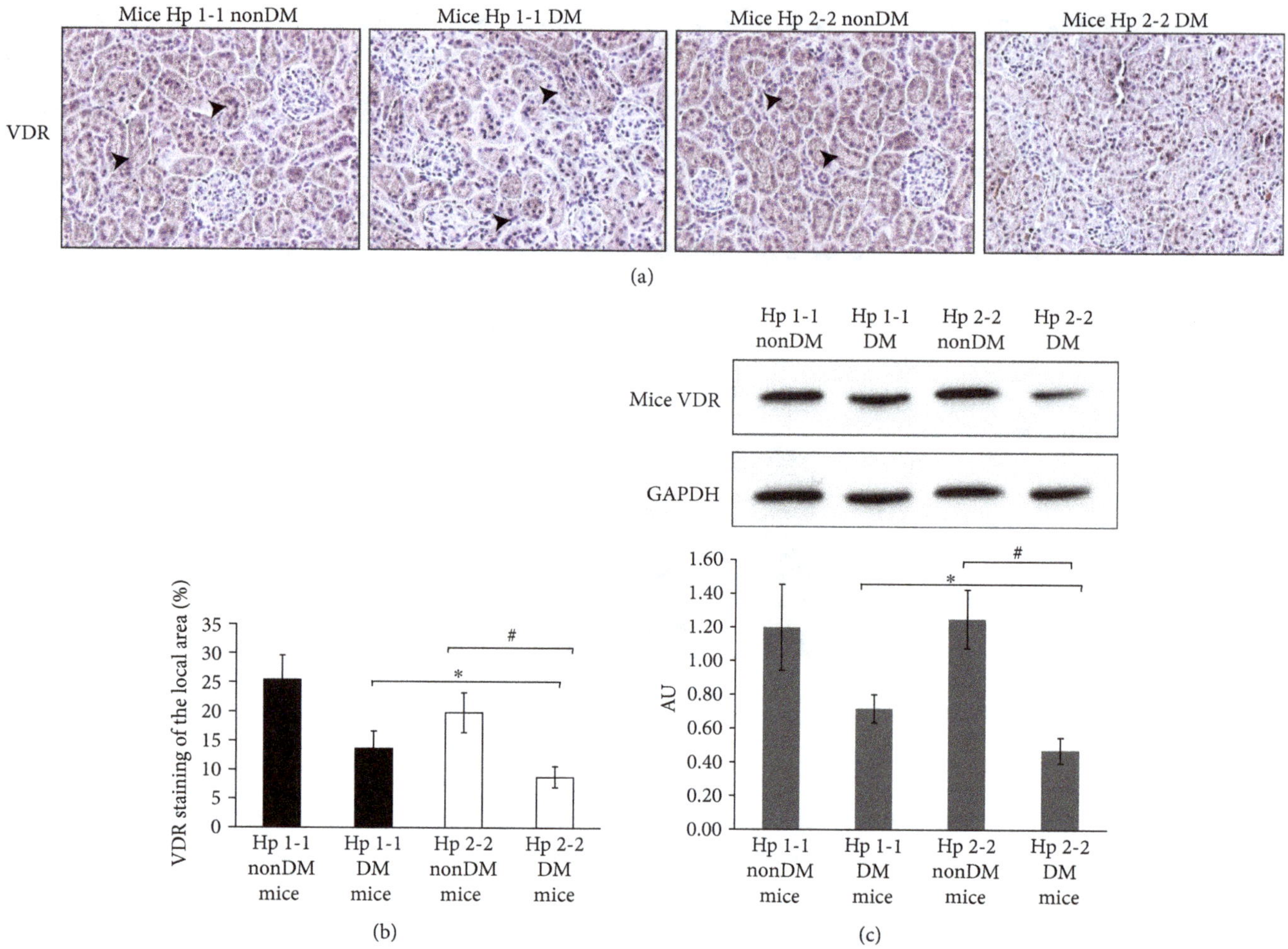

FIGURE 5: Renal vitamin D receptor (VDR) expression in nondiabetic (nonDM) and diabetic (DN) mice. (a) Renal sections from Hp 1-1 and 2-2 mice were subjected to IHC of VDR (brown, indicated by arrowheads). (b) There was a significant decrease in the percentage of the VDR-stained area in the tubules of Hp 2-2 DM renal sections compared with Hp 1-1 DM ($^{*}p < 0.05$) or with nonDM Hp 2-2 renal sections ($^{\#}p < 0.05$). (c) Western blot analysis of VDR with the mice renal lysate. Proteins were detected by immunoblotting with antibodies against VDR and GAPDH. The values represent the mean ± SEM for 3 independent experiments subjected to 2-tailed, 2-sampled unequal variance Student's t-test, with $^{*}p = 0.001$ compared with Hp 2-2 nonDM and $^{\#}p = 0.005$ compared with Hp 1-1DM. AU: arbitrary units.

0.08 AU) compared with Hp 1-1 DM mice (0.72 ± 0.08 AU; $p = 0.005$) or with Hp 2-2 nonDM mice (1.25 ± 0.17 AU; $p = 0.001$).

The renal expression of VDR was decreased also in human's renal sections. VDR staining in human's sections was mainly in the nucleus. As shown in Figures 6(a) and 6(b), the percentage of stained nuclei significantly decreased in CKD Hp 2-2 DN renal sections (29.5 ± 6.61%) compared with DM Hp 1-1 sections (37.44 ± 4.35%, $p < 0.001$) or compared with nonDM Hp 2-2 sections (59.9 ± 9.55%, $p < 0.001$).

Contrary to the decreased expression of VDR that was observed in DM mice and in patients with Hp 2-2 genotype, renal expression of 1-α-hydroxylase was increased in these mice and patients (Figures 7(a) and 8(a)). 1-α-Hydroxylase staining in mice showed a significant decrease in the percentage of the stained area of 1-α-hydroxylase in DN Hp 2-2 mice (18.64 ± 2.87%) compared with DM Hp 1-1 sections (9.1 ± 1.45%, $p < 0.05$) but insignificant compared with nonDM Hp 2-2 sections (17.26 ± 2.62%, $p = 0.611$, Figure 7(b)).

Western blot analysis with the mice renal lysates (Figure 7(c)) supports these observations. As shown in Figure 7(c), there was a significant increase in 1-α-hydroxylase expression in Hp 2-2 DN mice (0.84 ± 0.08 AU) compared with DM Hp 1-1 genotype (0.55 ± 0.12 AU, $p = 0.008$) but insignificant compared with Hp 2-2 nonDM mice (0.67 ± 0.1 AU).

Similar to mice results, 1-α-hydroxylase staining in human renal sections also showed a significant decrease in the percentage of the stained area in DN Hp 2-2 sections (16.22 ± 2.84%) compared with DM Hp 1-1 sections (11 ± 0.98%, $p < 0.05$) but insignificant compared with nonDM Hp 2-2 sections (12.21 ± 2.37%, $p = 0.67$, Figures 8(a) and 8(b)).

4. Discussion

Oxidative stress is an important possible causative factor of DN [33]. Hence, the Hp genotype is a major determinant of DN progression [3–5]. The Hp 2 protein is inferior to

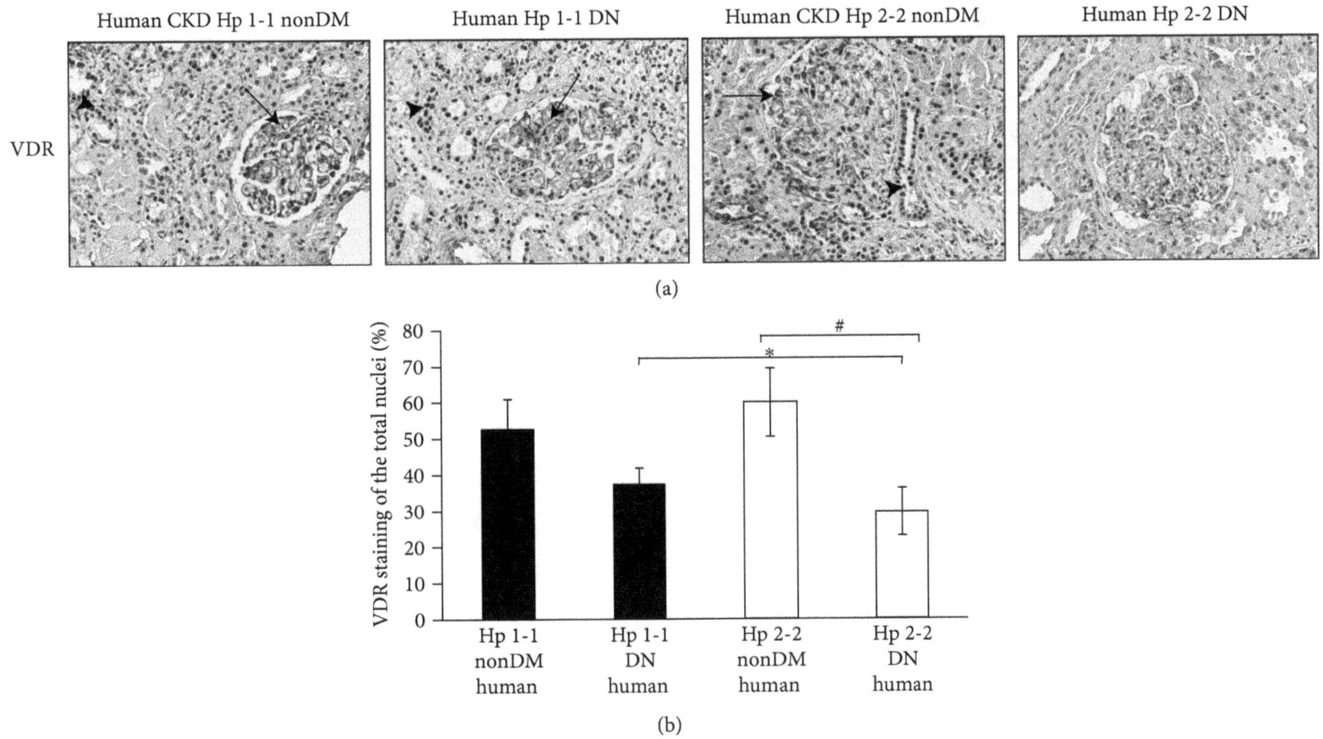

Figure 6: Renal vitamin D receptor (VDR) expression in nondiabetic (nonDM) and diabetic (DN) patients. (a) Renal biopsies from Hp 1-1 and 2-2 CKD patients were subjected to IHC of VDR. There was a significant decrease in VDR expression (brown) in the tubules (indicated by arrowheads) and in the glomerulus (indicated by black arrows) of Hp 2-2 DM renal sections compared with Hp 1-1 DM or with nonDM Hp 2-2 renal sections. (b) Quantification of VDR staining shows a significant decrease in the percentage of stained nuclei of Hp 2-2 DM sections compared with DM Hp 1-1 sections ($^{*}p < 0.001$) or compared with the nonDM Hp 2-2 genotype ($^{\#}p < 0.001$).

the Hp 1 protein in binding to free Hb and neutralizing its oxidative potential [6–8], and this difference is exaggerated in the diabetic state. We have previously demonstrated a correlation between the Hp 2-2 genotype and the accumulation of iron deposits in the lysosomes of the renal PCT in mice, which results in lysosomal membrane injury and renal cells damage caused by oxidative stress [13, 14]. The source of excess PCT iron in Hp 2-2 DN is Hb [8]. In Hp 2-2 DM, the normal clearance mechanism via the CD163 receptor for the Hp-Hb complex is severely impaired with approximately a 5-fold increase in the half-life of the complex [14, 34]. Furthermore, iron is known to enhance organ damage induced by oxidants to generate highly toxic hydroxyl radicals. Thus, it is possible that the deposition of renal iron leads to a decrease in α-klotho renal expression by inducing oxidative stress [35, 36].

In this study, we set out to explore the hypothesis that the excess iron deposition in DN individuals and mice with Hp 2-2 genotype leads to downstream effects on the α-klotho-VDR axis that consequently leads to renal PCT injury. We have shown significantly increased iron deposits in the PCT of Hp 2-2 DN mice and patients that were associated with decreased α-klotho and VDR renal expression. We further found out that in the Hp 2-2 genotype, α-klotho renal expression is gradually reduced with the progression in CKD stages, and this decrease is more prominent in the diabetic state. This association is in agreement with previous studies that have shown that renal *α-klotho* gene expression is regulated by pathophysiological conditions including hypertension, diabetes, and chronic renal failure in animal models and in humans [16, 17, 20, 29–32].

It is known that CKD patients suffer from a vitamin D-deficient state, but the precise mechanism of the renal injury and the impairment of vitamin D activation remain elusive. Since normal renal expression of the α-klotho protein is required for normal 1,25-dihyroxyvitamin D homeostasis via downregulation of 1-α-hydroxylase and upregulation of 24-hydroxylase [37], we further explored whether the decreased α-klotho renal expression in Hp 2-2 DN genotype affects the expression of renal VDR and 1-α-hydroxylase. We found out that in DN Hp 2-2 patients and mice, while the expression of VDR was decreased, 1-α-hydroxylase renal expression was increased probably as a compensation mechanism.

In the kidney, active vitamin D is important for maintaining podocyte integrity and suppressing renin gene expression and inflammation [38]. Therefore, vitamin D has the potential to have a favorable impact on DN severity in Hp 2-2 phenotype via kidney protection from oxidative stress injury [39–41]. The beneficial effects of vitamin D on renal fibrosis in DN are mediated by VDR via restoration of α-klotho expression. Furthermore, α-klotho deficiency in combination with hyperglycemia can aggravate the oxidative damage that contributes to the exacerbation of DN. The klotho protein also has endogenous antifibrotic function via antagonism of Wnt/β-catenin signaling, suggesting that loss

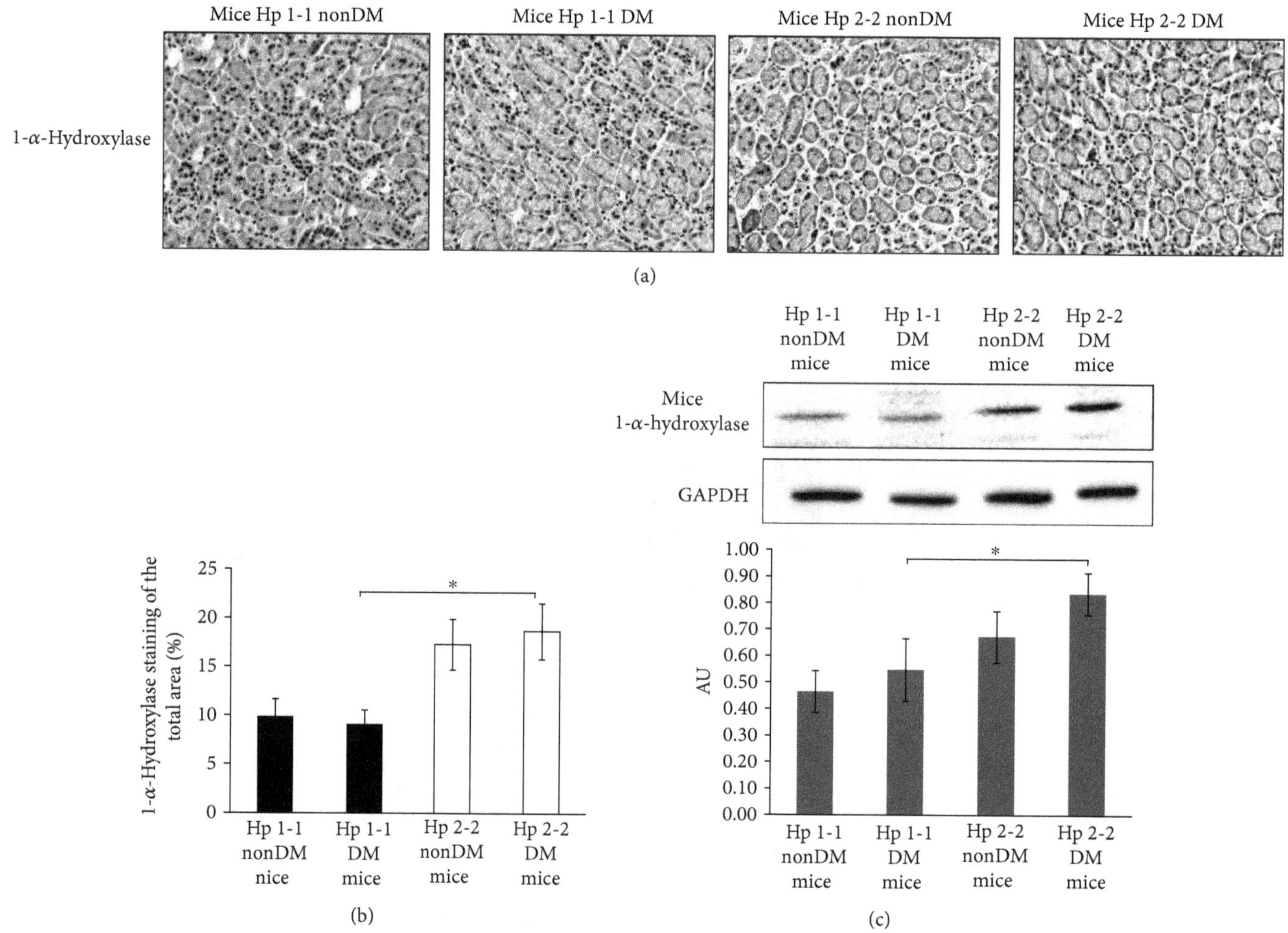

FIGURE 7: 1-α-Hydroxylase expression in diabetic and nondiabetic (nonDM) mice. (a) Slides from mice renal biopsies were subjected to IHC of 1-α-hydroxylase. (b) There was a significant increase in the percentage of the stained area of 1-α-hydroxylase in the tubules of Hp 2-2 DM renal sections compared with Hp 1-1 DM sections ($^{*}p < 0.05$) but insignificant compared with nonDM Hp 2-2 genotype. (c) Western blot analysis of 1-α-hydroxylase with the mice renal lysate. Proteins were detected by immunoblotting with antibodies against 1-α-hydroxylase and GAPDH. The values represent the mean ± SEM for 3 independent experiments subjected to 2-tailed, 2-sampled unequal variance Student's t-test, with $^{\#}p = 0.008$ compared with Hp 1-1DM. AU: arbitrary units.

of α-klotho may contribute to the progression of DN by accelerated fibrogenesis [42]. In addition, suppressive effects of α-klotho on the insulin-like growth factor pathway may be associated with inhibitory action on renal fibrosis and cardio-renal protection in high oxidative stress conditions such as diabetes and its complications [42, 43].

Hence, the potential utility of the α-klotho-VDR axis in clinical practice is anticipated to be at least twofold. First, α-klotho has the potential to serve as an early and sensitive biomarker of DN. However, its specificity and its prognostic value and differential diagnostic value in human disease remain to be examined. Second, α-klotho exogenous supplementation and/or upregulation or restoration of α-klotho by reducing the iron levels via chelating agent or dietary iron restriction may provide novel therapy for DN patients with Hp 2-2 genotype to retard or block its progression to advanced CKD by arresting or slowing progression as well as by preventing and reversing complications [33].

It is important to note that the current study has some limitations. The prevalence of the Hp 2-2 genotype in Western societies including Israel is 35–50% while the prevalence of Hp 1-1 is only 10–15%. Furthermore, since the Hp 2-2 genotype is associated with the development of reduced GFR and increased development of diabetic complications, combined with the fact that the biopsies that we used in the study were taken only for clinical reasons, most of our DN patients have the Hp 2-2 genotype. Hence, we have a limited number of Hp 1-1 biopsies compared with Hp 2-2 biopsies. However, in this study, we explored our hypothesis by using the genetically engineered Hp 2-2 mouse model that represents the human DN, and we strengthened our observations with the human experiments. The STZ-induced type 1 diabetes C57B1/6 mouse has been widely used as a model for DN since this mouse model has the spectrum of micro- and macrovascular complications similar to human disease including hyper-filtration, glomerular hypertrophy, and albuminuria [13, 44].

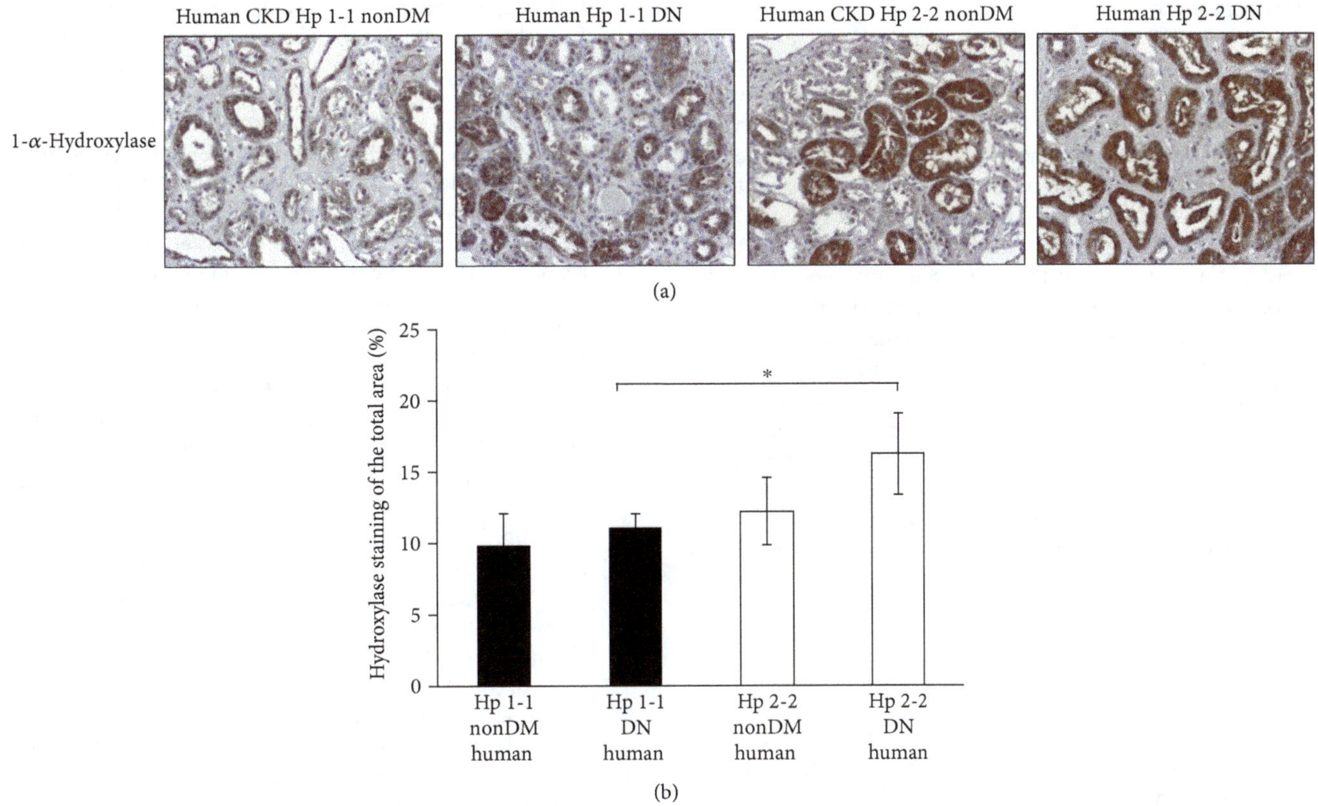

FIGURE 8: 1-α-Hydroxylase expression in diabetic and nondiabetic (nonDM) CKD patients. (a) Slides from human's renal biopsies were subjected to IHC of 1-α-hydroxylase. (b) There was a significant increase in the percentage of the stained area of 1-α-hydroxylase in the tubules of Hp 2-2 DM renal sections compared with Hp 1-1 DM sections ($^*p < 0.05$) but insignificant compared with the nonDM Hp 2-2 genotype.

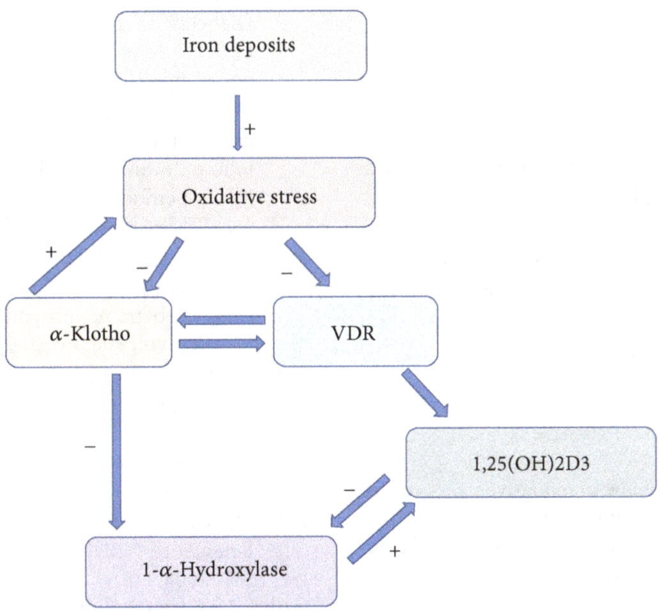

FIGURE 9: Suggested mechanism for the renal proximal convoluted tubule (PCT) injury in Hp 2-2 DN. The increased iron deposits in the PCT of the Hp 2-2 genotype generate a prooxidative environment in the kidney, leading to reduced renal expression of α-klotho and VDR proteins accompanied by an increased level of PCT injury. This subsequently interferes with vitamin D activation by 1-α-hydroxylase in the PCT, thereby increasing the kidney injury and the incidence of DN and its complications.

5. Conclusion

We conclude that the iron-klotho-VDR axis is a key player in the mechanism contributing to iron-mediated PCT injury in DN mice and patients with Hp 2-2 genotype. Based on our observations, we suggest a novel pathophysiological mechanism explaining why DN patients with Hp 2-2 genotypes suffer from severe renal PCT injury as well as why the progression to end-stage renal disease is increased in these patients. We propose that the increased iron deposits in the PCT of the Hp 2-2 genotype generate a prooxidative environment in the kidney, leading to reduced renal expression of α-klotho and VDR proteins, accompanied with a high level of PCT injury. It subsequently interferes with vitamin D activation by 1-α-hydroxylase in the PCT, thereby increasing the kidney injury and the incidence of DN or its complications among Hp 2-2 genotype patients (Figure 9). We believe that targeting the iron-klotho-vitamin D axis especially in DM Hp 2-2 patients may open the way for new ideas regarding the pathogenesis and treatment of early stages of DN [33].

Disclosure

The current manuscript was presented as a poster at The 6th World Congress on Controversies to Consensus in Diabetes, Obesity, and Hypertension.

Conflicts of Interest

The authors declare that the institution of Andrew Levy owns rights to a patent on haptoglobin phenotype prediction of diabetic complications.

Acknowledgments

This work was funded in part by the Israel Science Foundation grant to Andrew P. Levy and by Migal, Galilee Research Institute grant to Farid Nakhoul. Authors also acknowledge Professor Edmond Sabo for his helpful advises and his technical help during IHC quantification and Sophia Tehawkho, Tina Ashmoz, Remah Abbas, and Sagi Gleitman for their technical help during the experiments.

References

[1] J. Makuc and D. Petrovic, "A review of oxidative stress related genes and new antioxidant therapy in diabetic nephropathy," *Cardiovascular & Hematological Agents in Medicinal Chemistry*, vol. 9, no. 4, pp. 253–261, 2011.

[2] A. P. Levy, J. E. Levy, S. Kalet-Litman et al., "Haptoglobin genotype is a determinant of iron, lipid peroxidation, and macrophage accumulation in the atherosclerotic plaque," *Arteriosclerosis, Thrombosis, and Vascular Biology*, vol. 27, no. 1, pp. 134–140, 2007.

[3] I. Dahan, N. Thauho, F. Nakhoul, N. Nakhoul, H. Jabaly, and E. Farber, "Haptoglobin polymorphism as an independent predictor of diabetic nephropathy and retinopathy," *Harefuah*, vol. 155, no. 7, pp. 439–442, 2016.

[4] D. M. Nathan and for the DCCT/EDIC Research Group, "The diabetes control and complications trial/epidemiology of diabetes interventions and complications study at 30 years: overview," *Diabetes Care*, vol. 37, no. 1, pp. 9–16, 2014.

[5] T. J. Orchard, W. Sun, P. A. Cleary et al., "Haptoglobin genotype and the rate of renal function decline in the diabetes control and complications trial/epidemiology of diabetes interventions and complications study," *Diabetes*, vol. 62, no. 9, pp. 3218–3223, 2013.

[6] M. Melamed-Frank, O. Lache, B. I. Enav et al., "Structure-function analysis of the antioxidant properties of haptoglobin," *Blood*, vol. 98, no. 13, pp. 3693–3698, 2001.

[7] A. P. Levy, R. Asleh, S. Blum et al., "Haptoglobin: basic and clinical aspects," *Antioxidants & Redox Signaling*, vol. 12, no. 2, pp. 293–304, 2010.

[8] R. Asleh, J. Guetta, S. Kalet-Litman, R. Miller-Lotan, and A. P. Levy, "Haptoglobin genotype- and diabetes-dependent differences in iron-mediated oxidative stress in vitro and in vivo," *Circulation Research*, vol. 96, no. 4, pp. 435–441, 2005.

[9] T. Costacou, R. E. Ferrell, and T. J. Orchard, "Haptoglobin genotype: a determinant of cardiovascular complication risk in type 1 diabetes," *Diabetes*, vol. 57, no. 6, pp. 1702–6, 2008.

[10] A. P. Levy, I. Hochberg, K. Jablonski et al., "Haptoglobin phenotype is an independent risk factor for cardiovascular disease in individuals with diabetes: the Strong Heart Study," *Journal of the American College of Cardiology*, vol. 40, no. 11, pp. 1984–1990, 2002.

[11] T. J. Orchard, J. C. Backlund, T. Costacou et al., "Haptoglobin 2-2 genotype and the risk of coronary artery disease in the Diabetes Control and Complications Trial/Epidemiology of Diabetes Interventions and Complications study (DCCT/EDIC)," *Journal of Diabetes and its Complications*, vol. 30, no. 8, pp. 1577–1584, 2016.

[12] I. Dahan, E. Farber, N. Thauho et al., "Interaction between the haptoglobin 2 phenotype and diabetes mellitus on systolic pulmonary arterial pressure and nitric oxide bioavailability in hemodialysis patients," *Journal of Diabetes Research*, vol. 2015, Article ID 613860, 7 pages, 2015.

[13] F. Nakhoul, N. Nakhoul, R. Asleh, R. Miller-Lotan, and A. P. Levy, "Is the Hp 2-2 diabetic mouse model a good model to study diabetic nephropathy?," *Diabetes Research and Clinical Practice*, vol. 100, no. 3, pp. 289–297, 2013.

[14] R. Asleh, F. M. Nakhoul, R. Miller-Lotan et al., "Poor lysosomal membrane integrity in proximal tubule cells of haptoglobin 2-2 genotype mice with diabetes mellitus," *Free Radical Biology & Medicine*, vol. 53, no. 4, pp. 779–786, 2012.

[15] M. Kuro-o, "Klotho as a regulator of oxidative stress and senescence," *Biological Chemistry*, vol. 389, no. 3, pp. 233–241, 2008.

[16] I. M. Kacso, C. I. Bondor, and G. Kacso, "Soluble serum klotho in diabetic nephropathy: relationship to VEGF-A," *Clinical Biochemistry*, vol. 45, no. 16-17, pp. 1415–1420, 2012.

[17] S. Devaraj, B. Syed, A. Chien, and I. Jialal, "Validation of an immunoassay for soluble klotho protein: decreased levels in

diabetes and increased levels in chronic kidney disease," *American Journal of Clinical Pathology*, vol. 137, no. 3, pp. 479–485, 2012.

[18] S. S. Kim, S. H. Song, I. J. Kim et al., "Decreased plasma α-klotho predict progression of nephropathy with type 2 diabetic patients," *Journal of Diabetes and its Complications*, vol. 30, no. 5, pp. 887–892, 2016.

[19] N. Koh, T. Fujimori, S. Nishiguchi et al., "Severely reduced production of klotho in human chronic renal failure kidney," *Biochemical and Biophysical Research Communications*, vol. 280, no. 4, pp. 1015–1020, 2001.

[20] F. Nie, D. Wu, H. Du et al., "Serum klotho protein levels and their correlations with the progression of type 2 diabetes mellitus," *Journal of Diabetes and its Complications*, vol. 31, no. 3, pp. 594–598, 2017.

[21] Y. Wang and Z. Sun, "Current understanding of klotho," *Ageing Research Reviews*, vol. 8, no. 1, pp. 43–51, 2009.

[22] M. C. Hu, M. Kuro-o, and O. W. Moe, "Renal and extrarenal actions of klotho," *Seminars in Nephrology*, vol. 33, no. 2, pp. 118–129, 2013.

[23] M. C. Hu, K. Shiizaki, M. Kuro-o, and O. W. Moe, "Fibroblast growth factor 23 and klotho: physiology and pathophysiology of an endocrine network of mineral metabolism," *Annual Review of Physiology*, vol. 75, no. 1, pp. 503–533, 2013.

[24] W. Al-Badr and K. J. Martin, "Vitamin D and kidney disease," *Clinical Journal of the American Society of Nephrology*, vol. 3, no. 5, pp. 1555–1560, 2008.

[25] Y. Wang, M. L. Borchert, and H. F. Deluca, "Identification of the vitamin D receptor in various cells of the mouse kidney," *Kidney International*, vol. 81, no. 10, pp. 993–1001, 2012.

[26] Y. Wang, D. K. Deb, Z. Zhang et al., "Vitamin D receptor signaling in podocytes protects against diabetic nephropathy," *Journal of the American Society of Nephrology*, vol. 23, no. 12, pp. 1977–1986, 2012.

[27] R. Agarwal, "Vitamin D, proteinuria, diabetic nephropathy, and progression of CKD," *Clinical Journal of the American Society of Nephrology*, vol. 4, no. 9, pp. 1523–1528, 2009.

[28] W. Koch, W. Latz, M. Eichinger et al., "Genotyping of the common haptoglobin Hp 1/2 polymorphism based on PCR," *Clinical Chemistry*, vol. 48, no. 9, pp. 1377–1382, 2002.

[29] A. Inci, F. Sari, M. Coban et al., "Soluble klotho and fibroblast growth factor 23 levels in diabetic nephropathy with different stages of albuminuria," *Journal of Investigative Medicine*, vol. 64, no. 6, pp. 1128–1133, 2016.

[30] J. Miranda, R. Romero, S. J. Korzeniewski et al., "The anti-aging factor α-klotho during human pregnancy and its expression in pregnancies complicated by small-for-gestational-age neonates and/or preeclampsia," *The Journal of Maternal-Fetal & Neonatal Medicine*, vol. 27, no. 5, pp. 449–457, 2013.

[31] R. Nagai, Y. Saito, Y. Ohyama et al., "Endothelial dysfunction in the klotho mouse and downregulation of klotho gene expression in various animal models of vascular and metabolic diseases," *Cellular and Molecular Life Sciences*, vol. 57, no. 5, pp. 738–746, 2000.

[32] F. Sari, A. Inci, S. Dolu, H. Y. Ellidag, R. Cetinkaya, and F. F. Ersoy, "High serum soluble α-klotho levels in patients with autosomal dominant polycystic kidney disease," *Journal of Investigative Medicine*, vol. 65, no. 2, pp. 358 362, 2016.

[33] Y. Ikeda, H. Enomoto, S. Tajima et al., "Dietary iron restriction inhibits progression of diabetic nephropathy in db/db mice," *American Journal of Physiology-Renal Physiology*, vol. 304, no. 7, pp. F1028–F1036, 2013.

[34] R. Asleh, S. Blum, S. Kalet-Litman et al., "Correction of HDL dysfunction in individuals with diabetes and the haptoglobin 2-2 genotype," *Diabetes*, vol. 57, no. 10, pp. 2794–2800, 2008.

[35] M. Mitobe, T. Yoshida, H. Sugiura, S. Shirota, K. Tsuchiya, and H. Nihei, "Oxidative stress decreases klotho expression in a mouse kidney cell line," *Nephron Experimental Nephrology*, vol. 101, no. 2, pp. e67–e74, 2005.

[36] K. Saito, N. Ishizaka, H. Mitani, M. Ohno, and R. Nagai, "Iron chelation and a free radical scavenger suppress angiotensin II-induced downregulation of klotho, an anti-aging gene, in rat," *FEBS Letters*, vol. 551, no. 1–3, pp. 58–62, 2003.

[37] D. K. Deb, T. Sun, K. E. Wong et al., "Combined vitamin D analog and AT1 receptor antagonist synergistically block the development of kidney disease in a model of type 2 diabetes," *Kidney International*, vol. 77, no. 11, pp. 1000–1009, 2010.

[38] M. Hamzawy, S. A. A. Gouda, L. Rashid, M. Attia Morcos, H. Shoukry, and N. Sharawy, "The cellular selection between apoptosis and autophagy: roles of vitamin D, glucose and immune response in diabetic nephropathy," *Endocrine*, vol. 58, no. 1, pp. 66–80, 2017.

[39] Y. C. Li, "Podocytes as target of vitamin D," *Current Diabetes Reviews*, vol. 7, no. 1, pp. 35–40, 2011.

[40] T. K. Thethi, M. A. Bajwa, H. Ghanim et al., "Effect of paricalcitol on endothelial function and inflammation in type 2 diabetes and chronic kidney disease," *Journal of Diabetes and its Complications*, vol. 29, no. 3, pp. 433–437, 2015.

[41] J. Guo, C. Lu, F. Zhang et al., "VDR activation reduces proteinuria and high-glucose-induced injury of kidneys and podocytes by regulating Wnt signaling pathway," *Cellular Physiology and Biochemistry*, vol. 43, no. 1, pp. 39–51, 2017.

[42] H. Sugiura, T. Yoshida, S. Shiohira et al., "Reduced klotho expression level in kidney aggravates renal interstitial fibrosis," *American Journal of Physiology-Renal Physiology*, vol. 302, no. 10, pp. F1252–F1264, 2012.

[43] C. Rüster, S. Franke, S. Reuter, R. Mrowka, T. Bondeva, and G. Wolf, "Vitamin D3 partly antagonizes advanced-glycation endproducts-induced NFκB activation in mouse podocytes," *Nephron*, vol. 134, no. 2, pp. 105–116, 2016.

[44] M. D. Breyer, E. Böttinger, Brosius FC 3rd et al., "Mouse models of diabetic nephropathy," *Journal of the American Society of Nephrology*, vol. 16, no. 1, pp. 27–45, 2005.

8

Association between *MYH9* and *APOL1* Gene Polymorphisms and the Risk of Diabetic Kidney Disease in Patients with Type 2 Diabetes in a Chinese Han Population

Hailing Zhao,[1] Liang Ma,[2] Meihua Yan,[1] Yan Wang,[1,3] Tingting Zhao,[1] Haojun Zhang,[1] Peng Liu,[1,3] Yanzhen Liu,[1] and Ping Li[1]

[1]*Beijing Key Lab for Immune-Mediated Inflammatory Diseases, Institute of Clinical Medical Science, China-Japan Friendship Hospital, Beijing, China*
[2]*Clinical Laboratory, China-Japan Friendship Hospital, Beijing, China*
[3]*Graduate School of Peking Union Medical College, Chinese Academy of Medical Science and Peking Union Medical College, Beijing, China*

Correspondence should be addressed to Ping Li; lp8675@163.com

Academic Editor: Secundino Cigarran

Single-nucleotide polymorphisms (SNPs) in *MYH9-APOL1* gene regions have been reported to be associated with diabetic kidney disease (DKD) in the American population. We examined the association between polymorphisms in *MYH9-APOL1* and DKD susceptibility in a Chinese Han population. *MYH9* rs3752462 (T>C) and *APOL1* rs136161 (C>G) were genotyped in 303 DKD patients and 364 type 2 diabetes mellitus (T2DM) patients without kidney disease using the TaqMan SNP genotyping assay. Chi-squared test and multivariate logistic regression were used to evaluate the association. We observed that only *MYH9* rs3752462 was associated with DKD (genotype, $P = 0.004$; allele, $P = 0.002$). Genetic model analysis revealed that rs3752462 was associated with increased risk of DKD under a dominant model adjusted by age and sex (adjusted odds ratio (aOR), 1.675; 95% CI 1.225–2.289; $P = 0.001$) and an additive model (TC versus TT: aOR, 1.649; 95% CI 1.187–2.290; CC versus TT: aOR, 1.817; 95% CI 0.980–3.367; $P = 0.005$). The combined effect of rs3752462 TC + rs136161 CC genotype showed an association of DKD adjusted by age and sex (aOR, 1.732; 95% CI 1.128–2.660; $P = 0.012$). After a Holm-Bonferroni correction for multiple tests, the C allele frequencies of the rs3752462 and the TC + CC genotype in the dominant model were considered statistically significant with a markedly increased risk of DKD ($P < 0.00208$; $P < 0.002$). Our results suggest that *MYH9* rs3752462 is significantly associated with an increased risk of DKD in Chinese Han individuals.

1. Introduction

Diabetic kidney disease (DKD) is a common and serious microvascular complication of diabetes mellitus (DM), which is characterized by an elevated urinary albumin excretion rate, elevated blood pressure, and declined renal function. Approximately 30–40% of DM patients will develop DKD, which is the leading cause of end-stage renal disease (ESRD) and renal failure [1]. Genetic factors appear critical in its pathogenesis based upon the evidence including aggregation in families, variable incidence rates of DKD between different races, and the highly heritable nature of diabetic renal clinic and histologic changes [2]. Compared to the Caucasian population, the Asia populations are more likely to suffer from DKD [3]. Identification of potentially susceptible genes and loci is needed to facilitate earlier identification and prevention of DKD, particularly in China.

The *MYH9* gene located on chromosome 22 q12.3-13.2 encodes nonmuscle myosin IIA. The approximately 224 kDa protein is widely expressed in most cells in the body [4, 5]. Polymorphisms in *MYH9* have been strongly associated with ESRD according to genome-wide association studies (GWAS), including human immunodeficiency virus- (HIV-) associated nephropathy in African Americans and idiopathic focal segmental glomerulosclerosis in European Americans and Hispanic Americans. Multiple common single-nucleotide polymorphisms (SNPs) in *MYH9* are associated with a greater risk for nondiabetic ESRD [6–8]. The *APOL1* gene, which is also located on chromosome 22, encodes apolipoprotein L-1. This gene has been associated with kidney disease in African Americans [9]. *APOL1* gene polymorphisms have also been more intensely associated with the risk of kidney disease previously attributed to *MYH9* [10]. The two genes cosegregate in many populations, which makes it difficult to differentiate between the two association signals.

A few studies reported the association of *MYH9* or *APOL1* with DKD. A GWAS and transethnic meta-analysis established the significant associations of *MYH9* and *APOL1* on chromosome 22 q12.3 with DKD in European American, African American, and American Indian populations. Furthermore, *MYH9* (rs5750250)-*APOL1* (rs136161) contributed the strongest association with DKD in African American populations [11]. Another study reported the association of four *MYH9* SNPs (rs4821480, rs2032487, rs4281481, and rs3752462) with T2DM-ESRD susceptibility in European Americans [8]. However, among them, only *MYH9* rs3752462 and *APOL1* rs136161 present genetic polymorphisms in Chinese Han individuals.

The susceptibility of *MYH9* and *APOL1* polymorphisms with DKD in Chinese populations has not been well studied. Considering the strong ethnic heterogeneity for gene polymorphisms, we evaluated the association of *MYH9* rs3752462 (T>C) and *APOL1* rs136161 (C>G) with DKD in a Chinese Han population.

2. Materials and Methods

2.1. Subjects. The clinic-based, case-control study recruited a total of 667 volunteers with T2DM. Among them, 303 patients with a history of DKD were defined as the case group. The remaining 364 participants, who had been diagnosed as T2DM for at least 7 years and had no history of DKD, were defined as the control group, regardless of age and sex.

Type 2 diabetes patients were diagnosed according to the 2012 American Diabetes Association diagnostic criteria; DKD patients were defined by the National Kidney Foundation Kidney Disease Outcomes Quality Initiative (NKF K-DOQI) guidelines.

This study was approved by the institutional ethics committee of the China-Japan Friendship Hospital (Beijing, China), and written informed consent was obtained from all individuals.

2.2. DNA Isolation and Genotyping. Genomic DNA was extracted from peripheral blood using the QIAamp DNA Blood Mini Kit (Qiagen, Hilden, Germany) in accordance with the manufacturer's protocol and quantified using a NanoDrop 1000 spectrophotometer (Thermo Scientific, Waltham, MA, USA). Genotyping was confirmed using the TaqMan SNP genotyping assay (Applied Biosystems, Waltham, MA, USA) and the ABI PRISM 7500 Sequence Detection System (Applied Biosystems).

Polymerase chain reaction (PCR) amplification was performed in a 25 μL reaction mixture containing 50 ng DNA, 12.5 μL of Premix Ex Taq (Takara, Shiga, Japan), 5 pmol of each primer (Applied Biosystems), and 3 pmol of each probe (Applied Biosystems). The amplification conditions consisted of 40 cycles of 95°C for 10 min, 92°C for 15 seconds, and 60°C for 1 min. The primers used to detect SNPs were synthesized by Applied Biosystems.

To verify genotypes, the PCR products were randomly selected for DNA sequencing analysis by TsingKe Biological Technology (Beijing, China) and the results were compared with the results of TaqMan genotyping. The primers used for the PCR were rs3752462, 5′-AAGACACCTCCACAAC CAACAC-3′ (forward) and 5′-GCTCTTCAACCACACCAT GTTC-3′ (reverse), and rs136161, 5′-CTCTCTTGCTG GCT TATGGAA-3′ (forward) and 5′-GCTGTGATGTGGGACT TGTTT-3′ (reverse).

2.3. Statistical Analyses. Clinical data, including age, gender, body mass index (BMI), blood pressure, duration of diabetes, A1C, total cholesterol (TC), high-density lipoprotein cholesterol (HDL-C), low-density lipoprotein cholesterol (LDL-C), triglyceride (TG), and homocysteine (Hcy), were non-Gaussian distributed. Wilcoxon signed-rank test was used to analyze the differences in clinical characteristics of the DKD and diabetic groups, and the data are presented as median (interquartile range). The Hardy-Weinberg equilibrium analysis of both SNPs was conducted using the Chi-squared test. The genotype and allelic frequencies of SNPs were also assessed by the Chi-squared test.

Multivariate logistic regression was carried out to analyze the association between each SNP and susceptibility to DKD after adjustment for age and gender in the additive, recessive, or dominant models. Multivariate logistic regression was also used for the combined effect of both *MYH9* rs3752462 and *APOL1* rs136161 polymorphism on DKD. An example to define these genetic models is the rs3752462 SNP, where C is the minor allele. For the dominant model, CC and TC were coded as 1 and TT was coded as 0. For the recessive model, CC was coded as 1 and TC and TT were coded as 0. For the additive model, CC, TC, and TT were coded as 2, 1, and 0, respectively. For SNP rs136161, G is the minor allele.

The Holm-Bonferroni correction was started by ordering the P values (from lowest to highest) as $P_{(1)} \ldots P_{(m)}$ and let the associated hypotheses be $H_{(1)} \ldots H_{(m)}$. For a given significance level α, let κ be the minimal index such that $P > \alpha/(m + 1 - \kappa)$. Reject the null hypotheses $H_{(1)} \ldots H_{(\kappa-1)}$ and reject $H_{(\kappa)} \ldots H_{(m)}$. In present research, association analysis was performed for 26 times, $m = 26$.

3. Results

3.1. Subjects. A total of 667 T2DM participants were included, including 303 patients with a history of DKD and 364 patients without a history of kidney disease. The clinical characteristics of the participants are listed in Table 1.

Table 1: Demographics and clinical characteristics of T2DM patients with and without kidney diseases.

Variables	DKD ($n = 303$)[a]	DM ($n = 364$)[a]	P
Age (y)	63.0 (55.0, 72.0)	61.0 (54.0, 68.0)	0.002
Sex, male (%)	63.4 (192/303)	58.0 (211/364)	0.156
BMI (kg/m^2)	25.82 (24.0, 28.23)	25.29 (23.2, 27.78)	0.008
Duration of diabetes (y)	15.0 (9.0, 21.0)	13.0 (10.0, 18.0)	0.039
History of hypertension (%)	77.56 (235/303)	48.08 (175/364)	<0.001
Current smoking (%)	33.0 (100/303)	26.6 (97/364)	0.073
SBP (mmHg)	138.0 (125.0, 150.0)	126.0 (120.0, 139.8)	<0.001
DBP (mmHg)	80.0 (75.0, 84.0)	80.0 (70.0, 80.0)	0.026
A1C (%)	8.0 (6.7, 9.35)	7.5 (6.5, 9.2)	0.037
Hcy (μmol/L)	13.89 (11.09, 17.22)	11.49 (9.54, 13.62)	<0.001
TC (mmol/L)	4.21 (3.49, 5.06)	4.17 (3.55, 4.92)	0.51
HDL-C (mmol/L)	0.96 (0.78, 1.18)	1.02 (0.85, 1.24)	0.004
LDL-C (mmol/L)	2.34 (1.86, 3.05)	2.38 (1.91, 2.96)	0.74
TG (mmol/L)	1.74 (1.22, 2.57)	1.43 (1.0, 2.17)	<0.001

Abbreviations: A1C, hemoglobin A1C; BMI, body mass index; DBP, diastolic blood pressure; Hcy, homocysteine; HDL-C, high-density lipoprotein cholesterol; LDL-C, low-density lipoprotein cholesterol; SBP, systolic blood pressure; TC, total cholesterol; TG, triglyceride. [a]Data are shown as median (interquantile range) or %. $P < 0.05$ indicates statistical significance.

There were no significant differences in gender, smoking, TC, and LDL-C between the two groups. However, there were significant differences in age, BMI, duration of diabetes, blood pressure, A1C, Hcy, HDL-C, and TG between the DKD and T2DM groups.

3.2. Genotype and Allele Distributions of MYH9 rs3752462 and APOL1 rs136161 Polymorphisms. The genotype and allele frequencies of the rs3752462 and rs136161 polymorphisms in DKD and T2DM groups are shown in Table 2. Both SNPs were in Hardy-Weinberg equilibrium ($P > 0.05$), and their minor allele frequencies were >5%. The genotype and allele frequencies of the rs3752462 were different between DKD and T2DM groups (genotype, $P = 0.004$; allele, $P = 0.002$). A significant association with the increased risk of DKD remained for the minor allele C after a Holm-Bonferroni correction ($P < 0.00208$). However, there was no significant differences in the genotype and allele frequencies of the rs136161 between the two groups (genotype, $P = 0.944$; allele, $P = 0.751$).

3.3. Association of MYH9 rs3752462 and APOL1 rs136161 Polymorphisms with DKD. Different genetic models were applied to verify the associations of *MYH9* rs3752462 and *APOL1* rs136161 polymorphisms with DKD (Table 3). We assumed that the minor alleles of both SNPs were the risk factors compared to the common alleles. In the dominant model, multivariate logistic regression analysis revealed that when the rs3752462 TT genotype was used as the reference, the TC + CC genotype was associated with a high risk of DKD (TC + CC versus TT: odds ratio (OR), 1.690; 95% CI 1.240–2.303; $P = 0.001$). In the additive model, when the rs3752462 TT homozygote genotype was used as the reference, the TC and CC genotypes were associated with a decreased risk of DKD (TC versus TT: OR, 1.684; 95% CI 1.216–2.332; CC versus TT: OR, 1.720; 95% CI 0.935–3.162; $P = 0.004$). In the recessive model, when the rs3752462 TT + TC genotype was used as the reference, the CC genotype was not associated with the risk of DKD (CC versus TT + TC: OR, 1.398; 95% CI 0.772–2.533; $P = 0.269$). The results were remained similar after adjusted by age and sex. After the Holm-Bonferroni correction, only the TC + CC genotype showed significant association with an increased risk of DKD ($P < 0.002$). There was no significant association between *APOL1* rs136161 and the risk of DKD under these genetic models, which was remained similar after adjustment for age and sex (Table 3).

3.4. Combined Effect of MYH9 rs3752462 and APOL1 rs136161 Polymorphisms on DKD. Multivariate logistic regression analysis was applied to analyze the combined effect of both SNPs on DKD (Table 4). When the rs3752462 TT + rs136161 CC genotype was used as the reference, we found that the patients with rs3752462 TC + rs136161 CC genotype showed a higher risk of DKD (OR, 1.734; 95% CI 1.134–2.652; $P = 0.011$). The combined effect of other genotypes of rs3752462 and rs136161 was also examined; however, no difference was found. After adjustment by age and sex, the results were similar (Table 4). However, there was no significant association after Holm-Bonferroni correction.

4. Discussion

DKD is one of the most frequent microvascular complications of diabetes and is the leading cause of ESRD worldwide. Genetic heterogeneity and gene-gene or gene-environment interactions are frequently hypothesized as being important in this complex genetic disorder [12]. In the present study, 667 participants (303 DKD patients and 364 DM patients) were enrolled to investigate associations of *MYH9* rs3752462 and *APOL1* rs136161 with the risk of DKD in a

TABLE 2: Genotype and allele frequency of SNPs rs3752462 and rs136161 between DKD patients ($n = 303$) and DM controls ($n = 364$).

	Genotypes, n (%)					Alleles, n (%)		
rs3752462	TT	TC	CC	HWE P value	P	T	C	P
DM	227 (62.4%)	115 (31.6%)	22 (6.0%)	0.155	0.004*	569 (57.1%)	159 (42.9%)	**0.002***,Δ
DKD	150 (49.5%)	128 (42.2%)	25 (8.3%)	0.752		428 (70.6%)	178 (29.4%)	
rs136161	CC	CG	GG	HWE P value	P	C	G	P
DM	213 (58.5%)	126 (34.6%)	25 (6.9%)	0.287	0.944	552 (75.8%)	176 (24.2%)	0.751
DKD	180 (59.4%)	104 (34.3%)	19 (6.3%)	0.449		464 (76.6%)	142 (23.4%)	

*$P < 0.05$; Δ indicates statistical significance by Holm-Bonferroni correction; HWE: Hardy-Weinberg equilibrium.

TABLE 3: Genetic model analyses of the association between the SNPs and DKD with adjustment for age and gender.

	Genetic models	Genotypes	DKD	DM	Without adjustment OR (95% CI)	P	With adjustment OR (95% CI)	P
rs3752462	Additive	TT	150 (49.5%)	227 (62.4%)	1#		1#	
		TC	128 (42.2%)	115 (31.6%)	1.684 (1.216–2.332)	0.004*	1.649 (1.187–2.290)	0.005*
		CC	25 (8.3%)	22 (6.0%)	1.720 (0.935–3.162)		1.817 (0.980–3.367)	
	Dominant	TT	150 (49.5%)	227 (62.4%)	1#	0.001*,Δ	1#	0.001*,Δ
		TC + CC	153 (50.5%)	137 (37.6%)	1.690 (1.240–2.303)		1.675 (1.225–2.289)	
	Recessive	TT + TC	278 (91.8%)	342 (94.0%)	1#	0.269	1#	0.193
		CC	25 (8.2%)	22 (6.0%)	1.398 (0.772–2.533)		1.493 (0.817–2.728)	
rs136161	Additive	CC	180 (59.4%)	213 (58.5%)	1#		1#	
		CG	104 (34.3%)	126 (34.6%)	0.977 (0.704–1.354)	0.944	1.011 (0.726–1.407)	0.901
		GG	19 (6.3%)	25 (6.9%)	0.899 (0.480–1.686)		0.869 (0.460–1.644)	
	Dominant	CC	180 (59.4%)	213 (58.5%)	1#	0.816	1#	0.933
		CG + GG	123 (40.6%)	151 (41.5%)	0.964 (0.707–1.314)		0.987 (0.721–1.350)	
	Recessive	CC + CG	284 (93.7%)	339 (93.1%)	1#	0.757	1#	0.652
		GG	19 (6.3%)	25 (6.9%)	0.907 (0.489–1.681)		0.866 (0.463–1.618)	

Abbreviations: ORs, odds ratios; CI, confidence interval. #Reference category (odds ratio, 1.0); *P value < 0.05; Δ indicates statistical significance by Holm-Bonferroni correction.

TABLE 4: The combined effect of *MYH9* rs3752462 and *APOL1* rs136161 polymorphisms on DKD.

Genotypes rs3752462	rs136161	DKD 303	DM 364	Without adjustment OR (95% CI)	P	With adjustment¶ OR (95% CI)	P
TT	CC	89	134	1#	—	1#	—
TT	CG + GG	61	93	0.988 (0.649–1.503)	0.953	1.039 (0.679–1.588)	0.861
TC	CC	76	66	1.734 (1.134–2.652)	0.011*	1.732 (1.128–2.660)	0.012*
TC	CG + GG	52	49	1.598 (0.995–2.565)	0.052	1.596 (0.989–2.575)	0.055
CC	CC	15	13	1.737 (0.789–3.826)	0.170	1.923 (0.864–4.283)	0.109
CC	CG + GG	10	9	1.673 (0.654–4.281)	0.283	1.736 (0.669–4.503)	0.257

#Reference category (odds ratio, 1.0); ¶Adjustment for age and gender; *P value < 0.05.

Chinese Han population. Our results indicate that the minor allele of SNP rs3752462 is associated with an increased risk of DKD, while *APOL1* rs136161 was not significantly associated with DKD. The results suggest that *MYH9* rs3752462 might play an important role in the risk of DKD in the Chinese Han population.

The first association study of *MYH9* with kidney disease was observed in the patients with the giant platelet syndromes, a group of diseases caused by *MYH9* mutations and with a spectrum of abnormalities including low platelet count, hearing loss, giant platelets, and cataract may present focal segmental glomerular sclerosis (FSGS) [7]. *APOL1* is a neighbor gene presenting very strong cosegregation with *MYH9* in African descendants. Two studies reported stronger association with CKD of *APOL1* than *MYH9*, being the marker possibly responsible for the effect previously attributed to *MYH9* [9, 13]. Previous studies suggested that common polymorphisms in *MYH9* were strongly associated with nondiabetic kidney diseases in several ethnic populations [14–16]. However, polymorphisms in *MYH9* have been proven to be associated with diabetic nephropathy in 1963 European Americans, including 536 cases with T2DM-ESRD and 1427 nonnephropathy controls [8]. A recent GWAS and transethnic meta-analysis showed that SNPs in the *MYH9-APOL1* gene region showed the strongest association with DKD in African Americans, which provided suggestive evidence for association with DKD, although it did not reach genome-wide significance ($P < 5 \times 10^{-8}$) [11]. Our results indicated that *MYH9* rs3752462 was strongly associated with clinically diagnosed DKD in a Chinese Han population, and the minor allele C contributed to the increased risk of DKD, which might be due to genetic heterogeneity. Although the genotype and allele frequencies of *APOL1* rs136161 were not associated with DKD, SNP rs136161 CC genotype combined with SNP rs3752462 TC genotype showed association with the risk of DKD, providing further evidence that single genetic abnormalities were rarely the only cause of complex disease.

MYH9 encodes the nonmuscle myosin heavy chain 9, which forms myosin II with other subunits. Myosin II, a motor protein, binds actin to regulate cellular motility. *MYH9* is mainly expressed in the podocytes, as well as in mesangial cells and arteriolar and peritubular capillaries in kidneys. As a motor protein, abnormal *MYH9* expression, localization, or function change will lead to cytoskeleton damage, further causing proteinuria or renal failure in patients with CKD [17–19]. Classical deletion of *Myh9* in mice results in embryonic lethality due to the loss of cell-cell adhesion and cell movement during gastrulation [20, 21]. Podocytespecific deletion of *Myh9* in C57BL/6 mice causes significant susceptibility to experimental doxorubicin hydrochloride glomerulopathy [22]. A common missense mutation in MYH9 (E1841K) alters podocyte cytoskeletal structure and renders podocytes more susceptible to injury after a damaging stimulus [23]. However, the mechanisms responsible for them have not been defined. Wasik et al. found that the activity of myosin II was reduced by septin 7, which could hinder GLUT4 storage vesicle and fusion with the plasma membrane, reduce glucose uptake into podocytes, and further cause insulin resistance [24]. Fan et al. showed that NM-IIA activity was also inhibited by SLIT2/ROBO2 signaling, which could reduce podocyte adhesion in kidney glomeruli and aggravate the injuries of the glomerular filtration barrier in patients with CKD [25].

SNP rs3752462 is located in intron 13 of *MYH9*, and the functional effect has not been reported. One possibility was that the mutation in noncoding areas modulated gene transcription or pre-mRNA splicing. Furthermore, *MYH9* rs3752462 might directly regulate gene expression or on a more distant gene (such as *APOL1*). It has been reported that the strongest kidney disease association was mapped to the region of introns 13–15 by genotyping 79 *MYH9* SNPs in a total of 2496 cases (FSGS, HIV-associated nephropathy, and ESRD attributed to hypertension) and healthy controls [26]. Therefore, SNP rs3752462 in *MYH9* might be a functional variation or just a tag SNP in strong linkage disequilibrium with the causal functional SNP. This hypothesis needs confirmation in a future study.

Recently, *MYH9* rs3752462 was associated with cerebrovascular blood flow (CBF) in patients with type 2 diabetes [27]. Both cerebrovascular disease and DKD were the main vascular complications of T2DM, which implies similar molecular mechanisms in the association of *MYH9* rs3752462 with cerebrovascular disease and DKD. In addition, the T allele of SNP rs3752462 was associated with an excess risk for high blood pressure in patients with CKD in a Chinese population. It was also revealed that SNP rs3752462 was an independent predictor of a reduced glomerular filtration rate in the Spanish RENASTUR cohort population [28]. Therefore, blood pressure or glomerular filtration rate might be involved in the risk of *MYH9* rs3752462 on DKD.

The association of *MYH9-APOL1* is very interesting in DKD. It could provide the genetic tool to identify DM patients with increased risk of progressing to DKD, at least in populations in whom the mutations are known to be prevalent variations. Comprehension of the biological mechanisms determining proteinuria and CKD in patients presenting these mutations can create opportunity for new therapeutic targets and measures.

In conclusion, our study suggests that *MYH9* SNP rs3752462 is significantly associated with DKD in patients with DM and confirms the minor allele C as a risk factor of DKD. *APOL1* rs136161 was not related to the risk of DKD in our sample, but the result can be related to our small sample size. It will be a current challenge to explore the biological mechanisms underlying this association in future research.

Conflicts of Interest

The authors declare that they have no conflicts of interest.

Authors' Contributions

Hailing Zhao and Liang Ma contributed equally to this work.

Acknowledgments

This study was supported by the National Natural Science Foundation of China (Grant nos. 81503418 and 8162010803) and a Project of International Collaboration in Science and Technology Grant, China (Grant no. 2011DFA31860).

References

[1] A. J. Collins, B. Kasiske, C. Herzog et al., "United States Renal Data System 2006 annual data report abstract," *American Journal of Kidney Diseases*, vol. 49, Supplement 1, pp. A6–A7, 2007.

[2] B. I. Freedman, M. Bostrom, P. Daeihagh, and D. W. Bowden, "Genetic factors in diabetic nephropathy," *Clinical Journal of the American Society of Nephrology*, vol. 2, no. 6, pp. 1306–1316, 2007.

[3] R. Gupta and A. Misra, "Epidemiology of microvascular complications of diabetes in South Asians and comparison with other ethnicities," *Journal of Diabetes*, vol. 8, no. 4, pp. 470–482, 2016.

[4] C. Arrondel, N. Vodovar, B. Knebelmann et al., "Expression of the nonmuscle myosin heavy chain IIA in the human kidney and screening for *MYH9* mutations in Epstein and Fechtner syndromes," *Journal of the American Society of Nephrology*, vol. 13, no. 1, pp. 65–74, 2002.

[5] S. P. Fukuda, T. S. Matsui, T. Ichikawa et al., "Cellular force assay detects altered contractility caused by a nephritis-associated mutation in nonmuscle myosin IIA," *Development, Growth & Differentiation*, vol. 59, no. 5, pp. 423–433, 2017.

[6] W. H. Linda Kao, M. J. Klag, L. A. Meoni et al., "*MYH9* is associated with nondiabetic end-stage renal disease in African Americans," *Nature Genetics*, vol. 40, no. 10, pp. 1185–1192, 2008.

[7] J. B. Kopp, M. W. Smith, G. W. Nelson et al., "*MYH9* is a major-effect risk gene for focal segmental glomerulosclerosis," *Nature Genetics*, vol. 40, no. 10, pp. 1175–1184, 2008.

[8] J. N. Cooke, M. A. Bostrom, P. J. Hicks et al., "Polymorphisms in *MYH9* are associated with diabetic nephropathy in European Americans," *Nephrology Dialysis Transplantation*, vol. 27, no. 4, pp. 1505–1511, 2012.

[9] B. I. Freedman, J. B. Kopp, C. D. Langefeld et al., "The apolipoprotein L1 (*APOL1*) gene and nondiabetic nephropathy in African Americans," *Journal of the American Society of Nephrology*, vol. 21, no. 9, pp. 1422–1426, 2010.

[10] G. A. Hawkins, D. J. Friedman, L. Lu et al., "Re-sequencing of the *APOL1-APOL4* and *MYH9* gene regions in African Americans does not identify additional risks for CKD progression," *American Journal of Nephrology*, vol. 42, no. 2, pp. 99–106, 2015.

[11] S. K. Iyengar, J. R. Sedor, B. I. Freedman et al., "Genome-wide association and trans-ethnic meta-analysis for advanced diabetic kidney disease: family investigation of nephropathy and diabetes (FIND)," *PLoS Genetics*, vol. 11, no. 8, article e1005352, 2015.

[12] G. Dorval, O. Gribouval, V. Martinez-Barquero et al., "Clinical and genetic heterogeneity in familial steroid-sensitive nephrotic syndrome," *Pediatric Nephrology*, vol. 33, no. 3, pp. 473–483, 2018.

[13] S. Tzur, S. Rosset, R. Shemer et al., "Missense mutations in the *APOL1* gene are highly associated with end stage kidney disease risk previously attributed to the *MYH9* gene," *Human Genetics*, vol. 128, no. 3, pp. 345–350, 2010.

[14] B. H. Keeling and B. R. Taylor, "Keloids and non-diabetic kidney disease: similarities and the *APOL1–MYH9* haplotype as a possible genetic link," *Medical Hypotheses*, vol. 81, no. 5, pp. 908–910, 2013.

[15] C. M. O'Seaghdha, R. S. Parekh, S. J. Hwang et al., "The *MYH9*/ *APOL1* region and chronic kidney disease in European-Americans," *Human Molecular Genetics*, vol. 20, no. 12, pp. 2450–2456, 2011.

[16] M. A. Bostrom, L. Lu, J. Chou et al., "Candidate genes for non-diabetic ESRD in African Americans: a genome-wide association study using pooled DNA," *Human Genetics*, vol. 128, no. 2, pp. 195–204, 2010.

[17] N. Singh, N. Nainani, P. Arora, and R. C. Venuto, "CKD in *MYH9*-related disorders," *American Journal of Kidney Diseases*, vol. 54, no. 4, pp. 732–740, 2009.

[18] D. B. Johnstone, O. Ikizler, J. Zhang, and L. B. Holzman, "Background strain and the differential susceptibility of podocyte-specific deletion of *Myh9* on murine models of experimental glomerulosclerosis and HIV nephropathy," *PLoS One*, vol. 8, no. 7, article e67839, 2013.

[19] T. Sekine, M. Konno, S. Sasaki et al., "Patients with Epstein–Fechtner syndromes owing to MYH9 R702 mutations develop progressive proteinuric renal disease," *Kidney International*, vol. 78, no. 2, pp. 207–214, 2010.

[20] A. N. Mhatre, Y. Li, N. Bhatia, K. H. Wang, G. Atkin, and A. K. Lalwani, "Generation and characterization of mice with Myh9 deficiency," *NeuroMolecular Medicine*, vol. 9, no. 3, pp. 205–215, 2007.

[21] J. Crish, M. A. Conti, T. Sakai, R. S. Adelstein, and T. T. Egelhoff, "Keratin 5-Cre-driven excision of nonmuscle myosin IIA in early embryo trophectoderm leads to placenta defects and embryonic lethality," *Developmental Biology*, vol. 382, no. 1, pp. 136–148, 2013.

[22] D. B. Johnstone, J. Zhang, B. George et al., "Podocyte-specific deletion of *Myh9* encoding nonmuscle myosin heavy chain 2A predisposes mice to glomerulopathy," *Molecular and Cellular Biology*, vol. 31, no. 10, pp. 2162–2170, 2011.

[23] S. Cechova, F. Dong, F. Chan, M. J. Kelley, P. Ruiz, and T. H. Le, "*MYH9* E1841K mutation augments proteinuria and podocyte injury and migration," *Journal of the American Society of Nephrology*, vol. 29, no. 1, pp. 155–167, 2018.

[24] A. A. Wasik, V. Dumont, J. Tienari et al., "Septin 7 reduces nonmuscle myosin IIA activity in the SNAP23 complex and hinders GLUT4 storage vesicle docking and fusion," *Experimental Cell Research*, vol. 350, no. 2, pp. 336–348, 2017.

[25] X. Fan, H. Yang, S. Kumar et al., "SLIT2/ROBO2 signaling pathway inhibits nonmuscle myosin IIA activity and destabilizes kidney podocyte adhesion," *JCI Insight*, vol. 1, no. 19, article e86934, 2016.

[26] G. W. Nelson, B. I. Freedman, D. W. Bowden et al., "Dense mapping of *MYH9* localizes the strongest kidney disease associations to the region of introns 13 to 15," *Human Molecular Genetics*, vol. 19, no. 9, pp. 1805–1815, 2010.

[27] C. Ling, C. Y. Cai, B. C. Chang et al., "*MYH9* gene polymorphisms may be associated with cerebrovascular blood flow in patients with type 2 diabetes," *Genetics and Molecular Research*, vol. 14, no. 1, pp. 1008–1016, 2015.

[28] B. Tavira, E. Coto, J. Gómez et al., "Association between a *MYH9* polymorphism (rs3752462) and renal function in the Spanish RENASTUR cohort," *Gene*, vol. 520, no. 1, pp. 73–76, 2013.

9

Role of Epigenetic Histone Modifications in Diabetic Kidney Disease Involving Renal Fibrosis

Jing Sun, Yangwei Wang, Wenpeng Cui, Yan Lou, Guangdong Sun, Dongmei Zhang, and Lining Miao

Department of Nephrology, Second Hospital of Jilin University, Changchun 130041, China

Correspondence should be addressed to Lining Miao; miaolining55@163.com

Academic Editor: Wei J. Liu

One of the commonest causes of end-stage renal disease is diabetic kidney disease (DKD). Renal fibrosis, characterized by the accumulation of extracellular matrix (ECM) proteins in glomerular basement membranes and the tubulointerstitium, is the final manifestation of DKD. The TGF-β pathway triggers epithelial-to-mesenchymal transition (EMT), which plays a key role in the accumulation of ECM proteins in DKD. DCCT/EDIC studies have shown that DKD often persists and progresses despite glycemic control in diabetes once DKD sets in due to prior exposure to hyperglycemia called "metabolic memory." These imply that epigenetic factors modulate kidney gene expression. There is evidence to suggest that in diabetes and hyperglycemia, epigenetic histone modifications have a significant effect in modulating renal fibrotic and ECM gene expression induced by TGF-β1, as well as its downstream profibrotic genes. Histone modifications are also implicated in renal fibrosis through its ability to regulate the EMT process triggered by TGF-β signaling. In view of this, efforts are being made to develop HAT, HDAC, and HMT inhibitors to delay, stop, or even reverse DKD. In this review, we outline the latest advances that are being made to regulate histone modifications involved in DKD.

1. Introduction

One of the main causes of end-stage renal disease is diabetic kidney disease (DKD) [1]. Approximately 20% to 40% of diabetic patients eventually develop DKD. Although the exact cause of DKD is unknown, several factors including genetic, environmental, and hemodynamic factors; high blood glucose; high blood lipids; hypertension; and proteinuria contribute to its development [2]. All these factors appear to modulate the production and action of various growth factors/cytokines and reactive oxygen species (ROS), which will give rise to podocyte damage and interstitial inflammation that participate in the pathogenesis of DKD. This complex set of events ultimately leads to glomerular dysfunction and renal failure due to the deposition of excess extracellular matrix (ECM) proteins and increase in renal glomerulosclerosis [2, 3]. Chronic and relentless fibrosis in both glomerular and tubulointerstitial compartments are characterized by ECM accumulation and an increase in the deposition of collagen, fibronectin, and laminin in mesangial matrix, glomerular basement membranes, and tubulointerstitium, which are pathologic manifestations of DKD [4]. It is known that even after control of hyperglycemia, diabetic patients may continue to develop renal complication with glomerular and tubulointerstitial fibrosis, eventually leading to renal failure [5]. These evidences suggest that epigenetics may have a significant role in the pathobiology of DKD [6].

2. Role of Renal Fibrosis in Diabetic Kidney Disease

The accumulation of ECM proteins is the hallmark of DKD [4, 7]. This is supported by observation that collagens, fibronectin, and laminin are deposited in increased amounts in the glomerular basement membrane and mesangial extracellular matrix, even in the early stages of DKD (microalbuminuria stage), leading to the occurrence of diabetic diffuse glomerulosclerosis [4, 8–10]. In the late stages of diabetic glomerulosclerosis, which is called Kimmelstiel-Wilson lesion, the deposition of type I and III collagens increase severely [11, 12]. Type IV collagen in both serum and urine have been demonstrated to increase in the early and established stages of DKD [13–15]. Thus, it can be seen that accumulation of ECM proteins work throughout the whole process of the renal fibrosis in DKD.

TGF-β1, a broad-spectrum cytokine [16, 17], which could be induced by hyperglycemia, advanced glycation end-products, mitogen-activated protein kinase (MAPK), and protein kinase C (PKC) pathway [18], plays a crucial role in the progression of glomerular enlargement and the excess deposition of ECM in DKD [19, 20]. Hyperlycemia-induced increase in the deposition of matrix proteins that result in glomerulosclerosis is due to the increased expression and activation of TGF-β1 in glomerular cells, podocytes [21], and mesangial cells [22]. In addition, it can also stimulate α-smooth muscle actin (α-SMA), collagen type I expression, and cell hypertrophy [23, 24]. Connective tissue growth factor (CTGF) appears to be a downstream molecule of TGF-β1, ultimately leading to renal fibrosis after activation [25–27]. It has been shown that the profibrotic action of TGF-β1 could be blocked by CTGF antisense oligonucleotides [28]. It is investigated that after activation, CTGF can increase the expression of fibronectin and collagens IV, III, and I and facilitate the deposition and assembly of ECM proteins [29, 30].

It has been shown that activated myofibroblasts are the principal effector cells, and its number could be correlated with the excess deposition of interstitial ECM in DKD [31]. However, the precise origin and activation procedure of myofibroblasts in fibrotic kidneys remains unclear. Studies by Galichon and Hertig [32] revealed that myofibroblasts might arise from tubular epithelial cells through epithelial-to-mesenchymal transition (EMT) in the process of renal fibrosis. In general, it is believed that the transformation of impaired tubular epithelial cells into mesenchymal cells is the most probable mechanism associated with the development of fibrosis in DKD [31]. Both in vitro and in vivo studies revealed that EMT could be triggered by a number of agents, in which profibrotic element transforming growth factor-β1 (TGF-β1) appears to be a major player [33, 34].

3. Diabetes Nephropathy and Metabolic Memory

It is known that despite achieving glycemic control, patients with diabetes, who experienced prior exposure to high glucose levels, continue to develop diabetic complications including DKD. This manifestation is known as "metabolic memory." In the Diabetes Control and Complications Trial (DCCT), wherein conventional versus intensive insulin therapy were compared in type I diabetic patients, it was observed that intensive insulin regimen reduced the incidence or severity of diabetic renopathy, peripheral neuropathy, and retinopathy compared to patients who were on nonintensive insulin therapy [35]. When the DCCT cohort was examined annually for the next eight years, as part of the follow-up to understand the long-term consequences of therapies instituted, referred to as Epidemiology of Diabetes Interventions and Complications (EDIC) study, it was noted that patients who maintained strict glycemic control during the DCCT had a sustained benefit in postponing the advancement of DKD. It was also observed that DKD progression was much less aggressive in the strict glycemic control group compared to the conventional group, even though HbA1c levels did not substantially differ between these two groups during the EDIC phase [36]. In support of these results, it was reported that type 2 diabetic patients, who were under intensive glycemic control, exhibited long-term benefits in the form of a decrease in both macro and microvascular complications, which was referred to as the "legacy effect" [37].

Furthermore, studies performed in experimental animal models also provided additional support to this concept of "metabolic memory." For instance, Li et al. [38] manifested that vascular smooth muscle cells obtained from the aortas of db/db mice (type 2 diabetes) exhibited upregulated proinflammatory responses compared to controls (db/+ mice that were nondiabetic). Similarly, type 1 diabetic rats that had hyperglycemia for several weeks prior to inducing normoglycemia revealed the progression of DKD [39]. Homologous evidence with diabetic rats confirmed that despite islet transplantation (that lasted for at least 12 weeks), which had their hyperglycemia reverted to normoglycemia after six weeks of diabetes, progression of diabetic retinopathy is continuously shown [40]. Previous observations confirm that "metabolic memory" plays a key role in the development of diabetic complications, which calls for more in depth and intense studies to determine the molecular mechanisms underlying this process. These evidences led to the belief that epigenetic factors may have an effect in the pathobiology of "metabolic memory" and diabetic complications.

4. Epigenetics and Histone Modifications

Waddington [41] originally defined epigenetics as being responsible for programmed changes during embryonic development, as a result of "the causal interaction(s) between genes and their products that brings in a change in phenotype." The epigenome acts as a bridge between genetics and the environment, and the epigenetic code modifies gene expression to determine the final phenotype without alterations in DNA sequences [42]. Epigenetic modifications could change disease phenotype by affecting the target gene directly, as a reply to environmental signals and pathologic states such as diet, exercise, toxins, oxidative stress, inflammation, and metabolic changes [43]. Epigenetic alterations of gene(s) have an important effect in the formation and development of embryo, X-chromosome inactivation, genomic imprinting, cell differentiation and identity, stable inheritance of gene expression, function of immune cells, plasticity of stem cells, and cellular responses to environmental signals [44, 45]. Histone modifications and DNA methylation, along with noncoding RNAs, are collectively known as epigenetic modifications that contain the epigenetic information needed for the stable heredity of gene expression prototypes in differentiated cells [45]. Recent investigations have revealed that epigenetic mechanisms play a significant role in the pathobiology of diabetes mellitus and DKD.

Histone modifications, in essence termed posttranslational modifications of histone in chromatin, are an important part of the epigenetic layer that maintains normal cellular transcriptional patterns [46]. Histone modifications mostly occur in the exposed histone amino-terminal tails such as lysine acetylation (Kac), lysine methylation (Kme), and ubiquitination, as well as threonine and serine phosphorylation and arginine methylation [47]. These produce modifications in histone tails and chromatin structure changes that lead to changes in the binding of transcription agents to their respective core promoter elements, resulting in the activation or suppression of special genes [48]. Recently, it was reported that histone modifications, especially histone acetylation and histone methylation modifications, seem to be important in the pathobiology of DKD, which would be discussed in this review.

Histone acetylation, the acetylation of the N-terminal tails of H3K and H4K, is a reversible dynamic process [49]. In general, histone acetylation of the lysine site (such as H3K14ac, H3K9ac, and H4K5ac) of gene promoters stimulates transcriptional activation, while the removal of acetylation is relevant to gene repression [50] (Figure 1). Histone acetylation states are determined both by histone acetyltransferases (HATs) and histone deacetylases (HDACs). P300/CBP (CREB-binding protein), one of the predominant histone acetyltransferases catalyzed lysine acetylation, is a chromatin marker that results in gene activation. In another way, HDACs modulate the removal of acetylation and act as a repressor of gene transcription [45] (Figure 1). Furthermore, HDACs can be assorted into four classes, depending on their sequence similarity and cofactor interactions: class I (HDACs 1, 2, 3, and 8) is nuclear enzymes, extensively expressed in diverse tissue types; class II (HDACs 4, 5, 6,7, 9, and 10) and class IV (HDAC 11), which are chiefly located in the cytoplasm, are expressed in specific tissues; and class III embraces the sirtuin family (SIRT1–7) [51, 52]. The expression of the different family members of HDACs varies from tissue to tissue and exhibits different biological effects. In adult kidneys, all of class I and II HDAC members are expressed [52].

Histone methylation, in contrast to acetylation, is more constant and long-standing [48]. Histone methylation takes place on both arginine and lysine residues, which may be mono-, di-, or trimethylated. Histone methylation could be manifested as gene repression or activation depending upon the residue modified [53]. In general, H3K36me2/3, H3K4me1/2/3, and H3K79me2 are relevant to the activation of gene transcription. However, H3K9me2/3, H3K27me3, and H4K20me3 are considered as repressive chromatin markers [54] (Figure 1). Despite being relatively stable, histone methylation could be dynamically modified through the concerted action of histone methyltransferases (HMTs) and histone demethylases (HDMs) [55]. Due to varying specificities of numerous HDMs, their potential role in various diseases is currently being evaluated.

5. Histone Modifications Participate in the Progression of Diabetic Kidney Disease

Accumulating evidences show that epigenetic histone modification plays a significant role in modulating kidney gene expression under diabetic circumstances (Figure 1). In both in vitro and in vivo investigations related to diabetes, it has been demonstrated that histone lysine methylation and acetylation patterns changed, along with the recruitment of HATs/HDACs or HMTs at gene promoters [6, 48, 56, 57]. Histone hyperacetylation and increased H3K4me are implicated in the modification of islet-specific insulin gene expression in response to changing glucose levels, which correlated with p300 HAT and HMT SET7/9 recruitment [58, 59]. Knockdown of Jhdm2a gene, the H3K9me2 demethylase, has been reported to lead to obesity and hyperlipidemia, implying an important role of histone modifications in diabetes [60]. Monocytes from T1D and T2D patients have been found to have increased H3K9/14Ac in company with the recruitment of HAT p300/CBP at promoters of inflammatory genes TNF-α and COX-2, which resulted in the upregulation of the expression of these inflammatory genes [61]. It was reported that renal mesangial cells induced the transcription of fibrotic genes in reply to TGF-β1, and high glucose is due to the enrichment of active chromatin marks (H3K4me1/2/3, H3K9/14Ac) and the decrease of repressive markers (H3K9me2/me3) at promoters of these genes, along with the histone lysine acetyltransferase (p300/CBP) and histone lysine methyltransferase (SET7) occupancies at fibrotic gene promoters [62, 63]. On the other hand, these effects were significantly reversed by the HAT domain mutations of p300/CBP or SET7/9 gene silencing. Studies in animal models have also revealed epigenetic histone modifications in DKD. Global histone changes associated with the transcription of fibrotic genes related to DKD have also been described [44]. In type 1 diabetic mice, diabetes-induced increases in histone acetylation and HAT activity, as well as the enrichment of H3K9/14Ac and HAT p300/CBP at the fibrotic gene promoters contributed to the upregulation of the expression of fibrotic genes that were significantly and persistently attenuated by a novel curcumin analog C66 treatment [64]. These studies emphasize the critical role played by epigenetic histone modifications in the pathogenesis of diabetic kidney disease. A better apprehension of these variations in histone lysine acetylation and methylation may aid in the identification of new biomarkers and significant therapeutic targets for DKD.

6. Histone Modifications Involve Renal Fibrosis of DKD

A key element in DKD is the excess accumulation of ECM proteins comprising fibronectin, collagens, and laminin in the kidney [65]. It has been widely believed that EMT is triggered by TGF-β1, which is an outstanding mechanism in the progression of fibrosis due to DKD [66], and this can be countered and reversed by BMP-7 [34]. It has been demonstrated that the TGF-β1 has an important role in triggering EMT and the accumulation of ECM proteins

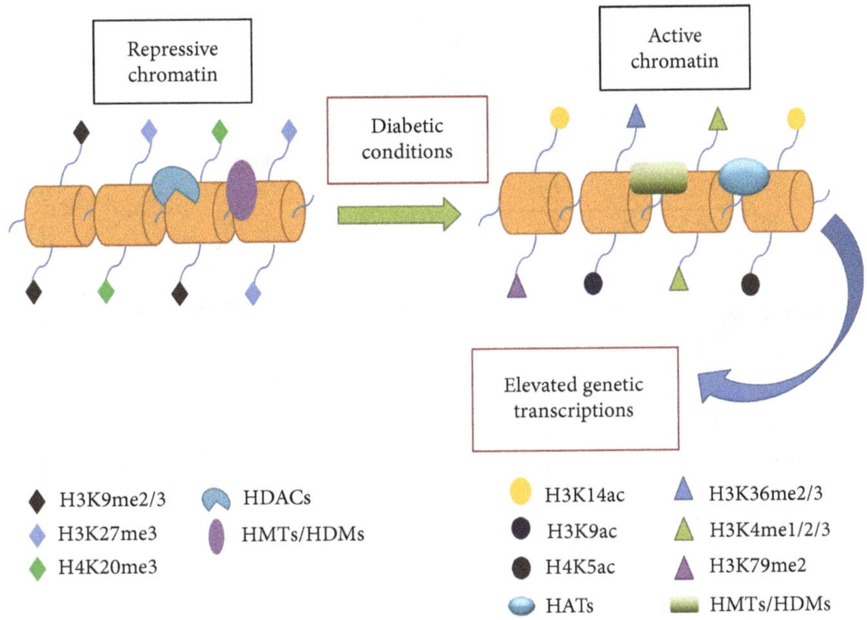

FIGURE 1: Histone modifications stimulate the gene expressions in diabetic conditions. In normal conditions, histone deacetylases (HDACs) and histone methyltransferases (HMTs)/histone demethylases (HDMs) recruit at the gene promoters, leading to the removal of acetylation and the accumulation of repressive chromatin markers (such as H3K9me2/3, H3K27me3, and H4K20me3) at the gene promoters and inhibiting the initiation of genetic transcriptions. While in diabetic conditions, the repressive histone modifications are cleared away and are replaced by the enrichment of active chromatin marks (histone acetylations and H3K36me2/3, H3K4me1/2/3, and H3K79me2), resulting in the upregulation of the expression of inflammatory and fibrotic genes and ultimately promoting the progress of diabetic renal complications. HDACs, histone deacetylases; HATs, histone acetyltransferase; HMTs, histone methyltransferase; HDMs, histone demethylases.

in DKD [18, 67]. Histone modifications also influence the expression and regulation of pathways known to mediate renal fibrosis in DKD.

7. Histone Modifications Promote the Expression of Profibrotic Factors

The profibrotic cytokines such as plasminogen activator inhibitor 1 (PAI-1), connective tissue growth factor (CTGF), and p21 play a significant role in the progression of excess deposition of ECM in DKD. A lot of studies demonstrated that the expressions of profibrotic cytokines were regulated by the histone modifications in diabetic condition (Figure 2). In cultured rat mesangial cell, high glucose and TGF-β1 induced elevation of active Kme marks (H3K4me1, 2, and 3) and decrease of inhibitive marks (H3K9me2 and 3) at PAI-1 and CTGF gene promoters, accompanied with the accumulation of HMT SET7/9 to fibrotic and ECM gene promoters, resulting in the increased expression of these profibrotic proteins [63]. Similarly, in TGF-β1 and high-glucose-treated rat mesangial cells, the enrichment of H3K9/14Ac and HAT p300/CBP at promoters of PAI-1 and p21 gene promoted the facilitation of PAI-1 and p21 production [62]. In a study using type 1 diabetic mice, renal CTGF and PAI-1 gene expressions were augmented by the activation of histone acetylation and HAT activity, as well as the enrichment of H3K9/14Ac and HAT p300/CBP at the promoters of CTGF and PAI-1 gene [64].

8. Histone Modifications Accelerate the Accumulation of ECM Proteins

ECM proteins such as collagen, laminin, and fibronectin, accumulated in mesangial matrix, glomerular basement membranes, and the tubulointerstitium, are pathologic features of DKD. Epigenetic histone modifications may involve in the progression of renal fibrosis of DKD by means of regulating the gene transcription of ECM proteins (Figure 2).

In both in vitro and in vivo diabetic kidney disease, collagen gene expressions can be regulated by histone modifications through the recruitment of HATs/HDACs and HMTs at collagen gene promoters, and histone lysine methylation and acetylation patterns changed. Several studies revealed that histone acetyltransferase p300 accelerates COL1A1/COL1A2 expression in numerous physiological and pathological cellular processes [57, 68–70]. Cultured tubular epithelial cells in diabetic conditions and kidneys of diabetic mice revealed an increased expression of myocardin-related transcription factor A (MRTF-A), which led to the recruitment of p300 and WDR5 to collagen promoters, resulting in transcriptional activation [71]. In contrast, MRTF-A silencing notably resulted in the disappearance of acetylated histone H3K18/K27 and trimethylated histone H3K4 indicative of transcriptional activation. Sun et al. [63] found that in mesangial cells of rat, TGF-β1 and high-glucose treatment increased the levels of positive chromatin marks, such as H3K4me1, H3K4me2, and H3K4me3, and reduced the levels of inhibitive marks including H3K9me2

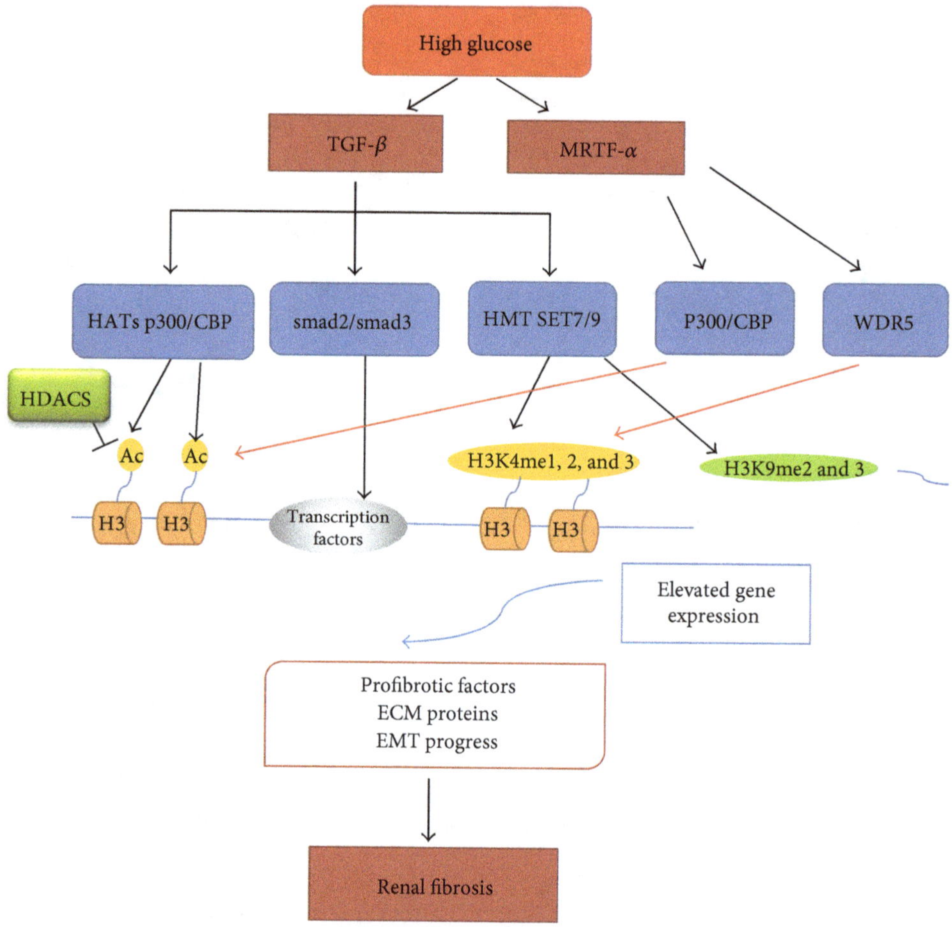

FIGURE 2: Histone modifications regulate gene transcription involving renal fibrosis of diabetic kidney disease. TGF-β signaling pathway, activated by high glucose, will stimulate two types of epigenetic histone mechanisms including histone acetylation and histone methylation. TGF-β1 activates the histone acetyltransferase (HAT) p300/CBP, followed by the enrichment of H3K9/14Ac and HAT p300/CBP at the promoters of renal fibrotic genes, and then increases the transcriptions of fibrotic genes and EMT progress. After induced by TGF-β1, the methyltransferase SET7/9 enriches at fibrotic gene promoters, leading to increases of positive chromatin marks, such as H3K4me1, H3K4me2, and H3K4me3, and reductions of inhibitive marks including H3K9me2 and H3K9me3, at promoters of fibrotic genes. Eventually, the expressions of renal fibrotic genes are upregulated, which will result in the progression of DKD. Another pathway, myocardin-related transcription factor A (MRTF-A), also can be activated by high glucose. MRTF-A can regulate the histone acetylation and histone methylation of renal fibrotic genes by accelerating the recruitment of HAT p300/CBP and HMT WDR5 to fibrotic gene promoters, resulting in transcriptional activation. DKD, diabetic kidney disease; TGF-β, transforming growth factor β; MRTF-A, myocardin-related transcription factor A; HAT, histone acetyltransferase; HDAC, histone deacetylase; HMT, histone methyltransferase; Smad, mothers against decapentaplegic homologue; ECM, excess extracellular matrix; EMT, epithelial-to-mesenchymal transition.

and H3K9me3, at collagen-α1 gene promoters. These changes were found to be associated with the recruitment of H3K4 methyltransferase SET7/9 to collagen-α1 gene promoters, which eventually led to the upregulation of collagen-α1 gene expression. Through siRNA studies, it has been shown that SET7/9 gene silencing attenuates collagen-α1 gene expression induced by TGF-β1. In rat mesangial cells cultured in diabetic conditions or pretreated with TGF-β1, expressions of a methyltransferase SET7 increased, along with the enrichment of SET7 at fibrotic gene Col1a1/Col4a1 promoters. Contrarily, SET7 gene silencing suppressed Col1a1/Col4a1 gene expression [72].

In addition, in high-glucose-treated mesangial cells and diabetic animals, histone modifications stimulated the transcription of fibronectin gene and ECM accumulation, ultimately promoted the progression of renal fibrosis. This is supported by the observation that in rat mesangial cells pretreated TGF-β1 and high glucose, the H3K9/14Ac and HAT p300/CBP assembled at promoters of fibronectin-1 (FN-1) gene, which will bring about the facilitation of FN-1 expression [62]. In another study, it was noted that renal fibronectin-1 (FN-1) gene expression in type 1 diabetic mice was augmented by the enrichment of H3K9/14Ac and HAT p300/CBP at the promoters of the FN-1 gene, which would lead to the development of renal fibrosis and expression of DKD [64].

Both cell culture and animal studies lent support to the effect for HDACs in the regulation of ECM collection and renal fibrosis in DKD [73]. Moreover, a recent study revealed the expression of various HDACs in kidneys of patients with diabetes and streptozotocin- (STZ-) induced diabetic rats, which prove that HDAC4 plays a considerable role in the progression of DKD [74].

9. Histone Modifications Stimulate EMT Progress

EMT is widely recognized as an important mechanism that could result in the transformation of injured renal tubular cells into mesenchymal cells. This transition from renal tubular cells to mesenchymal cells may result in the renal dysfunction all throughout the nephron in chronic renal failure including DKD [18, 31]. Histone modification is similarly involved in kidney fibrosis through the progression of EMT. Yoshikawa et al. [75] reported the global reduction of heterochromatin marker H3K9Me2, increase of euchromatin marker H3K4Me3, and increase of the transcriptional marker H3K36Me3 during the EMT progress, which are mostly dependent upon lysine-specific deaminase-1 (Lsd1). Studies in a unilateral urethral obstruction model revealed that TGF-β1-induced EMT in rat tubular epithelial cells could be blocked by trichostatin A (TSA), a nonselective HDAC inhibitor, leading to the suppression of fibronectin and α-SMA gene expression in the kidney [76]. Additionally, TSA inhibited TGF-β1-stimulated EMT in human proximal convoluted epithelial cells [75]. Similar results have also been reported in STZ-induced diabetes and TGF-β1-intervened tubular epithelial cells from normal rat kidney (NRK52-E), indicating that HDAC-2 has an important role in the progression of DKD [77].

10. TGF-β Signaling Pathway Regulates the Histone Modifications

TGF-β signaling is considerable in the stimulation of the expression of fibrotic and ECM genes associated with changes in posttranscriptional histone modifications in diabetes or hyperglycemia conditions. TGF-β1 regulates fibrotic gene expression by activating transcription factors including Smad2, Smad3, and Smad4, collaborating with HATs and chromatin remodeling factors. This viewpoint is supported by the observation that TGF-β1 and high-glucose treatment led to the enrichment of H3K9/14Ac and HAT p300/CBP interaction with Sp1 and Smad binding sites at promoters of PAI-1 and p21 gene in rat mesangial cells, along with the enhancement of the interaction between p300 and Smad2/3 and Sp1, as well as the increase of Smad2/3 acetylation, followed by the facilitation of PAI-1 and p21 production [62]. In a rat mesangial cell culture model, the increased expression of Col1a1, PAI-1, and CTGF genes induced by TGF-β1 was associated with elevated levels of active Kme marks (H3K4me1, 2, and 3) and reduced levels of inhibitive marks (H3K9me2 and 3) at their promoters and was accompanied with the accumulation of HMT SET7/9 to fibrotic and ECM gene promoters [63]. Conversely, increased fibrotic and ECM levels induced by hyperglycemia and changes in promoter H3Kac and H3Kme, as well as SET7 recruitment, were
ficantly blocked by TGF-β1 antibody treatment, empha-
he significant role of TGF-β1 in hyperglycemia-
igenetic histone modifications [62, 63]. A
ease in HDAC-2 activity has been reported
tic rats induced by STZ and db/db mice,
ated NRK52-E cells [77]. In addition, MS-275, a selective inhibitor of class I HDAC, reversed to a significant degree of fibrosis in DKD by inhibiting TGF-β signaling and renal fibroblast activation [78]. Thus, TGF-β1-induced EMT progress and histone modification seem to have a significant role in the accumulation of ECM and tubular interstitial fibrosis [75–77, 79]. These indicate that histone modification modulates renal fibrotic and ECM gene expression under diabetic conditions through TGF-β signaling (Figure 2).

11. Epigenetic Therapies in Diabetic Kidney Disease to Suppress Renal Fibrosis

In view of the evidences discussed in the preceding section, attempts are being made to inhibit the activities of HAT, HDAC, and HMT, in order to suppress DKD (Table 1). Curcumin, a HAT p300 inhibitor, prevented high-glucose-induced changes in gene transcription levels associated with the downregulation of histone acetylation [80, 81], although further studies revealed that curcumin failed to attenuate albuminuria associated with diabetes mellitus [82]. In contrast, curcumin analog C66 significantly and persistently prevented renal fibrotic gene expression in diabetic mice by inhibiting diabetes-associated increases in p300/CBP expression, HAT activities, and histone acetylation [64]. Furthermore, emerging evidences have shown that HDAC inhibitors with protective effects on kidneys could serve as potential antifibrotic molecules in DKD (Table 1). However, it remains unclear whether the effects of HDACs are due to the inhibition of epigenetics or nonepigenetics [73]. Valproic acid (VPA), an antiepileptic and antimigraine drug, is a nonspecific HDAC inhibitor. A recent study revealed that VPA treatment significantly suppressed histological alterations and fibrosis in diabetic rat kidneys and decreased the fibrotic gene expression and accumulation of ECM proteins [83]. In kidneys of STZ-induced diabetic rats, TSA suppressed the mRNA and protein expression of the constituents of the ECM and ameliorated the EMT progress [77]. Similar beneficial actions were observed in NRK52-E cells in vitro with VPA and class I HDAC-selective inhibitor SK-7041. Due to the complexity of histone methylations and the multiplicity of HMTs, the effects of HMT inhibitors in the renal fibrosis of DKD remain unclear. However, a recent study revealed that histone demethylase JMJDA2A inhibition achieved by chemical inhibitor 2,4-PDCA and siRNA suppressed VSMC migration, proliferation, and inflammation caused by hyperglycemia in vitro and mitigated neointimal formation in balloon-injured diabetic rats [84].

12. Conclusion

The pathogenesis of DKD is complex, in which interactions among injury factors, growth factors/cytokines, ROS, inflammation and fibrosis participate in several signal transduction pathways. Chronic, relentless renal fibrosis and ECM accumulation are pathologic features of DKD. At present, it is widely believed that the TGF-β pathway, which triggers EMT progress, plays a significant role in the accumulation of ECM proteins in DKD. A number of investigations have

Table 1: Effects of HDAC inhibitors on diabetic kidney disease.

HDAC inhibitors	Selectivity	Experimental model	Effects	Mechanism	References
Valproic acid	HDAC I/II	STZ-induced diabetic rat kidneys and TGF-β1-treated NRK52-E cells	Decreases ECM components and prevents EMT	Suppresses TGF-β1-induced activation of HDAC-2	[77]
		STZ-induced diabetic kidneys	Alleviates the renal damage and fibrosis	Repressing the myofibroblast transformation and fibrogenesis	[83]
TSA	HDAC I/II	STZ-induced diabetic rat kidneys and TGF-β1-treated NRK52-E cells	Decreases ECM components and prevents EMT	Suppresses TGF-β1-induced activation of HDAC-2	[77]
		TGF-β1-treated RMCs	Further increased TGF-β1-stimulated PAI-1 gene transcriptional capability and expression	Further amplified TGF-β1-motivated H3K9/14Ac levels	[62]
SK7041	HDAC I	STZ-induced diabetic rat kidneys and TGF-β1-treated NRK52-E cells	Decreases ECM components and prevents EMT	Suppresses TGF-β1-induced activation of HDAC-2	[77]
Vorinostat	HDAC I/II	Cultured proximal tubule cells and STZ-induced diabetic kidneys	Attenuated cellular proliferation, suppressed glomerular hypertrophy	Downregulated EGFR expression	[85]
		STZ-diabetic mice	Decreased oxidative stress, albuminuria, and collagen IV deposition	Interplay between eNOS activity and oxidative stress	[86]
Sodium butyrate (NaB)	Pan HDAC inhibitor	STZ-induced diabetic kidneys	Ameliorated renal function and relieved histological alterations, apoptosis, fibrosis, and DNA damage	NA	[87]

confirmed the presence of "metabolic memory" in the progression of diabetic complications including DKD. Over the past years, epigenetic factors have been implicated in "metabolic memory" and diabetic complications, as described above. Accumulating evidence suggests that in diabetes and hyperglycemia conditions, epigenetic histone modifications play a considerable role in modulating kidney gene expression, which contributes to renal fibrosis and ECM accumulation. Histone modification is likewise involved in kidney fibrosis through the regulation of EMT progress. In addition, TGF-β signaling can stimulate the expression of fibrotic and ECM genes correlated with changes in posttranscriptional histone modifications induced by diabetes or hyperglycemia. As histone modifications are implicated in the progression of kidney fibrosis, several HDAC, HAT, and HMT inhibitors are currently being advanced for the management of DKD, which could attenuate fibrogenesis. Hence, it is imperative to understand the consequences of variations in histone lysine acetylation and methylation, in order to explore novel biomarkers and therapeutic directions for DKD.

Abbreviations

α-SMA: α-Smooth muscle actin
BMP-7: Bone morphogenic protein 7
CTGF: Connective tissue growth factor
DKD: Diabetic kidney disease
ECM: Excess extracellular matrix
EMT: Epithelial-to-mesenchymal transition
FN-1: Fibronectin-1
HAT: Histone acetyltransferase
HDAC: Histone deacetylase
HMT: Histone methyltransferase
MRTF-A: Myocardin-related transcription factor A
PAI-1: Plasminogen activator inhibitor 1
Smad: Mothers against decapentaplegic homologue
STZ: Streptozotocin
TGF-β1: Transforming growth factor β1
TSA: Trichostatin A.

Conflicts of Interest

The authors declare that they have no conflicts of interest.

Acknowledgments

This work was funded in part by the National Natural Science Foundation of China (no. 81600572 and no. 81570652), Science and Technology Development Program funded project of Jilin Province, China (no. 20130206056SF and no. 20150520034JH), Chinese Society of Nephrology (no. 14050440581), and Administration of Traditional Chinese Medicine of Jilin Province funded project (no. 2014-ZP35).

References

[1] Y. S. Kanwar, L. Sun, P. Xie, F. Y. Liu, and S. Chen, "A glimpse of various pathogenetic mechanisms of diabetic nephropathy," *Annual Review of Pathology*, vol. 6, pp. 395–423, 2011.

[2] F. P. Schena and L. Gesualdo, "Pathogenetic mechanisms of diabetic nephropathy," *Journal of the American Society of Nephrology*, vol. 16, Supplement 1, pp. S30–S33, 2005.

[3] G. Wolf, "New insights into the pathophysiology of diabetic nephropathy: from haemodynamics to molecular pathology," *European Journal of Clinical Investigation*, vol. 34, no. 12, pp. 785–796, 2004.

[4] C. R. Ban and S. M. Twigg, "Fibrosis in diabetes complications: pathogenic mechanisms and circulating and urinary markers," *Vascular Health and Risk Management*, vol. 4, no. 3, pp. 575–596, 2008.

[5] L. M. Villeneuve, M. A. Reddy, and R. Natarajan, "Epigenetics: deciphering its role in diabetes and its chronic complications," *Clinical and Experimental Pharmacology & Physiology*, vol. 38, no. 7, pp. 451–459, 2011.

[6] L. M. Villeneuve and R. Natarajan, "Epigenetic mechanisms," *Contributions to Nephrology*, vol. 170, pp. 57–65, 2011.

[7] C. Hu, L. Sun, L. Xiao et al., "Insights into the mechanisms involved in the expression and regulation of extracellular matrix proteins in diabetic nephropathy," *Current Medicinal Chemistry*, vol. 22, no. 24, pp. 2858–2870, 2015.

[8] E. C. Tsilibary, "Microvascular basement membranes in diabetes mellitus," *The Journal of Pathology*, vol. 200, no. 4, pp. 537–546, 2003.

[9] Y. Liu, Z. Wang, W. Yin et al., "Severe insulin resistance and moderate glomerulosclerosis in a minipig model induced by high-fat/ high-sucrose/ high-cholesterol diet," *Experimental Animals*, vol. 56, no. 1, pp. 11–20, 2007.

[10] B. Olgemoller and E. Schleicher, "Alterations of glomerular matrix proteins in the pathogenesis of diabetic nephropathy," *The Clinical Investigator*, vol. 71, 5 Supplement, pp. S13–S19, 1993.

[11] M. B. Stokes, S. Holler, Y. Cui et al., "Expression of decorin, biglycan, and collagen type I in human renal fibrosing disease," *Kidney International*, vol. 57, no. 2, pp. 487–498, 2000.

[12] L. Schaefer, I. Raslik, H. J. Grone et al., "Small proteoglycans in human diabetic nephropathy: discrepancy between glomerular expression and protein accumulation of decorin, biglycan, lumican, and fibromodulin," *The FASEB Journal*, vol. 15, no. 3, pp. 559–561, 2001.

[13] A. Matheson, M. D. Willcox, J. Flanagan, and B. J. Walsh, "Urinary biomarkers involved in type 2 diabetes: a review," *Diabetes/Metabolism Research and Reviews*, vol. 26, no. 3, pp. 150–171, 2010.

[14] K. Tashiro, I. Koyanagi, I. Ohara et al., "Levels of urinary matrix metalloproteinase-9 (MMP-9) and renal injuries in patients with type 2 diabetic nephropathy," *Journal of Clinical Laboratory Analysis*, vol. 18, no. 3, pp. 206–210, 2004.

[15] C. Granier, K. Makni, L. Molina, B. Jardin-Watelet, H. Ayadi, and F. Jarraya, "Gene and protein markers of diabetic nephropathy," *Nephrology, Dialysis, Transplantation*, vol. 23, no. 3, pp. 792–799, 2008.

[16] C. E. Hills, R. Bland, J. Bennett, P. M. Ronco, and P. E. Squires, "TGF-beta1 mediates glucose-evoked up-regulation of connexin-43 cell-to-cell communication in HCD-cells," *Cellular Physiology and Biochemistry*, vol. 24, no. 3-4, pp. 177–186, 2009.

[17] E. P. Bottinger and M. Bitzer, "TGF-beta signaling in renal disease," *Journal of the American Society of Nephrology*, vol. 13, no. 10, pp. 2600–2610, 2002.

[18] C. E. Hills and P. E. Squires, "TGF-beta1-induced epithelial-to-mesenchymal transition and therapeutic intervention in diabetic nephropathy," *American Journal of Nephrology*, vol. 31, no. 1, pp. 68–74, 2010.

[19] J. M. Veeneman, P. E. de Jong, R. M. Huisman, and D. J. Reijngoud, "Re: Adey et al. Reduced synthesis of muscle proteins in chronic renal failure. Am J Physiol Endocrinol Metab 278: E219-E225, 2000," *American Journal of Physiology. Endocrinology and Metabolism*, vol. 280, no. 1, pp. E197–E198, 2001.

[20] K. Sharma, F. N. Ziyadeh, B. Alzahabi et al., "Increased renal production of transforming growth factor-beta1 in patients with type II diabetes," *Diabetes*, vol. 46, no. 5, pp. 854–859, 1997.

[21] H. S. Lee, "Pathogenic role of TGF-beta in the progression of podocyte diseases," *Histology and Histopathology*, vol. 26, no. 1, pp. 107–116, 2011.

[22] H. S. Lee and C. Y. Song, "Differential role of mesangial cells and podocytes in TGF-beta-induced mesangial matrix synthesis in chronic glomerular disease," *Histology and Histopathology*, vol. 24, no. 7, pp. 901–908, 2009.

[23] C. Dai and Y. Liu, "Hepatocyte growth factor antagonizes the profibrotic action of TGF-beta1 in mesangial cells by stabilizing Smad transcriptional corepressor TGIF," *Journal of the American Society of Nephrology*, vol. 15, no. 6, pp. 1402–1412, 2004.

[24] C. E. Hills, N. Al-Rasheed, N. Al-Rasheed, G. B. Willars, and N. J. Brunskill, "C-peptide reverses TGF-beta1-induced changes in renal proximal tubular cells: implications for treatment of diabetic nephropathy," *American Journal of Physiology. Renal Physiology*, vol. 296, no. 3, pp. F614–F621, 2009.

[25] C. Tikellis, M. E. Cooper, S. M. Twigg, W. C. Burns, and M. Tolcos, "Connective tissue growth factor is up-regulated in the diabetic retina: amelioration by angiotensin-converting enzyme inhibition," *Endocrinology*, vol. 145, no. 2, pp. 860–866, 2004.

[26] P. Roestenberg, F. A. van Nieuwenhoven, J. A. Joles et al., "Temporal expression profile and distribution pattern indicate a role of connective tissue growth factor (CTGF/CCN-2) in diabetic nephropathy in mice," *American Journal of Physiology. Renal Physiology*, vol. 290, no. 6, pp. F1344–F1354, 2006.

[27] T. Umezono, M. Toyoda, M. Kato et al., "Glomerular expression of CTGF, TGF-beta 1 and type IV collagen in diabetic nephropathy," *Journal of Nephrology*, vol. 19, no. 6, pp. 751–757, 2006.

[28] B. S. Weston, N. A. Wahab, and R. M. Mason, "CTGF mediates TGF-beta-induced fibronectin matrix deposition by upregulating active alpha5beta1 integrin in human mesangial cells," *Journal of the American Society of Nephrology*, vol. 14, no. 3, pp. 601–610, 2003.

[29] H. M. Kok, L. L. Falke, R. Goldschmeding, and T. Q. Nguyen, "Targeting CTGF, EGF and PDGF pathways to prevent progression of kidney disease," *Nature Reviews. Nephrology*, vol. 10, no. 12, pp. 700–711, 2014.

[30] D. Tampe and M. Zeisberg, "Potential approaches to reverse or repair renal fibrosis," *Nature Reviews. Nephrology*, vol. 10, no. 4, pp. 226–237, 2014.

[31] I. Loeffler and G. Wolf, "Epithelial-to-mesenchymal transition in diabetic nephropathy: fact or fiction?" *Cell*, vol. 4, no. 4, pp. 631–652, 2015.

[32] P. Galichon and A. Hertig, "Epithelial to mesenchymal transition as a biomarker in renal fibrosis: are we ready for the bedside?" *Fibrogenesis Tissue Repair*, vol. 4, 11 pages, 2011.

[33] M. Fragiadaki and R. M. Mason, "Epithelial-mesenchymal transition in renal fibrosis - evidence for and against," *International Journal of Experimental Pathology*, vol. 92, no. 3, pp. 143–150, 2011.

[34] M. Zeisberg, J. Hanai, H. Sugimoto et al., "BMP-7 counteracts TGF-beta1-induced epithelial-to-mesenchymal transition and reverses chronic renal injury," *Nature Medicine*, vol. 9, no. 7, pp. 964–968, 2003.

[35] W. T. D. E. R. Group, "Effect of intensive therapy on the microvascular complications of type 1 diabetes mellitus," *Jama*, vol. 287, no. 19, pp. 2563–2569, 2002.

[36] Writing Team for the Diabetes Control and Complications Trial/Epidemiology of Diabetes Interventions and Complications Research Group, "Sustained effect of intensive treatment of type 1 diabetes mellitus on development and progression of diabetic nephropathy: the Epidemiology of Diabetes Interventions and Complications (EDIC) study," *Jama*, vol. 290, no. 16, pp. 2159–2167, 2003.

[37] G. Schernthaner, "Diabetes and cardiovascular disease: is intensive glucose control beneficial or deadly? Lessons from ACCORD, ADVANCE, VADT, UKPDS, PROactive, and NICE-SUGAR," *Wiener Medizinische Wochenschrift (1946)*, vol. 160, no. 1-2, pp. 8–19, 2010.

[38] S. L. Li, M. A. Reddy, Q. Cai et al., "Enhanced proatherogenic responses in macrophages and vascular smooth muscle cells derived from diabetic db/db mice," *Diabetes*, vol. 55, no. 9, pp. 2611–2619, 2006.

[39] R. A. Kowluru, S. N. Abbas, and S. Odenbach, "Reversal of hyperglycemia and diabetic nephropathy: effect of reinstitution of good metabolic control on oxidative stress in the kidney of diabetic rats," *Journal of Diabetes and Its Complications*, vol. 18, no. 5, pp. 282–288, 2004.

[40] H. P. Hammes, I. Klinzing, S. Wiegand, R. G. Bretzel, A. M. Cohen, and K. Federlin, "Islet transplantation inhibits diabetic retinopathy in the sucrose-fed diabetic Cohen rat," *Investigative Ophthalmology & Visual Science*, vol. 34, no. 6, pp. 2092–2096, 1993.

[41] C. H. Waddington, "The epigenotype. 1942," *International Journal of Epidemiology*, vol. 41, no. 1, pp. 10–13, 2012.

[42] P. W. Franks and J. A. Nettleton, "Invited commentary: gene X lifestyle interactions and complex disease traits—inferring cause and effect from observational data, sine qua non," *American Journal of Epidemiology*, vol. 172, no. 9, pp. 992–997, 2010, discussion 998-999.

[43] M. R. Wing, A. Ramezani, H. S. Gill, J. M. Devaney, and D. S. Raj, "Epigenetics of progression of chronic kidney disease: fact or fantasy?" *Seminars in Nephrology*, vol. 33, no. 4, pp. 363–374, 2013.

[44] M. A. Reddy, J. Tak Park, and R. Natarajan, "Epigenetic modifications in the pathogenesis of diabetic nephropathy," *Seminars in Nephrology*, vol. 33, no. 4, pp. 341–353, 2013.

[45] T. Kouzarides, "Chromatin modifications and their function," *Cell*, vol. 128, no. 4, pp. 693–705, 2007.

[46] R. Bonasio, S. Tu, and D. Reinberg, "Molecular signals of epigenetic states," *Science*, vol. 330, no. 6004, pp. 612–616, 2010.

[47] V. W. Zhou, A. Goren, and B. E. Bernstein, "Charting histone modifications and the functional organization of

mammalian genomes," *Nature Reviews. Genetics*, vol. 12, no. 1, pp. 7–18, 2011.

[48] L. M. Villeneuve and R. Natarajan, "The role of epigenetics in the pathology of diabetic complications," *American Journal of Physiology. Renal Physiology*, vol. 299, no. 1, pp. F14–F25, 2010.

[49] R. Murr, "Interplay between different epigenetic modifications and mechanisms," *Advances in Genetics*, vol. 70, pp. 101–141, 2010.

[50] M. A. Reddy and R. Natarajan, "Epigenetics in diabetic kidney disease," *Journal of the American Society of Nephrology*, vol. 22, no. 12, pp. 2182–2185, 2011.

[51] X. J. Yang and E. Seto, "HATs and HDACs: from structure, function and regulation to novel strategies for therapy and prevention," *Oncogene*, vol. 26, no. 37, pp. 5310–5318, 2007.

[52] A. J. de Ruijter, A. H. van Gennip, H. N. Caron, S. Kemp, and A. B. van Kuilenburg, "Histone deacetylases (HDACs): characterization of the classical HDAC family," *The Biochemical Journal*, vol. 370, Part 3, pp. 737–749, 2003.

[53] S. Jorgensen, G. Schotta, and C. S. Sorensen, "Histone H4 lysine 20 methylation: key player in epigenetic regulation of genomic integrity," *Nucleic Acids Research*, vol. 41, no. 5, pp. 2797–2806, 2013.

[54] G. D. Sun, W. P. Cui, Q. Y. Guo, and L. N. Miao, "Histone lysine methylation in diabetic nephropathy," *Journal of Diabetes Research*, vol. 2014, Article ID 654148, 9 pages, 2014.

[55] M. Wegner, D. Neddermann, M. Piorunska-Stolzmann, and P. P. Jagodzinski, "Role of epigenetic mechanisms in the development of chronic complications of diabetes," *Diabetes Research and Clinical Practice*, vol. 105, no. 2, pp. 164–175, 2014.

[56] S. Tonna, A. El-Osta, M. E. Cooper, and C. Tikellis, "Metabolic memory and diabetic nephropathy: potential role for epigenetic mechanisms," *Nature Reviews. Nephrology*, vol. 6, no. 6, pp. 332–341, 2010.

[57] M. C. Thomas, "Epigenetic mechanisms in diabetic kidney disease," *Current Diabetes Reports*, vol. 16, no. 3, p. 31, 2016.

[58] C. Ling and L. Groop, "Epigenetics: a molecular link between environmental factors and type 2 diabetes," *Diabetes*, vol. 58, no. 12, pp. 2718–2725, 2009.

[59] S. K. Chakrabarti, J. Francis, S. M. Ziesmann, J. C. Garmey, and R. G. Mirmira, "Covalent histone modifications underlie the developmental regulation of insulin gene transcription in pancreatic beta cells," *The Journal of Biological Chemistry*, vol. 278, no. 26, pp. 23617–23623, 2003.

[60] M. A. Reddy and R. Natarajan, "Epigenetic mechanisms in diabetic vascular complications," *Cardiovascular Research*, vol. 90, no. 3, pp. 421–429, 2011.

[61] F. Miao, I. G. Gonzalo, L. Lanting, and R. Natarajan, "In vivo chromatin remodeling events leading to inflammatory gene transcription under diabetic conditions," *The Journal of Biological Chemistry*, vol. 279, no. 17, pp. 18091–18097, 2004.

[62] H. Yuan, M. A. Reddy, G. Sun et al., "Involvement of p300/CBP and epigenetic histone acetylation in TGF-beta1-mediated gene transcription in mesangial cells," *American Journal of Physiology. Renal Physiology*, vol. 304, no. 5, pp. F601–F613, 2013.

[63] G. Sun, M. A. Reddy, H. Yuan, L. Lanting, M. Kato, and R. Natarajan, "Epigenetic histone methylation modulates fibrotic gene expression," *Journal of the American Society of Nephrology*, vol. 21, no. 12, pp. 2069–2080, 2010.

[64] Y. Wang, Y. Wang, M. Luo et al., "Novel curcumin analog C66 prevents diabetic nephropathy via JNK pathway with the involvement of p300/CBP-mediated histone acetylation," *Biochimica et Biophysica Acta*, vol. 1852, no. 1, pp. 34–46, 2015.

[65] S. O. Kolset, F. P. Reinholt, and T. Jenssen, "Diabetic nephropathy and extracellular matrix," *The Journal of Histochemistry and Cytochemistry*, vol. 60, no. 12, pp. 976–986, 2012.

[66] F. C. Brosius 3rd, "New insights into the mechanisms of fibrosis and sclerosis in diabetic nephropathy," *Reviews in Endocrine & Metabolic Disorders*, vol. 9, no. 4, pp. 245–254, 2008.

[67] M. K. Diamond-Stanic, Y. H. You, and K. Sharma, "Sugar, sex, and TGF-beta in diabetic nephropathy," *Seminars in Nephrology*, vol. 32, no. 3, pp. 261–268, 2012.

[68] A. K. Ghosh, S. Bhattacharyya, R. Lafyatis et al., "p300 is elevated in systemic sclerosis and its expression is positively regulated by TGF-beta: epigenetic feed-forward amplification of fibrosis," *The Journal of Investigative Dermatology*, vol. 133, no. 5, pp. 1302–1310, 2013.

[69] Y. Kanamaru, A. Nakao, Y. Tanaka et al., "Involvement of p300 in TGF-beta/Smad-pathway-mediated alpha2(I) collagen expression in mouse mesangial cells," *Nephron. Experimental Nephrology*, vol. 95, no. 1, pp. e36–e42, 2003.

[70] M. Fang, X. Kong, P. Li et al., "RFXB and its splice variant RFXBSV mediate the antagonism between IFNgamma and TGFbeta on COL1A2 transcription in vascular smooth muscle cells," *Nucleic Acids Research*, vol. 37, no. 13, pp. 4393–4406, 2009.

[71] H. Xu, X. Wu, H. Qin et al., "Myocardin-related transcription factor a epigenetically regulates renal fibrosis in diabetic nephropathy," *Journal of the American Society of Nephrology*, vol. 26, no. 7, pp. 1648–1660, 2015.

[72] H. Yuan, M. A. Reddy, S. Deshpande et al., "Epigenetic histone modifications involved in profibrotic gene regulation by 12/15-lipoxygenase and its oxidized lipid products in diabetic nephropathy," *Antioxidants & Redox Signaling*, vol. 24, no. 7, pp. 361–375, 2016.

[73] H. B. Lee, H. Noh, J. Y. Seo, M. R. Yu, and H. Ha, "Histone deacetylase inhibitors: a novel class of therapeutic agents in diabetic nephropathy," *Kidney International. Supplement*, vol. 73, no. 106, pp. S61–S66, 2007.

[74] X. Wang, J. Liu, J. Zhen et al., "Histone deacetylase 4 selectively contributes to podocyte injury in diabetic nephropathy," *Kidney International*, vol. 86, no. 4, pp. 712–725, 2014.

[75] M. Yoshikawa, K. Hishikawa, T. Marumo, and T. Fujita, "Inhibition of histone deacetylase activity suppresses epithelial-to-mesenchymal transition induced by TGF-beta1 in human renal epithelial cells," *Journal of the American Society of Nephrology*, vol. 18, no. 1, pp. 58–65, 2007.

[76] M. Pang, J. Kothapally, H. Mao et al., "Inhibition of histone deacetylase activity attenuates renal fibroblast activation and interstitial fibrosis in obstructive nephropathy," *American Journal of Physiology. Renal Physiology*, vol. 297, no. 4, pp. F996–F1005, 2009.

[77] H. Noh, E. Y. Oh, J. Y. Seo et al., "Histone deacetylase-2 is a key regulator of diabetes- and transforming growth factor-beta1-induced renal injury," *American Journal of Physiology. Renal Physiology*, vol. 297, no. 3, pp. F729–F739, 2009.

[78] N. Liu, S. He, L. Ma et al., "Blocking the class I histone deacetylase ameliorates renal fibrosis and inhibits renal fibroblast

activation via modulating TGF-beta and EGFR signaling," *PloS One*, vol. 8, no. 1, article e54001, 2013.

[79] O. G. McDonald, H. Wu, W. Timp, A. Doi, and A. P. Feinberg, "Genome-scale epigenetic reprogramming during epithelial-to-mesenchymal transition," *Nature Structural & Molecular Biology*, vol. 18, no. 8, pp. 867–874, 2011.

[80] S. Chen, B. Feng, B. George, R. Chakrabarti, M. Chen, and S. Chakrabarti, "Transcriptional coactivator p300 regulates glucose-induced gene expression in endothelial cells," *American Journal of Physiology. Endocrinology and Metabolism*, vol. 298, no. 1, pp. E127–E137, 2010.

[81] J. M. Yun, I. Jialal, and S. Devaraj, "Epigenetic regulation of high glucose-induced proinflammatory cytokine production in monocytes by curcumin," *The Journal of Nutritional Biochemistry*, vol. 22, no. 5, pp. 450–458, 2011.

[82] J. Ma, L. Phillips, Y. Wang et al., "Curcumin activates the p38MPAK-HSP25 pathway in vitro but fails to attenuate diabetic nephropathy in DBA2J mice despite urinary clearance documented by HPLC," *BMC Complementary and Alternative Medicine*, vol. 10, p. 67, 2010.

[83] S. Khan, G. Jena, and K. Tikoo, "Sodium valproate ameliorates diabetes-induced fibrosis and renal damage by the inhibition of histone deacetylases in diabetic rat," *Experimental and Molecular Pathology*, vol. 98, no. 2, pp. 230–239, 2015.

[84] H. Qi, Z. Jing, W. Xiaolin et al., "Histone demethylase JMJD2A inhibition attenuates neointimal hyperplasia in the carotid arteries of balloon-injured diabetic rats via transcriptional silencing: inflammatory gene expression in vascular smooth muscle cells," *Cellular Physiology and Biochemistry*, vol. 37, no. 2, pp. 719–734, 2015.

[85] R. E. Gilbert, Q. Huang, K. Thai et al., "Histone deacetylase inhibition attenuates diabetes-associated kidney growth: potential role for epigenetic modification of the epidermal growth factor receptor," *Kidney International*, vol. 79, no. 12, pp. 1312–1321, 2011.

[86] A. Advani, Q. Huang, K. Thai et al., "Long-term administration of the histone deacetylase inhibitor vorinostat attenuates renal injury in experimental diabetes through an endothelial nitric oxide synthase-dependent mechanism," *The American Journal of Pathology*, vol. 178, no. 5, pp. 2205–2214, 2011.

[87] S. Khan and G. Jena, "Sodium butyrate, a HDAC inhibitor ameliorates eNOS, iNOS and TGF-beta1-induced fibrogenesis, apoptosis and DNA damage in the kidney of juvenile diabetic rats," *Food and Chemical Toxicology*, vol. 73, pp. 127–139, 2014.

10

Urinary Excretion of Kidney Aquaporins as Possible Diagnostic Biomarker of Diabetic Nephropathy

Luigi Rossi,[1] Maria Celeste Nicoletti,[2] Monica Carmosino,[2] Lisa Mastrofrancesco,[2] Antonella Di Franco,[1] Francesca Indrio,[1] Rossella Lella,[1] Luigi Laviola,[1] Francesco Giorgino,[1] Maria Svelto,[2] Loreto Gesualdo,[1] and Giuseppe Procino[2]

[1] *DETO, University of Bari, Bari, Italy*
[2] *Department of Biosciences, Biotechnologies and Biopharmaceutics, University of Bari, Bari, Italy*

Correspondence should be addressed to Giuseppe Procino; giuseppe.procino@uniba.it

Academic Editor: Paolo Fiorina

Diabetic nephropathy (DN) is a microangiopathic complication of diabetes mellitus (DM) affecting one-third of diabetic patients. The large variability in the clinical presentation of renal involvement in patients with DM makes kidney biopsy a prerequisite for a correct diagnosis. However, renal biopsy is an invasive procedure associated with risk of major complications. Numerous studies aimed to identify a noninvasive biomarker of DN but, so far, none of these is considered to be sufficiently specific and sensitive. Water channel aquaporins (AQPs), expressed at the plasma membrane of epithelial tubular cells, are often dysregulated during DN. In this work, we analyzed the urine excretion of AQP5 and AQP2 (uAQP5 and uAQP2), *via* exosomes, in 35 diabetic patients: 12 normoalbuminuric with normal renal function (DM), 11 with proteinuric nondiabetic nephropathy (NDN), and 12 with histological diagnosis and classification of DN. ELISA and WB analysis independently showed that uAQP5 was significantly increased in DN patients. Interestingly, linear regression analysis showed a positive correlation between uAQP5 and the histological class of DN. The same analysis, focusing on uAQP2, showed comparable results. Taken together, these data suggest a possible use of AQP5 and AQP2 as novel noninvasive biomarkers to help in classifying the clinical stage of DN.

1. Introduction

Diabetes mellitus (DM) affects over 350 million people worldwide and its prevalence and incidence are growing, thus suggesting the concept of a *diabetic pandemic*. Diabetic patients have twice the risk of dying of cardiovascular complication compared to nondiabetic subjects of the same age [1, 2].

Diabetic nephropathy (DN) is a slow, progressive loss of kidney function caused by long-standing DM, both type I and type II. DN affects only one-third of diabetic patients, suggesting the concomitant involvement of environmental and genetic factors contributing to the initiation and progression of diabetic kidney disease [3, 4].

It is very important to emphasize the concept that DN is only one of the possible forms of kidney damage occurring in diabetic patients. In fact, renal damage in these patients may be due to other causes that can coexist with the diabetic damage or even represent the only pathogenic factor in over 40% of diabetic patients [5]. DN is classified into four hierarchical glomerular lesions with a separate evaluation for degrees of interstitial and vascular involvement [6, 7].

In renal diseases, except those due to congenital abnormalities and obstructions, only kidney biopsy allows an etiologic diagnosis. This is clearly an invasive method and, for this reason, its use is limited to selected cases. Currently, microalbuminuria is the only, early, noninvasive marker of endothelial dysfunction in kidney. Microalbuminuria is defined as small quantities of albumin in the urine, ranging from 30 to 300 mg/day. This value is very well accepted in both type I and type II DM not only as diagnostic biomarker but also as prognostic and pathogenic factor [8–10].

However, microalbuminuria has important limits: first of all it does not allow an etiologic diagnosis of DN, because it is just a marker of endothelial damage; secondly, it does not relate type and amount of kidney damage; finally, it is not an essential condition associated with DN: in fact, it is known that some diabetic patients worsen to renal failure without showing albuminuria [11, 12].

Other proteins than albumin have been proposed as diagnostic marker of DN: β2 microglobulin (β2MG) and ubiquitin [13]. Nevertheless, these proteins have also limitations: β2MG is a marker of tubular damage, and until now there are no studies comparing urinary β2MG excretion in diabetic versus nondiabetic nephropathy patients. Also ubiquitin relevance as diagnostic marker is limited by the lack of correlation between its urinary levels and histologic classification of DN.

The majority of the studies, undertaken to identify novel urinary biomarkers, focused on the analysis of soluble proteins in the urine; more recently, the possibility to search for novel biomarkers associated with nanoscale vesicles known as exosomes, released into the urinary space, is emerging. This approach opens new perspective for better understanding the molecular mechanisms leading to renal damage and to discover new biomarkers [14, 15].

Novel ideal biomarkers of DN should be characterized by sensitivity, specificity, early appearance, and low invasiveness. The water channels aquaporins (AQPs) may have a relevant role in the establishment and maintenance of DN because of their role in the regulation of fluid balance in the kidney and since polyuria is a very early clinical sign of diabetes.

Among the 13 isoforms cloned in humans, at least 9 are expressed in the kidney: AQP1-8 and AQP11 [16, 17].

AQP1 [18] is highly expressed in the glomerular capillaries at the plasma membrane of proximal tubule epithelial cells [19]. AQP2 [20] is expressed at the apical plasma membrane of principal cells (PC) of collecting duct (CD) during antidiuretic hormone (ADH) stimulation [17]. We previously showed that, under physiological conditions, AQP5 is expressed in the intercalated β-cells of the CD [21].

Early reports showed that renal AQPs might be dysregulated in diabetic patients and in DN [22–24]. Wu et al. showed that AQP5 is upregulated in kidney biopsies from DN patients [25]. On the basis of this evidence, in this work, we analyzed the urinary excretion of AQP1, AQP2, and AQP5 in three groups of patients: 12 diabetic with no sign of nephropathy (DM), 12 diabetic with histologic diagnosis of diabetic nephropathy (DN), and 11 diabetic with nondiabetic nephropathy (NDN).

In this pilot investigation, we found that urine excretion of AQP2 and AQP5, but not AQP1, was dramatically higher in DN patients compared to DM and NDN patients and positively correlated with the progression of the DN, according to the histologic classification.

Taken together, these data support a possible application of urinary excreted AQP2 and AQP5 as ideal biomarkers for the diagnosis of DN.

2. Materials and Methods

2.1. Study Participants. In this study, we enrolled 35 patients to evaluate urinary excretion of AQP2, AQP5, AQP1, and NKCC2. All patients were affected by type 2 diabetes mellitus. The main demographic, clinical, and laboratory features are summarized in Table 1.

Seven healthy (nondiabetic) volunteers were also recruited as controls. They were not hospitalized and provided urine samples.

The following four groups entered the study:

(1) 7 control healthy patients with normal glycemia, GFR, blood pressure, and albuminuria (CTR)

(2) 12 diabetic patients with no apparent sign of nephropathy, normal GFR, and normoalbuminuria (DM)

(3) 12 diabetic patients with biopsy-proven diabetic nephropathy (DN), classified according to the criteria proposed by Tervaert et al. [7] and reported in Table 2

(4) 11 diabetic patients with nondiabetic nephropathy (NDN) described in Table 2.

2.2. Ethics Statements. The design of the study was observational, since no additional intervention was planned apart from routine medical care. Samples were collected after the patients gave their written informed consent and the study was reviewed and approved by the Institutional Review Board of the Polyclinic Hospital, University of Bari Medical School, Bari (Italy) (study number ST 3325, prot. 823 approved on 20 July 2009), and it was carried out in accordance with the Helsinki Declaration of 1975 (as revised in 2000). No individual patient data are reported in this article.

2.3. Urine and Tissue Collection. All samples from all patients and healthy volunteers enrolled in this study were collected at the Nephrology, Dialysis and Transplant Department of the University Hospital "Policlinico di Bari," Bari (Italy). First morning urine samples were supplemented with Protease Inhibitor Cocktail Tablets (Roche Diagnostics GmbH), centrifuged at 3,000 rpm for 10 minutes at 4°C to remove cellular debris, and stored at −80°C. Urine creatinine was quantified by the Jaffe reaction.

Patients diagnosed with diabetic nephropathy and nondiabetic nephropathy underwent kidney biopsy. Control human kidneys samples were obtained from the normal-appearing renal cortex harvested from a nondiabetic patient diagnosed with renal carcinoma and undergoing a nephrectomy with approval of the local ethics committee. At time of biopsy, all patients were clinically stable regarding water balance and blood pressure. All patients gave signed consent for the use of their tissue for research purposes at the time of biopsy or radical nephrectomy.

2.4. Antibodies. Rabbit affinity purified polyclonal antibody against amino acids 251–265 of rat AQP5 (cat.# AQP5-005) was from Alomone Labs (http://www.alomone.com). The antibody is designed to cross-react also with human AQP5. We tested the absence of cross-reaction of the anti-AQP5 antibody with AQP2 (data not shown). Rabbit polyclonal antibody against human AQP2 was previously described [26]. Rabbit anti-AQP1 antibody (cat.# SC-20810) and rabbit anti-flotillin-1 antibody (cat.# sc-25506) were from Santa Cruz

TABLE 1: Demographic and clinical characteristics of 12 diabetic patients (DM), 11 diabetic patients with nondiabetic nephropathy (NDN), and 12 patients with diabetic nephropathy (DN). Data are expressed as the mean ± standard error of the mean (SEM). Statistical analysis was performed using one-way ANOVA followed by Newman-Keuls multiple comparison test. P values < 0.05 were considered statistically significant.

	Diabetes mellitus (DM)	Nondiabetic nephropathy (NDN)	Diabetic nephropathy (DN)	P value	
Number of patients	12	11	12		
Sex (female/male)	2/10	4/7	2/10		
Age (years)	56 ± 4	58 ± 5	63 ± 4	DM versus NDN	$P = 0.88$
				DM versus DN	$P = 0.25$
				NDN versus DN	$P = 0.38$
uCr (mg/dL)	188 ± 20	81 ± 14	89 ± 22	DM versus NDN	$P = 0.0003$
				DM versus DN	$P = 0.0028$
				NDN versus DN	$P = 0.75$
CKD EPI	99 ± 5	64 ± 13	42 ± 9	DM versus NDN	$P = 0.016$
				DM versus DN	$P < 0.0001$
				NDN versus DN	$P = 0.17$
uACR (mg/g)	23 ± 14	1156 ± 402	2580 ± 677	DM versus NDN	$P = 0.0076$
				DM versus DN	$P = 0.001$
				NDN versus DN	$P = 0.092$
MAP (mmHg)	92 ± 4	95 ± 4	100 ± 4	DM versus NDN	$P = 0.61$
				DM versus DN	$P = 0.12$
				NDN versus DN	$P = 0.27$
Plasma TG (mg/dL)	117 ± 22	216 ± 31	253 ± 41	DM versus NDN	$P = 0.015$
				DM versus DN	$P = 0.0076$
				NDN versus DN	$P = 0.49$
Total CHO (mg/dL)	157 ± 10	164 ± 12	165 ± 11	DM versus NDN	$P = 0.64$
				DM versus DN	$P = 0.61$
				NDN versus DN	$P = 0.98$
BMI (kg/m^2)	29 ± 2	27 ± 1	30 ± 1	DM versus NDN	$P = 0.37$
				DM versus DN	$P = 0.69$
				NDN versus DN	$P = 0.10$
Antidiabetic agents	Insulin = 6 ADO = 6	Insulin = 3 ADO = 8	Insulin = 5 ADO = 6 None = 1		

uCr, urine creatinine; CKD-EPI (Chronic Kidney Disease Epidemiology Collaboration), estimated glomerular filtration rate; uACR, urine albumin/urine creatinine; MAP, mean arterial pressure; Plasma TG, plasma triglyceride levels; Total CHO, total plasma cholesterol levels; BMI, body mass index.

Biotechnology (http://www.scbt.it). Rabbit anti-NKCC2 polyclonal antibody (cat.# AB3562P) and monoclonal anti-Na^+/K^+-ATPase (cat.# 05-369) were from Millipore (http://www.merckmillipore.com). Anti-rabbit IgG (whole molecule)-peroxidase antibody (cat.# A0545) was from Sigma-Aldrich (http://www.sigmaaldrich.com).

2.5. Immunofluorescence. Human kidney samples were fixed in 4% paraformaldehyde in PBS at 4°C, embedded in paraffin wax, and cut into 5 μm sections with a microtome. Antigen retrieval was performed by boiling sections in citrate buffer (10 mM sodium citrate, 0,05% Tween 20, pH 6) for 30 minutes. Nonspecific binding sites were blocked with 1% BSA in PBS for 30 min. Sections were then incubated with rabbit anti-AQP2 antibody (1:1000) followed by incubation with Alexa Fluor-conjugated secondary antibody (http://www.lifetechnologies.com). Confocal images were obtained with a confocal laser-scanning microscope (Leica TSC-SP2, Mannheim, Germany).

2.6. Purification of Urine Exosomes and Western Blotting Analysis. Isolation of exosomes from urine was performed using a two-step differential centrifugation method [27]. Briefly, an equal volume of urine samples (1 mL) was centrifuged at 17,000 ×g for 10 min at 4°C to remove urinary sediment and supernatants were ultracentrifuged at 200,000 ×g for 1 hour

TABLE 2: Histologic classification of patients according to criteria proposed by Tervaert et al. [7].

(a) Patients with diabetic nephropathy (DN)

Patient	K-DOQI stage (CKD-EPI)	Histologic class of DN	Interstitial fibrosis and tubular atrophy	Interstitial inflammation	Arteriolar hyalinosis	Large vessels arteriosclerosis
1	4	IV	3	1	2	1
2	5	IV	3	2	2	1
3	3	IIa	2	1	1	2
4	5	IV	3	1	1	1
5	3	III	2	1	2	1
6	1	IIa	2	1	2	1
7	3	III	2	1	2	1
8	4	III	2	1	1	1
9	3	III	3	2	2	1
10	3	IIb	2	1	2	1
11	1	IIb	1	1	1	1
12	3	III	3	1	1	1

(b) Patients with nondiabetic nephropathy (NDN)

Patient	K-DOQI stage (CKD-EPI)	Histologic diagnosis	Interstitial fibrosis and tubular atrophy	Interstitial inflammation	Arteriolar hyalinosis	Large vessels arteriosclerosis
1	1	Nephroangiosclerosis	2	0	1	1
2	3	FSGS (NOS)	1	0	1	0
3	1	Lupus GN (V)	2	0	0	0
4	5	Interstitial GN	3	1	1	1
5	5	Endocapillary and extracapillary GN	2	1	1	1
6	4	Nephroangiosclerosis	2	2	2	1
7	1	Membranous GN II	1	0	2	1
8	1	FSGS (perihilar)	2	1	1	1
9	2	Membranous GN I	2	0	1	1
10	2	Membranous GN II	1	0	1	1
11	3	FSGS (NOS)	2	2	2	1

at 4°C. The resulting exosome-enriched pellets were resuspended in 60 μL of Laemmli's buffer and denatured for 10 min at 60°C.

Ten microliters of each sample was resolved on 12% SDS-PAGE and electroblotted onto Immobilon-P PVDF membrane (http://www.merckmillipore.com). After blocking with 3% BSA in Tris buffer saline/Tween 20 (TBS-T), blots were incubated overnight at 4°C with the following primary antibodies: anti-flotillin-1 (1.200), anti-Na^+/K^+-ATPase (1:5000), anti-AQP5 (1:1000), anti-AQP2 (2 μg/mL), anti-AQP1 (1:500), and anti-NKCC2 (1:1000). Membranes were washed and incubated with the anti-rabbit IgG peroxidase antibody (1:10000). Reactive proteins were revealed with SuperSignal™ West Pico Chemiluminescent Substrate (https://www.thermofisher.com) and chemiluminescence was detected with ChemiDoc XRS (Bio-Rad) equipped with Image Lab™ software for image acquisition. Densitometry analysis was performed with ImageJ software (NIH, Bethesda, MD).

2.7. ELISA Test for uAQP5 and uAQP2. Quantitation of urinary AQP5 (uAQP5) and AQP2 (uAQP2) was performed using a standard ELISA protocol originally established by Umenishi et al., [28] with some modifications [29]. Synthetic peptides reproducing the last 15 amino acids of the C-terminal region of the rat AQP5 and human AQP2 were used as internal standard for AQP5 and AQP2 assay, respectively. Urinary AQ5 and AQP2 excretion was normalized to urinary creatinine and expressed as fmol/mg urine creatinine.

2.8. Statistical Analysis. Data were expressed as mean ± standard error (SE) of the mean. Statistical analysis was performed using a nonparametric Kruskal-Wallis one-way ANOVA test, linear regression test, and Spearman's rank-order correlation. P values < 0.05 were considered statistically significant. For statistical analysis, GraphPad Prism 5 software was used. Data were obtained from at least three independent experiments for each experimental condition.

3. Results

3.1. Urinary AQP5 Excretion. An ELISA assay was designed and carried out to quantify uAQP5 excretion between the four groups of patients previously described. Results are reported in Figure 1(a) and expressed as fmol AQP5/mg uCr.

uAQP5-to-creatinine *ratio* was the highest in patients with diabetic nephropathy (DN) compared to patients with nondiabetic nephropathy (NDN) and diabetic subjects (DM) and healthy nondiabetic volunteers (CTR). No statistically significant difference in uAQP5 excretion was observed between CTR and DM and NDN groups.

We next investigated whether the increase in uAQP5 excretion was related with the progression of DN. To this end, we performed a post hoc subanalysis of uAQP5 excretion after grouping all DN patients according to stages II, III, and IV of DN, performed as described in Materials and Methods.

As shown in Figure 1(b), uAQP5 excretion progressively increased in parallel with the histological class of DN. uAQP5 was significantly higher in DN patients at stage II compared to CTR and DM and NDN groups. uAQP5 did not further increase in DN patients at stage III but almost doubled in DN patients at stage IV. Linear regression analysis (Figure 1(c)) showed a strong, positive association between uAQP5 and the progression of DN ($r^2 = 0.56$; $P = 0.0051$).

Exosome-associated proteins were isolated from equal volumes (1 mL) of urine from all patients, separated by standard SDS-PAGE and analyzed by Western blotting. The results showed the presence of the exosome marker flotillin-1 [30] and the absence of the basolateral membrane marker Na^+/K^+-ATPase (see supplemental Figure 1 in Supplementary Material available online at https://doi.org/10.1155/2017/4360357). The Western blotting analysis also confirmed the marked increase in uAQP5 in patients with DN.

As reported in Figure 1(d), a strong band of approximately 27 kDa for AQP5 was detected in almost all urine exosomes isolated from the DN group, while a faint band was immunodetected only in six out of the eleven NDN patients. Exosomes isolated from the CTR and DM groups showed no detectable signal for AQP5. The densitometry analysis of uAQP5 bands, normalized to uCr (Figure 1(e)), indicated that uAQP5 was dramatically increased in the DN subjects when compared to CTR and DM and NDN groups.

When DN patients were grouped according to the stage of DN (Figure 1(f)), the analysis showed a tendency to a progressive increase of uAQP5 excretion with the progression of the DN, although linear regression analysis did not show a statistical significant correlation (Figure 1(g); $r^2 = 0.33$; $P = 0.05$). Spearman's rank-order correlation between uAQP5 and uACR or glomerular filtration rate (GFR), calculated as CKD-EPI, is reported in supplemental Figure 2. In both NDN and DN patients, uAQP5 did not correlate with uACR (supplemental Figure 2, C, E). Only DN patients showed a significant, negative correlation between uAQP5 and CKD-EPI (supplemental Figure 2F).

3.2. Urinary AQP2 Excretion. We next evaluated whether also uAQP2 was altered in DN patients using the ELISA test as described above.

Similar to uAQP5, uAQP2-to-creatinine *ratio* was maximal in patients with ND compared to both CTR and DM and NDN groups (Figure 2(a)) and there was no statistically significant difference between CTR and DM and NDN patients.

A further analysis, performed after grouping DN patients according to the histological classification of DN, indicated that the most severe stages (III and IV) were characterized by a significantly higher uAQP2 excretion compared to CTR and DM and NDN subjects (Figure 2(b)). In contrast, uAQP2 in DN subjects at stage II was comparable to that of CTR and DM and NDN groups. Linear regression analysis showed a positive relationship between uAQP2 and the progression of DN (Figure 2(c); $r^2 = 0.58$; $P = 0.0038$).

Semiquantitative Western blotting analysis of the uAQP2 abundance in urinary exosomes gave results in line with those obtained by ELISA. In fact, a protein band of approximately 29 kDa, corresponding to AQP2, was significantly more abundant in patients with DN compared to the three reference groups (Figures 2(d) and 2(e)). The post hoc statistical analysis performed on DN patients showed that uAQP2 progressively increased with the class of DN (Figure 2(f)). Compared to CTR subjects, all three classes of DN patients showed a progressive increase of uAQP2. Compared to DM and NDN patients, only DN patients assigned to classes III and IV showed higher uAQP2 excretion. Linear regression analysis confirmed that uAQP2 abundance positively correlated with the severity of DN (Figure 1(g); $r^2 = 0.64$; $P = 0.0031$). Spearman's rank-order correlation between uAQP2 and uACR or glomerular filtration rate (GFR), calculated as CKD-EPI, is reported in supplemental Figure 3. In both NDN and DN patients, uAQP2 did not correlate with uACR (supplemental Figure 3, C, E). Only DN patients showed a significant, negative correlation between uAQP2 and CKD-EPI (supplemental Figure 3F).

Importantly, both uAQP5 and uAQP2 were correlated neither with blood pressure nor with plasma cholesterol (total, HDL, and LDL) nor with antihypertensive or antidiabetic drugs, including statins.

3.3. AQP2 Abundance and Subcellular Localization in Kidney Biopsies. AQP2 was also immunolocalized in sections of renal cortex biopsies from DN and NDN patients. As control, we used normal kidney tissue obtained as explained in Materials and Methods. Figure 3 shows representative confocal pictures of AQP2 staining taken in the cortical collecting ducts of normal kidney, kidneys of patients with classes II, III, and IV DN, and kidneys of NDN patients. In control tissue, AQP2 was mainly localized in intracellular storage vesicles accumulated at the subapical region (magnified ×2 in the insets). In contrast, in tissues from all DN patients, AQP2 staining was brighter and progressively accumulated at the luminal plasma membrane in parallel with the histologic classification of DN (see magnified ×2 insets). AQP2 staining in different forms of NDN showed a predominant subapical localization similar to that observed in control samples.

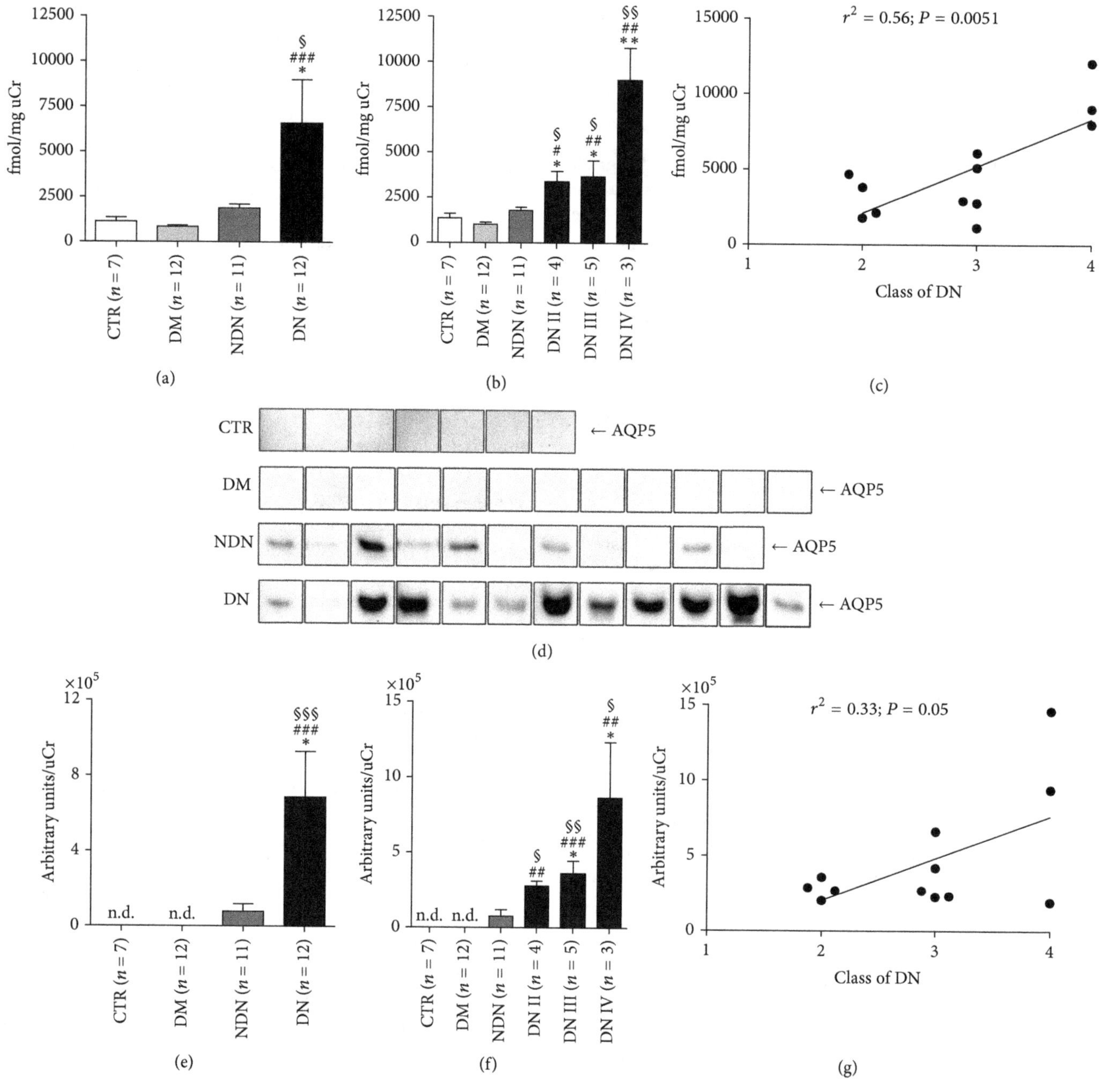

FIGURE 1: The urinary excretion of AQP5 dramatically increases in DN patients and positively correlates with the clinical severity of DN. (a) Urinary AQP5 excretion was measured by ELISA in urine samples of healthy subjects (CTR, $n = 7$), patients with DM ($n = 12$), patients with NDN ($n = 11$), and patients with DN ($n = 12$) and expressed as fmol/mg urine creatinine. All data are reported as mean ± SEM. $^{\$}P < 0.05$ versus CTR, $^{\#\#\#}P < 0.001$ versus DM, and $^{*}P < 0.05$ versus NDN, obtained by Kruskal-Wallis one-way ANOVA test. (b) DN patients were grouped according to the histological changes evaluated by kidney biopsy: DN stage II ($n = 4$), DN stage III ($n = 5$), and DN stage IV ($n = 3$) and uAQP5 at each stage compared to uAQP5 in CTR and DM and NDN patients. All data are reported as mean ± SEM. $^{\$\$}P < 0.01$ and $^{\$}P < 0.05$ versus CTR, $^{\#\#}P < 0.01$ and $^{\#}P < 0.05$ versus DM, and $^{**}P < 0.01$ and $^{*}P < 0.05$ versus NDN, obtained by Kruskal-Wallis one-way ANOVA test. (c) Linear regression analysis of uAQP5 abundance, as measured by ELISA, with the class of DN ($r^2 = 0.56$; $P = 0.0051$). (d) Exosomes were isolated from urine of healthy subjects (CTR, $n = 7$), patients with DM ($n = 12$), patients with NDN ($n = 11$), and patients with DN ($n = 12$) using the two-step differential centrifugation method. Total exosome proteins were resolved on 12% SDS-PAGE and analyzed by Western blotting for AQP5 abundance. (e) Densitometry analysis of the uAQP5 band intensities was normalized for uCr and reported as means ± SEM. $^{\$\$\$}P < 0.001$ versus CTR, $^{\#\#\#}P < 0.001$ versus DM, and $^{*}P < 0.05$ versus NDN, obtained by Kruskal-Wallis one-way ANOVA test. n.d.: nondetectable. (f) DN patients were grouped according to the histological changes evaluated by kidney biopsy: DN stage II ($n = 4$), DN stage III ($n = 5$), and DN stage IV ($n = 3$) and densitometry analysis of uAQP5 at each stage compared to uAQP5 in CTR and DM and NDN patients. All data are reported as mean ± SEM. $^{\$\$}P < 0.01$ and $^{\$}P < 0.05$ versus CTR, $^{\#\#}P < 0.01$ and $^{\#\#\#}P < 0.001$ versus DM, and $^{*}P < 0.05$ versus NDN, obtained by Kruskal-Wallis one-way ANOVA test. (g) Linear regression analysis of uAQP5 abundance, as semiquantified by Western blotting, with the class of DN ($r^2 = 0.33$; $P = 0.05$).

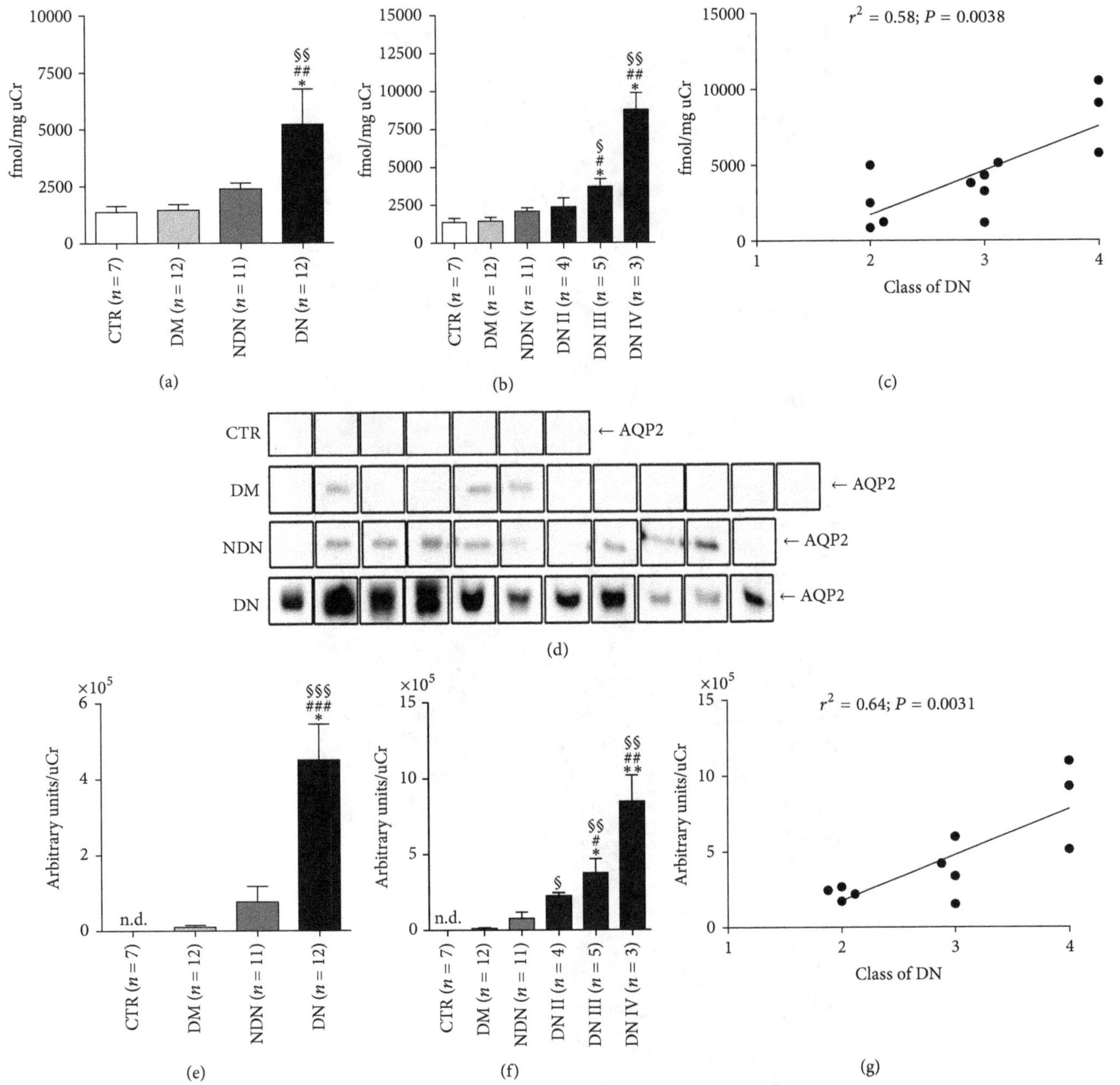

FIGURE 2: The urinary excretion of AQP2 dramatically increases in DN patients and positively correlates with the clinical severity of DN. (a) Urinary AQP2 excretion was measured by ELISA in urine samples of healthy subjects (CTR, $n = 7$), patients with DM ($n = 12$), patients with NDN ($n = 11$), and patients with DN ($n = 12$) and expressed as fmol/mg urine creatinine. All data are reported as mean ± SEM. $^{\S\S}P < 0.01$ versus CTR, $^{\#\#}P < 0.01$ versus DM, and $^{*}P < 0.05$ versus NDN, obtained by Kruskal-Wallis one-way ANOVA test. (b) DN patients were grouped according to the histological changes evaluated by kidney biopsy: DN stage II ($n = 4$), DN stage III ($n = 5$), and DN stage IV ($n = 3$) and uAQP2 at each stage compared to uAQP2 in DM and NDN patients. All data are reported as mean ± SEM. $^{\S\S}P < 0.01$ and $^{\S}P < 0.05$ versus CTR, $^{\#\#}P < 0.01$ and $^{\#}P < 0.05$ versus DM, and $^{*}P < 0.05$ versus NDN, obtained by Kruskal-Wallis one-way ANOVA test. (c) Linear regression analysis of uAQP2 abundance, as measured by ELISA, with the class of DN ($r^2 = 0.58$; $P = 0.0038$). (d) Exosomes were isolated from urine of healthy subjects (CTR, $n = 7$), patients with DM ($n = 12$), patients with NDN ($n = 11$), and patients with DN ($n = 11$) using the two-step differential centrifugation method. Total exosome proteins were resolved on 12% SDS-PAGE and analyzed by Western blotting for AQP2 abundance. (e) Densitometry analysis of the uAQP2 band intensities was normalized for uCr and reported as means ± SEM. $^{\S\S\S}P < 0.001$ versus CTR, $^{\#\#\#}P < 0.001$ versus DM, and $^{*}P < 0.05$ versus NDN, obtained by Kruskal-Wallis one-way ANOVA test. (f) DN patients were grouped according to the histological changes evaluated by kidney biopsy: DN stage II ($n = 4$), DN stage III ($n = 4$), and DN stage IV ($n = 3$) and densitometry analysis of uAQP2 at each stage compared to uAQP2 in CTR and DM and NDN patients. All data are reported as mean ± SEM. $^{\S\S}P < 0.01$ and $^{\S}P < 0.05$ versus CTR, $^{\#\#}P < 001$ and $^{\#}P < 0.05$ versus DM, and $^{**}P < 0.01$ and $^{*}P < 0.05$ versus NDN, obtained by Kruskal-Wallis one-way ANOVA test. (g) Linear regression analysis of uAQP2 abundance, as semiquantified by Western blotting, with the class of DN ($r^2 = 0.64$; $P = 0.0031$).

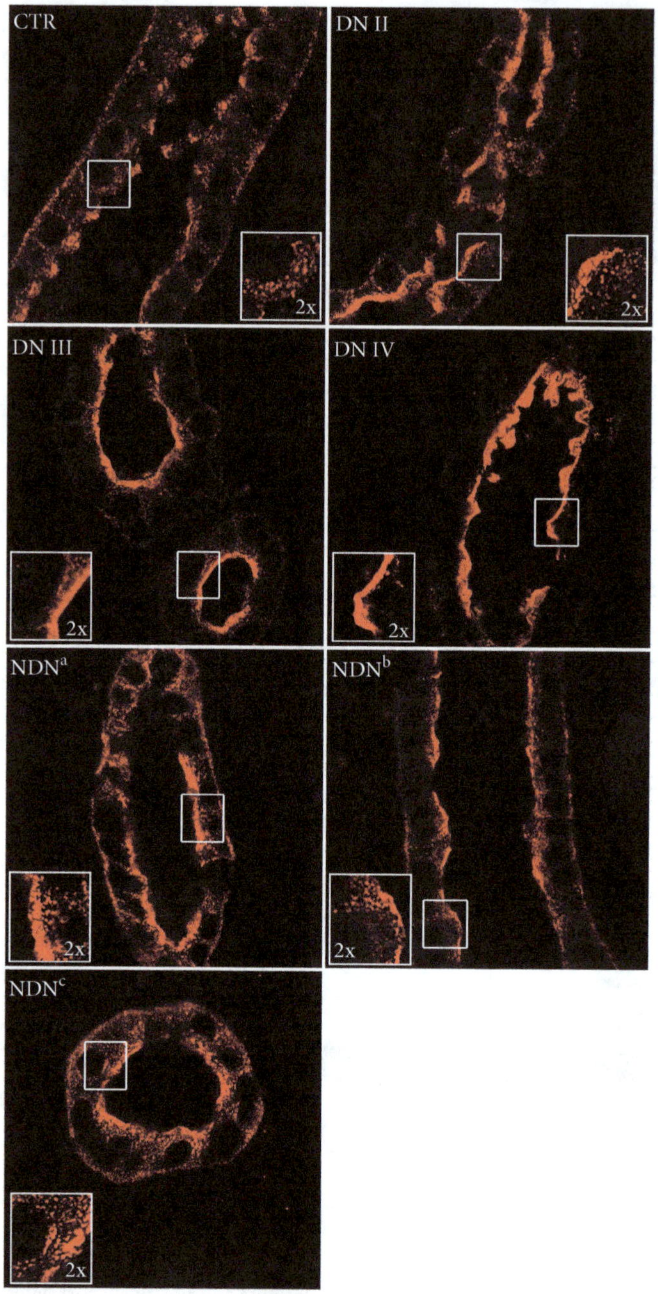

FIGURE 3: AQP2 plasma membrane localization increases in DN patients and with the clinical severity of DN. Human kidney biopsies from control kidney (CTR), DN, and NDN patients were subjected to immunofluorescence analysis of AQP2 subcellular localization. AQP2 immunostaining, shown in red, was visualized in the *xy* apical confocal plan. Confocal pictures are representative of AQP2 staining in the cortical collecting duct of normal kidney (CTR), kidneys of patients with class II (DN II), class III (DN III), and class IV (DN IV) DN, and kidneys of NDN patients. NDN[a] is a patient with membranous nephropathy and angiosclerosis, NDN[b] is a patient with chronic interstitial nephritis, and NDN[c] is a patient with endocapillary/extracapillary glomerulonephritis. Similar results were obtained in three patients per each group.

3.4. Urinary AQP1 and NKCC2 Excretion. We next analyzed the urine excretion of AQP1 and NKCC2 in the three groups of patients.

The amounts of uAQP1 and uNKCC2, excreted through the exosomes pathway, were analyzed by Western blotting (Figures 4(a)–5(a)).

As indicated by the densitometry analysis (Figure 4(b)), uAQP1, normalized for the uCr, was significantly increased in DN compared to CTR and DM patients. As for uNKCC2, densitometric analysis (Figure 5(b)) revealed that both DN and NDN patients has a significant higher uNKCC2 excretion compared only to DM patients. However, excretion of both

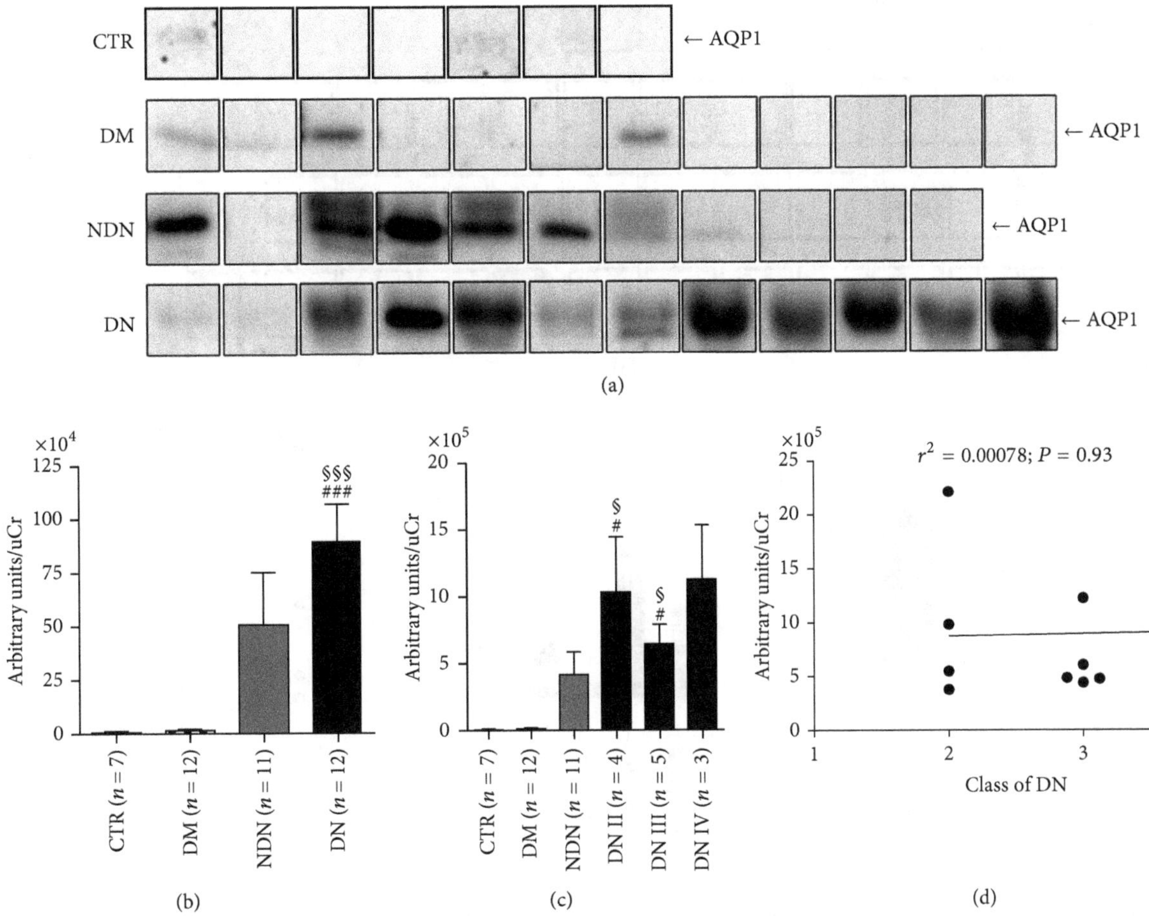

FIGURE 4: The urinary excretion of AQP1 increases in both DN and NDN patients and does not correlate with the clinical severity of DN. (a) Exosomes were isolated from urine of healthy subjects (CTR, $n = 7$), patients with DM ($n = 12$), patients with NDN ($n = 11$), and patients with DN ($n = 12$) using the two-step differential centrifugation method. Total exosome proteins were resolved on 12% SDS-PAGE and analyzed by Western blotting for AQP1 abundance. (b) Densitometry analysis of the uAQP1 band intensities was normalized for uCr and reported as means ± SEM. $^{§§§}P < 0.001$ versus CTR and $^{###}P < 0.001$ versus DM, obtained by Kruskal-Wallis one-way ANOVA test. (c) DN patients were grouped according to the histological changes evaluated by kidney biopsy: DN stage II ($n = 4$), DN stage III ($n = 5$), and DN stage IV ($n = 3$) and densitometry analysis of uAQP1 at each stage compared to uAQP1 in CTR and DM and NDN patients. All data are reported as mean ± SEM. $^{§}P < 0.05$ versus CTR and $^{#}P < 0.05$ versus DM, obtained by Kruskal-Wallis one-way ANOVA test. (d) Linear regression analysis of uAQP1 abundance, as semiquantified by Western blotting, with the class of DN ($r^2 = 0.00078$; $P = 0.93$).

uAQP1 and uNKCC2 was not statistically different between DN and NDN patients.

The post hoc analysis, performed after grouping DN patients according to the class of DN (Figure 4(c)), showed that AQP1 was higher in classes II and III of DN compared with CTR and DM but not with NDN. DN patients in class IV did not show a significant higher uAQP1 excretion compared with the three reference groups. Moreover, the linear regression analysis (Figure 4(d)) showed that uAQP1 did not correlate with DN stage.

As for NKCC2, patients with class II DN showed significantly higher uNKCC2 only compared with DM patients but not with CTR or DN (Figure 5(c)). Linear regression analysis did not show positive or negative relationship between uNKCC2 and the progression of DN (Figure 5(d)).

4. Discussion

A number of biomarkers have been exploited in the last decades as tools for early detection of DN [31, 32], yet, to date, none have outperformed microalbuminuria in larger scale, prospective longitudinal studies [33]. However, a number of evidences indicate that albuminuria may not be an optimal marker for the early detection of DN. In fact, about 10–25% of diabetic patients follow the "normoalbuminuria pathway," showing a progressive decline of GFR without worsening proteinuria [34]. In addition, moderate increases in albumin excretion are associated with a variety of other conditions, including obesity, posture, exercise, diet, smoking, gender, puberty, infection, and inflammation. Therefore, changes in albuminuria may reflect a modification of another disease process that might not be causally related to the development

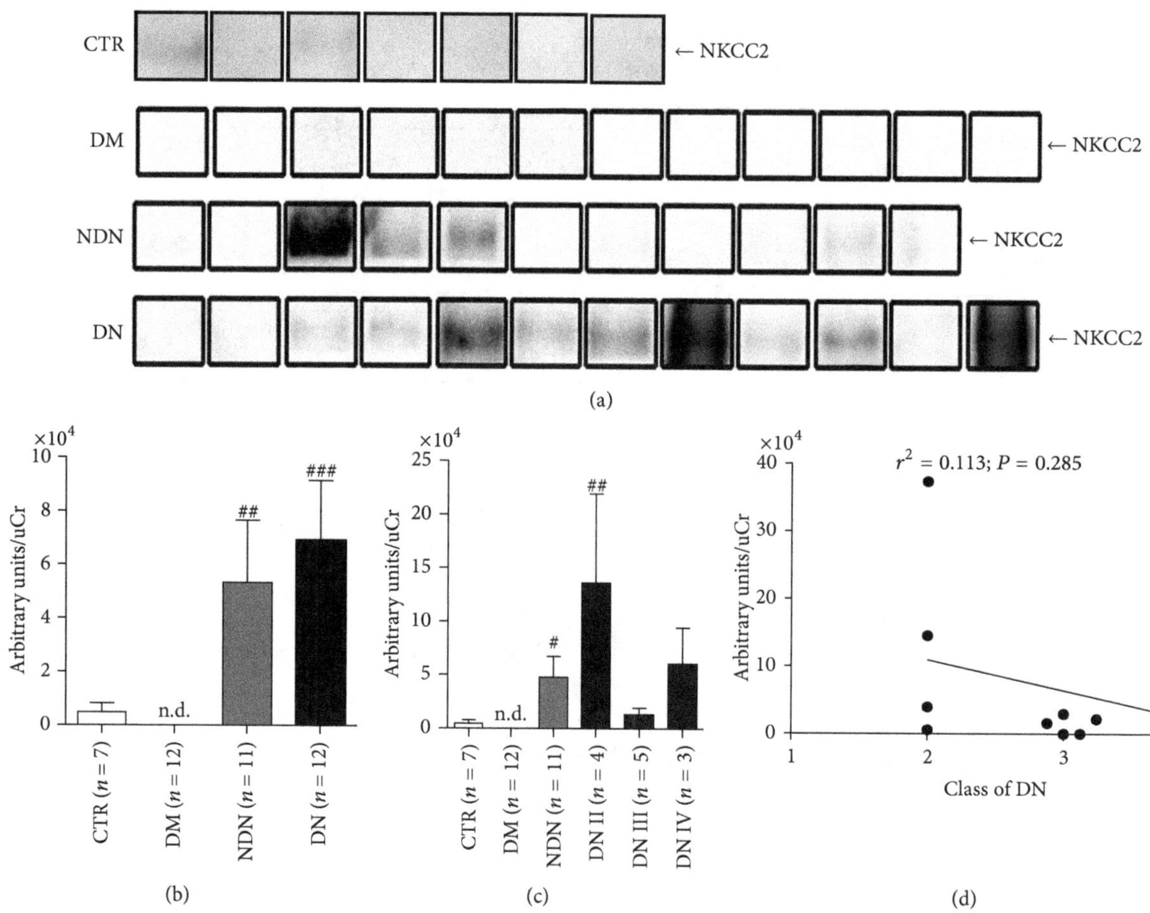

Figure 5: The urinary excretion of NKCC2 increases in both DN and NDN patients and does not correlate with the clinical severity of DN. (a) Exosomes were isolated from urine of healthy subjects (CTR, $n = 7$), patients with DM ($n = 12$), patients with NDN ($n = 11$), and patients with DN ($n = 12$) using the two-step differential centrifugation method. Total exosome proteins were resolved on 10% SDS-PAGE and analyzed by Western blotting for NKCC2 abundance. (b) Densitometry analysis of the uNKCC2 band intensities was normalized for uCr and reported as means ± SEM. $^{###}P < 0.001$ and $^{##}P < 0.01$ versus DM, obtained by Kruskal-Wallis one-way ANOVA test. n.d.: nondetectable. (c) DN patients were grouped according to the histological changes evaluated by kidney biopsy: DN stage II ($n = 4$), DN stage III ($n = 5$), and DN stage IV ($n = 3$) and densitometry analysis of uNKCC2 at each stage compared to uNKCC2 in CTR and DM and NDN patients. All data are reported as mean ± SEM. $^{##}P < 0.01$ and $^{#}P < 0.05$ versus DM, obtained by Kruskal-Wallis one-way ANOVA test. (d) Linear regression analysis of uNKCC2 abundance, as semiquantified by Western blotting, with the class of DN ($r^2 = 0.113$; $P = 0.285$).

of DN [35]. In the present study, we investigated the possible use of renal aquaporins as biomarkers of tubular damage in patients with histologically proven diagnosis of DN. Recently, studies have shown that not only glomerular damage but also tubulointerstitial damage is an important factor in the progression of DN [36]. Markers of tubular damage could, therefore, be potentially useful in the evaluation of prognosis and for monitoring the effectiveness of treatment in DN. Given the pivotal role of renal AQPs in regulating the fluid balance in the kidney [37], we thought that they might be dysregulated in DN.

The first important finding of this study is that both uAQP5 and uAQP2 were dramatically and selectively upregulated in DN but not in DM and NDN patients. This result likely indicates that increased excretion of uAQP5 and uAQP2 is not a common feature of all forms of chronic kidney disease but rather specific for DN. Both proteins were found to be more abundant in the untreated urine and in the exosome fraction isolated from the urine of DN patients, compared with the three control groups. Two independent experimental approaches were used, an ELISA test on slow-speed urine supernatants and a Western blotting analysis on an ultra-speed sediment, enriched in urine exosomes. Interestingly, the supernatant of the ultra-speed centrifugation did not contain measurable amounts of AQP2 or AQP5 as assessed by ELISA test (data not shown), indicating that both AQP5 and AQP2 in the urine are bound to membrane structures. Regardless of the method used, measurements were normalized for the uCr content. Strikingly, we also demonstrated a strong positive relationship between the abundance of both biomarkers and the progression of DN. Interestingly, the higher sensitivity of the ELISA test, compared to WB, could detect an increase of uAQP5 in DN patients in class II, compared to the three control groups. Patients in class III

DN, analyzed by both methods, showed a tendency, although not statistically significant, to a further increase of uAQP5, compared with class II DN. Eventually, patients in class IV showed a dramatic increase of uAQP5. In our study, uAQP2 showed a similar tendency to increase in DN patients in parallel with the progression of the disease. In addition, we confirmed in human kidney biopsies from DN patients that the higher excretion of AQP2 corresponded to a substantial increase of AQP2 at the plasma membrane of principal cells of the collecting ducts. It is well acknowledged that AQP2 enters the apical exosome pathway [27] and the amount of AQP2 excreted into the urine is proportional to that expressed at the apical plasma membrane in a number of physiopathological conditions [38–41].

The concomitant increase of uAQP5 and uAQP2 excretion in DN patients prompted us to investigate the urinary excretion of other membrane proteins expressed in the kidney tubule and involved in the maintenance of the hydroelectrolytes homeostasis. AQP1 and NKCC2 are apically expressed in the proximal tubule and thick ascending limb, respectively [19, 42], and are increased in various types of nephropathy [43, 44]. We showed here that urinary excretion of AQP1 and NKCC2 increased in both DN and NDN patients but this phenomenon was neither positively nor negatively related to the progression of DN. Thus, quantitation of uAQP1 and uNKCC2 would not allow a differential diagnosis between nephropathies and is not useful to classify different stages of DN.

Our results about the upregulation of uAQP5 in DN patients are in line with previous findings from Wu et al. [25] who reported that AQP5 was expressed in the collecting ducts of patients with DN. During the preparation of this manuscript, the same authors demonstrated, with a similar approach, that uAQP5 is upregulated in the urine of DN patients and positively correlated with the stage of DN [45]. In their study, however, they classified DN patients to stages III, IV, and V on the basis of microalbuminuria and macroalbuminuria and increased serum creatinine and limited their analysis to uAQP5 alone. In the present study, we focused our analysis only on patients with histologic-proven diagnosis and staging of DN and analyzed a larger panel of urinary biomarkers. None of the patients enrolled in the present study showed microalbuminuria; thus we could not establish a relationship between AQP5 or AQP2 excretion and this parameter. We also validated the results obtained with the ELISA test on urine samples with a Western blotting analysis on the urine exosome fraction. Our analysis also suggests that, in analogy with AQP2, AQP5 is excreted into the urine through exosomes.

The molecular mechanism responsible for increased expression and excretion of AQP5 and AQP2 in DN patients is unknown and is out of the scope of the present study. However, at least for AQP2, we could hypothesize that AVP might have a key role in this process. Animal studies reported a marked increase of AVP secretion in streptozotocin-induced DM rats and a compensatory increase of AQP2 [46, 47]. Higher AVP levels were also measured in patients with type 2 DM [48] even before they show advanced diabetic complications [49]. From a renal perspective, high AVP levels may be beneficial in early DM by limiting the amount of water required for the excretion of high amount of glucose [46, 50]. In the long term, however, AVP might cause adverse outcomes by aggravating the fluid overload observed in macroalbuminuric DN patients. The adverse effect of AVP on chronic kidney disease (CKD) and DN is well reviewed by Bankir et al. [51]. Most of the work has been done in diabetic animals, which, however, might not be a suitable model to compare with humans. Anyway, the contribution of AVP to DN in humans is supported by several observations: (i) infusion of the AVP analogue desmopressin strongly increases urine albumin excretion in healthy individuals but not in patients with loss-of-function mutations of the type 2 vasopressin receptor [52]; (ii) in epidemiological studies, the percentage of patients with microalbuminuria increased with increasing plasma concentrations of copeptin, a surrogate marker of AVP [53]. Although in the present work we did not measure AVP or copeptin plasma levels in our patients, we can hypothesize that they have sustained levels of circulating AVP which might account for the increased expression/urine excretion of AQP2.

An intriguing hypothesis might be the fact that AVP also regulates AQP5 expression and excretion in the kidney of DN patients. Interestingly, it has been demonstrated that, in human chromosome band 12q13, AQP2 and AQP5 have a closely spaced tandem arrangement [54]. Moreover, in nasal and lung epithelia, cAMP, acting through a PKA/CREB element, upregulated AQP5 expression [55]. Although this mechanism needs to be demonstrated in renal cells, it would nicely fit with the finding presented here.

5. Conclusions

Taken together, the results of this pilot investigation demonstrate that urinary excretion of AQP2 and AQP5 might represent a novel urine proteomic signature able to reliably identify diabetic patients with DN using a noninvasive approach. In particular, uAQP5 levels seem to better discriminate DN from NDN patients and may represent a potential novel noninvasive biomarker for the diagnosis and follow-up of DN patients. The ELISA assay showed higher sensitivity, strong specificity, and higher throughput. Besides, it requires a few microliters of unprocessed urine to detect uAQP5. Although our results were obtained on a small cohort of patients, we obtained a strong positive relationship between uAQP5 and the histologic class of DN. A further study, on a larger group of patients, including those with class I DN, would also help to establish how early AQP5 appears in the urine of patients with subclinical signs of DN and to better discriminate between patients in class II and class III of DN.

Disclosure

The abstract of this work has been previously presented at the Kidney Week Meeting of the American Society of Nephrology (San Diego, CA, 3–8 November 2015) and at the Experimental Biology Meeting (San Diego, CA, 2–6 April 2016) and published in the FASEB Journal, vol. 30 number

1 Supplement, April 2016 (http://www.fasebj.org/content/30/1_Supplement/968.20.short). There is no full-text article associated with this abstract published in the FASEB Journal.

Competing Interests

The authors declare that they have no competing interests.

Authors' Contributions

Luigi Rossi and Maria Celeste Nicoletti equally contributed to the manuscript and should be considered first authors.

References

[1] G. Danaei, M. M. Finucane, Y. Lu et al., "National, regional, and global trends in fasting plasma glucose and diabetes prevalence since 1980: systematic analysis of health examination surveys and epidemiological studies with 370 country-years and 2•7 million participants," *The Lancet*, vol. 378, no. 9785, pp. 31–40, 2011.

[2] N. J. Morrish, S.-L. Wang, L. K. Stevens et al., "Mortality and causes of death in the WHO multinational study of vascular disease in diabetes," *Diabetologia*, vol. 44, no. 2, pp. S14–S21, 2001.

[3] E. Bonora, S. Kiechl, J. Willeit et al., "Population-based incidence rates and risk factors for type 2 diabetes in white individuals: the Bruneck study," *Diabetes*, vol. 53, no. 7, pp. 1782–1789, 2004.

[4] A. J. Collins, R. N. Foley, B. Chavers et al., "United States Renal Data System 2011 annual data report: atlas of chronic kidney disease & end-stage renal disease in the United States," *American Journal of Kidney Diseases*, vol. 59, no. 1, supplement 1, article A7, pp. e1–e420, 2012.

[5] G. Mazzucco, T. Bertani, M. Fortunato et al., "Different patterns of renal damage in type 2 diabetes mellitus: a multicentric study on 393 biopsies," *American Journal of Kidney Diseases*, vol. 39, no. 4, pp. 713–720, 2002.

[6] M. Fiorentino, D. Bolignano, V. Tesar et al., "Renal biopsy in 2015—from epidemiology to evidence-based indications," *American Journal of Nephrology*, vol. 43, no. 1, pp. 1–19, 2016.

[7] T. W. Tervaert, A. L. Mooyaart, K. Amann et al., "Pathologic classification of diabetic nephropathy," *Journal of the American Society of Nephrology*, vol. 21, no. 4, pp. 556–563, 2010.

[8] M. Abbate, C. Zoja, and G. Remuzzi, "How does proteinuria cause progressive renal damage?" *Journal of the American Society of Nephrology*, vol. 17, no. 11, pp. 2974–2984, 2006.

[9] A. Schmitz and M. Vaeth, "Microalbuminuria: a major risk factor in non-insulin-dependent diabetes. A 10-year follow-up study of 503 patients," *Diabetic Medicine*, vol. 5, no. 2, pp. 126–134, 1988.

[10] G. C. Viberti, R. J. Jarrett, and H. Keen, "Microalbuminuria as predictor of nephropathy in diabetics," *The Lancet*, vol. 320, no. 8298, p. 611, 1982.

[11] R. J. MacIsaac, C. Tsalamandris, S. Panagiotopoulos, T. J. Smith, K. J. McNeil, and G. Jerums, "Nonalbuminuric renal insufficiency in type 2 diabetes," *Diabetes Care*, vol. 27, no. 1, pp. 195–200, 2004.

[12] G. Pugliese, A. Solini, C. Fondelli et al., "Reproducibility of albuminuria in type 2 diabetic subjects. Findings from the Renal Insufficiency and Cardiovascular Events (RIACE) Study," *Nephrology Dialysis Transplantation*, vol. 26, no. 12, pp. 3950–3954, 2011.

[13] M. Papale, S. Di Paolo, R. Magistroni et al., "Urine proteome analysis may allow noninvasive differential diagnosis of diabetic nephropathy," *Diabetes Care*, vol. 33, no. 11, pp. 2409–2415, 2010.

[14] E. J. Hoorn, T. Pisitkun, R. Zietse et al., "Prospects for urinary proteomics: exosomes as a source of urinary biomarkers," *Nephrology*, vol. 10, no. 3, pp. 283–290, 2005.

[15] F. Raimondo, S. Corbetta, L. Morosi et al., "Urinary exosomes and diabetic nephropathy: a proteomic approach," *Molecular BioSystems*, vol. 9, no. 6, pp. 1139–1146, 2013.

[16] S. Nielsen, T. Kwon, J. Frøkiær, and P. Agre, "Regulation and dysregulation of aquaporins in water balance disorders," *Journal of Internal Medicine*, vol. 261, no. 1, pp. 53–64, 2007.

[17] Y. Noda, E. Sohara, E. Ohta, and S. Sasaki, "Aquaporins in kidney pathophysiology," *Nature Reviews Nephrology*, vol. 6, no. 3, pp. 168–178, 2010.

[18] P. Agre, G. M. Preston, B. L. Smith et al., "Aquaporin CHIP: the archetypal molecular water channel," *American Journal of Physiology - Renal Fluid and Electrolyte Physiology*, vol. 265, no. 4, pp. F463–F476, 1993.

[19] A. B. Maunsbach, D. Marples, E. Chin et al., "Aquaporin-1 water channel expression in human kidney," *Journal of the American Society of Nephrology*, vol. 8, no. 1, pp. 1–14, 1997.

[20] K. Fushimi, S. Uchida, Y. Harat, Y. Hirata, F. Marumo, and S. Sasaki, "Cloning and expression of apical membrane water channel of rat kidney collecting tubule," *Nature*, vol. 361, no. 6412, pp. 549–552, 1993.

[21] G. Procino, L. Mastrofrancesco, F. Sallustio et al., "AQP5 is expressed in type-B intercalated cells in the collecting duct system of the rat, mouse and human kidney," *Cellular Physiology and Biochemistry*, vol. 28, no. 4, pp. 683–692, 2011.

[22] J. J. Bedford, J. P. Leader, and R. J. Walker, "Aquaporin expression in normal human kidney and in renal disease," *Journal of the American Society of Nephrology*, vol. 14, no. 10, pp. 2581–2587, 2003.

[23] T. Nakamura, T. Saito, I. Kusaka et al., "Decrease in urinary excretion of aquaporin-2 associated with impaired urinary concentrating ability in diabetic nephropathy," *Nephron*, vol. 92, no. 2, pp. 445–448, 2002.

[24] H. Andersen, U. G. Friis, P. B. L. Hansen, P. Svenningsen, J. E. Henriksen, and B. L. Jensen, "Diabetic nephropathy is associated with increased urine excretion of proteases plasmin, prostasin and urokinase and activation of amiloride-sensitive current in collecting duct cells," *Nephrology Dialysis Transplantation*, vol. 30, no. 5, pp. 781–789, 2015.

[25] H. Wu, L. Chen, X. Zhang et al., "Aqp5 is a new transcriptional target of Dot1a and a regulator of Aqp2," *PLoS ONE*, vol. 8, no. 1, Article ID e53342, 2013.

[26] G. Tamma, G. Procino, A. Strafino et al., "Hypotonicity induces aquaporin-2 internalization and cytosol-to-membrane translocation of ICln in renal cells," *Endocrinology*, vol. 148, no. 3, pp. 1118–1130, 2007.

[27] T. Pisitkun, R.-F. Shen, and M. A. Knepper, "Identification and proteomic profiling of exosomes in human urine," *Proceedings of the National Academy of Sciences of the United States of America*, vol. 101, no. 36, pp. 13368–13373, 2004.

[28] F. Umenishi, S. N. Summer, M. Cadnapaphornchai, and R. W. Schrier, "Comparison of three methods to quantify urinary aquaporin-2 protein," *Kidney International*, vol. 62, no. 6, pp. 2288–2293, 2002.

[29] G. Valenti, W. Fraszl, F. Addabbo et al., "Water immersion is associated with an increase in aquaporin-2 excretion in healthy volunteers," *Biochimica et Biophysica Acta—Biomembranes*, vol. 1758, no. 8, pp. 1111–1116, 2006.

[30] A. de Gassart, C. Géminard, B. Février, G. Raposo, and M. Vidal, "Lipid raft-associated protein sorting in exosomes," *Blood*, vol. 102, no. 13, pp. 4336–4344, 2003.

[31] R. Bassi, A. Fornoni, A. Doria, and P. Fiorina, "CTLA4-Ig in B7-1-positive diabetic and non-diabetic kidney disease," *Diabetologia*, vol. 59, no. 1, pp. 21–29, 2016.

[32] G. Currie and C. Delles, "Urinary proteomics for diagnosis and monitoring of diabetic nephropathy," *Current Diabetes Reports*, vol. 16, no. 11, article 104, 2016.

[33] G. Currie, "Biomarkers in diabetic nephropathy: present and future," *World Journal of Diabetes*, vol. 5, no. 6, pp. 763–776, 2014.

[34] R. J. MacIsaac and G. Jerums, "Diabetic kidney disease with and without albuminuria," *Current Opinion in Nephrology and Hypertension*, vol. 20, no. 3, pp. 246–257, 2011.

[35] R. J. MacIsaac, G. Jerums, and M. E. Cooper, "New insights into the significance of microalbuminuria," *Current Opinion in Nephrology and Hypertension*, vol. 13, no. 1, pp. 83–91, 2004.

[36] R. E. Gilbert and M. E. Cooper, "The tubulointerstitium in progressive diabetic kidney disease: more than an aftermath of glomerular injury?" *Kidney International*, vol. 56, no. 5, pp. 1627–1637, 1999.

[37] M. L. A. Kortenoeven and R. A. Fenton, "Renal aquaporins and water balance disorders," *Biochimica et Biophysica Acta (BBA)—General Subjects*, vol. 1840, no. 5, pp. 1533–1549, 2014.

[38] G. Valenti, A. Laera, G. Pace et al., "Urinary aquaporin 2 and calciuria correlate with the severity of enuresis in children," *Journal of the American Society of Nephrology*, vol. 11, no. 10, pp. 1873–1881, 2000.

[39] L. Murer, F. Addabbo, M. Carmosino et al., "Selective decrease in urinary aquaporin 2 and increase in prostaglandin E2 excretion is associated with postobstructive polyuria in human congenital hydronephrosis," *Journal of the American Society of Nephrology*, vol. 15, no. 10, pp. 2705–2712, 2004.

[40] K. Kanno, S. Sasaki, Y. Hirata et al., "Urinary excretion of aquaporin-2 in patients with diabetes insipidus," *New England Journal of Medicine*, vol. 332, no. 23, pp. 1540–1545, 1995.

[41] G. Valenti, A. Laera, S. Gouraud et al., "Low-calcium diet in hypercalciuric enuretic children restores AQP2 excretion and improves clinical symptoms," *American Journal of Physiology—Renal Physiology*, vol. 283, no. 5, pp. F895–F903, 2002.

[42] P. Igarashi, G. B. Vanden Heuvel, J. A. Payne, and B. Forbush III, "Cloning, embryonic expression, and alternative splicing of a murine kidney-specific Na-K-Cl cotransporter," *The American Journal of Physiology—Renal Fluid and Electrolyte Physiology*, vol. 269, no. 3, article 2, pp. F405–F418, 1995.

[43] J. M. Jensen, F. H. Mose, A.-E. O. Kulik, J. N. Bech, R. A. Fenton, and E. B. Pedersen, "Abnormal urinary excretion of NKCC2 and AQP2 in response to hypertonic saline in chronic kidney disease: an intervention study in patients with chronic kidney disease and healthy controls," *BMC Nephrology*, vol. 15, article 101, 2014.

[44] J. J. Morrissey and E. D. Kharasch, "The specificity of urinary aquaporin 1 and perilipin 2 to screen for renal cell carcinoma," *The Journal of Urology*, vol. 189, no. 5, pp. 1913–1920, 2013.

[45] Y. Lu, L. Chen, B. Zhao et al., "Urine AQP5 is a potential novel biomarker of diabetic nephropathy," *Journal of Diabetes and its Complications*, vol. 30, no. 5, pp. 819–825, 2016.

[46] M. Ahloulay, F. Schmitt, M. Déchaux, and L. Bankir, "Vasopressin and urinary concentrating activity in diabetes mellitus," *Diabetes & Metabolism*, vol. 25, no. 3, pp. 213–222, 1999.

[47] L. N. Nejsum, T.-H. Kwon, D. Marples et al., "Compensatory increase in AQP2, p-AQP2, and AQP3 expression in rats with diabetes mellitus," *American Journal of Physiology—Renal Physiology*, vol. 280, no. 4, pp. F715–F726, 2001.

[48] K. Kamoi, M. Ishibashi, and T. Yamaji, "Thirst and plasma levels of vasopressin, angiotensin II and atrial natriuretic peptide in patients with non-insulin-dependent diabetes mellitus," *Diabetes Research and Clinical Practice*, vol. 11, no. 3, pp. 195–202, 1991.

[49] Y. Iwasaki, K. Kondo, T. Murase, H. Hasegawa, and Y. Oiso, "Osmoregulation of plasma vasopressin in diabetes mellitus with sustained hyperglycemia," *Journal of Neuroendocrinology*, vol. 8, no. 10, pp. 755–760, 1996.

[50] L. Bankir, P. Bardoux, and M. Ahloulay, "Vasopressin and diabetes mellitus," *Nephron*, vol. 87, no. 1, pp. 8–18, 2001.

[51] L. Bankir, N. Bouby, and E. Ritz, "Vasopressin: a novel target for the prevention and retardation of kidney disease?" *Nature Reviews Nephrology*, vol. 9, no. 4, pp. 223–239, 2013.

[52] P. Bardoux, D. G. Bichet, H. Martin et al., "Vasopressin increases urinary albumin excretion in rats and humans: involvement of V2 receptors and the renin-angiotensin system," *Nephrology Dialysis Transplantation*, vol. 18, no. 3, pp. 497–506, 2003.

[53] E. Meijer, S. J. L. Bakker, N. Halbesma, P. E. de Jong, J. Struck, and R. T. Gansevoort, "Copeptin, a surrogate marker of vasopressin, is associated with microalbuminuria in a large population cohort," *Kidney International*, vol. 77, no. 1, pp. 29–36, 2010.

[54] T. Ma, B. Yang, F. Umenishi, and A. S. Verkman, "Closely spaced tandem arrangement of AQP2, AQP5, and AQP6 genes in a 27-kilobase segment at chromosome locus 12q13," *Genomics*, vol. 43, no. 3, pp. 387–389, 1997.

[55] W. Wang and M. Zheng, "Role of cAMP-PKA/CREB pathway in regulation of AQP 5 production in rat nasal epithelium," *Rhinology*, vol. 49, no. 4, pp. 464–469, 2011.

Research Progress on Mechanism of Podocyte Depletion in Diabetic Nephropathy

Haoran Dai,[1] Qingquan Liu,[1,2] and Baoli Liu[1,2]

[1]*Department of Nephrology, Shunyi Branch, Beijing Hospital of Traditional Chinese Medicine, Station East 5, Shunyi District, Beijing 101300, China*
[2]*Beijing Hospital of Traditional Chinese Medicine Affiliated to Capital Medical University, 23 Meishuguanhou Street, Dongcheng District, Beijing 100010, China*

Correspondence should be addressed to Qingquan Liu; liuqingquan2003@126.com and Baoli Liu; polyliu2000@sina.com

Academic Editor: Wei J. Liu

Diabetic nephropathy (DN) together with glomerular hyperfiltration has been implicated in the development of diabetic microangiopathy in the initial stage of diabetic diseases. Increased amounts of urinary protein in DN may be associated with functional and morphological alterations of podocyte, mainly including podocyte hypertrophy, epithelial-mesenchymal transdifferentiation (EMT), podocyte detachment, and podocyte apoptosis. Accumulating studies have revealed that disruption in multiple renal signaling pathways had been critical in the progression of these pathological damages, such as adenosine monophosphate-activated kinase signaling pathways (AMPK), wnt/β-catenin signaling pathways, endoplasmic reticulum stress-related signaling pathways, mammalian target of rapamycin (mTOR)/autophagy pathway, and Rho GTPases. In this review, we highlight new molecular insights underlying podocyte injury in the progression of DN, which offer new therapeutic targets to develop important renoprotective treatments for DN over the next decade.

1. Introduction

Diabetic nephropathy (DN), as the primary cause of end-stage renal failure, is one of the most serious complications in diabetic patients, which develops in up to 30%–40% of patients with types 1 or 2 diabetes mellitus [1]. An early sign of DN is an increased amount of urinary protein and characterized by mesangial nodular hyperplasia and thickening of the glomerular basement membrane (GBM). Microalbuminuria plays an important role in the change of the GBM. Additionally, a detailed renal biopsy data analysis regarding diabetics showed that diabetic kidney damage would include visceral epithelial cells and sertoli cell dysfunction [2, 3]. Although some researches demonstrated that podocyte injury had association with the development of DN [4], the mechanisms underlying this association are still not entirely understood and need to be further investigated.

2. Proteinuria and Podocyte Injury in DN

Glomerular epithelial cells, also called podocytes, are highly specialized cells, which are composed of cytoskeletal structure, joint connection, and branching foot processes circling the GBM. Podocytes, as terminal differentiation cells, are important functional cells in the glomerulus and can not regenerate when they suffer from injury. Their damage and apoptosis could result in the destruction of the glomerular filtration membrane and induce unfavorable factors in DN [5]. Foot processes are consisted of basal aspects, basolateral region and parietal region, which firmly adhere to the GBM through podoplanin protein. The basolateral region was found interdigitating with the neighboring basolateral region by slit diaphragm (SD) [6]. Furthermore, transmembrane proteins connect adapter proteins with actin cytoskeleton to maintain filtration barrier structure and function. In the podocyte parietal region, salivary proteins are used to maintain a filtration way among adjacent foot processes in the GBM through sufficient negatively charging [7]. Podocytes play an important role in pathological mechanisms underlying DN. Imasawa et al. [8] declared that structure and function in podocyte molecules transformed in high-glucose conditions, which resulted from suppression of myocyte-specific enhancer factor 2C (MEF2C) and myogenic factor 5 (MYF5) expressions through using a conditionally differentiating human podocyte cell line.

3. Pathomechanism of Podocyte Injury

3.1. Podocyte Hypertrophy. Although the pathophysiology of podocyte hypertrophy in the initial stage of DN is still ambiguous, animal and human studies have established that glomerular podocyte hypertrophy was associated with the development of DN [9, 10]. Previous researches indicated that MAPK, TGF-β, and AngII had different effects on mesangial matrices and cells, leading to glomerular hypertrophy in the progress of DN. However, elaborate mechanisms underlying podocyte hypertrophy were less reported [11]. Romero et al. [12] concluded that AngII increased expressions of parathyroid hormone-related protein (PTHrP), TGF-β1, and cell cycle regulatory protein-p27Kip, which promoted the aggravation of podocyte hypertrophy in high glucose. The mammalian target of rapamycin (mTOR) signaling mainly consisted of mTORC1 and mTORC2. Several studies suggested that mTORC1 was closely associated with the activation of podocyte hypertrophy which was induced by high glucose [13]. In the early stage of diabetes, it was obviously found that high filtration of glomerular is accompanied with podocyte hypertrophy. In general, mature podocytes had to expand the size of themselves in order to compensate for glomerular dilation, which contributed to cover the denuded region of the GBM, because they were terminal-differentiated cells, which no longer are proliferated [14, 15]. Jo et al. [16] declared that interleukin 6 (IL-6) and its downstream cascade signaling proteins, such as Gp130 signal transducer and activator of transcription 3 (STAT3) signal transducer, were key regulators related to podocyte hypertrophy in a high-glucose environment. In general, hyperglycemia induced the overexpression of nuclear STAT3 via the activation of upstream signal transduction element Gp130, which is eventually leading to podocyte hypertrophy. Kim et al. [17] found that TCTP, as a mediating signal of cell growth, was overexpressed with high percentage in the glomeruli of diabetic mice and gave rise to podocyte hypertrophy. Fluorescent double-labeling method indicated that TCTP was mainly observed in podocytes. Studies showed that TCTP could activate the mTORC1 signal pathway and promote high expression of CKIs, which caused podocyte cycle arrest and hypertrophy. On the contrary, overexpression of mTORC1 and CKIs could be inhibited by gene knockout of TCTP, to make the podocyte bodies smaller. Meanwhile, in vitro experiments indicated that TCTP inhibitor could downregulate the expression of CKIs, ameliorating podocyte hypertrophy caused by high glucose. Kim et al. [18] showed that AngII could also upregulate protein expressions of kinases ERK1/2 and Akt/PKB, which contributed to podocyte hypertrophy. Hence, it has been shown that all ERK1/2, Akt/PKB, IL-6/JAK2/STAT3, and mTOR signal-pathway activities had important roles in podocyte hypertrophy (Figure 1).

3.2. Podocyte Epithelial-Mesenchymal Transition. Previous studies have shown a connection between podocyte apoptosis and proteinuria. However, more and more studies have demonstrated that normal epithelial cells showed phenotype conversion of a variety of nephropathies [19]. Cells lost their original features when the pathological process of EMT occurred, which induced disappeared cell contact, damaged cell polarity, and recaptured characteristics of the mesenchymal markers, such as vimentin, α-smooth muscle actin (α-SMA), and fibroblast-specific protein 1 (FSP1). FSP1 is one of the important members of calcium-binding protein S100 family and also a fibroblast-specific protein without epithelial cells [20]. Many studies showed that renal tubular epithelial cells and podocytes were activated after acute (48–72 h) exposure of cells to elevated glucose levels or other stimulations of diabetes, which resulted in less protein expressions of E-cadherin and ZO-1. Conversely, expressions of transdifferentiation proteins, such as α-SMA and vimentin, were immediately increased after these stimulation [21–23]. In the initial stage of STZ-induced diabetes, morphology of podocytes were damaged, accompanied with increased expression of the podocyte marker, nephrin protein, and a fall in the mesenchymal marker, desmin protein [24]. Yamaguchi et al. [25] found that FSP1-positive cells were significantly increased in urinary sediment and approximately attached to 86 percent of total podocytes in 109 type 2 diabetes patients. 43 of these patients with massive proteinuria in this study experienced kidney biopsy. The FSP1 positive cells selectively expressed Snail and ILK preferentially, which played pivotal roles in inducing EMT. Xing et al. [26] demonstrated that podocyte incubated in elevated glucose levels for 48 h could trigger activation of the PI3K/AKT pathway and elevate protein expressions of α-SMA and desmin. Whereas, protein expressions of podocalyxin and nephrin were suppressed. Functionally, it is apparently speculated that podocyte EMT may be tightly related to the PI3K/AKT signal pathway. Li et al. [27] found that the elevated glucose level upregulated protein expression of Snail and suppressed protein expressions of P-cadherin and nephrin in vitro. The change above decreased podocyte-related proteins of nephrin and ZO-1, elevated expressions of desmin, MMP9, and FSP1 in sequence. As shown in Figure 2, podocyte EMT widely participated in the early stage of podocyte deletion in diabetes mellitus via leading to podocyte detachment or podocyte apoptosis [28].

3.3. Podocyte Detachment. Podocytes and the glomerular basement membrane (GBM) are closely connected and then prevent the excretion of proteinuria via sustaining the glomerular filtration barrier. Researches showed that not only dead podocytes but also normal podocytes were found in the urinary sediment of patients with kidney disease. Furthermore, it had been concluded that podocytes could be cultured from urine of a healthy person [22]. One study

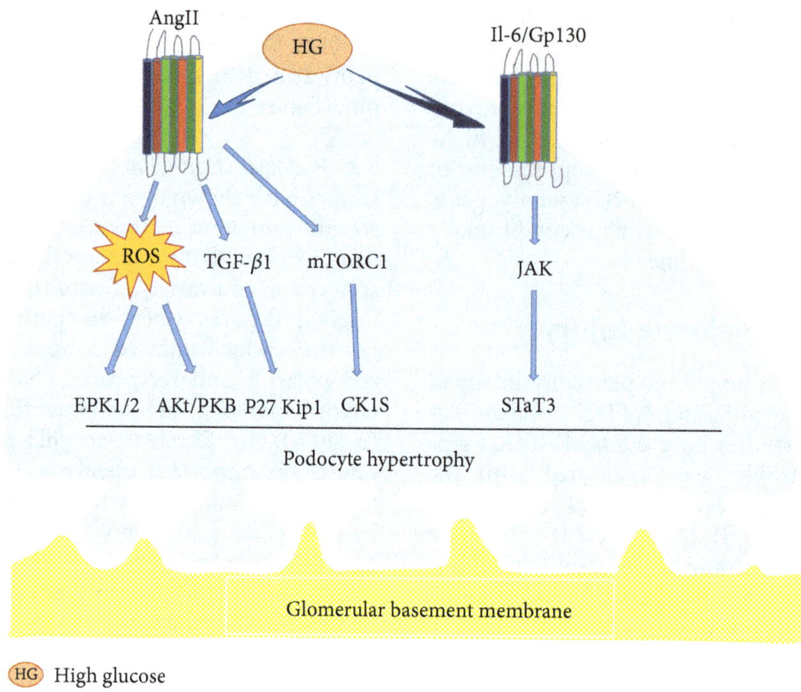

FIGURE 1: Podocyte hypertrophy. In elevated glucose levels, AngII could elevate protein expressions of kinases ERK1/2 and Akt/PKB through ROS, trigger activation of p27Kip1 via TGF-β1 signal pathway, or upregulate protein expression of CKIs by activating mTORC1, which eventually resulted in glomerular podocyte hypertrophy. Additionally, high glucose also induced podocyte hypertrophy via activation of the IL-6/Gp130-JAK/STAT3 signal pathway.

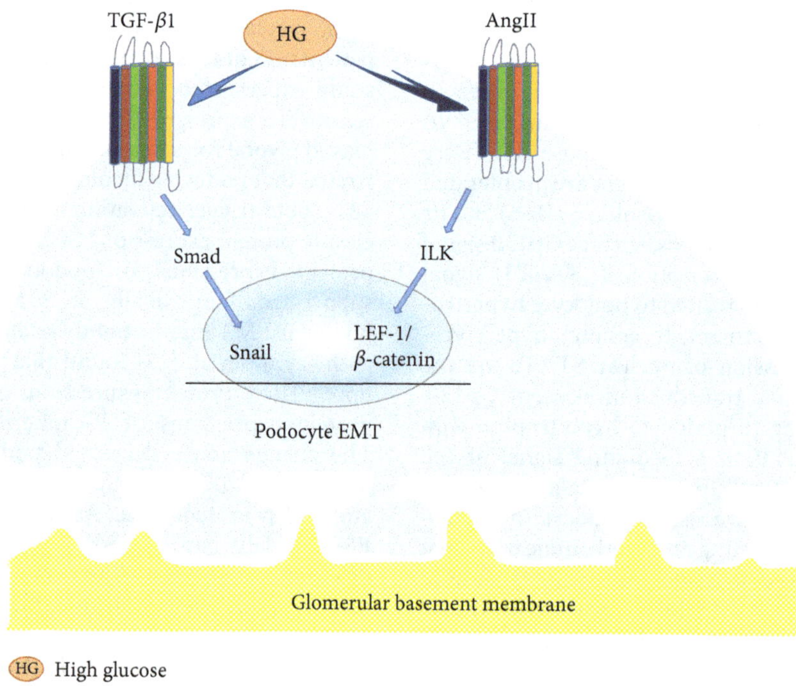

FIGURE 2: Podocyte EMT. In elevated glucose levels, the TGF-β1/Smad signal pathway resulted in increased protein expression of Snail in cultured podocytes, which induced podocyte EMT. Additionally, AngII promoted translocation of β-catenin/LEF-1 complexes into the nucleus through the enhancement of ILK in transitioning epithelia, where they downregulated CD2AP expression via promoting EMT transcription in podocytes.

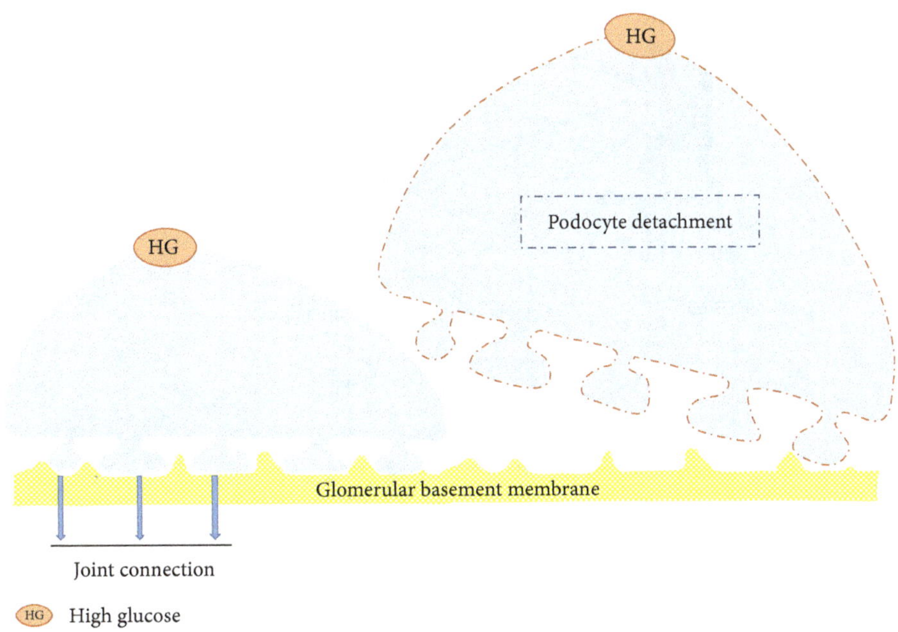

Figure 3: Podocyte detachment. Some podocytes became hypertrophic and stripped from the basement membrane in sequence, while the others tightly combined with basement membrane at the same stage of DN, which seems to be more related to podocyte EMT.

displayed that urinary podocyte might be used as an earlier biomarker of DN than proteinuria albuminuria in respect of renal injury [29]. It was generally known that integrin $\alpha3\beta1$ was an important receptor which could tightly connect podocyte with the GBM [30]. Jim et al. [31] drew a conclusion that the expressions of podocyte marker proteins in the diabetic kidney, such as synaptopodin, podocin, and nephrin, were significantly decreased, which could result in podocyte cytoskeleton disorder, damaged sufficient adhesion, and separation between podocyte and the basement membrane. Hyperglycemia could downregulate expression of integrin $\alpha3\beta1$ in both human and rat, as well as trigger activation of integrin-linked kinase (ILK). In addition, recent researches suggested that $\alpha3\beta1$ participated in the adhesion function of podocyte [32, 33]. Experimental researches on animals displayed that podocytes could break away from the glomerulus basement membrane in an artificial diabetic rat induced by streptozotocin (STZ) [34]. It was also suggested that both podocyte detachment and podocyte early changed in DN. However, whether podocyte detachment or podocyte hypertrophy appeared earlier was still difficult to distinguish [35]. It was obviously found that podocyte loss contributed to the development of DN. In the progression of disease, we found that in the same stage of DN, some podocytes became hypertrophy and detached from the basement membrane. Whereas, the others tightly combined with the basement membrane [36] (Figure 3).

3.4. Podocyte Apoptosis. Apoptosis pathway is involved in cellular growth and differentiation in many diseases, such as DN and IgA nephropathy. There are some evidences that podocyte apoptosis played a role in reduction in density and number of glomerular. Susztak et al. [37] found that mitochondria could activate nicotinamide adenine dinucleotide phosphate (NADPH) oxidase and reactive oxygen species (ROS) in high glucose, improve the expressions of p38 protein kinase and caspase 3 at the same time, then led to podocyte apoptosis, and produced much proteinuria. Glycosylation end products activated transcription factor FOXO4, which also induced podocyte apoptosis via p38 protein kinase signaling pathways [38]. In addition, the cytochrome P450 family raised hydroxyl and reduced coenzyme II twenty-four carbon olefine acid oxidase in high glucose, which increased the active oxygen class produces and prompting podocyte apoptosis [39]. Notch1 signal-dependent activation of p53 is a new podocyte apoptosis pathway [40]. A recent study found that podocyte apoptosis was closely related to the expression level of Notch, which then induced proteinuria and glomerular sclerosis. The activation of Notch signaling pathway may be included in DN all-acquired common mechanism of kidney disease [41]. Experiment with STZ-induced diabetes mouse displayed that the expressions of Jag, Notch, and ICN1 were increased immediately and the downstream component, such as Hesl and Heyl, were activated. It is also shown that the expressions of Bcl-2 and p53 were provoked, and the process eventually induced podocyte apoptosis [42]. Under normal circumstances, apoptosis-promoting and anti-apoptosis signaling pathways coexisted in a same condition which maintained dynamic balance and guaranteed the stability environment. In general, phosphatidylinositol-3 kinase/protein kinase in podocyte plays a crucial role in inhibition of podocyte apoptosis signaling pathways. The experiment also suggested that protein kinase phosphorylation reduced in db/db mice, which may be an important inducement for podocyte apoptosis [43]. Liu et al. [44] found that podocyte apoptosis was associated with the disorder of cytoskeleton. Nestin is a VI intermediate filament protein related cell cytoskeleton which expressed in podocyte. The protein expression

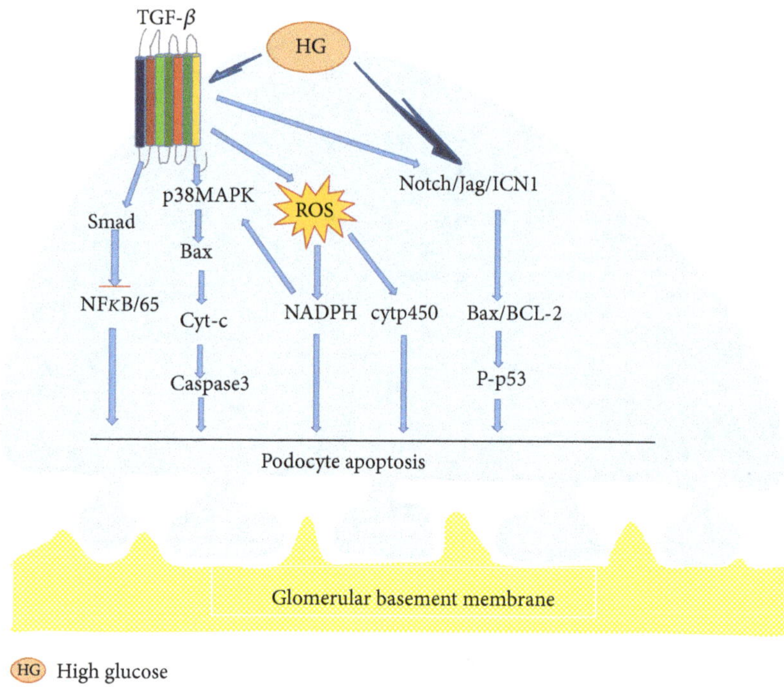

FIGURE 4: Podocyte detachment. In elevated glucose levels, TGF-β provoked p38 MAPK, Smad signal pathway and NADPH, and cytp450 to increase the protein expressions of Bax, cytochrome C, and caspase-3, which resulted from overproduction of ROS. All of the above processes could result in podocyte apoptosis. They also stimulated the Notch/Jag/ICN1 signal pathway, which activated the Bcl-2 and p53 apoptotic pathways and induced podocyte apoptosis.

of nestin reduced in high glucose, however, podocyte apoptosis rate increased. TGF-β1 could directly activate Smad7, which inhibit the activity of NF-kB and resulted in podocyte apoptosis. It also could provoke p38 MAP kinase, enhance the protein expressions of Bax and produce cytochrome C, which activated caspase-3 apoptosis pathway in sequence [45]. Liu et al. [46] demonstrated that metadherin was a potent modulator of podocyte apoptosis, which represented the target of miR-30 miRNAs, facilitating podocyte apoptosis via activating the HG-induced p38 MAPK-dependent pathway. Yao et al. [47] concluded that AS-IV inhibited podocyte apoptosis induced by high glucose, which reduced the expressions of TRPC6 and impaired the crosstalk of intracellular Ca2+ in podocytes. More and more evidences [48] indicated that AS-IV could protect the kidney from DN, including reduced podocyte damages and suppressed podocyte apoptosis through antioxidative stress and anti-inflammatory signaling pathways (Figure 4).

4. Main Signaling Pathways of Podocyte Injury Mechanism in DN

Many studies [49] suggested that DN podocyte injury was induced by the association of multiple factors, including mechanical stress, inflammatory reaction, oxidative stress, TGF-β1 induction, renin angiotensin aldosterone system (RAAS) activation, and AGEs accumulation. And there are lots of signaling pathways involved in the regulation mTOR signaling pathways mediated by autophagy, adenosine monophosphate-activated kinase (AMPK) signaling pathway, Wnt/β-catenin signaling pathway, and so on.

4.1. Adenosine Monophosphate-Activated Kinase Signaling Pathways (AMPK) in DN. AMPK is not only a serine protein kinase [50] playing a vital role in cells and tissues metabolisms of the diabetes progression but also one of the important metabolic emergency protein kinases. AMPK pathway is an autophagy-related signaling pathway composed of subunit heterologous proteins α, β, and γ, which was activated as lack of energy in cells [51]. In the activation process, it could combine calmodulin-dependent kinase β (CaMKK) and transform-activated kinase 1 (TAK-l). Then, it also effectively mediated intracellular calcium concentration and triggered the activation of the AMPK pathway to induce autophagy [52]. Conversely, AMPK could inhibit mTORCl activity and induce autophagy through TSCl/2-Rheb signaling pathways and/or phosphorus acidification of raptor-related regulatory protein [53]. Meanwhile, AMPK also directly launch the phosphorylation of Ulkl/2 and induction of autophagy [54]. In addition, Sharma et al. [55] reported that adiponectin attenuated the induction of oxidative stress, reduced the synthesis of NADPH in podocyte, and simultaneously reduced albuminuria excretion in adiponectin-knockout mouse which could activate the AMPK pathway.

4.2. Wnt/β-Catenin Signaling Pathways in DN. Wnt protein is one kind of secreted glycoprotein, containing a signal peptide and 23 or 24 conserved cysteine residues. It was activated via binding to ligand proteins and the Frizzled protein family. Wnts triggered a cascade of downstream reaction protein including axin, Disheveled, adenomatous polyposis coli (APC), and glycogen synthase kinase- (GSK-) 3β, which gave rise to phosphorylation of β-catenin in nuclei [56]. Researches showed that Wnt signaling pathway had effects on the differentiation, hyperplasia, maturation, and viability of cells [57]. It had been declared to be induced in DN, which played a crucial role in apoptosis and EMT formation of mesangial cells, podocyte, and tubular cells [58]. However, Dickkopf-related protein 1 (DKK1) is a secreted protein consisted of two cysteine abundant regions, which could reduce podocyte injury, decrease albuminuria, and protect the kidney by specific blocking Wnt/β-catenin signal pathways [59, 60]. Liu et al. [61] found that curcumin could prevent glomerular podocyte injury by inhibiting activated Wnt family members and β-catenin downstream effectors in obesity-related glomerular disease model. Zhang et al. [62, 63] demonstrated that ubiquitin carboxy-terminal hydrolase-1 (UCH-L1) is abnormally expressed in injury podocytes, especially in immune-mediated disease. They also proved that the Wnt/β-catenin signal pathway is promptly activated in podocyte, coinciding with overexpression of UCH-L1 induced by high glucose meanwhile [64]. Li et al. [65] announced that podocyte incubated in high glucose underwent injury, which attributed to the upregulation of transient receptor potential cation channel 6 (TRPC6) protein triggered by the classic Wnt/β-catenin pathway.

4.3. Endoplasmic Reticulum Stress-Related Signaling Pathways in DN. Recent studies suggested that endoplasmic reticulum stress was closely relevant to the injury of podocytes, endothelial cells, and mesangial cells in DN. It could induce glomerular obstacle of podocyte structure and function, participate in a variety of kidney diseases, and also lead to glomerular sclerosis [66]. Continuous endoplasmic reticulum stress had effects on the function of endoplasmic reticulum and could launch apoptosis signaling pathways which were mediated by endoplasmic reticulum stress at the same time and then activated the downstream apoptotic signaling molecules [67]. In patients with diabetes, hyperglycemia can motivate endoplasmic reticulum stress through a variety of ways, then cause cellular damage [68]. As important factors of DN, advanced glycation end products (AGE) could upregulate the protein expressions of glucose-regulated protein 78 (GRP78) and induce endoplasmic reticulum stress depending on its dosage and time, eventually inducing apoptosis of podocyte [69]. In addition, high glucose and free fatty acids could induce endoplasmic reticulum stress as well as the occurrence of apoptosis in podocyte of rats, which could be inhibited via exogenous endoplasmic reticulum molecular chaperone [70]. Endoplasmic reticulum stress may aggravate podocyte dysfunction in the early stage of DN [71]. The relationship between endoplasmic reticulum stress and podocyte injury could be summarized as follows: both hyperglycemia and AGE could initiate endoplasmic reticulum stress and activate mTORC-1 protein. Furthermore, continuous injury will contribute to podocyte apoptosis by the caspase-12 pathway, while AGE could act on collagen type IV, leading to podocytes loss or dysfunction [15, 72].

4.4. mTOR Signaling Pathways Mediated by Autophagy in DN. Studies have shown that intervention in the activity of the mTOR signaling pathway is likely to aggravate podocyte injury in DN renal tissue [73]. Activated podocytes in mTORC1 could result in dislocation of nephrin protein, ZO-1 (skeleton protein) disorders, and podocyte EMT, which could eventually lead to podocyte detachment, foot process fusion and disappearance, and other podocyte injuries in Inoki knockout PcKO Tsc1 mouse. In conclusion, mTORC1 activity has a key regulatory role in podocyte injury on the DN model of rats [15]. In addition, many pharmacological studies of mTOR inhibitors have further elucidated the importance of mTOR in mediating DN podocyte injury from another perspective such as rapamycin-protected podocytes [15, 74]. Recent researches have indicated that autophagy, a protective mechanism of podocyte, was used to against damage in a variety of pathological factors. On the contrary, autophagy defects not only led to podocyte injury and proteinuria but also aggravated glomerular sclerosis [54, 75, 76]. Rapamycin, as the mTOR inhibitor, acted on the autophagy pathway and protected the podocyte [55]. In conclusion, there were two kinds of defense mechanism that the autophagy/mTOR signal pathway is using to protect podocytes from further injury. The pathway of mTORC1 is activated and the protective autophagy is inhibited when podocyte is in a high-glucose environment. Specifically, mTORC1 inhibited the autophagosome by initiating the activity of UNC-51-like kinase 1 (ULK1) [13, 77]. In addition, rapamycin could upregulate the protein expression of 1A/1B light chain 3 (LC3) in vitro and improved podocyte autophagy disorders in sequence [78].

4.5. Rho/ROCK Signaling Pathway in DN. The Rho family is mainly composed of RhoA, Rac1, and Cdc42. They were the vital mediators of the actin cytoskeleton protein structure [79]. RhoA/ROCK pathway was the important process in the progression of DN and could induce downstream signaling element cell apoptosis, migration, and differentiation [80]. Immoderate activities of Rac1, a key element in the Rho GTPases family, could cause macroalbuminuria quickly with focal foot process effacement, indicating podocyte apoptosis and slit diaphragm protein expression reductions in high glucose [81, 82]. Wang et al. [83] found that Drp1 at serine 600, as a substrate of Rho signal pathway, not only initiated mitochondrial ROS and podocyte apoptosis in high glucose but also was phosphorylated in ROCK1 knock-out mouse. RhoA played an important role in glomerular filtration barrier integrity, and its overexpression could damage the structure and function of the barrier [84, 85]. Phosphatase and tensin homolog (PTEN) could inhibit the activation of the RhoA/Rac1/Cdc42 signaling pathway, which contributed to reverse the cytoskeletal rebuilding and prevent the development of DN [86, 87]. Previous studies demonstrated that Rho-GTPase family elements were probably activated to induce the downstream cascade reaction when they were exposed in the environment of diabetics, such as AGEs,

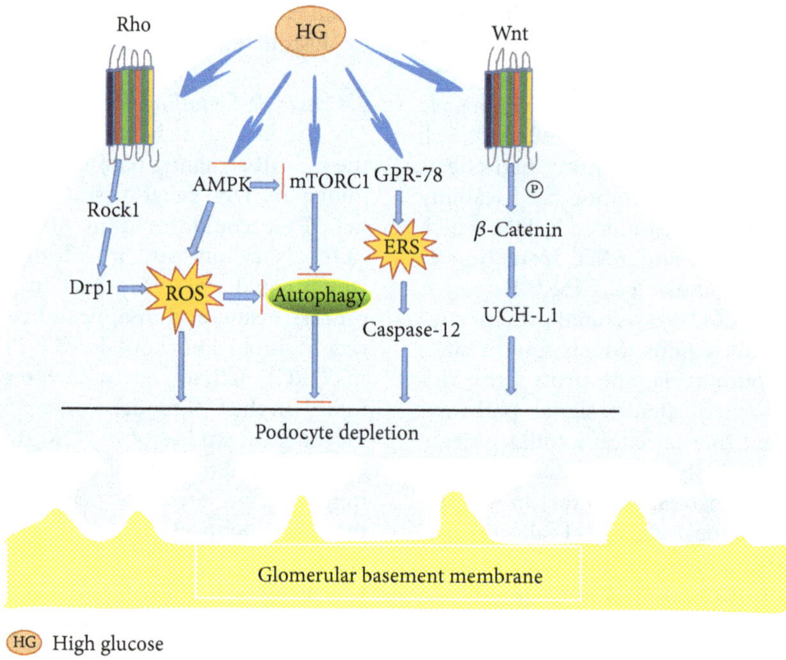

FIGURE 5: Signaling pathways underlying podocyte injury in DN. Hyperglycemia induced podocyte injury through the Rho/ROCK1 and AMPK signal pathways. Part elements of the signal pathway initiated autophagy that protects from podocyte injury through ROS or mTORC1 participation in the active process. Additionally, GPR-78 activated ERS to induce podocyte apoptosis based on the caspase-12 signal pathway, and the Wnt/β-catenin signal pathway may have similar changes in podocyte injury, which could induce podocyte depletion via upregulating expression of UCH-L1 in high glucose.

hyperglycemia, oxidized LDL, and ROS [88, 89]. Xie et al. [90] suggested that Berberine not only inhibited RhoA/ROCK to improve DN but also regulated Rho GTPases to reduce oxidative stress.

5. Conclusion

Podocyte injury is an important factor in DN progression. Several studies implied that the process of albuminuria development in DN was complicated, which presumably included four phases in sequence as follows: podocyte hypertrophy, podocyte EMT, podocyte detachment, and podocyte apoptosis, serving as the warning mark of GFR in DN [91]. More and more signal pathways which induced podocyte injury have been discovered [92], such as Wnt/β-catenin signaling pathways, Rho-GTPase signaling pathways, mTOR signaling pathways, and endoplasmic reticulum stress-related signaling pathways (Figure 5). People have understood the multiple pathogenesis mechanisms of podocyte injury in DN, but the complex clinical manifestations of that tell us that there is still potential knowledge required to study and discuss.

Conflicts of Interest

The authors confirm that there is no conflict of interests.

Acknowledgments

This work was supported by grants from the National Science and Technology Major Project (no. 81673907) and Beijing Municipal Science & Technology Project (no. Z161100000516024).

References

[1] L. Gnudi, R. J. Coward, and D. A. Long, "Diabetic nephropathy: perspective on novel molecular mechanisms," *Trends in Endocrinology and Metabolism*, vol. 27, no. 11, pp. 820–830, 2016.

[2] K. Drummond, M. Mauer, and International Diabetic Nephropathy Study Group, "The early natural history of nephropathy in type 1 diabetes. II. Early renal structural changes in type 1 diabetes," *Diabetes*, vol. 51, no. 5, pp. 1580–1587, 2002.

[3] M. E. Pagtalunan, P. L. Miller, S. Jumping-Eagle et al., "Podocyte loss and progressive glomerular injury in type II diabetes," *The Journal of Clinical Investigation*, vol. 99, no. 2, pp. 342–348, 1997.

[4] M. Dalla Vestra, A. Masiero, A. M. Roiter, A. Saller, G. Crepaldi, and P. Fioretto, "Is podocyte injury relevant in diabetic nephropathy? Studies in patients with type 2 diabetes," *Diabetes*, vol. 52, no. 4, pp. 1031–1035, 2003.

[5] Y. Maezawa, M. Takemoto, and K. Yokote, "Cell biology of diabetic nephropathy: roles of endothelial cells, tubulointerstitial cells and podocytes," *Journal of Diabetes Investigation*, vol. 6, no. 1, pp. 3–15, 2015.

[6] D. B. Johnstone and L. B. Holzman, "Clinical impact of research on the podocyte slit diaphragm," *Nature Clinical Practice Nephrology*, vol. 2, no. 5, pp. 271–282, 2006.

[7] T. Takeda, "Podocyte cytoskeleton is connected to the integral membrane protein podocalyxin through Na+/H+-exchanger

regulatory factor 2 and ezrin," *Clinical and Experimental Nephrology*, vol. 7, no. 4, pp. 260–269, 2003.

[8] T. Imasawa, E. Obre, N. Bellance et al., "High glucose repatterns human podocyte energy metabolism during differentiation and diabetic nephropathy," *The FASEB Journal*, vol. 31, no. 1, pp. 294–307, 2016.

[9] J. S. Lin and K. Susztak, "Podocytes: the weakest link in diabetic kidney disease," *Current Diabetes Reports*, vol. 16, no. 5, p. 45, 2016.

[10] N. Herbach, I. Schairer, A. Blutke et al., "Diabetic kidney lesions of GIPRdn transgenic mice: podocyte hypertrophy and thickening of the GBM precede glomerular hypertrophy and glomerulosclerosis," *American Journal of Physiology - Renal Physiology*, vol. 296, no. 4, pp. 819–829, 2009.

[11] N. H. Kim, "Podocyte hypertrophy in diabetic nephropathy," *Nephrology (Carlton)*, vol. 10, Supplement, pp. S14–S16, 2005.

[12] M. Romero, A. Ortega, A. Izquierdo, P. López-Luna, and R. J. Bosch, "Parathyroid hormone-related protein induces hypertrophy in podocytes via TGF-β1 and p27Kip1: implications for diabetic nephropathy," *Nephrology, Dialysis, Transplantation*, vol. 25, no. 8, pp. 2447–2457, 2010.

[13] M. K. Lu, X. G. Gong, and K. L. Guan, "mTOR in podocyte function: is rapamycin good for diabetic nephropathy?," *Cell Cycle*, vol. 10, no. 20, pp. 3415-3416, 2011.

[14] M. Gödel, B. Hartleben, N. Herbach et al., "Role of mTOR in podocyte function and diabetic nephropathy in humans and mice," *The Journal of Clinical Investigation*, vol. 121, no. 6, pp. 2197–2209, 2011.

[15] K. Inoki, H. Mori, J. Wang et al., "mTORC1 activation in podocytes is a critical step in the development of diabetic nephropathy in mice," *The Journal of Clinical Investigation*, vol. 121, no. 6, pp. 2181–2196, 2011.

[16] H. A. Jo, J. Y. Kim, S. H. Yang et al., "The role of local IL6/JAK2/STAT3 signaling in high glucose-induced podocyte hypertrophy," *Kidney Research Clinical Practice*, vol. 35, no. 4, pp. 212–218, 2016.

[17] D. K. Kim, B. Y. Nam, J. J. Li et al., "Translationally controlled tumour protein is associated with podocyte hypertrophy in a mouse model of type 1 diabetes," *Diabetologia*, vol. 55, no. 4, pp. 1205–1217, 2012.

[18] N. H. Kim, H. Rincon-Choles, B. Bhandari, G. G. Choudhury, H. E. Abboud, and Y. Gorin, "Redox dependence of glomerular epithelial cell hypertrophy in response to glucose," *American Journal of Physiology - Renal Physiology*, vol. 290, no. 3, pp. 741–751, 2006.

[19] Y. Liu, "Epithelial to mesenchymal transition in renal fibrogenesis: pathologic significance molecular mechanism, and therapeutic intervention," *Journal of the American Society Nephrology*, vol. 15, no. 1, pp. 1–12, 2004.

[20] J. P. Thiery and J. P. Sleeman, "Complex networks orchestrate epithelial-mesenchymal transitions," *Nature Reviews Molecular Cell Biology*, vol. 7, no. 2, pp. 131–142, 2006.

[21] Q. Lu, X. J. Ji, Y. X. Zhou et al., "Quercetin inhibits the mtorc1/p70s6k signaling-mediated renal tubular epithelial-mesenchymal transition and renal fibrosis in diabetic nephropathy," *Pharmacological Research*, vol. 99, pp. 237–247, 2015.

[22] I. Loeffler and G. Wolf, "Epithelial-to-mesenchymal transition in diabetic nephropathy: fact or fiction?," *Cell*, vol. 4, no. 4, pp. 631–652, 2015.

[23] L. Liu, W. Fu, J. Xu, L. Shao, and Y. Wang, "Effect of bmp7 on podocyte transdifferentiation and smad7 expression induced by hyperglycemia," *Clinical Nephrology*, vol. 84, no. 2, pp. 95–99, 2015.

[24] H. Y. Dai, M. Zheng, R. N. Tang et al., "Effects of angiotensin receptor blocker on phenotypic alterations of podocytes in early diabetic nephropathy," *The American Journal of the Medical Sciences*, vol. 341, no. 3, pp. 207–214, 2011.

[25] Y. Yamaguchi, M. Iwano, D. Suzuki et al., "Epithelial-mesenchymal transition as a potential explanation for podocyte depletion in diabetic nephropathy," *American Journal Kidney Diseases*, vol. 54, no. 4, pp. 653–664, 2009.

[26] L. Xing, Q. Liu, S. Fu et al., "PTEN inhibits high glucose-induced phenotypic transition in podocytes," *Journal of Cellular Biochemistry*, vol. 116, no. 8, pp. 1776–1784, 2015.

[27] Y. Li, Y. S. Kang, C. Dai, L. P. Kiss, X. Wen, and Y. Liu, "Epithelial-to-mesenchymal transition is a potential pathway leading to podocyte dysfunction and proteinuria," *The American Journal of Pathology*, vol. 172, no. 2, pp. 299–308, 2008.

[28] S. U. Vogelmann, W. J. Nelson, B. D. Myers, and K. V. Lemley, "Urinary excretion of viable podocytes in health and renal disease," *American Journal of Physiology - Renal Physiology*, vol. 285, no. 1, pp. F40–F48, 2003.

[29] D. Yu, A. Petermann, U. Kunter, S. Rong, S. J. Shankland, and J. Floege, "Urinary podocyte loss is a more specific marker of ongoing glomerular damage than proteinuria," *Journal of the American Society of Nephrology*, vol. 16, no. 6, pp. 1733–1741, 2005.

[30] S. Mathew, X. Chen, A. Pozzi, and R. Zent, "Integrins in renal development," *Pediatric Nephrology*, vol. 27, no. 6, pp. 891–900, 2012.

[31] B. Jim, M. Ghanta, A. Qipo et al., "Dysregulated nephrin in diabetic nephropathy of type 2 diabetes: a cross sectional study," *PLoS One*, vol. 7, no. 5, article e36041, 2012.

[32] J. Chen, D. Gui, Y. Chen, L. Mou, Y. Liu, and J. Huang, "Astragaloside IV improves high glucose-induced podocyte adhesion dysfunction via alpha3beta1 integrin upregulation and integrin-linked kinase inhibition," *Biochemical Pharmacology*, vol. 76, no. 6, pp. 796–804, 2008.

[33] H. C. Chen, C. A. Chen, J. Y. Guh, J. M. Chang, S. J. Shin, and Y. H. Lai, "Altering expression of alpha3beta1 integrin on podocytes of human and rats with diabetes," *Life Sciences*, vol. 67, no. 19, pp. 2345–2353, 2000.

[34] M. Regoli and M. Bendayan, "Alterations in the expression of the alpha 3 beta 1 integrin in certain membrane domains of the glomerular epithelial cells (podocytes) in diabetes mellitus," *Diabetologia*, vol. 40, no. 1, pp. 15–22, 1997.

[35] M. Miyauchi, M. Toyoda, K. Kobayashi et al., "Hypertrophy and loss of podocytes in diabetic nephropathy," *Internal Medicine*, vol. 48, no. 18, pp. 1615–1620, 2009.

[36] W. Kriz, B. Hähnel, H. Hosser, S. Rösener, and R. Waldherr, "Structural analysis of how podocytes detach from the glomerular basement membrane under hypertrophic stress," *Front Endocrinol (Lausanne)*, vol. 5, p. 207, 2014.

[37] K. Susztak, A. C. Raff, M. Schiffer, and E. P. Böttinger, "Glucose-induced reactive oxygen species cause apoptosis of podocytes and podocyte depletion at the onset of diabetic nephropathy," *Diabetes*, vol. 55, no. 1, pp. 225–233, 2006.

[38] P. Y. Chuang, Q. Yu, W. Fang, J. Uribarri, and J. C. He, "Advanced glycation endproducts induce podocyte apoptosis by activation of the FOXO4 transcription factor," *Kidney International*, vol. 72, no. 8, pp. 965–976, 2007.

[39] A. A. Eid, Y. Gorin, B. M. Fagg et al., "Mechanisms of podocyte injury in diabetes: role of cytochrome P450 and NADPH oxidases," *Diabetes*, vol. 58, no. 5, pp. 1201–1211, 2009.

[40] T. Niranjan, B. Bielesz, A. Gruenwald et al., "The Notch pathway in podocytes plays a role in the development of glomerular disease," *Nature Medicine*, vol. 14, no. 3, pp. 290–298, 2008.

[41] R. Bonegio and K. Susztak, "Notch signaling in diabetic nephropathy," *Experimental Cell Research*, vol. 318, no. 9, pp. 986–992, 2012.

[42] F. Gao, M. Yao, Y. Cao, S. Liu, Q. Liu, and H. Duan, "Valsartan ameliorates podocyte loss in diabetic mice through the Notch pathway," *International Journal of Molecular Medicine*, vol. 37, no. 5, pp. 1328–1336, 2016.

[43] T. Tejada, P. Catanuto, A. Ijaz et al., "Failure to phosphorylate AKT in podocytes from mice with early diabetic nephropathy promotes cell death," *Kidney International*, vol. 73, no. 12, pp. 1385–1393, 2008.

[44] W. Liu, Y. Zhang, J. Hao et al., "Nestin protects mouse podocytes against high glucose-induced apoptosis by a Cdk5-dependent mechanism," *Journal of Cellular Biochemistry*, vol. 113, no. 10, pp. 3186–3196, 2012.

[45] J. H. Li, X. R. Huang, H. J. Zhu et al., "Advanced glycation end products activate Smad signaling via TGF-beta-dependent and independent mechanisms: implications for diabetic renal and vascular disease," *The FASEB Journal*, vol. 18, no. 1, pp. 176–178, 2004.

[46] W. T. Liu, F. F. Peng, H. Y. Li et al., "Metadherin facilitates podocyte apoptosis in diabetic nephropathy," *Cell Death & Disease*, vol. 7, no. 11, article e2477, 2016.

[47] X. M. Yao, Y. J. Liu, Y. M. Wang, H. Wang, and B. B. Zhu, "Astragaloside IV prevents high glucose-induced podocyte apoptosis via downregulation of TRPC6," *Molecular Medicine Reports*, vol. 13, no. 6, pp. 5149–5156, 2016.

[48] D. Gui, J. Huang, Y. Guo et al., "Astragaloside IV ameliorates renal injury in streptozotocin-induced diabetic rats through inhibiting NF-κB-mediated inflammatory genes expression," *Cytokine*, vol. 61, no. 3, pp. 970–977, 2013.

[49] D. Kawanami, K. Matoba, and K. Utsunomiya, "Signaling pathways in diabetic nephropathy," *Histology and Histopathology*, vol. 31, no. 10, pp. 1059–1067, 2016.

[50] Y. Kim and C. W. Park, "Adenosine monophosphate-activated protein kinase in diabetic nephropathy kidney," *Kidney Research and Clinical Practice*, vol. 35, no. 2, pp. 69–77, 2016.

[51] S. Kume, M. C. Thomas, and D. Koya, "Nutrient sensing, autophagy, and diabetic nephropathy," *Diabetes*, vol. 61, no. 1, pp. 23–29, 2012.

[52] S. Alers, A. S. Lffler, S. Wesselborg, and B. Stork, "Role of AMPK-mTOR-UIk1/2 in the regulation of autophagy: cross talk, shortcuts and feedbacks," *Molecular and Cellular Biology*, vol. 32, no. 1, pp. 2–11, 2012.

[53] J. Kim, M. Kundu, B. Viollet, and K. L. Guan, "AMPK and mTOR regulate autophagy through direct phosphorylation of UIk1," *Nature Cell Bio1ogy*, vol. 13, no. 2, pp. 132–141, 2011.

[54] Y. Tanaka, S. Kume, M. Kitada et al., "Autophagy as a therapeutic target in diabetic nephropathy," *Experimental Diabetes Research*, vol. 2012, Article ID 628978, 12 pages, 2012.

[55] K. Sharma, S. RamachandraRao, G. Qiu et al., "Adiponectin regulates albuminuria and podocyte function in mice," *The Journal of Clinical Investigation*, vol. 118, no. 5, pp. 1645–1656, 2008.

[56] H. Levers and R. Nusse, "Wnt/β-catenin signaling and disease," *Cell*, vol. 149, no. 6, pp. 1192–1205, 2012.

[57] I. Matsui, T. Ito, H. Kurihara, E. Imai, T. Ogihara, and H. M. Snail, "Snail, a transcriptional regulator, represses nephrin expression in glomerular epithelial cells of nephrotic rats," *Laboratory Investigation*, vol. 87, no. 3, pp. 273–283, 2007.

[58] L. Xiao, M. Wang, S. Yang, F. Liu, and L. Sun, "A glimpse of the pathogenetic mechanisms of Wnt/β-catenin signaling in diabetic nephropathy," *BioMed Research International*, vol. 2013, Article ID 987064, 7 pages, 2013.

[59] H. Kato, A. Gruenwald, J. H. Suh et al., "Wnt/β-catenin pathway in podocytes integrates cell adhesion, differentiation, and survival," *The Journal of Biological Chemistry*, vol. 286, no. 29, pp. 26003–26015, 2011.

[60] W. He, Y. S. Kang, C. Dai, and Y. Liu, "Blockade of Wnt/β-catenin signaling by paricalcitol ameliorates proteinuria and kidney injury," *Journal of American Society of Nephrology*, vol. 22, no. 1, pp. 90–103, 2011.

[61] B. L. Liu, Y. P. Chen, H. Cheng et al., "The protective effects of curcumin on obesity-related glomerulopathy are associated with inhibition of wnt/β-catenin signaling activation in podocytes," *Evidence-Based Complementary and Alternative Medicine*, vol. 2015, Article ID 827472, 12 pages, 2015.

[62] H. Zhang, X. Mao, Y. Sun et al., "NF-κB upregulates ubiquitin C-terminal hydrolase 1 in diseased podocytes in glomerulonephritis," *Molecular Medicine Reports*, vol. 12, no. 2, pp. 2893–2901, 2015.

[63] H. Zhang, Y. Sun, R. Hu et al., "The regulation of the UCH-L1 gene by transcription factor NF-κB in podocytes," *Cellular Signalling*, vol. 25, no. 7, pp. 1574–1585, 2013.

[64] H. Zhang, W. Luo, Y. Sun, Y. Qiao, and L. Zhang, "Wnt/β-catenin signaling mediated-UCH-L1 expression in podocytes of diabetic nephropathy," *International Journal of Molecular Sciences*, vol. 17, no. 9, article E1404, 2016.

[65] Z. Li, J. Xu, P. Xu, S. Liu, and Z. Yang, "Wnt/β-catenin signalling pathway mediates high glucose induced cell injury through activation of TRPC6 in podocytes," *Cell Proliferation*, vol. 46, no. 1, pp. 76–85, 2013.

[66] Y. Yuan, X. Xu, C. Zhao et al., "The roles of oxidative stress, endoplasmic reticulum stress, and autophagy in aldosterone mineralocorticoid receptor-induced podocyte injury," *Laboratory Investigation*, vol. 95, no. 12, pp. 1374–1386, 2015.

[67] G. Rong, X. Tang, T. Guo et al., "Advanced oxidation protein products induce apoptosis in podocytes through induction of endoplasmic reticulum stress," *Journal of Physiology and Biochemistry*, vol. 71, no. 3, pp. 455–470, 2015.

[68] Y. Cao, Y. Hao, H. Li et al., "Role of endoplasmic reticulum stress in apoptosis of differentiated mouse podocytes induced by high glucose," *International Journal of Molecular Medicine*, vol. 33, no. 4, pp. 809–816, 2014.

[69] Y. Chen, C. P. Liu, K. F. Xu et al., "Effect of taurine-conjugated ursodeoxycholic acid on endoplasmic reticulum stress and apoptosis induced by advanced glycation end products in cultured mouse podocytes," *American Journal of Nephrology*, vol. 28, no. 6, pp. 1014–1022, 2008.

[70] S. M. Colgan, A. A. Hashimi, and R. C. Austin, "Endoplasmic reticulum stress and lipid dysregulation," *Expert Reviews in Molecular Medicine*, vol. 13, article e4, 2011.

[71] A. Zhuang and J. M. Forbes, "Stress in the kidney is the road to pERdition: is endoplasmic reticulum stress a pathogenic mediator of diabetic nephropathy?," *The Journal of Endocrinology*, vol. 222, no. 3, pp. R97–R111, 2014.

[72] M. Sakaguchi, M. Isono, K. Isshiki, T. Sugimoto, D. Koya, and A. Kashiwagi, "Inhibition of mTOR signaling with rapamycin attenuates renal hypertrophy in the early diabetic mice," *Biochemical and Biophysical Research Communications*, vol. 340, no. 1, pp. 296–301, 2006.

[73] M. Pourghasem, H. Shafi, and Z. Babazadeh, "Histological changes of kidney in diabetic nephropathy," *Caspian Journal of Internal Medicine*, vol. 6, no. 3, pp. 120–127, 2015.

[74] L. Wu, Z. Feng, S. Cui et al., "Rapamycin upregulates autophagy by inhibiting the mTOR-ULK1 pathway, resulting in reduced podocyte injury," *PLoS One*, vol. 8, no. 5, article e63799, 2013.

[75] B. Hartleben, M. Gödel, C. Meyer-Schwesinger et al., "Autophagy influences glomerular disease susceptibility and maintains podocyte homeostasis in aging mice," *The Journal of Clinical Investigation*, vol. 120, no. 4, pp. 1084–1096, 2010.

[76] Y. Ding and M. E. Choi, "Autophagy in diabetic nephropathy," *The Journal of Endocrinology*, vol. 224, no. 1, pp. R15–R30, 2015.

[77] N. Hosokawa, T. Hara, T. Kaizuka et al., "Nutrient-dependent mTORC1 association with the ULK1-Atg13-FIP200 complex required for autophagy," *Molecular Biology of the Cell*, vol. 20, no. 7, pp. 1981–1991, 2009.

[78] T. Xiao, X. Guan, L. Nie et al., "Rapamycin promotes podocyte autophagy and ameliorates renal injury in diabetic mice," *Molecular and Cellular Biochemistry*, vol. 394, no. 1-2, pp. 145–154, 2014.

[79] S. M. Blattner, J. B. Hodgin, M. Nishio et al., "Divergent functions of the Rho GTPases Rac1 and Cdc42 in podocyte injury," *Kidney International*, vol. 84, no. 5, pp. 920–930, 2013.

[80] R. Komers, "Rho kinase inhibition in diabetic kidney disease," *British Journal of Clinical Pharmacology*, vol. 76, no. 4, pp. 551–559, 2013.

[81] H. Yu, H. Suleiman, A. H. Kim et al., "Rac1 activation in podocytes induces rapid foot process effacement and proteinuria," *Molecular and Cellular Biology*, vol. 33, no. 23, pp. 4755–4764, 2013.

[82] M. Ishizaka, T. Gohda, M. Takagi et al., "Podocyte-specific deletion of Rac1 leads to aggravation of renal injury in STZ-induced diabetic mice," *Biochemical and Biophysical Research Communications*, vol. 467, no. 3, pp. 549–555, 2015.

[83] W. Wang, Y. Wang, J. Long et al., "Mitochondrial fission triggered by hyperglycemia is mediated by rock1 activation in podocytes and endothelial cells," *Cell Metabolism*, vol. 15, no. 2, pp. 186–200, 2012.

[84] K. Asanuma, E. Yanagida-Asanuma, C. Faul, Y. Tomino, K. Kim, and P. Mundel, "Synaptopodin orchestrates actin organization and cell motility via regulation of RhoA signalling," *Nature Cell Biology*, vol. 8, no. 5, pp. 485–491, 2006.

[85] L. Wang, M. J. Ellis, J. A. Gomez, W. Eisner, and W. Fennell, "Mechanisms of the proteinuria induced by Rho GTPases," *Kidney International*, vol. 81, no. 11, pp. 1075–1085, 2012.

[86] J. S. Lin, Y. Shi, H. Peng et al., "Loss of PTEN promotes podocyte cytoskeletal rearrangement, aggravating diabetic nephropathy," *The Journal of Pathology*, vol. 236, no. 1, pp. 30–40, 2015.

[87] H. Y. Gee, P. Saisawat, S. Ashraf, T. W. Hurd, and V. Vega-Warner, "ARHGDIA mutations cause nephrotic syndrome via defective RHO GTPase signaling," *The Journal of Clinical Investigation*, vol. 123, no. 8, pp. 3243–3253, 2013.

[88] F. Peng, D. Wu, B. Gao, A. J. Ingram, and B. Zhang, "RhoA/Rho-kinase contribute to the pathogenesis of diabetic renal disease," *Diabetes*, vol. 57, no. 6, pp. 1683–1692, 2008.

[89] G. I. Welsh, L. J. Hale, V. Eremina, M. Jeansson, and Y. Maezawa, "Insulin signaling to the glomerular podocyte is critical for normal kidney function," *Cell Metabolism*, vol. 12, no. 4, pp. 329–340, 2010.

[90] X. Xie, X. Chang, L. Chen, K. Huang, and J. Huang, "Berberine ameliorates experimental diabetes-induced renal inflammation and fibronectin by inhibiting the activation of RhoA/ROCK signaling," *Molecular and Cellular Endocrinology*, vol. 381, no. 1-2, pp. 56–65, 2013.

[91] S. S. Guhr, M. Sachs, A. Wegner, J. U. Becker, and T. N. Meyer, "The expression of podocyte-specific proteins in parietal epithelial cells is regulated by protein degradation," *Kidney International*, vol. 84, no. 3, pp. 532–544, 2013.

[92] F. C. Brosius, C. C. Khoury, C. L. Buller, and S. Chen, "Abnormalities in signaling pathways in diabetic nephropathy," *Expert Review of Endocrinology and Metabolism*, vol. 5, no. 1, pp. 51–64, 2010.

12

Serotonin and Its Receptor as a New Antioxidant Therapeutic Target for Diabetic Kidney Disease

Yu Yang,[1] Hui Huang,[1,2] Zheng Xu,[2,3] and Jun-kai Duan[4]

[1]*Department of Endocrinology, Metabolism, and Genetics, Jiangxi Provincial Children's Hospital, Nanchang, Jiangxi, China*
[2]*Pediatric Research Institute, Department of Pediatrics, University of Louisville, Louisville, KY, USA*
[3]*Department of Cardiovascular Disorders, The First Hospital of Jilin University, Changchun, China*
[4]*Department of Cardiovascular Disorders, Jiangxi Provincial Children's Hospital, Nanchang, Jiangxi, China*

Correspondence should be addressed to Yu Yang; yyhhjxey@gmail.com

Academic Editor: Robertina Giacconi

Diabetic kidney disease (DKD) is a widespread chronic microvascular complication of diabetes mellitus (DM), affects almost 30–50% of patients, and represents a leading cause of death of DM. Serotonin or 5-hydroxytryptamine (5-HT) is a multifunctional bioamine that has crucial roles in many physiological pathways. Recently, emerging evidence from experimental and clinical studies has demonstrated that 5-HT is involved in the pathogenesis of diabetic vascular complications. The 5-HT receptor (5-HTR) antagonists exert renoprotective effects by suppressing oxidative stress, suggesting that 5-HTR can be used as a potential target for treating DKD. In this review, therefore, we summarize the published information available for the involvement of 5-HT and 5-HTR antagonists in the pathogenesis of various diabetic complications with a particular focus of DKD. We conclude that 5-HTR is a potential therapeutic target for treating DKD, as it has been successfully applied in animal models and has currently being investigated in randomized and controlled clinical trials.

1. Introduction

Diabetic kidney disease (DKD) is one of the most epidemic chronic microvascular complications of diabetes mellitus (DM), and it is prevalent in approximately 30–50% of patients with diabetes [1–5]. DKD is the leading cause of chronic and end-stage renal diseases worldwide, and in the past few decades, it has been associated with high morbidity and mortality [6–11].

The pathogenesis of DKD remains not completely understood; however, there is strong experimental evidence that prolonged hyperglycemia leads to the mitochondrial production of reactive oxygen species (ROS), resulting in oxidative stress, which plays a key role in DKD [12–16]. Inflammation induced and exacerbated by oxidative stress is closely associated with the development and progression of DKD.

5-Hydroxytryptamine (5-HT) is a potent vasoactive amine that plays pivotal roles in insulin secretion [17–19], energy metabolism [20], mitochondrial biogenesis [21], the immune system [22, 23], and vascular inflammation [24–27]. However, the functions of 5-HT have not been elucidated yet. Recently, several studies have shown that 5-HT and 5-HT receptors (5-HTR) are involved in the pathogenesis of diabetic vascular complications [17, 28–31]. 5-HTR antagonists have a renoprotective effect by suppressing oxidative stress and inflammatory cytokines [32–35], suggesting that 5-HTR antagonists could be used to treat DKD. This review assesses and describes the current understanding of 5-HT's involvement in the pathogenesis of DKD and the potential use of 5-HTR antagonists in the clinical treatment of DKD.

2. 5-HT Synthesis and Metabolism and 5-HT Receptors

5-HT is a monoamine neurotransmitter and hormone mainly produced by enterochromaffin cells of the gastrointestinal tract [21]. 5-HT is derived from tryptophan and predominantly stored in circulating platelets, and it is distributed throughout the body to regulate the hormones of

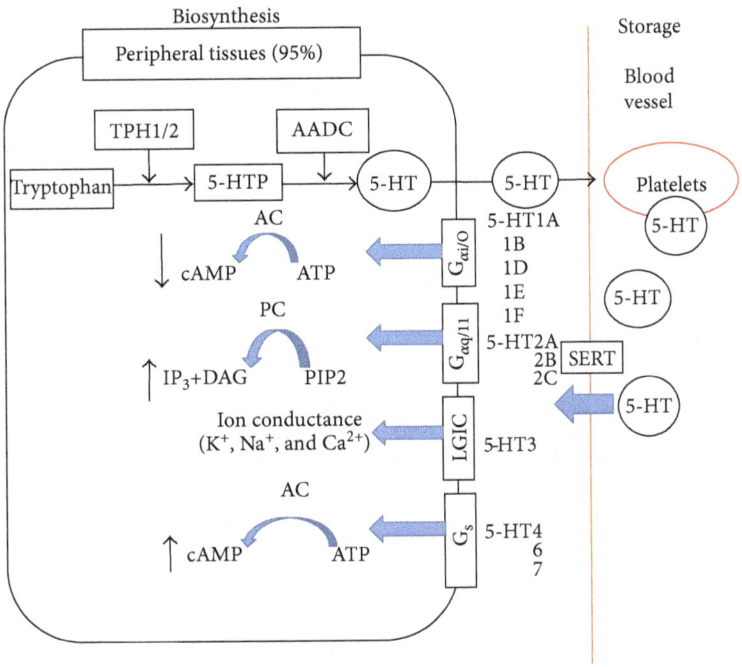

FIGURE 1: A model of 5-HT biosynthesis and metabolism in peripheral tissues. 5-HT synthesis is dependent on the enzyme tryptophan hydroxylase (TPH); the released 5-HT is controlled by the autonomous nervous system and released locally into the circulatory system, and most of them are stored in platelets. Reuptake of 5-HT is mediated by SERT. The effects of 5-HT are mediated through 14 serotonergic receptors that have been grouped into seven broad families. All 5-HTRs are G protein-coupled receptors (GPCRs), except 5-HT_3 that is a ligand-gated cationic channel. 5-HT GPCRs were coupled to all three canonical signaling pathways through $G_{\alpha i/O}$, $G_{\alpha q/11}$, and G_s that are involved in the cAMP pathway and allow this receptor family to modulate several biochemical signaling pathways.

several main physiological parameters, such as cardiovascular function [36], insulin secretion [17], energy homeostasis [20], and appetite [37].

5-HT synthesis is dependent on the enzyme tryptophan hydroxylase (TPH), which is encoded by two different genes: tryptophan hydroxylase 1 (Tph1) and Tph2, which are expressed in the peripheral tissues and brain, respectively. Peripheral 5-HT is presumed to be unable to cross the blood-brain barrier. The majority of the peripheral 5-HT is stored in platelets and also present in other tissues and many cells. The released 5-HT is controlled by the autonomous nervous system and released locally into the circulatory system, where it is used for the aggregation of platelets through various stimuli, including atherosclerosis [26, 38]. 5-HT is primarily inactivated by the reuptake of serotonergic neurons that secrete it; this reuptake is mediated by the highly selective plasmalemma 5-HT transporter (5-HTT), which is also known as the serotonin transporter (SERT) [39] (Figure 1).

5-HT produces a myriad of physiological and pathological effects in humans, which are mediated through 14 serotonergic (5-HTergic) receptors that have been grouped into seven broad families (5-HT_1, 5-HT_2, 5-HT_3, 5-HT_4, 5-HT_5, 5-HT_6, and 5-HT_7). All 5-HTRs are G protein-coupled receptors (GPCRs), except 5-HT_3 that is a ligand-gated cationic channel. 5-HT GPCR was coupled to all three canonical signaling pathways through $G_{\alpha i}/_O$, $G_{\alpha q/11}$, and G_s that are involved in the cAMP pathway and allow this receptor family to modulate several biochemical signaling pathways [40].

3. 5-HT in Diabetes and Diabetic Complications

Pancreatic β-cells synthesize and store 5-HT, which is coreleased with insulin [41]. An increased plasma level of 5-HT is a biomarker for diabetic complications, and positive correlations have been established between the plasma 5-hydroxyindoleacetic acid (5-HIAA; the main 5-HT metabolite) level and coronary heart disease [36, 42–45]. Selective serotonergic functional alterations have shown therapeutic relevance in diabetic rats [29, 30, 46]. These studies and their findings have been summarized in the subsequent sections and suggest that 5-HT plays a role in DM.

3.1. 5-HT and Gestational Diabetes. In pregnant mice, prolactin (PRL) stimulates islet prolactin receptors (PRLRs) to trigger a strong upregulation of both isoforms of TPH. TPH upregulation activates 5-HT synthesis in some pancreatic β-cells, which in turn induce glucose-stimulated insulin secretion (GSIS) [47, 48]. The insulin secretion is upregulated by the 5-HT_{2B} receptor (5-HT_{2B}R) and downregulated by the 5-HT_{1D} receptor (5-HT_{1D}R) in β-cells, making 5-HT a paracrine regulator of β-cell proliferation. 5-HT_{3A}R channels in wild-type animals allow a 5-HT-mediated influx of

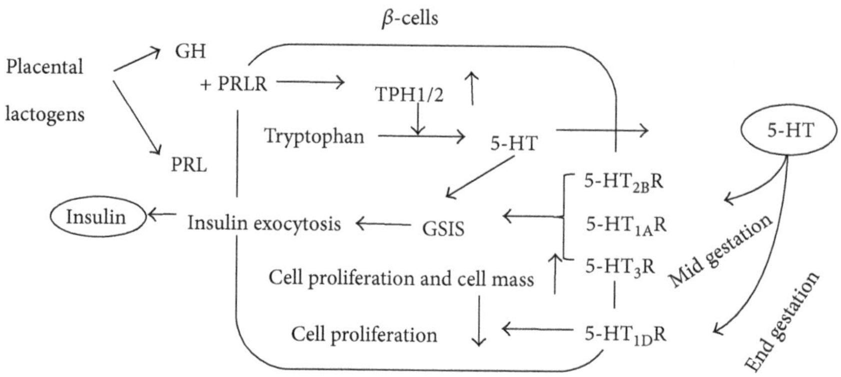

FIGURE 2: Mechanism of 5-HT in the mouse pancreatic beta-cells during pregnancy. In pregnant mice, prolactin (PRL) stimulates islet prolactin receptors (PRLRs) to trigger a strong upregulation of both isoforms of TPH. TPH upregulation activates 5-HT synthesis in some pancreatic β-cells, which in turn induce GSIS. The insulin secretion is upregulated by the 5-HT_{2B} receptor ($5\text{-HT}_{2B}R$) and downregulated by the 5-HT_{1D} receptor ($5\text{-HT}_{1D}R$) in β-cells, making 5-HT a paracrine regulator of β-cell proliferation. $5\text{-HT}_{3A}R$ channels in wild-type animals allow a 5-HT-mediated influx of cations, depolarizing the resting membrane potential and lowering the threshold for glucose-induced insulin exocytosis.

cations, depolarizing the resting membrane potential and lowering the threshold for glucose-induced insulin exocytosis [19, 49], as illustrated in Figure 2. Disrupting this balance can result in gestational diabetes.

3.2. 5-HTR and Type 2 DM. Type 2 DM (T2DM) describes a group of metabolic disorders characterized by defects in insulin secretion and insulin sensitivity. Impaired insulin secretion from pancreatic β-cells is an important factor in the etiology of T2DM. However, the complex regulation and mechanism of insulin secretion from β-cells have not been completely elucidated.

High plasma levels of 5-HT have been reported in patients with T2DM, although its potential effect on insulin secretion is unclear. The release of 5-HT from activated platelets is enhanced, decreasing intraplatelet 5-HT content and resulting in increased plasma levels of 5-HT in patients with diabetes [44].

3.2.1. $5\text{-HT}_{2C}R$. $5\text{-HT}_{2C}R$-deficient mice are overweight, exhibit an abnormal feeding behavior, show insulin resistance, and have significantly higher blood glucose concentrations, suggesting that 5-HT may affect glucose and lipid metabolism [17, 20, 50]. Insulin secretion is affected by $5\text{-HT}_{2C}R$, which is indicative of the possibility that an aberrant 5-HT system could also affect the regulation of energy metabolism. Increased expression of $5\text{-HT}_{2C}R$ in both the hypothalamus and β-cells could mediate a protective strategy to prevent excess energy intake. As illustrated in Figure 3, $5\text{-HT}_{2C}R$-expressing pro-opiomelanocortin neurons are required to control energy and glucose homeostasis [51].

Although, in human T2DM islet cells, the expression of $5\text{-HT}_{2C}R$ has not been observed [31], the $5\text{-HT}_{2C}R$ agonist Belviq (lorcaserin) is the first FDA-approved drug to treat obesity in 15 years [52], and central serotonin 2C receptors regulated glucose homeostasis and may represent a rational target for type 2 diabetes (T2DM) treatment [53, 54]. The $5\text{-HT}_{2C}R$ agonist m-chlorophenylpiperazine (mCPP) improves glucose homeostasis and insulin sensitivity, and antagonists or genetic loss of $5\text{-HT}_{2C}R$ impairs glucose homeostasis [55, 56].

3.2.2. $5\text{-HT}_{1D}R$ and $5\text{-HT}_{1A}R$. Bennet et al. [31] reported that $5\text{-HT}_{1D}R$ and $5\text{-HT}_{1A}R$ messenger RNA expression was increased in human T2DM islets. 5-HT inhibits both basal- and glucose-induced insulin secretions, and the selective $5\text{-HT}_{1D}R$ agonist (PNU142633) inhibits GSIS in nondiabetic human islets, whereas the $5\text{-HT}_{1D}R$ antagonist (LY310762) stimulates GSIS. Interestingly, upon stimulation with 5-HT in isolated islets from patients with T2DM, the inhibitory effect of 5-HT was completely lost (both in basal and stimulatory conditions of glucose); instead, the stimulation of insulin secretion was observed. This indicated that 5-HT acts through increased signaling through the $5\text{-HT}_{2A}R$ in diabetic conditions. The $5\text{-HT}_{2A}R$ antagonist (sarpogrelate hydrochloride) markedly decreased the glycated hemoglobin A1c level. The expression of $5\text{-HT}_{1D}R$ had a negative correlation with somatostatin (SST) and SST receptors (SSTR) 1–5, whereas the expression of $5\text{-HT}_{2A}R$ did not have any correlation with either SST or any of the SSTRs; this suggests that increased expression of $\text{HT}_{1D}R$ in human islet cells, as observed in T2DM islet cells, leads to decreased expression of SST and its receptors (Figure 4).

3.3. 5-HT as an Immunomodulator in DM. Although several physiological causes that lead to DM remain unknown, evidence suggests that autoimmunity plays an important role in DM and diabetic complications. There is an increasingly collective perspective regarding the association of 5-HT with the activation of immunoinflammatory pathways and the onset of autoimmune reactions. Almost all the circulating 5-HT are found in platelets and released following platelet activation, on contact with damaged endothelium or induced by ischemia, indicating that 5-HT also contributes to the innate and adaptive immune responses [22, 57]. 5-HT

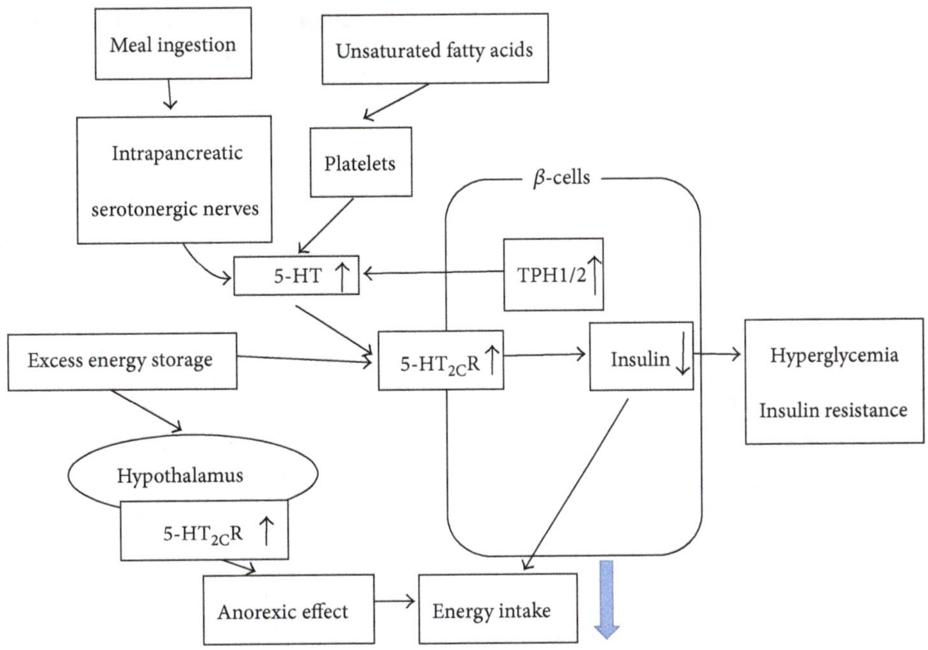

FIGURE 3: Model showing the modulation of 5-HT2cR in DM. 5-HT2CR-deficient mice showed that 5-HT may affect glucose and lipid metabolism. Insulin secretion is affected by 5-HT2CR, which is indicative of the possibility that an aberrant 5-HT system could also affect the regulation of energy metabolism. Increased expression of 5-HT2CR in both the hypothalamus and β-cells could mediate a protective strategy to prevent excess energy intake. 5-HT2CR-expressing pro-opiomelanocortin neurons are required to control energy and glucose homeostasis.

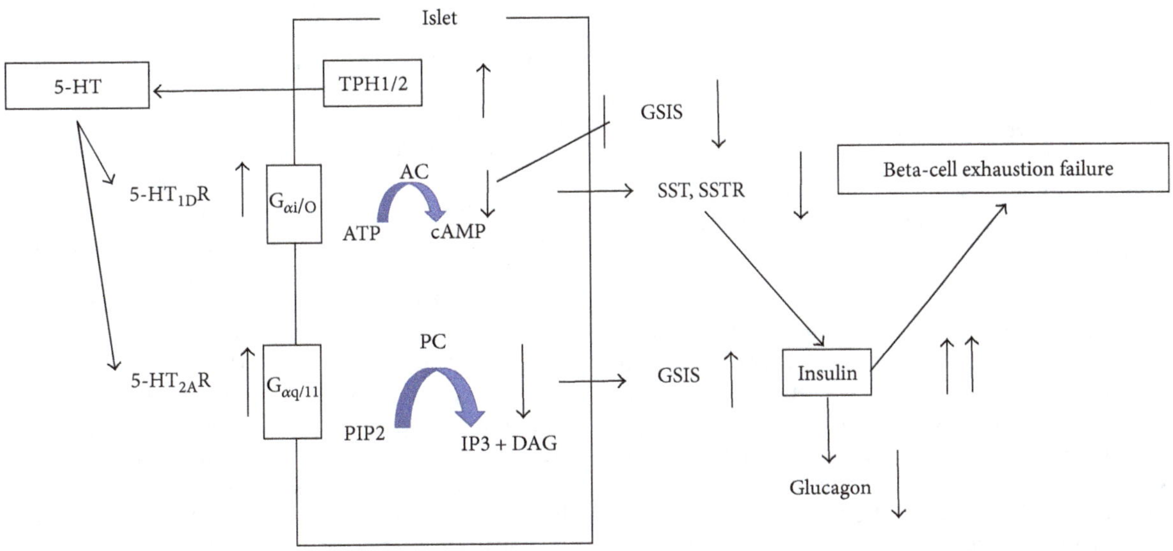

FIGURE 4: Illustration to show the mechanism of 5-HT1D and 5-HT2AR in human T2DM. 5-HT1DR and 5-HT1AR messenger RNA expression was increased in human T2DM islets. The 5-HT2AR antagonist (sarpogrelate hydrochloride) markedly decreased the glycated hemoglobin A1c level. The expression of 5-HT1DR had a negative correlation with somatostatin (SST) and SST receptors (SSTR), whereas the expression of 5-HT2AR did not have any correlation with either SST or any of the SSTRs; this suggests that increased expression of HT1DR in human islet cells, as observed in T2DM islet cells, leads to decreased expression of SST and its receptors.

stimulation increases murine peritoneal macrophage production of proinflammatory cytokines [25]. The expression of 5-HTRs has been identified in rodent and human innate immune cells, which include neutrophils, eosinophils, monocytes, macrophages, dendritic cells, mast cells, and natural killer cells [58].

5-HT was identified as an immunomodulator owing to its ability to stimulate or inhibit inflammation.

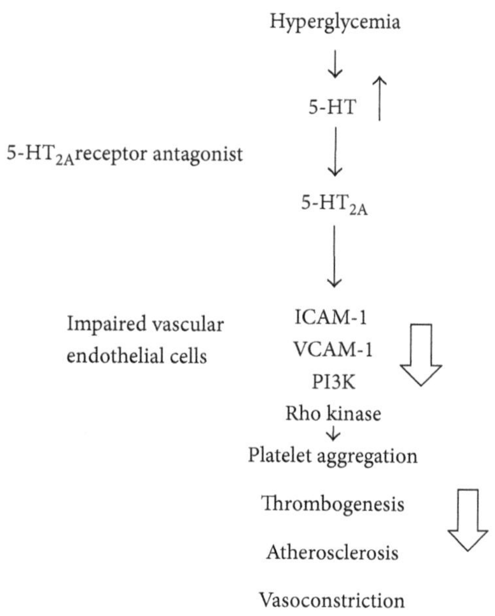

FIGURE 5: Mechanisms of 5-HT_{2A} receptor antagonist contributing to DM-induced cardiovascular complications. Sarpogrelate, a 5-HT2AR antagonist, has been shown to attenuate diabetes-induced cardiovascular complications, which decrease the blood glucose level, inhibit the release of intercellular adhesion molecule-1 (ICAM-1) and vascular cell adhesion molecule-1 (VCAM-1), and reduce 5-HT-induced contraction in aortas through the PI3K and Rho kinase pathway.

Moreover, 5-HT has immunomodulatory effects that are induced by activating 5-HTR and SERT, which are differentially expressed in many leukocytes. Arthritis [59], systemic sclerosis [38, 60], lung fibrosis [61], and allergic asthma [62] are all associated with changes in the serotonergic system, which is associated with leukocytes.

3.4. $5\text{-HT}_{2A}R$ and DM-Induced Vascular Complications. 5-HT is a potent vasoactive amine in the cardiovascular system. Cardiovascular disorders of diabetes can be characterized by atherosclerosis [63]. There is strong evidence that impaired vascular endothelial and smooth muscle functions play important roles in the process of DM-induced cardiovascular complications [63, 64]. 5-HT, induced by impaired vascular endothelial cells, is involved in the pathological process of platelet aggregation [45], thrombogenesis [65], contraction of carotid arteries [66], and arteriogenesis [67] in DM-induced vascular complications through $5\text{-HT}_{2A}R$.

Sarpogrelate, a 5-HT2AR antagonist, has been shown to attenuate diabetes-induced cardiovascular complications, which decrease the blood glucose level [66], inhibit the release of intercellular adhesion molecule-1(ICAM-1) and vascular cell adhesion molecule-1(VCAM-1) [68], and reduce 5-HT-induced contraction in aortas through the PI3K [66] and Rho kinase [69] pathway, as illustrated in Figure 5.

4. Mechanism of the 5-HTR Antagonist for Treating DKD

DKD is a main microvascular complication of diabetes and the most common cause of end-stage renal disease strongly associated with cardiovascular morbidity and mortality, which cause an enormous burden on affected patients and health care systems [70]. Histopathological changes associated with DKD are characterized by thickening of the glomerular basement membrane; podocyte effacement and hypertrophy; accumulation of extracellular matrix and proteins, such as collagen and fibronectin; and the hyalinization of afferent and efferent glomerular arterioles [71, 72].

Studies have indicated that inflammation is an important mechanism in the pathogenesis of DKD that triggers a complex network of pathophysiological events that modulate intracellular signaling pathways involving protein kinase C [73–75] and ROS [76–78] and act in a concerted manner to induce transcription factors, cytokines, chemokines, and growth factors during hyperglycemia [13–15, 79–81]. Although many factors have been implicated in the pathogenesis of DKD, inflammation is believed to play a fundamental role in the early development and progression of DKD [14, 71, 78, 80, 82]. Drugs with anti-inflammatory effects have been used as a new clinical approach for treating DKD.

Previous reports have indicated that the increased plasma concentrations of 5-HT or its metabolite (5-HIAA) are valuable biomarkers for estimating the DKD-associated risk during the early stages of the disease [35, 83, 84]. 5-HT has been shown to enhance the production of type IV collagen by human mesangial cells, and its production is mediated by the activation of protein kinase C and a subsequent increase in active transforming growth factor-β (TGF-β) [85]. Stimulation of $5\text{-HT}_{2A}Rs$ by 5-HT induces the expression of TGF-β through extracellular signal-regulated kinases, a key mediator of proliferative and fibrotic signals in mesangial cells [86–89], as illustrated in Figure 6.

Studies have shown that 5-HTR antagonists are effective in preventing diabetic nephropathy. Sarpogrelate, a 5-HT2 subtype 2A antagonist [33, 34], reduced albuminuria in the early stages of DKD by improving glomerular endothelial function through the reduction in glomerular platelet activation and an increase in serum adiponectin concentrations in a diabetic animal model. Ogawa et al. [90] and Park et al. [91] found that sarpogrelate can reduce albuminuria and plasma and urinary monocyte chemoattractant protein-1 levels in patients with DKD. Tropisetron, a 5-HT_3 receptor antagonist, can attenuate early DM through calcineurin inhibition and by suppressing oxidative stress and some inflammatory cytokines in streptozotocin-induced diabetic rats [32].

5. Conclusions

There is an increasing repertoire of evidence supporting 5-HT as a causative agent for increased ROS generation in DM. Since 5-HT mediates accelerated atherosclerosis in diabetes, pharmacological inhibition of the 5-HT receptor presents an attractive therapeutic strategy for

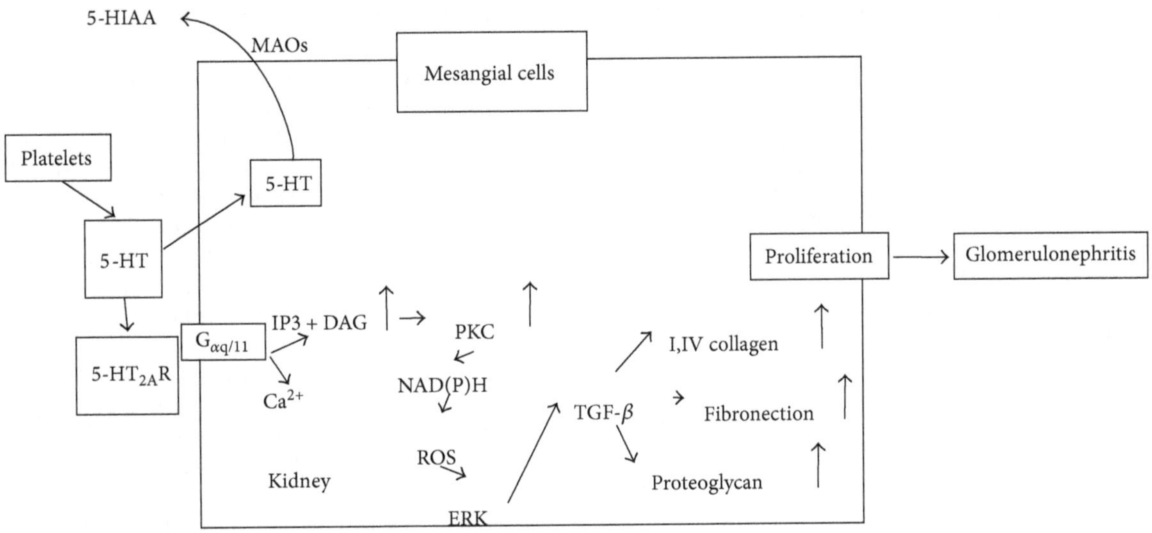

Figure 6: Illustration to show the mechanism of $5\text{-}HT_{2A}R$ in mesangial cells. 5-HT has been shown to enhance the production of type IV collagen by human mesangial cells, and its production is mediated by the activation of protein kinase C and a subsequent increase in active TGF-β. Stimulation of 5-HT2ARs by 5-HT induces the expression of TGF-β through extracellular signal-regulated kinases.

patients with diabetes to attenuate the development of nephropathy and macrovascular complications. A better understanding of the role of these new receptor targets in the context of DKD will facilitate the development of novel therapeutic strategies that can be successfully translated into clinical applications.

Abbreviations

5-HT:	5-Hydroxytryptamine
TPH:	Tryptophan hydroxylase
AADC:	Unbiquitous aromatic L-amino acid decarboxylase
5-HTT:	5-HT transporter
Cys-loop LGICs:	Cys-loop ligand-gated ion channels
5-HTT (SERT):	5-Hydroxytryptamine transporter
GPCRs:	G protein-coupled receptors
AC:	Adenylyl cyclase
cAMP:	Cyclic adenosine monophosphate
PIP2:	Phosphatidylinositol 4,5-bisphosphate
IP3:	Inositol trisphosphate
DAG:	Diacylglycerol
PRL:	Prolactin
PRLR:	Islet prolactin receptors
GSIS:	Glucose-stimulated insulin secretion
SST:	Somatostatin
SSTR:	SST receptors
Rho:	Ras homolog gene family member
ICAM-1:	Intercellular adhesion molecule-1
VCAM-1:	Vascular cell adhesion molecule-1
TGF-β:	Transforming growth factor-β
PKC:	Protein kinase C
ROS:	Reactive oxygen species
NADP:	Nicotinamide adenine dinucleotide phosphate
ERK:	Extracellular signal-regulated kinases.

Conflicts of Interest

The authors declare that there is no conflict of interest regarding the publication of this article.

Acknowledgments

This work was supported in part by the National Key Research and Development Program of China (2016YFC1305301) and the National Natural Science Foundation of China (no. 81460501).

References

[1] I. H. de Boer, T. C. Rue, Y. N. Hall, P. J. Heagerty, N. S. Weiss, and J. Himmelfarb, "Temporal trends in the prevalence of diabetic kidney disease in the United States," *The Journal of the American Medical Association*, vol. 305, pp. 2532–2539, 2011.

[2] S. P. Silveiro, G. N. Araujo, M. N. Ferreira, F. D. Souza, H. M. Yamaguchi, and E. G. Camargo, "Chronic kidney disease epidemiology collaboration (ckd-epi) equation pronouncedly underestimates glomerular filtration rate in type 2 diabetes," *Diabetes Care*, vol. 34, pp. 2353–2355, 2011.

[3] A. S. Krolewski, "Progressive renal decline: the new paradigm of diabetic nephropathy in type 1 diabetes," *Diabetes Care*, vol. 38, pp. 954–962, 2015.

[4] R. Amin, B. Widmer, A. T. Prevost et al., "Risk of microalbuminuria and progression to macroalbuminuria in a cohort with childhood onset type 1 diabetes: prospective observational study," *British Medical Journal*, vol. 336, pp. 697–701, 2008.

[5] A. Kowalski, A. Krikorian, and E. V. Lerma, "Diabetes and chronic kidney disease," *Disease-a-Month*, vol. 61, pp. 378–386, 2015.

[6] J. J. Liu, S. C. Lim, L. Y. Yeoh et al., "Ethnic disparities in risk of cardiovascular disease, end-stage renal disease and

all-cause mortality: a prospective study among Asian people with type 2 diabetes," *Diabetic Medicine*, vol. 33, pp. 332–339, 2016.

[7] C. C. Lim, B. W. Teo, P. G. Ong et al., "Chronic kidney disease, cardiovascular disease and mortality: a prospective cohort study in a multi-ethnic Asian population," *European Journal of Preventive Cardiology*, vol. 22, pp. 1018–1026, 2015.

[8] K. R. Tuttle, G. L. Bakris, R. W. Bilous et al., "Diabetic kidney disease: a report from an ADA Consensus Conference," *Diabetes Care*, vol. 37, pp. 2864–2883, 2014.

[9] E. T. Rosolowsky, J. Skupien, A. M. Smiles et al., "Risk for ESRD in type 1 diabetes remains high despite renoprotection," *Journals of the American Society of Nephrology*, vol. 22, pp. 545–553, 2011.

[10] R. Saran, Y. Li, B. Robinson et al., "US renal data system 2015 annual data report: epidemiology of kidney disease in the United States," *American Journal of Kidney Diseases*, vol. 67, pp. A7–A8, 2016.

[11] S. B. Ghaderian, F. Hayati, S. Shayanpour, and S. S. Beladi Mousavi, "Diabetes and end-stage renal disease; a review article on new concepts," *Journal of Renal Injury Prevention*, vol. 4, pp. 28–33, 2015.

[12] H. B. Lee, "Reactive oxygen species-regulated signaling pathways in diabetic nephropathy," *Journal of the American Society of Nephrology*, vol. 14, pp. 241S–245S, 2003.

[13] K. Susztak, A. C. Raff, M. Schiffer, and E. P. Bottinger, "Glucose-induced reactive oxygen species cause apoptosis of podocytes and podocyte depletion at the onset of diabetic nephropathy," *Diabetes*, vol. 55, pp. 225–233, 2006.

[14] L. E. Fridlyand and L. H. Philipson, "Oxidative reactive species in cell injury: mechanisms in diabetes mellitus and therapeutic approaches," *Annals of the New York Academy of Sciences*, vol. 1066, pp. 136–151, 2005.

[15] G. Al-Kafaji, M. A. Sabry, and C. Skrypnyk, "Time-course effect of high-glucose-induced reactive oxygen species on mitochondrial biogenesis and function in human renal mesangial cells," *Cell Biology International*, vol. 40, pp. 36–48, 2016.

[16] L. Sun, R. K. Dutta, P. Xie, and Y. S. Kanwar, "Myo-inositol oxygenase overexpression accentuates generation of reactive oxygen species and exacerbates cellular injury following high glucose ambience: a new mechanism relevant to the pathogenesis of diabetic nephropathy," *The Journal of Biological Chemistry*, vol. 291, pp. 5688–5707, 2016.

[17] K. Kim, C. M. Oh, M. Ohara-Imaizumi et al., "Functional role of serotonin in insulin secretion in a diet-induced insulin-resistant state," *Endocrinology*, vol. 156, pp. 444–452, 2015.

[18] Q. Zhang, Y. Zhu, W. Zhou, L. Gao, L. Yuan, and X. Han, "Serotonin receptor 2c and insulin secretion," *PLoS One*, vol. 8, article e54250, 2013.

[19] Y. Ohta, Y. Kosaka, N. Kishimoto et al., "Convergence of the insulin and serotonin programs in the pancreatic beta-cell," *Diabetes*, vol. 60, pp. 3208–3216, 2011.

[20] C. M. Oh, J. Namkung, Y. Go et al., "Regulation of systemic energy homeostasis by serotonin in adipose tissues," *Nature Communications*, vol. 6, p. 6794, 2015.

[21] K. A. Rasbach, J. A. Funk, T. Jayavelu, P. T. Green, and R. G. Schnellmann, "5-Hydroxytryptamine receptor stimulation of mitochondrial biogenesis," *The Journal of Pharmacology and Experimental Therapeutics*, vol. 332, pp. 632–639, 2010.

[22] R. Arreola, E. Becerril-Villanueva, C. Cruz-Fuentes et al., "Immunomodulatory effects mediated by serotonin," *Journal of Immunology Research*, vol. 2015, Article ID 354957, 21 pages, 2015.

[23] G. P. Ahern, "5-HT and the immune system," *Current Opinion in Pharmacology*, vol. 11, pp. 29–33, 2011.

[24] G. A. Ramirez, S. Franchini, P. Rovere-Querini, M. G. Sabbadini, A. A. Manfredi, and N. Maugeri, "The role of platelets in the pathogenesis of systemic sclerosis," *Frontiers in Immunology*, vol. 3, p. 160, 2012.

[25] M. de Las Casas-Engel and A. L. Corbi, "Serotonin modulation of macrophage polarization: inflammation and beyond," *Advances in Experimental Medicine and Biology*, vol. 824, pp. 89–115, 2014.

[26] M. Idzko, S. Pitchford, and C. Page, "Role of platelets in allergic airway inflammation," *The Journal of Allergy and Clinical Immunology*, vol. 135, pp. 1416–1423, 2015.

[27] J. J. Worthington, "The intestinal immunoendocrine axis: novel cross-talk between enteroendocrine cells and the immune system during infection and inflammatory disease," *Biochemical Society Transactions*, vol. 43, pp. 727–733, 2015.

[28] T. Sugiura, Y. Dohi, S. Yamashita, Y. Hirowatari, S. Fujii, and N. Ohte, "Serotonin in peripheral blood reflects oxidative stress and plays a crucial role in atherosclerosis: novel insights toward holistic anti-atherothrombotic strategy," *Atherosclerosis*, vol. 246, pp. 157–160, 2016.

[29] K. Nonogaki and T. Kaji, "Mosapride, a selective serotonin 5-HT4 receptor agonist, and alogliptin, a selective dipeptidyl peptidase-4 inhibitor, exert synergic effects on plasma active glp-1 levels and glucose tolerance in mice," *Diabetes Research and Clinical Practice*, vol. 110, pp. e18–e21, 2015.

[30] F. Montastruc, A. Palmaro, H. Bagheri, L. Schmitt, J. L. Montastruc, and M. Lapeyre-Mestre, "Role of serotonin 5-HT2c and histamine h1 receptors in antipsychotic-induced diabetes: a pharmacoepidemiological-pharmacodynamic study in vigibase," *European Neuropsychopharmacology*, vol. 25, pp. 1556–1565, 2015.

[31] H. Bennet, A. Balhuizen, A. Medina et al., "Altered serotonin (5-HT) 1D and 2A receptor expression may contribute to defective insulin and glucagon secretion in human type 2 diabetes," *Peptides*, vol. 71, pp. 113–120, 2015.

[32] A. Barzegar-Fallah, H. Alimoradi, F. Asadi, A. R. Dehpour, M. Asgari, and M. Shafiei, "Tropisetron ameliorates early diabetic nephropathy in streptozotocin-induced diabetic rats," *Clinical and Experimental Pharmacology & Physiology*, vol. 42, pp. 361–368, 2015.

[33] S. Kobayashi, M. Satoh, T. Namikoshi et al., "Blockade of serotonin 2A receptor improves glomerular endothelial function in rats with streptozotocin-induced diabetic nephropathy," *Clinical and Experimental Nephrology*, vol. 12, pp. 119–125, 2008.

[34] T. Takahashi, M. Yano, J. Minami et al., "Sarpogrelate hydrochloride, a serotonin2A receptor antagonist, reduces albuminuria in diabetic patients with early-stage diabetic nephropathy," *Diabetes Research and Clinical Practice*, vol. 58, pp. 123–129, 2002.

[35] K. Hara, Y. Hirowatari, Y. Shimura, and H. Takahashi, "Serotonin levels in platelet-poor plasma and whole blood in people with type 2 diabetes with chronic kidney disease," *Diabetes Research and Clinical Practice*, vol. 94, pp. 167–171, 2011.

[36] S. Watanabe, T. Matsumoto, M. Oda et al., "Insulin augments serotonin-induced contraction via activation of the IR/PI3K/PDK1 pathway in the rat carotid artery," *Pflügers Archiv-European Journal of Physiology*, vol. 468, no. 4, pp. 667–677, 2016.

[37] C. M. Oh, S. Park, and H. Kim, "Serotonin as a new therapeutic target for diabetes mellitus and obesity," *Diabetes & Metabolism Journal*, vol. 40, pp. 89–98, 2016.

[38] K. Hara, Y. Hirowatari, M. Yoshika, Y. Komiyama, Y. Tsuka, and H. Takahashi, "The ratio of plasma to whole-blood serotonin may be a novel marker of atherosclerotic cardiovascular disease," *The Journal of Laboratory and Clinical Medicine*, vol. 144, pp. 31–37, 2004.

[39] B. A. Davis, A. Nagarajan, L. R. Forrest, and S. K. Singh, "Mechanism of paroxetine (paxil) inhibition of the serotonin transporter," *Scientific Reports*, vol. 6, article 23789, 2016.

[40] J. D. McCorvy and B. L. Roth, "Structure and function of serotonin G protein-coupled receptors," *Pharmacology & Therapeutics*, vol. 150, pp. 129–142, 2015.

[41] G. Jaim-Etcheverry and L. M. Zieher, "Electron microscopic cytochemistry of 5-hydroxytryptamine (5-HT) in the beta cells of guinea pig endocrine pancreas," *Endocrinology*, vol. 83, pp. 917–923, 1968.

[42] A. Hameed, M. Ajmal, M. Nasir, and M. Ismail, "Genetic association analysis of serotonin transporter polymorphism (5-HTTLPR) with type 2 diabetes patients of Pakistani population," *Diabetes Research and Clinical Practice*, vol. 108, pp. 67–71, 2015.

[43] D. R. Gehlert and J. Shaw, "5-Hydroxytryptamine 1A (5HT1A) receptors mediate increases in plasma glucose independent of corticosterone," *European Journal of Pharmacology*, vol. 745, pp. 91–97, 2014.

[44] E. Ezzeldin, W. A. Souror, T. El-Nahhas, A. N. Soudi, and A. A. Shahat, "Biochemical and neurotransmitters changes associated with tramadol in streptozotocin-induced diabetes in rats," *BioMed Research International*, vol. 2014, Article ID 238780, 9 pages, 2014.

[45] Y. Hasegawa, A. Suehiro, S. Higasa, M. Namba, and E. Kakishita, "Enhancing effect of advanced glycation end products on serotonin-induced platelet aggregation in patients with diabetes mellitus," *Thrombosis Research*, vol. 107, pp. 319–323, 2002.

[46] K. V. Derkach, V. M. Bondareva, O. V. Chistyakova, L. M. Berstein, and A. O. Shpakov, "The effect of long-term intranasal serotonin treatment on metabolic parameters and hormonal signaling in rats with high-fat diet/low-dose streptozotocin-induced type 2 diabetes," *International Journal of Endocrinology*, vol. 2015, Article ID 245459, 17 pages, 2015.

[47] L. Goyvaerts, A. Schraenen, and F. Schuit, "Serotonin competence of mouse beta cells during pregnancy," *Diabetologia*, vol. 59, no. 7, pp. 1356–1363, 2016.

[48] M. Ohara-Imaizumi, H. Kim, M. Yoshida et al., "Serotonin regulates glucose-stimulated insulin secretion from pancreatic beta cells during pregnancy," *Proceedings of the National Academy of Sciences of the United States of America*, vol. 110, pp. 19420–19425, 2013.

[49] N. Paulmann, M. Grohmann, J. P. Voigt et al., "Intracellular serotonin modulates insulin secretion from pancreatic beta-cells by protein serotonylation," *PLoS Biology*, vol. 7, article e1000229, 2009.

[50] J. D. Crane, R. Palanivel, E. P. Mottillo et al., "Inhibiting peripheral serotonin synthesis reduces obesity and metabolic dysfunction by promoting brown adipose tissue thermogenesis," *Nature Medicine*, vol. 21, pp. 166–172, 2015.

[51] E. D. Berglund, C. Liu, J. W. Sohn et al., "Serotonin 2C receptors in pro-opiomelanocortin neurons regulate energy and glucose homeostasis," *The Journal of Clinical Investigation*, vol. 123, pp. 5061–5070, 2013.

[52] E. Colman, J. Golden, M. Roberts, A. Egan, J. Weaver, and C. Rosebraugh, "The FDA's assessment of two drugs for chronic weight management," *The New England Journal of Medicine*, vol. 367, pp. 1577–1579, 2012.

[53] O. J. Marston, A. S. Garfield, and L. K. Heisler, "Role of central serotonin and melanocortin systems in the control of energy balance," *European Journal of Pharmacology*, vol. 660, pp. 70–79, 2011.

[54] D. D. Lam and L. K. Heisler, "Serotonin and energy balance: molecular mechanisms and implications for type 2 diabetes," *Expert Reviews in Molecular Medicine*, vol. 9, pp. 1–24, 2007.

[55] J. Qiu, C. Xue, M. A. Bosch et al., "Serotonin 5-hydroxytryptamine2C receptor signaling in hypothalamic proopiomelanocortin neurons: role in energy homeostasis in females," *Molecular Pharmacology*, vol. 72, pp. 885–896, 2007.

[56] J. M. Wade, P. Juneja, A. W. MacKay et al., "Synergistic impairment of glucose homeostasis in ob/ob mice lacking functional serotonin 2C receptors," *Endocrinology*, vol. 149, pp. 955–961, 2008.

[57] G. Csaba, "Hormones in the immune system and their possible role. A critical review," *Acta Microbiologica et Immunologica Hungarica*, vol. 61, pp. 241–260, 2014.

[58] S. Zheng, S. Coventry, L. Cai et al., "Renal protection by genetic deletion of the atypical chemokine receptor ACKR2 in diabetic OVE mice," *Journal of Diabetes Research*, vol. 2016, Article ID 5362506, 11 pages, 2016.

[59] Y. Chabbi-Achengli, T. Coman, C. Collet et al., "Serotonin is involved in autoimmune arthritis through th17 immunity and bone resorption," *The American Journal of Pathology*, vol. 186, pp. 927–937, 2016.

[60] D. Hirigoyen, P. I. Burgos, V. Mezzano et al., "Inhibition of angiogenesis by platelets in systemic sclerosis patients," *Arthritis Research & Therapy*, vol. 17, p. 332, 2015.

[61] P. R. Pereira, M. C. Oliveira-Junior, B. MacKenzie et al., "Exercise reduces lung fibrosis involving serotonin/Akt signaling," *Medicine and Science in Sports and Exercise*, vol. 48, no. 7, pp. 1276–1284, 2016.

[62] G. Ahangari, S. E. Koochak, L. M. Amirabad, and G. D. Deilami, "Investigation of 5-HT2A gene expression in PBMCs of patients with allergic asthma," *Inflammation & Allergy Drug Targets*, vol. 14, pp. 60–64, 2015.

[63] J. M. Forbes and M. E. Cooper, "Mechanisms of diabetic complications," *Physiological Reviews*, vol. 93, pp. 137–188, 2013.

[64] K. E. Porter and K. Riches, "The vascular smooth muscle cell: a therapeutic target in type 2 diabetes?," *Clinical Science (London, England: 1979)*, vol. 125, pp. 167–182, 2013.

[65] K. Yamada, H. Niki, H. Nagai, M. Nishikawa, and H. Nakagawa, "Serotonin potentiates high-glucose-induced endothelial injury: the role of serotonin and 5-HT2A receptors in promoting thrombosis in diabetes," *Journal of Pharmacological Sciences*, vol. 119, pp. 243–250, 2012.

[66] T. Matsumoto, S. Watanabe, K. Taguchi, and T. Kobayashi, "Mechanisms underlying increased serotonin-induced contraction in carotid arteries from chronic type 2 diabetic Goto-Kakizaki rats," *Pharmacological Research*, vol. 87, pp. 123–132, 2014.

[67] S. C. Bir, M. Fujita, A. Marui et al., "New therapeutic approach for impaired arteriogenesis in diabetic mouse hindlimb ischemia," *Circulation Journal: Official Journal of the Japanese Circulation Society*, vol. 72, pp. 633–640, 2008.

[68] Y. Su, N. Mao, M. Li et al., "Sarpogrelate inhibits the expression of ICAM-1 and monocyte-endothelial adhesion induced by high glucose in human endothelial cells," *Molecular and Cellular Biochemistry*, vol. 373, pp. 195–199, 2013.

[69] P. M. Nelson, J. S. Harrod, and K. G. Lamping, "5HT(2a) and 5HT(2b) receptors contribute to serotonin-induced vascular dysfunction in diabetes," *Experimental Diabetes Research*, vol. 2012, Article ID 398406, 11 pages, 2012.

[70] E. R. Seaquist, "Addressing the burden of diabetes," *The Journal of the American Medical Association*, vol. 311, pp. 2267-2268, 2014.

[71] C. Mora-Fernandez, V. Dominguez-Pimentel, M. M. de Fuentes, J. L. Gorriz, A. Martinez-Castelao, and J. F. Navarro-Gonzalez, "Diabetic kidney disease: from physiology to therapeutics," *The Journal of Physiology*, vol. 592, pp. 3997–4012, 2014.

[72] G. Wolf, "New insights into the pathophysiology of diabetic nephropathy: from haemodynamics to molecular pathology," *European Journal of Clinical Investigation*, vol. 34, pp. 785–796, 2004.

[73] J. Wang, F. Qin, A. Deng, and L. Yao, "Different localization and expression of protein kinase C-beta in kidney cortex of diabetic nephropathy mice and its role in telmisartan treatment," *American Journal of Translational Research*, vol. 7, pp. 1116–1125, 2015.

[74] J. Yang and J. Zhang, "Influence of protein kinase C (PKC) on the prognosis of diabetic nephropathy patients," *International Journal of Clinical and Experimental Pathology*, vol. 8, pp. 14925–14931, 2015.

[75] K. Zhu, T. Kakehi, M. Matsumoto et al., "NADPH oxidase NOX1 is involved in activation of protein kinase C and premature senescence in early stage diabetic kidney," *Free Radical Biology & Medicine*, vol. 83, pp. 21–30, 2015.

[76] J. C. Jha, V. Thallas-Bonke, C. Banal et al., "Podocyte-specific NOX4 deletion affords renoprotection in a mouse model of diabetic nephropathy," *Diabetologia*, vol. 59, pp. 379–389, 2016.

[77] Y. Gorin, R. C. Cavaglieri, K. Khazim et al., "Targeting NADPH oxidase with a novel dual NOX1/NOX4 inhibitor attenuates renal pathology in type 1 diabetes," *American Journal of Physiology Renal Physiology*, vol. 308, pp. F1276–F1287, 2015.

[78] A. B. Bhatti and M. Usman, "Drug targets for oxidative podocyte injury in diabetic nephropathy," *Cureus*, vol. 7, article e393, 2015.

[79] S. C. Tang, W. H. Yiu, M. Lin, and K. N. Lai, "Diabetic nephropathy and proximal tubular damage," *Journal of Renal Nutrition: The Official Journal of the Council on Renal Nutrition of the National Kidney Foundation*, vol. 25, pp. 230–233, 2015.

[80] P. M. Garcia-Garcia, M. A. Getino-Melian, V. Dominguez-Pimentel, and J. F. Navarro-Gonzalez, "Inflammation in diabetic kidney disease," *World Journal of Diabetes*, vol. 5, pp. 431–443, 2014.

[81] L. Nalysnyk, M. Hernandez-Medina, and G. Krishnarajah, "Glycaemic variability and complications in patients with diabetes mellitus: evidence from a systematic review of the literature," *Diabetes, Obesity & Metabolism*, vol. 12, pp. 288–298, 2010.

[82] W. J. Ni, L. Q. Tang, and W. Wei, "Research progress in signalling pathway in diabetic nephropathy," *Diabetes/Metabolism Research and Reviews*, vol. 31, pp. 221–233, 2015.

[83] J. Saito, E. Suzuki, Y. Tajima, K. Takami, Y. Horikawa, and J. Takeda, "Increased plasma serotonin metabolite 5-hydroxyindole acetic acid concentrations are associated with impaired systolic and late diastolic forward flows during cardiac cycle and elevated resistive index at popliteal artery and renal insufficiency in type 2 diabetic patients with microalbuminuria," *Endocrine Journal*, vol. 63, no. 1, pp. 69–76, 2016.

[84] M. Fukui, E. Shiraishi, M. Tanaka et al., "Plasma serotonin is a predictor for deterioration of urinary albumin excretion in men with type 2 diabetes mellitus," *Metabolism: Clinical and Experimental*, vol. 58, pp. 1076–1079, 2009.

[85] M. Kasho, M. Sakai, T. Sasahara et al., "Serotonin enhances the production of type IV collagen by human mesangial cells," *Kidney International*, vol. 54, pp. 1083–1092, 1998.

[86] J. S. Grewal, L. M. Luttrell, and J. R. Raymond, "G protein-coupled receptors desensitize and down-regulate epidermal growth factor receptors in renal mesangial cells," *The Journal of Biological Chemistry*, vol. 276, pp. 27335–27344, 2001.

[87] J. S. Grewal, Y. V. Mukhin, M. N. Garnovskaya, J. R. Raymond, and E. L. Greene, "Serotonin 5-HT2A receptor induces TGF-beta1 expression in mesangial cells via ERK: proliferative and fibrotic signals," *The American Journal of Physiology*, vol. 276, pp. F922–F930, 1999.

[88] N. Pizzinat, J. P. Girolami, A. Parini, C. Pecher, and C. Ordener, "Serotonin metabolism in rat mesangial cells: involvement of a serotonin transporter and monoamine oxidase a," *Kidney International*, vol. 56, pp. 1391–1399, 1999.

[89] C. G. Nebigil, M. N. Garnovskaya, R. F. Spurney, and J. R. Raymond, "Identification of a rat glomerular mesangial cell mitogenic 5-HT2A receptor," *The American Journal of Physiology*, vol. 268, pp. F122–F127, 1995.

[90] S. Ogawa, T. Mori, K. Nako, T. Ishizuka, and S. Ito, "Reduced albuminuria with sarpogrelate is accompanied by a decrease in monocyte chemoattractant protein-1 levels in type 2 diabetes," *Clinical Journal of the American Society of Nephrology*, vol. 3, pp. 362–368, 2008.

[91] S. Y. Park, S. Y. Rhee, S. Oh et al., "Evaluation of the effectiveness of sarpogrelate on the surrogate markers for macrovascular complications in patients with type 2 diabetes," *Endocrine Journal*, vol. 59, pp. 709–716, 2012.

13

MicroRNA-22 Promotes Renal Tubulointerstitial Fibrosis by Targeting PTEN and Suppressing Autophagy in Diabetic Nephropathy

Yingying Zhang,[1,2] Siqi Zhao,[1,2] Depei Wu,[1,2] Xingmei Liu,[1,2] Mingjun Shi,[1,2] Yuanyuan Wang,[1,2] Fan Zhang,[1,2] Jing Ding,[1,2] Ying Xiao,[1,2] and Bing Guo[1,2]

[1]*Department of Pathophysiology, Guizhou Medical University, Guiyang, Guizhou 550025, China*
[2]*Laboratory of Pathogenesis Research, Drug Prevention and Treatment of Major Diseases, Guizhou Medical University, Guiyang, Guizhou 550025, China*

Correspondence should be addressed to Ying Xiao; yxhx20060725@126.com and Bing Guo; guobingbs@126.com

Academic Editor: Secundino Cigarran

Renal tubulointerstitial fibrosis (TIF) is a major feature of diabetic nephropathy (DN). There is increasing evidence demonstrating that microRNAs act as key players in the regulation of autophagy and are involved in DN. However, the exact link among microRNAs, autophagy, and TIF in DN is largely unknown. In this study, our results showed that TIF was observed in DN rats together with obvious autophagy suppression. Moreover, microRNA-22 (miR-22) was upregulated and associated with reduced expression of its target gene phosphatase and tensin homolog (PTEN) in both the kidneys of DN rats and high glucose-cultured NRK-52E cells. Intriguingly, induction of autophagy by rapamycin antagonized high glucose-induced collagen IV (Col IV) and α-SMA expression. In addition, ectopic expression of miR-22 suppressed autophagic flux and induced the expression of Col IV and α-SMA, whereas the inhibition of endogenous miR-22 effectively relieved high glucose-induced autophagy suppression and the expression of Col IV and α-SMA in NRK-52E cells. Overexpression of PTEN protectively antagonized high glucose- and miR-22-induced autophagy suppression and the expression of Col IV. Therefore, our findings indicated that miR-22 may promote TIF by suppressing autophagy partially via targeting PTEN and represents a novel and promising therapeutic target for DN.

1. Introduction

Renal tubulointerstitial fibrosis (TIF) frequently occurs in diabetic nephropathy (DN), which is a main cause of end-stage renal disease throughout the world [1, 2]. The degree of TIF is associated with declined renal function and it is characterized by tubular atrophy and excessive accumulation of extracellular matrix components, such as collagens and fibronectin. However, the mechanism by which TIF develops in DN warrants exploration. Autophagy is an important homoeostatic process that mediates the degradation of damaged organelles or protein aggregates. Although recent studies suggest that activation of autophagy may be a protective measure to suppress TIF and prevent the progression of DN [3, 4], the event that initiates this process remains unclear.

Increasing evidence has demonstrated that phosphatase and tensin homolog (PTEN) is closely related to renal fibrosis in DN [5, 6]. This phosphatase acts as a negative regulator of fibrosis, such as cardiac fibrosis, lung fibrosis, and liver fibrosis [7–9]. It can attenuate renal fibrosis by inhibiting the synthesis and accumulation of matrix protein and interacting with TGF-β and members of the Akt pathway [10–12]. Moreover, PTEN is a key regulator of autophagy. It can activate autophagy in a number of different disease models or cell types by inhibiting the PI3K/Akt/mTOR signaling pathway [13]. Therefore, exploring the regulation of PTEN may be a significant way to restrain the development of TIF and DN.

MicroRNAs (miRNAs) are a group of highly conserved, small noncoding RNAs that can modulate gene expression through posttranscriptional binding to the 3′UTR of their target genes [14]. They play an important role in autophagy and various pathological processes including diabetes and fibrosis [15–17]. Recently, the emerging roles of miRNAs in the pathogenesis of DN have been highlighted [18, 19]. However, to date, few miRNAs have been found to execute their biological functions in DN by targeting PTEN, such as miR-21, miR-214, and miR-217 [20–22]. Meanwhile, only a few miRNAs have been found to have an effect on DN by regulating autophagy [22]. Thus, it is becoming clear that miRNAs with the ability to regulate PTEN and autophagy may become a promising therapeutic target for DN.

In this study, we demonstrated that miR-22 promoted the expression of collagen IV (Col IV) and α-SMA by regulating the PTEN/Akt/mTOR pathway and suppressing autophagy in NRK-52E cells. Inhibition of the endogenous miR-22 increased autophagy and alleviated high glucose- (HG-) induced Col IV and α-SMA expression. Therefore, our results suggested that miR-22 might be a novel target for the treatment of TIF and DN.

2. Materials and Methods

2.1. Experimental Animals. Twenty healthy and specific pathogen-free (SPF) male Sprague-Dawley rats weighing 180 ± 20 g were provided by Beijing HFK Bioscience Co. Ltd. (Beijing, China). The animals were housed in a clean environment under a controlled temperature of 20–25°C in the animal center of Guizhou Medical University (Guizhou, China). All rats were randomly divided into a control group (NC group, $n = 10$) and a diabetic nephropathy group (DN group, $n = 10$). DN rats were induced by injecting streptozotocin (STZ; Sigma, MO, USA) in the tail vein at a dose of 55 mg/kg, while NC rats were injected with an equal volume of solvent. All rats were given a normal diet and unlimited drinking water. After 48 h, the high blood glucose level (fasting blood glucose ≥ 16.7 mM) indicated that the DN rat model was established successfully. Ten weeks after STZ or solvent injection, 24 h urine and femoral arterial blood from each rat was collected before the rats were sacrificed and urine protein and various biochemical indices were measured, respectively. All rats were anesthetized with intraperitoneal sodium pentobarbital (50 mg/kg) and were sacrificed by drawing-out all the blood from their hearts. The kidneys of each rat were harvested, one was fixed in 4% paraformaldehyde and the other one was immediately frozen in liquid nitrogen. The kidney index (KI) was calculated by right kidney weight (KW) and body weight (BW): KI = KW/BW. The study was conducted in accordance with the guidelines of the National Health and Medical Research Council of China's Code for the care and use of animals for scientific purpose.

2.2. Biochemical Assays. Blood glucose was measured by the oxidase method and 24 h urinary protein was measured by the Coomassie Brilliant Blue method. All tests were analyzed by a 1650 automatic biochemical analyzer (Beckman Instruments, CA, USA).

Table 1: The levels of kidney index (KI), blood glucose (BG), 24 h urine protein (24 h UP) in normal control (NC) group and diabetic nephropathy (DN) group (mean ± SEM. $n = 10$).

Group	KI (mg/g)	BG (mmol/l)	24 h UP (mg)
NC	7.70 ± 0.45	7.02 ± 1.39	39.64 ± 7.18
DN	11.86 ± 0.99*	28.55 ± 4.20*	261.75 ± 112.98*

*$P < 0.05$ versus control group.

2.3. Cell Culture. NRK-52E cells were cultured in Dulbeccos's modified Eagle's medium (DMEM; Hyclone, UT, USA) supplemented with 5% fetal bovine serum (FBS; Gibco, CA, USA) containing normal glucose (NG, 5.5 mM glucose) or HG (30 mM glucose). Cells in each group were seeded in 25 cm^2 culture flasks and cultured in the incubator with 5% CO_2 at 37°C for 24 h or 48 h for further study.

2.4. Histology and Immunohistochemistry. Renal tissue paraffin sections were subjected to hematoxylin-eosin (HE) staining, and renal tissue fibrosis was observed by Masson's trichrome. The biotin-streptavidin-peroxidase method (ZSBIO, Beijing, China) was applied to conduct immunohistochemistry. The primary antibody against Col IV (SAB4200500) was purchased from Sigma. Primary antibody (1 : 100) was diluted in phosphate-buffered saline (PBS) containing 1% bovine serum albumin (BSA), and the secondary antibodies used were affinity-purified biotinylated goat antimouse IgG. Sections incubated with PBS served as the negative control. Two blinded investigators observed all slides independently, and fifty fields of view were analyzed by Image-Pro plus 6.0.

2.5. Real-Time PCR Detection. Total RNA was extracted from renal tissues of NC or DN rats and NRK-52E cells using the TRIzol reagent (Invitrogen, CA, USA) according to manufacturer's protocol. For quantification of miR-22, the Bulge-Loop™ miRNA qRT-PCR primer kits (RiboBio, Guangzhou, China) were utilized following manufacturer's instructions. qPCR was performed using SuperReal PreMix (SYBR Green) (Tiangen, Beijing, China) with iQ SYBR Green SuperMix (Bio-Rad). The expression of miR-22 was defined from the threshold cycle (Ct), and relative expression levels were calculated using the $2^{-\Delta\Delta Ct}$ method after normalization with reference to the expression of U6 snRNA.

2.6. Western Blotting. Renal tissues and NRK-52E cells were lysed in RIPA lysis buffer (50 mM Tris-HCl, pH 7.4, 150 mM NaCl, 1% Triton X-100, 1% sodium deoxycholate, 0.1% SDS), supplemented with a complete protease inhibitor mixture (P0013B, Beyotime Shanghai, China). Subsequently, 30 μg protein samples were separated on an 8, 10, or 12.5% Tris-glycine gel and transferred onto a nitrocellulose membrane. The primary antibodies used for Western blotting were as follows: PTEN (Cell Signaling, 1 : 1000), Col IV (Sigma, 1 : 1000), LC3 (Cell Signaling, 1 : 1000), p62 (Cell Signaling, 1 : 2000), Akt (Cell Signaling, 1 : 1000), p-Akt (Cell Signaling, 1 : 1000), mTOR (Cell Signaling, 1 : 1000), p-mTOR (Cell Signaling, 1 : 1000), and β-actin (Actin; Abcam, 1 : 2000).

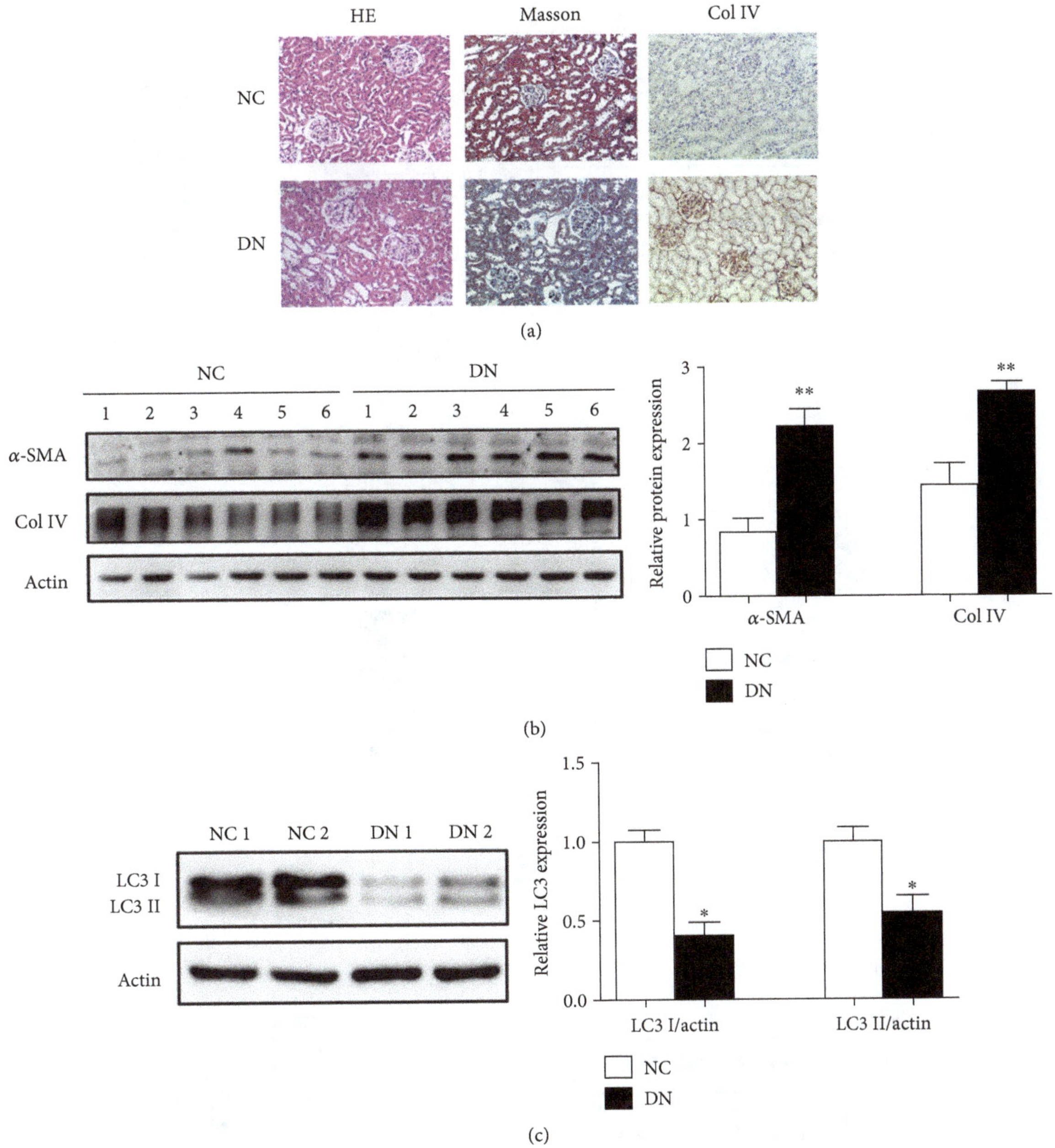

FIGURE 1: Developed renal fibrosis was accompanied by decreased autophagy in DN rats. (a) Representative photograph of histological changes and immunohistochemical staining for Col IV protein expression analysis of renal tissues in NC group and DN group. Figures were shown at ×200 magnification. For (b) and (c), Western blot assay was performed to detect the expression of Col IV, α-SMA, LC3-I, and LC3-II in renal tissues in NC group and DN group. ImageJ densitometric analysis of the level of Col IV, α-SMA, LC3-I, and LC3-II; data represent mean ± SEM, $n = 10$, $^*P < 0.05$ and $^{**}P < 0.01$.

2.7. Luciferase Reporter Assays. The fragment of the predicted miR-22 binding sequence or a mismatch sequence in the 3′UTR of PTEN mRNA, amplified from 293T genomic DNA, was cloned into the SpeI and HandIII restriction sites of the pMIR-REPORT plasmid (Invitrogen). The predicted target site was mutated by site-directed mutagenesis, and 50 nM miR-22 mimics or NC mimics (RiboBio, Guangzhou, China) were transfected into NRK-52E cells with 5 ng Renilla plasmid (Promega, Wisconsin, USA) and 100 ng of the WT or MUT plasmid that contain the 3′UTR of PTEN. Twenty-four hours before transfection, 5×10^4 cells were seeded in 24-well plates. A luciferase assay was performed 24 h after transfection using the dual-luciferase reporter assay system (Promega). The firefly luciferase activity was normalized to the Renilla luciferase activity.

2.8. Confocal Microscopy Analysis. NRK-52E cells were first transfected with pDsRed-LC3, and then they were transfected with NC mimics or miR-22 mimics for 24 h. Following

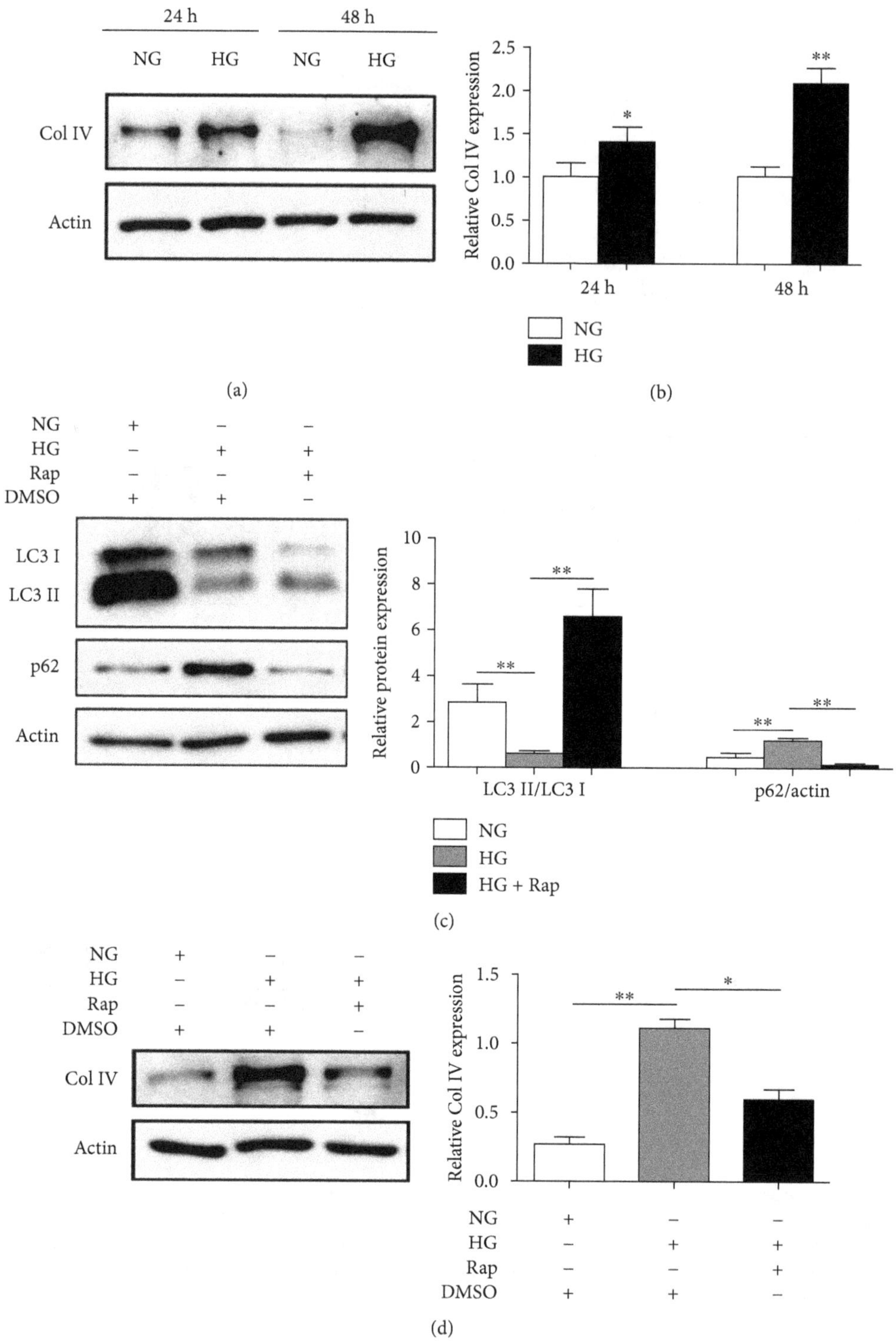

FIGURE 2: The function of autophagy on HG-induced expression of Col IV and α-SMA in NRK-52E cells. (a) NRK-52E cells were treated with NG or HG for 24 or 48 h; the protein level of Col IV was detected by Western blot. (b) ImageJ densitometric analysis of the protein level of Col IV; data represent mean ± SEM, $n = 3$, $^{*}P < 0.05$, $^{**}P < 0.01$. For (c) and (d), NRK-52E cells were treated with DMSO or 100 nM Rap and NG or HG for 48 h. The expression of LC3-I, LC3-II, p62, and Col IV was detected by Western blot. ImageJ densitometric analysis of the protein levels; data represent mean ± SEM, $n = 3$, $^{*}P < 0.05$, $^{**}P < 0.01$. Rap: rapamycin.

this incubation, cells were cultured with rapamycin (Rap) and NG or HG for another 24 h. The cells were then fixed and immediately analyzed by confocal microscopy (Olympus, FV1000, Japan). RFP-LC3 puncta formation and the localization of RFP-LC3 were observed.

2.9. Statistical Analysis. All experiments were repeated at least three times. The statistical significance between two groups was assessed using the Student's 2-tailed t-test. One-way ANOVA followed by a Bonferroni-Dunn test was used for the comparison of more than two groups. Data were

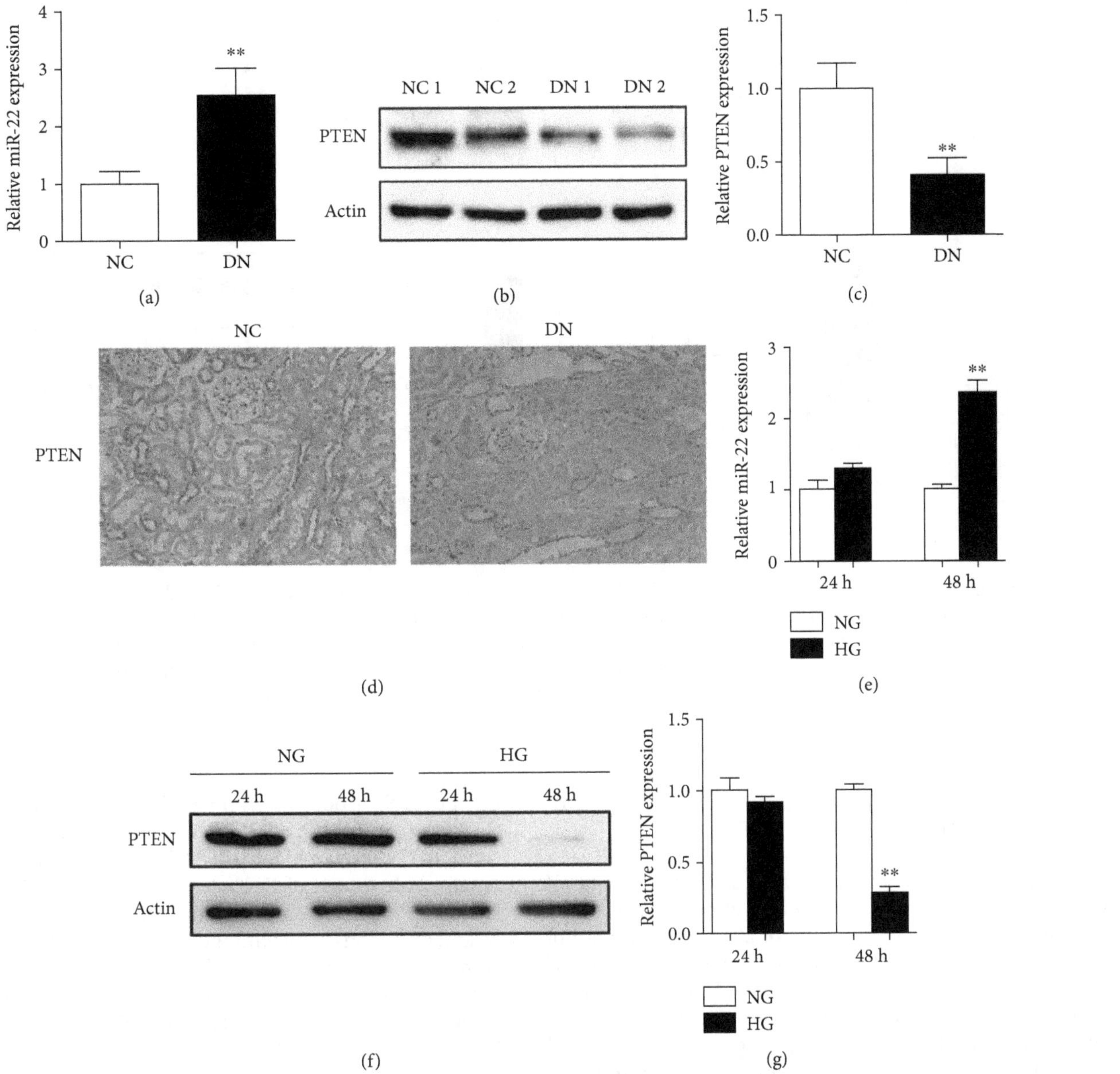

FIGURE 3: MiR-22 upregulated was associated with reduced PTEN in DN in vivo and in vitro. (a) The expression of miR-22 in renal tissues of NC group and DN group was analyzed by qPCR; data represent mean ± SEM, $n = 10$, $^{**}P < 0.01$. (b) The protein level of PTEN in renal tissues of NC group and DN group was detected by Western blot (c) and analyzed by ImageJ; data represent mean ± SEM, $n = 10$, $^{**}P < 0.01$. (d) Representative photograph of immunohistochemical staining for PTEN protein expression analysis of renal tissues in NC group and DN group. Figures were shown at ×200 magnification. (e) NRK-52E cells were treated with NG or HG for 24 or 48 h. The expression of miR-22 was analyzed by qPCR; data represent mean ± SEM, $n = 3$, $^{**}P < 0.01$. (f) The expression of PTEN was detected by Western blot (g) and analyzed by ImageJ; data represent mean ± SEM, $n = 3$, $^{**}P < 0.01$.

expressed as mean ± standard error of mean (SEM). $P < 0.05$ was considered significant.

3. Results

3.1. Decreased Autophagy Level Was Associated with Renal Fibrosis in DN Rats. In this study, our result showed that rats treated with STZ injection for 48 h presented a high blood glucose level. At the end of the study, KI, blood glucose, and 24 h urinary protein increased in DN rats as compared to healthy and SPF male Sprague-Dawley rats (Table 1). Histochemical staining was used to check and define the pathological changes in renal tissues. HE staining showed that the epithelial cells of the renal tubule emerged with mild vacuolar degeneration, and the renal tubules were distended with macrophages infiltrating the renal interstitium in the DN group (Figure 1(a)). The Masson stain revealed that the DN rats developed renal fibrosis and immunohistochemistry showed an upregulation of Col IV in renal tissues of DN rats under the light microscope (Figure 1(a)). Moreover, the expression of Col IV and α-SMA was upregulated, while LC-3I and LC-3II were decreased in renal tissues in DN

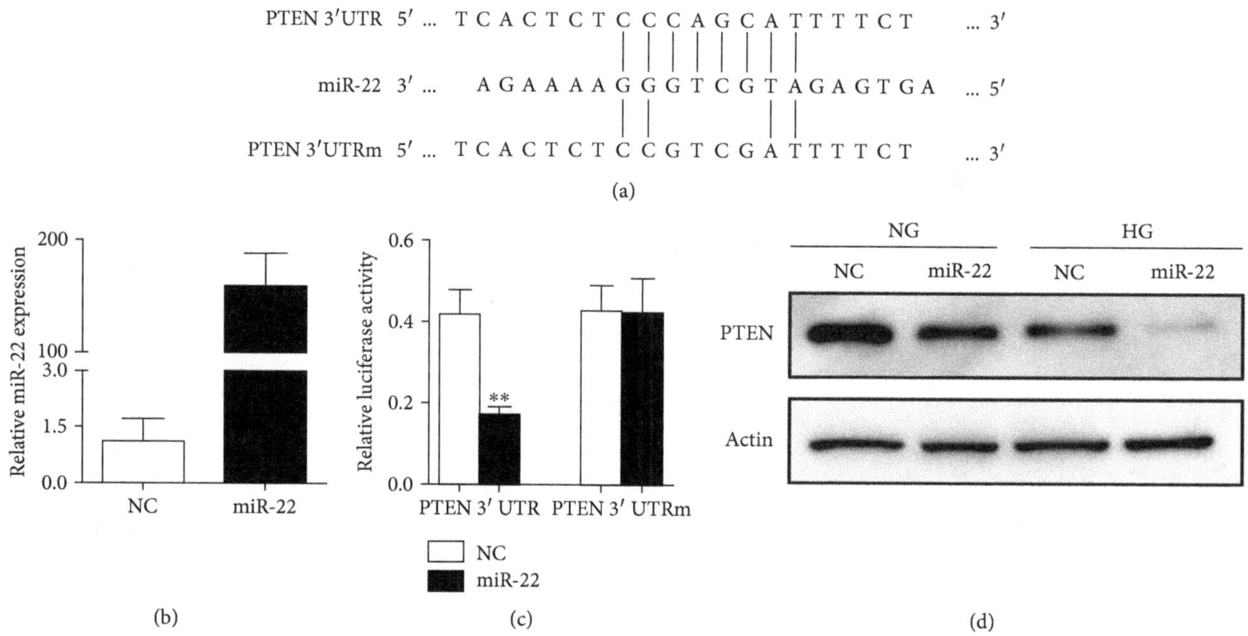

Figure 4: MiR-22 directly targets PTEN. (a) Predicted binding sequences and mutated site between miR-22 and seed site in 3′UTR of PTEN. (b) NRK-52E cells were transfected with miR-22 mimics or NC mimics for 24 h. qPCR was performed to detect the transfection efficiency of miR-22 mimics. (c) NRK-52E cells were cotransfected with 50 nM miR-22 mimics or NC mimics, 100 ng of the WT or MUT plasmid that contain 3′UTR of PTEN, and 5 ng Renilla plasmid; data represent mean ± SEM, $n = 3$, $^{**}P < 0.01$. (d) After transfected with miR-22 mimics or NC mimics for 24 h, NRK-52E cells were treated with NG or HG for another 48 h. The expression of PTEN was detected by Western blot.

group compared to control group as shown by Western blotting (Figures 1(b) and 1(c)).

3.2. Improving Autophagy Antagonized HG-Induced Col IV Expression. We next evaluate the effect of autophagy on the expression of Col IV *in vitro*. First of all, we used mannitol as a control, and the result showed that there had no obvious influence of mannitol on the expression of PTEN and α-SMA together with autophagy (Supplementary Figure 1). Western blots showed that Col IV levels were significantly increased after NRK-52E cells were treated with HG for 24 and 48 h as compared to the NG-treated group (Figures 2(a) and 2(b)). Then, NRK-52E cells were treated with DMSO or 100 nM Rap which is an autophagy agonist and NG or HG for 48 h. The conversion of LC3-I to LC3-II and the degradation of p62 were inhibited, and the expression of Col IV was upregulated after cells were treated with HG for 48 h as compared to the NG-treated group (Figures 2(c) and 2(d)). Moreover, as shown in Figures 2(c) and 2(d), Rap could effectively improve the conversion of LC3-I to LC3-II and the degradation of p62 and suppress the expression of Col IV. Therefore, autophagy may be a protective factor that inhibits the synthesis of Col IV and α-SMA, and thus, antagonizes TIF.

3.3. MiR-22 Was Upregulated and PTEN Was Downregulated in Renal Tissues of DN Rats and HG-Treated NRK-52E Cells. We further detected the expression of miR-22 and PTEN in renal tissues. The results showed a significantly increased expression of miR-22 and decreased expression of PTEN in the DN group as compared to the control group (Figure 3(a)–3(c)). In addition, immunohistochemistry indicated that the expression of PTEN was downregulated in renal tubule tissues of DN rats (Figure 3(d)). Subsequently, NRK-52E cells were cultured in NG or HG conditions for 24 and 48 h. Consistent with the results *in vivo*, the expression of miR-22 was upregulated and the protein level of PTEN was downregulated after HG treatment for 48 h, but there was no obvious differences in miR-22 and PTEN between NG- and HG-treated cells after 24 h (Figure 3(e)–3(g)).

3.4. PTEN Was a Direct Target of miR-22. For the dysregulation of miR-22 and PTEN in DN, we further explored their relationship in NRK-52E cells. By using TargetScan and miRanda bioinformatics tools, we found that miR-22 potentially targets PTEN (Figure 4(a)). Subsequently, we designed pMIR-reporter constructs containing either wild-type (WT) or mutated-type (Mut) miR-22 binding sites at the 3′UTR of PTEN. The expression of miR-22 was present at a high level after cells were transfected with miR-22 mimics for 24 h (Figure 4(b)). The luciferase reporter assay was performed 24 h after cotransfection with the WT or Mut PTEN 3′UTR clone and miR-22 or NC mimics. As shown in Figure 4(c), miR-22 mimics significantly reduced the luciferase activity of WT PTEN 3′UTR, but had no significant effect on Mut PTEN 3′UTR. Moreover, the protein expression of PTEN was downregulated by miR-22 after either NG or HG treatment for 48 h as compared with the negative controls in NRK-52E cells (Figure 4(d)).

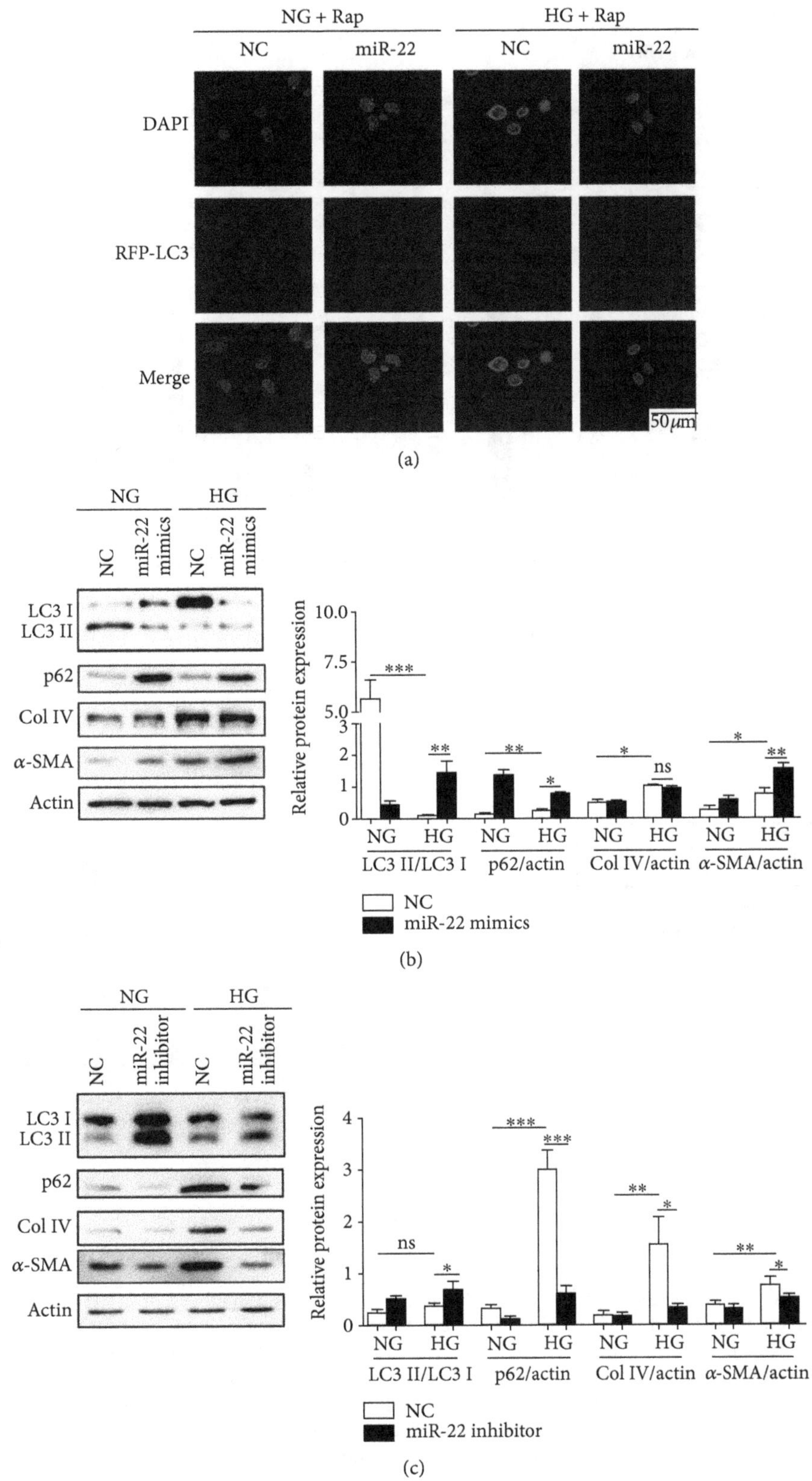

FIGURE 5: MiR-22 inhibited autophagy and mediated HG-induced Col IV and α-SMA expression. (a) After cotransfected with pDsRed-LC3 plasmid and miR-22 mimics or NC mimics for 24 h, NRK-52E cells were treated with NG or HG for another 48 h. NRK-52E cells were subsequently imaged using confocal microscopy. Scale bars represent 50 μm. Rap: rapamycin. For (b) and (c), after transfected with miR-22 mimics or NC mimics or miR-22 inhibitor or NC inhibitor for 24 h, NRK-52E cells were treated with NG or HG for another 48 h. The expression of LC3-I, LC3-II, p62, Col IV, and α-SMA was detected by Western blot. ImageJ densitometric analysis of the protein levels; data represent mean ± SEM, $n = 3$, $^{*}P < 0.05$, $^{**}P < 0.01$, $^{***}P < 0.001$, ns: not significant.

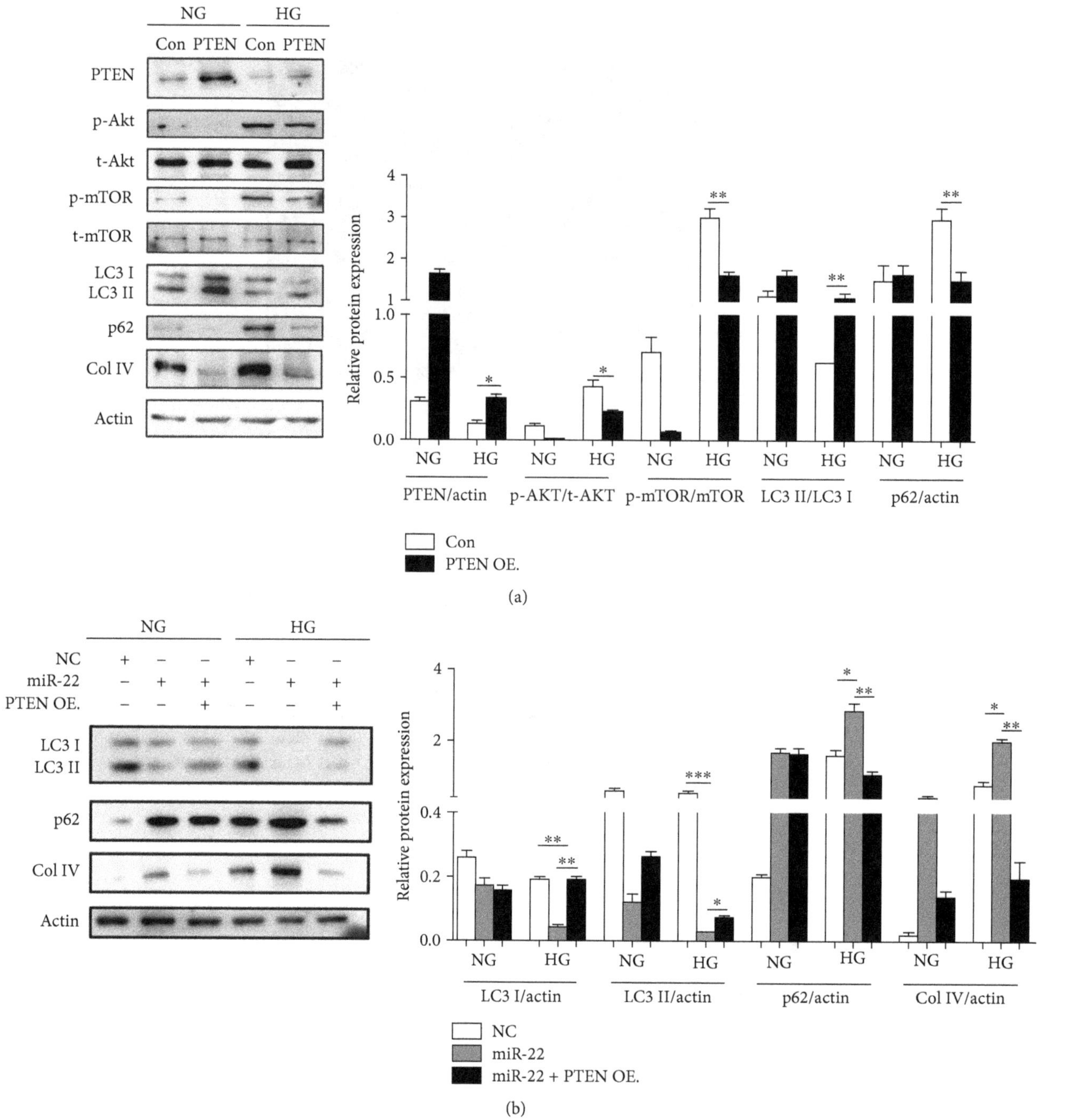

FIGURE 6: PTEN partially mediated the biological effect of miR-22 on autophagy and the synthesis of Col IV. (a) After transfected with PTEN overexpression plasmid or empty plasmid for 24 h, NRK-52E cells were cultured with NG or HG for another 48 h. The expression of PTEN, p-Akt, t-Akt, p-mTOR, t-mTOR, LC3-I, LC3-II, p62, and Col IV was detected by Western blot. p-Akt: phosphorylated Akt; t-Akt: total Akt; p-mTOR: phosphorylated mTOR; t-mTOR: total mTOR. ImageJ densitometric analysis of the protein levels; data represent mean ± SEM, $n = 3$, $^{*}P < 0.05$, $^{**}P < 0.01$. (b) After cotransfected with PTEN overexpression plasmid or empty plasmid and miR-22 mimics or NC mimics for 24 h, NRK-52E cells were treated with NG or HG for another 48 h. The expression of LC3-I, LC3-II, p62, and Col IV was detected by Western blot. ImageJ densitometric analysis of the protein levels; data represent mean ± SEM, $n = 3$, $^{*}P < 0.05$, $^{**}P < 0.01$, $^{***}P < 0.001$.

3.5. miR-22 Inhibited Autophagy and Promoted the Expression of Col IV and α-SMA. We next determined whether miR-22 had an effect on autophagy and fibrosis. pDsRed-LC3 plasmid and miR-22 or NC mimics were cotransfected into NRK-52E cells for 24 h, and then cells were treated with NG or HG for another 48 h. Confocal microscopy was used to analyze the samples, and the results showed decreased accumulation of pDsRed-LC3 puncta in the cytoplasm of miR-22 mimics-transfected and/or HG-treated cells (Figure 5(a)). Western blots revealed that miR-22 could suppress the conversion of LC3-I to LC3-II and the degradation of p62, meanwhile it promoted the expression of Col IV and α-SMA in NG- or HG-treated NRK-52E cells (Figure 5(b)). Moreover, a miR-22 inhibitor improved autophagic flux and suppressed the expression of Col IV and α-SMA as compared to the negative control (Figure 5(c)). Thus, inhibition of miR-22 may suppress TIF by the induction of autophagy.

3.6. miR-22 Regulation of Autophagy and the Expression of Col IV Were Partially through Targeting PTEN. As PTEN was a target for miR-22 in NRK-52E cells, it was tempting to speculate that PTEN might mediate the regulatory effects of miR-22 on autophagy and the synthesis of collagen. To test this hypothesis, NRK-52E cells were transfected with a PTEN overexpression plasmid or empty plasmid for 24 h before being treated with NG or HG for another 48 h. Western blots showed that forced expression of PTEN could suppress AKT-mTOR signaling, promote autophagic flux, and inhibit the expression of Col IV both in NG- and HG-treated cells (Figure 6(a)). Importantly, overexpression of PTEN could effectively antagonize miR-22-induced autophagy suppression and the expression of Col IV (Figure 6(b)).

4. Discussion

Several studies have demonstrated that miR-22 inhibition could attenuate the level of liver and cardiac fibrosis [23, 24]. Recently, it has been reported that miR-22 is upregulated in the kidney of STZ-induced DN mice [25]. However, little was known about the role and specific mechanism of miR-22 on TIF. The major findings of this study were that miR-22 acted as an inducer of TIF by suppressing autophagy in renal tubular epithelial cells and thus promoted the development of DN. miR-22 suppressed autophagy and induced the expression of Col IV partially by targeting PTEN. Suppression of miR-22 may be an effective measure in restraining TIF.

Autophagy that generated by various harmful factors contributes to maintenance of cell homeostasis. HG exposure induced neurotoxicity, promoted myocardial injury, and reduced angiogenic properties of human umbilical vein endothelial cells while suppressing autophagy. The induction of autophagy could effectively antagonize the cytotoxic effects of HG [26–28]. Moreover, several studies have suggested that autophagy may be a protective factor that antagonizes TIF and prevents the progression of DN [3, 4]. Furthermore, an increasing number of studies have indicated that miRNAs play an important role in autophagy and fibrosis. However, the relationship among miR-22, autophagy, and TIF in DN remains unclear. Therefore, DN rats and cell models were established and applied to investigate the function of miR-22 in TIF and determine the underlying mechanism. In the present study, we first showed that miR-22 was associated with autophagy in DN rats and it could induce the synthesis of Col IV and α-SMA by suppressing autophagy in renal tubular epithelial cells. On the contrary, miR-22 inhibition suppressed Col IV and α-SMA expression and thus represents a promising therapeutic target for DN. Nevertheless, the exact mechanism by which miR-22 works remains unclear.

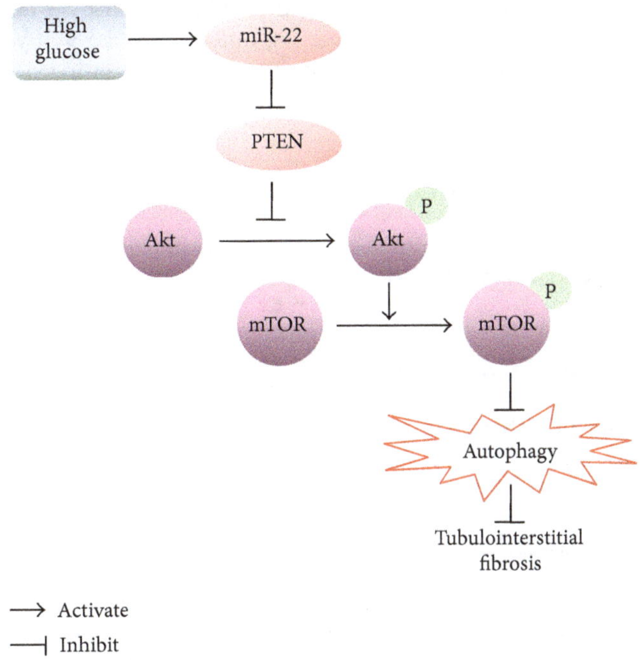

Figure 7: Principle signaling pathways involved in the effect of HG on autophagy and the expression of Col IV and α-SMA in NRK-52E cells. HG suppressed autophagy and in turn promoted Col IV and α-SMA expression via regulating PTEN/Akt/mTOR signaling pathway. By targeting PTEN, miR-22 mediated HG-inhibited autophagy and the synthesis of Col IV and α-SMA.

PTEN is known as a tumor suppressor but it also acted as an antifibrotic factor. Previous studies have demonstrated that PTEN was associated with renal fibrosis in DN [5, 6]. In addition, PTEN is a key activator of autophagy in various kinds of disease models or cell types by inhibiting the PI3K/AKT/mTOR signaling pathway. Thus, PTEN may play an important role in preventing the development of TIF by inducing autophagy in DN. Our data showed that PTEN could promote autophagic flux and inhibit Col IV expression by suppressing AKT-mTOR signaling both in NG- and HG-treated NRK-52E cells. This suggests that targeting PTEN may be an effective treatment for TIF. To date, only a few miRNAs were found to execute their biological functions in DN via targeting PTEN. Moreover, little is known about the effect of miRNAs on autophagy and TIF. Previous studies have indicated that PTEN was a potential target of miR-22 in cancer cells [29, 30]. However, whether PTEN mediated the biological effect of miR-22 in DN remained to be explored. Another key finding of the present study was that miR-22 suppressed autophagy and induced the expression of Col IV partially by targeting PTEN. Further research is needed to explore some of the other biological effects and targets of miR-22 in renal tubular epithelial cells as it would bring us a step closer to identifying the underlying mechanism in the pathogenesis of DN.

In summary, this study provides the novel finding that miR-22 was upregulated in renal tissues of DN rats and it exerted autophagy inhibition and profibrosis roles via targeting PTEN (Figure 7). Targeting miR-22 may be a novel and promising therapeutic approach in preventing the progression of DN.

Conflicts of Interest

The authors declare that there are no conflicts of interest regarding the publication of this paper.

Authors' Contributions

Yingying Zhang and Siqi Zhao contributed equally to this work.

Acknowledgments

This study was supported by the National Natural Science Foundation of China (no. 81360116), the Guizhou Province Science and Technology Foundation (no. (2014) 7006), and the Guiyang and Guizhou Medical University Joint Foundation (no. 20161001).

References

[1] K. Ina, H. Kitamura, S. Tatsukawa, T. Takayama, Y. Fujikura, and T. Shimada, "Transformation of interstitial fibroblasts and tubulointerstitial fibrosis in diabetic nephropathy," *Medical Electron Microscopy*, vol. 35, no. 2, pp. 87–95, 2002.

[2] K. R. Tuttle, G. L. Bakris, R. W. Bilous et al., "Diabetic kidney disease: a report from an ADA Consensus Conference," *American Journal of Kidney Diseases*, vol. 64, no. 4, pp. 510–533, 2014.

[3] H. Li, X. Peng, Y. Wang et al., "Atg5-mediated autophagy deficiency in proximal tubules promotes cell cycle G_2/M arrest and renal fibrosis," *Autophagy*, vol. 12, no. 9, pp. 1472–1486, 2016.

[4] N. Liu, L. Xu, Y. Shi, and S. Zhuang, "Podocyte autophagy: a potential therapeutic target to prevent the progression of diabetic nephropathy," *Journal of Diabetes Research*, vol. 2017, Article ID 3560238, 6 pages, 2017.

[5] A. D. McClelland, M. Herman-Edelstein, R. Komers et al., "*miR-21* promotes renal fibrosis in diabetic nephropathy by targeting PTEN and SMAD7," *Clinical Science*, vol. 129, no. 12, pp. 1237–1249, 2015.

[6] L. Zhu, S. Zhao, S. Liu, Q. Liu, F. Li, and J. Hao, "PTEN regulates renal extracellular matrix deposit via increased CTGF in diabetes mellitus," *Journal of Cellular Biochemistry*, vol. 117, no. 5, pp. 1187–1198, 2016.

[7] Y. Gao, M. Chu, J. Hong, J. Shang, and D. Xu, "Hypoxia induces cardiac fibroblast proliferation and phenotypic switch: a role for caveolae and caveolin-1/PTEN mediated pathway," *Journal of Thoracic Disease*, vol. 6, no. 10, pp. 1458–1468, 2014.

[8] Z. He, Y. Deng, W. Li et al., "Overexpression of PTEN suppresses lipopolysaccharide-induced lung fibroblast proliferation, differentiation and collagen secretion through inhibition of the PI3-K-Akt-GSK3beta pathway," *Cell & Bioscience*, vol. 4, no. 1, p. 2, 2014.

[9] Y. Cheng, Y. Tian, J. Xia et al., "The role of PTEN in regulation of hepatic macrophages activation and function in progression and reversal of liver fibrosis," *Toxicology and Applied Pharmacology*, vol. 317, pp. 51–62, 2017.

[10] X. Zhou, X. Zang, M. Ponnusamy et al., "Enhancer of Zeste homolog 2 inhibition attenuates renal fibrosis by maintaining Smad7 and phosphatase and tensin homolog expression," *Journal of the American Society of Nephrology*, vol. 27, no. 7, pp. 2092–2108, 2016.

[11] N. Dey, N. Ghosh-Choudhury, B. S. Kasinath, and G. G. Choudhury, "TGFβ-stimulated microRNA-21 utilizes PTEN to orchestrate AKT/mTORC1 signaling for mesangial cell hypertrophy and matrix expansion," *PLoS One*, vol. 7, no. 8, article e42316, 2012.

[12] T. Wu, Y. Liu, Z. Fan et al., "miR-21 modulates the immunoregulatory function of bone marrow mesenchymal stem cells through the PTEN/Akt/TGF-β1 pathway," *Stem Cells*, vol. 33, no. 11, pp. 3281–3290, 2015.

[13] J. H. Chen, P. Zhang, W. D. Chen et al., "ATM-mediated PTEN phosphorylation promotes PTEN nuclear translocation and autophagy in response to DNA-damaging agents in cancer cells," *Autophagy*, vol. 11, no. 2, pp. 239–252, 2015.

[14] D. Klein, R. Misawa, V. Bravo-Egana et al., "MicroRNA expression in alpha and beta cells of human pancreatic islets," *PLoS One*, vol. 8, no. 1, article e55064, 2013.

[15] J. Zhang, P. Wang, L. Wan, S. Xu, and D. Pang, "The emergence of noncoding RNAs as Heracles in autophagy," *Autophagy*, vol. 13, no. 6, pp. 1004–1024, 2017.

[16] I. V. Snowhite, G. Allende, J. Sosenko, R. L. Pastori, S. Messinger Cayetano, and A. Pugliese, "Association of serum microRNAs with islet autoimmunity, disease progression and metabolic impairment in relatives at risk of type 1 diabetes," *Diabetologia*, vol. 60, no. 8, pp. 1409–1422, 2017.

[17] S. K. Shetty, N. Tiwari, A. S. Marudamuthu et al., "p53 and miR-34a feedback promotes lung epithelial injury and pulmonary fibrosis," *The American Journal of Pathology*, vol. 187, no. 5, pp. 1016–1034, 2017.

[18] H. Wu, L. Kong, S. Zhou et al., "The role of microRNAs in diabetic nephropathy," *Journal of Diabetes Research*, vol. 2014, Article ID 920134, 12 pages, 2014.

[19] C. Zanchi, D. Macconi, P. Trionfini et al., "MicroRNA-184 is a downstream effector of albuminuria driving renal fibrosis in rats with diabetic nephropathy," *Diabetologia*, vol. 60, no. 6, pp. 1114–1125, 2017.

[20] M. Kölling, T. Kaucsar, C. Schauerte et al., "Therapeutic miR-21 silencing ameliorates diabetic kidney disease in mice," *Molecular Therapy*, vol. 25, no. 1, pp. 165–180, 2017.

[21] X. Wang, E. Shen, Y. Wang et al., "Cross talk between miR-214 and PTEN attenuates glomerular hypertrophy under diabetic conditions," *Scientific Reports*, vol. 6, no. 1, article 31506, 2016.

[22] J. Sun, Z. P. Li, R. Q. Zhang, and H. M. Zhang, "Repression of miR-217 protects against high glucose-induced podocyte injury and insulin resistance by restoring PTEN-mediated autophagy pathway," *Biochemical and Biophysical Research Communications*, vol. 483, no. 1, pp. 318–324, 2017.

[23] D. Ji, B. Li, Q. Shao, F. Li, Z. Li, and G. Chen, "MiR-22 suppresses BMP7 in the development of cirrhosis," *Cellular Physiology and Biochemistry*, vol. 36, no. 3, pp. 1026–1036, 2015.

[24] V. Jazbutyte, J. Fiedler, S. Kneitz et al., "MicroRNA-22 increases senescence and activates cardiac fibroblasts in the aging heart," *Age*, vol. 35, no. 3, pp. 747–762, 2013.

[25] R. Pofi, D. Fiore, R. De Gaetano et al., "Phosphodiesterase-5 inhibition preserves renal hemodynamics and function in mice with diabetic kidney disease by modulating miR-22 and BMP7," *Scientific Reports*, vol. 7, article 44584, 2017.

[26] Y. Li, Y. Zhang, L. Wang et al., "Autophagy impairment mediated by S-nitrosation of ATG4B leads to neurotoxicity in response to hyperglycemia," *Autophagy*, vol. 13, no. 7, pp. 1145–1160, 2017.

[27] B. Zhou, S. Lei, R. Xue, Y. Leng, Z. Xia, and Z. Y. Xia, "DJ-1 overexpression restores ischaemic post-conditioning-mediated cardioprotection in diabetic rats: role of autophagy," *Clinical Science*, vol. 131, no. 11, pp. 1161–1178, 2017.

[28] A. Rezabakhsh, M. Ahmadi, M. Khaksar et al., "Rapamycin inhibits oxidative/nitrosative stress and enhances angiogenesis in high glucose-treated human umbilical vein endothelial cells: role of autophagy," *Biomedicine & Pharmacotherapy*, vol. 93, pp. 885–894, 2017.

[29] S. S. Xia, G. J. Zhang, Z. L. Liu et al., "MicroRNA-22 suppresses the growth, migration and invasion of colorectal cancer cells through a Sp1 negative feedback loop," *Oncotarget*, vol. 8, no. 22, pp. 36266–36278, 2017.

[30] W. Fan, J. Huang, H. Xiao, and Z. Liang, "MicroRNA-22 is downregulated in clear cell renal cell carcinoma, and inhibits cell growth, migration and invasion by targeting PTEN," *Molecular Medicine Reports*, vol. 13, no. 6, pp. 4800–4806, 2016.

14

Tubulointerstitial Biomarkers for Diabetic Nephropathy

Bancha Satirapoj

Division of Nephrology, Department of Medicine, Phramongkutklao Hospital and College of Medicine, Bangkok, Thailand

Correspondence should be addressed to Bancha Satirapoj; satirapoj@yahoo.com

Academic Editor: Carlos Martinez Salgado

Patients with diabetic nephropathy have a higher risk of mortality, mostly from cardiovascular complications. Standard biomarkers including serum creatinine, estimated glomerular filtration rate, and albuminuria are imprecise, do not directly measure renal tissue injury, and are relatively insensitive to small changes in renal function. Thus, availability of novel biomarkers that are sensitive, specific, and precise as well as able to detect kidney injury and predict clinically significant outcomes would be widely useful in diabetic nephropathy. Novel biomarkers of the processes that induce tubulointerstitial changes may ultimately prove to better predict renal progression and prognosis in type 2 diabetes. Recently, certain biomarkers, which were initially identified in acute kidney injury, also have been reported to confer value in evaluating patients with chronic kidney disease. Biomarkers such as cystatin C, kidney injury molecule-1 (KIM-1), neutrophil gelatinase-associated lipocalin (NGAL), angiotensinogen, periostin, and monocyte chemoattractant protein-1 (MCP-1) reflect tubular injury. In this article, we focused on the potential applications of these biomarkers in diabetic nephropathy.

1. Introduction

In 2010, the worldwide adult population with diabetes mellitus was estimated to be about 285 million and by 2030 an increase by 54% to about 439 million is predicted, reflecting a remarkable increase in diabetes nephropathy [1]. Diabetic nephropathy develops along with generalized microvascular disease, most often concomitant with macrovascular disease including cardiovascular, cerebrovascular, and peripheral arterial diseases [2, 3]. Patients with diabetic nephropathy have a higher risk of mortality, mostly from cardiovascular complications, than diabetic patients without nephropathy [4]. According to the Thailand Renal Replacement Therapy (TRRT) Registry Report 2014, the most common cause of end-stage renal disease (ESRD) is diabetes mellitus.

Diabetic nephropathy is a multifactorial disease involving different pathogenic molecular processes and histopathological structure. A combination of renal tubulointerstitial biomarkers that could capture different pathogenic processes of renal injury may provide a more realistic picture of a patient's outcome. More recently, renal tubulointerstitium has been increasingly reported to play an integral role in the pathogenesis of diabetic nephropathy and correlates well with progressive renal function decline [5]. Novel biomarkers of the processes that induce tubulointerstitial changes might ultimately prove to be better predictors of renal progression and prognosis in type 2 diabetes (T2DM).

2. Standard Biomarkers of Diabetic Nephropathy

Blood urea nitrogen, serum creatinine, formulas to estimated glomerular filtration rate (GFR), proteinuria, and albuminuria are measures currently used to assess the presence and progress of diabetic nephropathy [2, 3]. However, these measures are imprecise, do not directly measure renal tissue injury, and are relatively insensitive to small changes in renal function. Thus, availability of novel biomarkers that are sensitive, specific, and precise as well as able to detect kidney injury and predict clinically significant outcomes would be widely useful in diabetic nephropathy [6].

Urinary albumin is filtered through the glomerulus and later reabsorbed by tubular cells through the megalin-cubilin pathway. Albuminuria is an important marker to predict the progression of diabetic nephropathy [7] and more severe and persistent albuminuria correlates with more rapid progression of diabetic nephropathy and cardiovascular disease among patients with T2DM. Screening for albuminuria should begin at 5-year diabetes duration among patients with type 1 diabetes and at the time of diagnosis among patients with T2DM based on the clinical practice guidelines for diabetic kidney disease outlined by the Kidney Disease Outcomes Quality Initiative (KDOQI) [8]. The preferred screening test is a urine albumin/creatinine ratio with a first-morning void spot collection. A renal biopsy may be necessary to confirm the clinical diagnosis when atypical features are present. Currently, 20–40% of patients with T2DM show GFR that declines before detecting albuminuria [9]. In addition, some studies have shown about 30–45% of diabetic patients with microalbuminuria progressed to macroalbuminuria in 10 years of follow-up; 30% regressed to normoalbuminuria, and 30–40% remained at microalbuminuria level [9]. For these reasons, investigations of new risk markers to predict progression of diabetic nephropathy are suggested.

3. Renal Pathology in Diabetic Nephropathy

Renal pathological changes are present among patients with long-standing diabetes before the onset of microalbuminuria [10]. The characteristic light microscopic features of diabetic nephropathy comprise three major lesions: thickened glomerular basement membranes (GBM) and tubular basement membranes, diffuse mesangial expansion, and hyalinosis of afferent and efferent arterioles. However, hyperglycemia-induced metabolic and hemodynamic stimuli are mediators of kidney injury [11, 12]. These activate inflammatory, pro-oxidant, ischemic, and fibrotic pathways leading to mesangial matrix accumulation; podocyte effacement and loss; GBM thickening; endothelial dysfunction; tubular atrophy, fibrosis, and dropout; tubulointerstitial inflammation; and renal arteriolar hyalinosis. Therefore, pathology in diabetic nephropathy affects all the renal cellular elements including the glomerular endothelium, mesangial cells, podocytes, and tubular epithelium.

Numerous relationships between tubulointerstitial change and functional outcomes have been reported. Interstitial fibrosis is often proportional to tubular atrophy and a strong predictor of the rate of progression from moderate to severe reduction in GFR [13, 14]. Urinary biomarker data in human beings support the view that tubule injury contributes in a primary way, rather than in a secondary manner, to the development of early diabetic nephropathy [6]. Novel tubular biomarkers related to renal injury in diabetic nephropathy could improve risk stratification and prediction.

4. Markers of Tubulointerstitial Injury

Many of the discovered biomarkers for diabetic nephropathy were identified by transcriptomic and proteomic analyses of renal tissues after injury. As such, a bias exists toward identifying markers from the renal tubulointerstitium, reflecting its greater mass compared with the vascular and glomerular compartments. Recently, certain biomarkers, which were initially identified in acute kidney injury (AKI), also have been reported to confer value in evaluating patients with CKD. Biomarkers such as cystatin C, kidney injury molecule-1 (KIM-1), neutrophil gelatinase-associated lipocalin (NGAL), angiotensinogen, periostin, and monocyte chemoattractant protein-1 (MCP-1) reflect tubular injury. In this article, we focused on the potential applications of these biomarkers in diabetic nephropathy as shown in Table 1.

4.1. Cystatin-C. Cystatin-C is produced from nucleated cells in the body. It has a molecular weight of 13 kDa, is easily filtered by the glomeruli, and is reabsorbed and catabolized by the proximal tubule. From a prospective observational study, urine cystatin C predicted the progression of T2DM with nephropathy [15]. T2DM with rapid renal progression had significantly increased levels of urine cystatin C when compared with the nonrapid renal progression group [16]. Urine cystatin C was an independent predictor of CKD progression in T2DM.

4.2. Neutrophil Gelatinase-Associated Lipocalin (NGAL). NGAL is a 24 kDa secreted glycoprotein. NGAL is expressed in the renal tubular epithelium, and a rise in urinary concentrations may provide an indication of acute renal injury that can be detected before the rise in serum creatinine concentration [17]. Models of acute kidney injury- (AKI-) to-chronic kidney disease (CKD) transition have implicated its role as a potential biomarker of a chronically injured kidney. In patients with CKD, overexpression of NGAL occurs in renal tubular cells, compared with its expression among non-CKD patients [18], and both serum and urinary NGAL represent a novel, independent renal predictor of the severity of renal disease and CKD progression [19]. In a related study carried out among patients with diabetic nephropathy, elevated urine NGAL level was reported to be associated with the progressive course of the disease leading to ESRD [20]. Similarly, in observational follow-up and our cohort study among patients with T2DM, high urine NGAL levels at baseline correlated with rapid decline of estimated GFR levels and increased serum creatinine [16, 20]. It has been postulated that in the setting of diabetic nephropathy, the rise in NGAL levels occurs independently of decreased GFR and reflects tubular injury and inflammation.

4.3. Kidney Injury Molecule-1 (KIM-1). KIM-1 is a type 1 membrane protein expressed on the apical membrane of proximal tubule cells. Its ectodomain is cleaved and released in the lumen of the tubule and finally appears in urine, which is stable [21]. This biomarker is undetected when the kidneys are normal. Thus, it serves as a specific and sensitive biomarker for proximal tubule damage. In an experimental animal model of tubulointerstitial damage from overload proteinuria, tubular KIM-1 expression was limited to areas with inflammation, fibrosis, and tubular damage [22]. One study also confirmed that KIM-1 was associated with tubulointerstitial inflammation and was overexpressed in the tubules of patients with proteinuric nephropathy, including diabetic nephropathy [23]. From a cross-sectional descriptive study, urine KIM-1 increased in T2DM with normoalbuminuria and mildly increased albuminuria [24]. Serum and urine KIM-1 predicted the rapid decline of GFR [16, 25].

Table 1: Biomarkers for diabetic nephropathy.

Biomarkers	Source cell	Description
Standard biomarkers		
Creatinine	Muscle cells	Glomerular filtration markers [8] Factors affecting creatinine generation (i) extremes of muscle mass, (ii) extremes of body size, (iii) diet and nutritional status: high protein diet and creatine supplements, (iv) muscle wasting diseases.
Albuminuria	—	Glomerular damage markers [8] 20–40% of diabetic patients with renal impairment exhibited normal albuminuria [9] No detection in tubulointerstitial injury [9]
Potential biomarkers		
Cystatin C	Nucleated cells/proximal tubular cells	Serum cystatin: glomerular filtration markers Urine cystatin: tubular markers Predicted the renal progression of type 2 diabetes [15, 16]
Neutrophil gelatinase-associated lipocalin (NGAL)	Neutrophils/distal tubular cells	Urine NGAL: distal tubular markers Increased in response to tubulointerstitial injury [17, 18] Predicted the renal progression of type 2 diabetes [16, 20]
Kidney injury molecule-1 (KIM-1)	Proximal tubular cells	Urine KIM-1: proximal tubular markers Increased in response to tubulointerstitial injury [22, 23] Predicted the renal progression of type 2 diabetes [16, 24–26]
Angiotensinogen	Proximal tubular cells	Urine angiotensinogen: proximal tubular markers Increased in response to renal RAAS activation [27, 29, 30] Predicted the renal progression of type 2 diabetes [16, 28, 31]
Periostin	Bone/distal tubular cells	Urine periostin: distal tubular markers Increased in response to renal fibrosis and inflammation [33, 34] Predicted the renal progression of type 2 diabetes [36]
Monocyte chemoattractant protein-1 (MCP-1)	Macrophages, glomerular and tubular cells	Urine MCP-1: glomerular and tubular markers Increased in response to renal inflammation [39–42] Predicted the albuminuria and renal progression of type 2 diabetes [47]

Urinary KIM-1 levels were also significantly higher among patients who progressed from macroalbuminuria to late-stage CKD, but it did not predict progression to end-stage renal disease independently of albuminuria [26]. Urinary KIM-1 excretion could become a noninvasive biomarker of tubulointerstitial injury in diabetic nephropathy. However, Mendelian randomization analysis indicated that the inverse association of increased KIM-1 levels with lower GFR was independent of AER and very likely to represent a causal link [26].

4.4. Angiotensinogen. Angiotensinogen is the only known substrate for renin. Changes in angiotensinogen could influence renin angiotensin aldosterone system (RAAS) activity and increase intrarenal RAAS components, parallel to the severity of fibrotic renal damage, and have been demonstrated in chronic progressive nephropathy [27, 28]. Renal angiotensinogen is formed primarily in proximal tubular cells and is secreted in tubular fluid. The activated intrarenal RAS was recently proposed to be involved in the progression of renal injury in multiple models of hypertension and in kidney diseases including diabetic nephropathy, immunoglobulin A (IgA) nephropathy, and radiation nephropathy [29, 30]. Urinary angiotensinogen level also correlates with intrarenal angiotensinogen levels and is independently associated with albuminuria and rapid GFR decline in T2DM [16, 28]. In diabetes with normoalbuminuria, urinary angiotensinogen was higher than in controls and demonstrated good performance in differentiating each stage of T2DM from controls [31]. Our research team proposed that angiotensinogen could serve as a potential urinary biomarker to diagnose diabetic nephropathy. It might be useful as an early biomarker of the activation of the RAAS in diabetic nephropathy.

4.5. Periostin. Periostin, osteoblast-specific factor 2, is an extracellular matrix protein firstly expressed in bone, is undetected in other main organs including the kidney [32], and is involved in the fibrosis process and tissue remodeling, kidney development, and tubular dedifferentiation in experimental models. Our study described, for the first time, the renal expression and urinary excretion of periostin in rats after CKD and in the kidneys of mice with diabetes [33]. Increased periostin expression in the glomeruli and tubular epithelium in diabetic renal pathology was observed. It serves as a marker of renal tubular injury and also correlates with worsening renal outcomes including serum creatinine, blood urea nitrogen, and estimated GFR in various chronic progressive kidney injuries [34, 35]. Urinary periostin levels were more significantly elevated among patients of normoalbuminuria, microalbuminuria, and macroalbuminuria compared with levels of healthy controls. Increased urine periostin level was significantly correlated with aging, high albuminuria, and decline of GFR [36]. The current study indicated that increased urine periostin levels could be detected among patients with T2DM before the onset of significant albuminuria and produced an associated renal derangement among patients with established diabetic nephropathy.

4.6. Monocyte Chemoattractant Protein-1 (MCP-1). The infiltration of inflammatory cells such as monocytes and macrophages in diseased kidneys is a hallmark of the progression of diabetic nephropathy [37]. MCP-1 as a member of the CC chemokine family is a major factor influencing macrophage accumulation in both animal and human models of renal damage [38]. MCP-1 is upregulated and expressed in the diabetic glomerular and renal tubular epithelium [39, 40], and a rise in urinary MCP-1 levels correlates with the extent of interstitial inflammatory infiltrate [41, 42]. In contrast, epidermal growth factor (EGF), a peptide growth factor, plays a protective role in progressive renal injury. EGF plays an important role in restoring barrier function in the healing phase of renal injury and is also a critical in vivo renal cell survival factor for developmentally mature kidneys [43, 44]. Urinary levels of EGF and EGF/MCP-1 ratios are inversely correlated with the extent of tubulointerstitial damage and determined renal prognosis in glomerulonephritis [45, 46]. Urinary levels of MCP-1 among patients with overt nephropathy were also more significantly elevated compared with levels among patients with normal albuminuria [47]. Our preliminary data found that urine MCP-1 and urine EGF/MCP-1 ratios were independently associated with renal progression among T2DM patients.

5. Conclusion

Novel biomarkers of the processes that induce tubulointerstitial changes may ultimately prove to be better predictors of renal progression and prognosis in T2DM. Our research integrated novel tubular biomarkers simultaneously and compared the performance of each tubular biomarker with standard urine albumin. High levels of urine tubular biomarkers such as urine cystatin C, angiotensinogen, KIM-1, and NGAL presented more rapid decline in renal function among Thai patients with T2DM [16]. This suggests that all novel tubular biomarkers would not be simple surrogate indexes of baseline estimated GFR, but markers on their own, predicting nephropathy progression beyond the information provided by serum creatinine and other conventional risk factors.

Conflicts of Interest

The author declares that no potential conflict of interests exists.

Acknowledgments

The author would like to thank the medical staff at the Division of Nephrology, Phramongkutklao Hospital and College of Medicine. This study was supported by a grant from Phramongkutklao Hospital and College of Medicine and the National Science and Technology Development Agency (NSTDA, P-13-00505), Bangkok, Thailand.

References

[1] G. Tramonti and Y. S. Kanwar, "Review and discussion of tubular biomarkers in the diagnosis and management of diabetic nephropathy," *Endocrine*, vol. 43, no. 3, pp. 494–503, 2013.

[2] B. Satirapoj and S. G. Adler, "Comprehensive approach to diabetic nephropathy," *Kidney Research and Clinical Practice*, vol. 33, no. 3, pp. 121–131, 2014.

[3] B. Satirapoj and S. G. Adler, "Prevalence and management of diabetic nephropathy in western countries," *Kidney Diseases*, vol. 1, no. 1, pp. 61–70, 2015.

[4] M. Afkarian, M. C. Sachs, B. Kestenbaum et al., "Kidney disease and increased mortality risk in type 2 diabetes," *Journal of the American Society of Nephrology*, vol. 24, no. 2, pp. 302–308, 2013.

[5] C. E. Hills and P. E. Squires, "The role of TGF-β and epithelial-to mesenchymal transition in diabetic nephropathy," *Cytokine & Growth Factor Reviews*, vol. 22, no. 3, pp. 131–139, 2011.

[6] B. Satirapoj, C. C. Nast, and S. G. Adler, "Novel insights into the relationship between glomerular pathology and progressive kidney disease," *Advances in Chronic Kidney Disease*, vol. 19, no. 2, pp. 93–100, 2012.

[7] H.-H. Parving, B. Oxenboll, P. A. Svendsen, J. S. Christiansen, and A. R. Andersen, "Early detection of patients at risk of developing diabetic nephropathy. A longitudinal study of urinary albumin excretion," *Acta Endocrinol*, vol. 100, no. 4, pp. 550–555, 1982.

[8] National Kidney Foundation, "KDOQI clinical practice guideline for diabetes and CKD: 2012 update," *American Journal of Kidney Diseases*, vol. 60, no. 5, pp. 850–886, 2012.

[9] P. Fioretto, M. W. Steffes, and M. Mauer, "Glomerular structure in nonproteinuric IDDM patients with various levels of albuminuria," *Diabetes*, vol. 43, no. 11, pp. 1358–1364, 1994.

[10] S. G. Adler, S. W. Kang, S. Feld et al., "Can glomerular mRNAs in human type 1 diabetes be used to predict transition from normoalbuminuria to microalbuminuria?," *American Journal of Kidney Diseases*, vol. 40, no. 1, pp. 184–188, 2002.

[11] B. Satirapoj, "Review on pathophysiology and treatment of diabetic kidney disease," *Journal of the Medical Association of Thailand*, vol. 93, Supplement 6, pp. S228–S241, 2010.

[12] B. Satirapoj, "Nephropathy in diabetes," *Advances in Experimental Medicine and Biology*, vol. 771, pp. 107–122, 2012.

[13] P. Fioretto, M. W. Steffes, D. E. Sutherland, and M. Mauer, "Sequential renal biopsies in insulin-dependent diabetic patients: structural factors associated with clinical progression," *Kidney International*, vol. 48, no. 6, pp. 1929–1935, 1995.

[14] S. Adler, L. J. Striker, G. E. Striker, D. T. Perkinson, J. Hibbert, and W. G. Couser, "Studies of progressive glomerular sclerosis in the rat," *The American Journal of Pathology*, vol. 123, no. 3, pp. 553–562, 1986.

[15] S. S. Kim, S. H. Song, I. J. Kim et al., "Urinary cystatin C and tubular proteinuria predict progression of diabetic nephropathy," *Diabetes Care*, vol. 36, no. 3, pp. 656–661, 2013.

[16] B. Satirapoj, K. Aramsaowapak, T. Tangwonglert, and O. Supasyndh, "Novel tubular biomarkers predict renal progression in type 2 diabetes mellitus: a prospective cohort study," *Journal of Diabetes Research*, vol. 2016, Article ID 3102962, 9 pages, 2016.

[17] J. Mishra, K. Mori, Q. Ma et al., "Amelioration of ischemic acute renal injury by neutrophil gelatinase-associated lipocalin," *Journal of the American Society of Nephrology*, vol. 15, no. 12, pp. 3073–3082, 2004.

[18] A. Viau, K. El Karoui, D. Laouari et al., "Lipocalin 2 is essential for chronic kidney disease progression in mice and humans," *Journal of Clinical Investigation*, vol. 120, no. 11, pp. 4065–4076, 2010.

[19] D. Bolignano, A. Lacquaniti, G. Coppolino et al., "Neutrophil gelatinase-associated lipocalin (NGAL) and progression of chronic kidney disease," *Clinical Journal of the American Society of Nephrology*, vol. 4, no. 2, pp. 337–344, 2009.

[20] Y. H. Yang, X. J. He, S. R. Chen, L. Wang, E. M. Li, and L. Y. Xu, "Changes of serum and urine neutrophil gelatinase-associated lipocalin in type-2 diabetic patients with nephropathy: one year observational follow-up study," *Endocrine*, vol. 36, no. 1, pp. 45–51, 2009.

[21] H. J. Bangstad, I. Seljeflot, T. J. Berg, and K. F. Hanssen, "Renal tubulointerstitial expansion is associated with endothelial dysfunction and inflammation in type 1 diabetes," *Scandinavian Journal of Clinical and Laboratory Investigation*, vol. 69, no. 1, pp. 138–144, 2009.

[22] M. M. van Timmeren, S. J. Bakker, V. S. Vaidya et al., "Tubular kidney injury molecule-1 in protein-overload nephropathy," *American Journal of Physiology-Renal Physiology*, vol. 291, no. 2, pp. F456–F464, 2006.

[23] M. M. van Timmeren, M. C. van den Heuvel, V. Bailly, S. J. Bakker, H. van Goor, and C. A. Stegeman, "Tubular kidney injury molecule-1 (KIM-1) in human renal disease," *The Journal of Pathology*, vol. 212, no. 2, pp. 209–217, 2007.

[24] J. A. de Carvalho, E. Tatsch, B. S. Hausen et al., "Urinary kidney injury molecule-1 and neutrophil gelatinase-associated lipocalin as indicators of tubular damage in normoalbuminuric patients with type 2 diabetes," *Clinical Biochemistry*, vol. 49, no. 3, pp. 232–236, 2016.

[25] S. E. Nielsen, H. Reinhard, D. Zdunek et al., "Tubular markers are associated with decline in kidney function in proteinuric type 2 diabetic patients," *Diabetes Research and Clinical Practice*, vol. 97, no. 1, pp. 71–76, 2012.

[26] N. M. Panduru, N. Sandholm, C. Forsblom et al., "Kidney injury molecule-1 and the loss of kidney function in diabetic nephropathy: a likely causal link in patients with type 1 diabetes," *Diabetes Care*, vol. 38, no. 6, pp. 1130–1137, 2015.

[27] M. L. Graciano, C. Cavaglieri Rde, H. Delle et al., "Intrarenal renin-angiotensin system is upregulated in experimental model of progressive renal disease induced by chronic inhibition of nitric oxide synthesis," *Journal of the American Society of Nephrology*, vol. 15, no. 7, pp. 1805–1815, 2004.

[28] S. S. Kim, S. H. Song, I. J. Kim et al., "Clinical implication of urinary tubular markers in the early stage of nephropathy with type 2 diabetic patients," *Diabetes Research and Clinical Practice*, vol. 97, no. 2, pp. 251–257, 2012.

[29] Y. Suzaki, Y. Ozawa, and H. Kobori, "Intrarenal oxidative stress and augmented angiotensinogen are precedent to renal injury in Zucker diabetic fatty rats," *International Journal of Biological Sciences*, vol. 3, no. 1, pp. 40–46, 2007.

[30] K. Miyata, N. Ohashi, Y. Suzaki, A. Katsurada, and H. Kobori, "Sequential activation of the reactive oxygen species/angiotensinogen/renin–angiotensin system axis in renal injury of type 2 diabetic rats," *Clinical and Experimental Pharmacology and Physiology*, vol. 35, no. 8, pp. 922–927, 2008.

[31] B. Satirapoj, N. Siritaweesuk, and O. Supasyndh, "Urinary angiotensinogen as a potential biomarker of diabetic nephropathy," *Clinical Kidney Journal*, vol. 7, no. 4, pp. 354–360, 2014.

[32] S. Takeshita, R. Kikuno, K. Tezuka, and E. Amann, "Osteoblast-specific factor 2: cloning of a putative bone adhesion protein with homology with the insect protein fasciclin I," *Biochemical Journal*, vol. 294, no. 1, pp. 271–278, 1993.

[33] B. Satirapoj, Y. Wang, M. P. Chamberlin et al., "Periostin: novel tissue and urinary biomarker of progressive renal injury induces a coordinated mesenchymal phenotype in tubular cells," *Nephrology Dialysis Transplantation*, vol. 27, no. 7, pp. 2702–2711, 2012.

[34] P. Wantanasiri, B. Satirapoj, M. Charoenpitakchai, and P. Aramwit, "Periostin: a novel tissue biomarker correlates with chronicity index and renal function in lupus nephritis patients," *Lupus*, vol. 24, no. 8, pp. 835–845, 2015.

[35] B. Satirapoj, R. Witoon, P. Ruangkanchanasetr, P. Wantanasiri, M. Charoenpitakchai, and P. Choovichian, "Urine periostin as a biomarker of renal injury in chronic allograft nephropathy," *Transplantation Proceedings*, vol. 46, no. 1, pp. 135–140, 2014.

[36] B. Satirapoj, S. Tassanasorn, M. Charoenpitakchai, and O. Supasyndh, "Periostin as a tissue and urinary biomarker of renal injury in type 2 diabetes mellitus," *PLoS One*, vol. 10, no. 4, article e0124055, 2015.

[37] T. Furuta, T. Saito, T. Ootaka et al., "The role of macrophages in diabetic glomerulosclerosis," *American Journal of Kidney Diseases*, vol. 21, no. 5, pp. 480–485, 1993.

[38] S. Segerer, P. J. Nelson, and D. Schlöndorff, "Chemokines, chemokine receptors, and renal disease: from basic science to pathophysiologic and therapeutic studies," *Journal of the American Society of Nephrology*, vol. 11, no. 1, pp. 152–176, 2000.

[39] T. Wada, K. Furuichi, N. Sakai et al., "Up-regulation of monocyte chemoattractant protein-1 in tubulointerstitial lesions of human diabetic nephropathy," *Kidney International*, vol. 58, no. 4, pp. 1492–1499, 2000.

[40] N. Banba, T. Nakamura, M. Matsumura, H. Kuroda, Y. Hattori, and K. Kasai, "Possible relationship of monocyte chemoattractant protein-1 with diabetic nephropathy," *Kidney International*, vol. 58, no. 2, pp. 684–690, 2000.

[41] G. Grandaliano, L. Gesualdo, E. Ranieri et al., "Monocyte chemotactic peptide-1 expression in acute and chronic human nephritides: a pathogenetic role in interstitial monocytes recruitment," *Journal of the American Society of Nephrology*, vol. 7, no. 6, pp. 906–913, 1996.

[42] B. H. Rovin, N. Doe, and L. C. Tan, "Monocyte chemoattractant protein-1 levels in patients with glomerular disease," *American Journal of Kidney Diseases*, vol. 27, no. 5, pp. 640–646, 1996.

[43] J. Lechner, N. A. Malloth, P. Jennings, D. Heckl, W. Pfaller, and T. Seppi, "Opposing roles of EGF in IFN-α-induced epithelial barrier destabilization and tissue repair," *American Journal of Physiology-Cell Physiology*, vol. 293, no. 6, pp. C1843–C1850, 2007.

[44] W. A. Kennedy 2nd, R. Buttyan, E. Garcia-Montes, C. A. Olsson, and I. S. Sawczuk, "Epidermal growth factor suppresses renal tubular apoptosis following ureteral obstruction," *Urology*, vol. 49, no. 6, pp. 973–980, 1997.

[45] S. Worawichawong, S. Worawichawong, P. Radinahamed et al., "Urine epidermal growth factor, monocyte chemoattractant protein-1 or their ratio as biomarkers for interstitial fibrosis and tubular atrophy in primary glomerulonephritis," *Kidney and Blood Pressure Research*, vol. 41, no. 6, pp. 997–1007, 2016.

[46] L. Gesualdo, S. Di Paolo, A. Calabró et al., "Expression of epidermal growth factor and its receptor in normal and diseased human kidney: an immunohistochemical and in situ hybridization study," *Kidney International*, vol. 49, no. 3, pp. 656–665, 1996.

[47] T. Morii, H. Fujita, T. Narita et al., "Association of monocyte chemoattractant protein-1 with renal tubular damage in diabetic nephropathy," *Journal of Diabetes and its Complications*, vol. 17, no. 1, pp. 11–15, 2003.

15

Urinary Proteome Analysis Identified Neprilysin and VCAM as Proteins Involved in Diabetic Nephropathy

Elena Guillén-Gómez[1,2] **Beatriz Bardají-de-Quixano,**[2,3] **Sílvia Ferrer,**[4] **Carlos Brotons,**[2,5] **Mark A. Knepper,**[6] **Montserrat Carrascal,**[7] **Joaquin Abian**[7] **José M. Mas,**[8] **Francesca Calero,**[2,9] **José A. Ballarín,**[2,9] **and Patricia Fernández-Llama**[2,9]

[1]*Molecular Biology Laboratory, Fundació Puigvert, Barcelona, Spain*
[2]*Universitat Autònoma de Barcelona, Institut d'Investigació Biomèdica Sant Pau (IIB Sant Pau), Barcelona, Spain*
[3]*Renal Transplantation Unit, Nephrology Department, Fundació Puigvert, Barcelona, Spain*
[4]*Maragall Primary Health Care Center, Barcelona, Spain*
[5]*Sardenya Primary Health Care Center, Barcelona, Spain*
[6]*Epithelial Systems Biology Laboratory, National Heart, Lung, and Blood Institute (NIH), Bethesda, MD, USA*
[7]*Proteomics Laboratory CSIC/UAB, Institut d'Investigacions Biomèdiques de Barcelona (IIBB-CSIC-IDIBAPS), Barcelona, Spain*
[8]*Anaxomics Biotech SL, Barcelona, Spain*
[9]*Hypertension Unit, Nephrology Department, Fundació Puigvert, Barcelona, Spain*

Correspondence should be addressed to Patricia Fernández-Llama; pfernandezllama@fundacio-puigvert.es

Academic Editor: Mark Yorek

Urinary proteome was analyzed and quantified by tandem mass tag (TMT) labeling followed by bioinformatics analysis to study diabetic nephropathy (DN) pathophysiology and to identify biomarkers of a clinical outcome. We included type 2 diabetic normotensive non-obese males with ($n = 9$) and without ($n = 11$) incipient DN (microalbuminuria). Sample collection included blood and urine at baseline (control and DN basal) and, in DN patients, after 3 months of losartan treatment (DN treated). Urinary proteome analysis identified 166 differentially abundant proteins between controls and DN patients, 27 comparing DN-treated and DN-basal patients, and 182 between DN-treated patients and controls. The mathematical modeling analysis predicted 80 key proteins involved in DN pathophysiology and 15 in losartan effect, a total of 95 proteins. Out of these 95, 7 are involved in both processes. VCAM-1 and neprilysin stand out of these 7 for being differentially expressed in the urinary proteome. We observed an increase of VCAM-1 urine levels in DN-basal patients compared to diabetic controls and an increase of urinary neprilysin in DN-treated patients with persistent albuminuria; the latter was confirmed by ELISA. Our results point to neprilysin and VCAM-1 as potential candidates in DN pathology and treatment.

1. Introduction

Diabetic nephropathy (DN) is the leading cause of end stage renal disease (ESRD) [1]. Incipient DN is characterized by the appearance of microalbuminuria that increases as the disease progresses and may lead to macroalbuminuria and renal failure. It is known that renin-angiotensin system (RAS) blockers, particularly angiotensin II (Ang II) antagonists such as losartan, can slow down the progression of ESRD [2].

Urine proteomics consists of a large-scale study in a single analysis to identify thousands of proteins and peptides. Urine proteomic investigations in DN identified potential biomarkers allowing an early detection of DN as well as prediction of normoalbuminuric diabetic patients prone to develop DN [3, 4]. Zürbig et al. also demonstrated the predictive value of urine proteomics for detection of progression to macroalbuminura [5]. Besides, the usefulness of urine proteomics to reveal potential biomarkers was evidenced by a multiple proteomic comparison researches in which several proteins differently abundant in patients with DN were identified. This was an important step forward to improve accurate diagnosis and understanding of the disease mechanisms [6, 7].

Despite this new progress, there is not yet an appropriate therapy to prevent DN. Moreover, it is common to find other clinical factors such as overweight, dyslipidemia, and hypertension in DN patients contributing to renal damage. In this work, we have studied incipient DN male patients before and after losartan treatment, and, in contrast with other studies, we have selected non-obese patients with a good blood pressure and lipid control, with the aim of improving the identification of factors closely related to the pathogenesis of DN.

2. Subjects and Methods

2.1. Patients. Twenty-one type 2 diabetic patients were enrolled in the study: 12 without DN (control patients) and 9 with incipient DN (DN basal). The inclusion criteria were (1) males ≥ 35 years old; (2) controlled hypertension by 24 h ambulatory blood pressure monitoring (ABPM) (24 h systolic BP (SBP) < 130 mmHg and 24 h diastolic BP (DBP) < 80 mmHg) [8]; and (3) absence (control cohort) or presence (DN patients) of persistent microalbuminuria: albumin/creatinine ratio from 2.26 mg/mmol to 22.6 mg/mmol at least in two out of three urine morning samples. The exclusion criteria were (1) estimated glomerular filtration rate (CKD-EPI) < 60 ml/min/1.73 m^2; (2) having taken a RAS inhibitor ≤ six months prior to inclusion; (3) any cardiovascular event during the past year; (4) serum potassium > 5.0 mmol/l; (5) serum LDL cholesterol > 3.0 mmol/l, triglyceride > 1.7 mmol/l, or glycated hemoglobin HbA1c > 7.5% (>58 mmol/mol); (6) body mass index (BMI) ≥ 35 kg/mm^2; (7) documented renal artery stenosis; (8) any condition that may alter the absorption, distribution, metabolism, or excretion of RAS inhibitor drugs; (9) history of malignancy in the last 5 years; (10) history or evidence of drug or alcohol abuse during the past year; (11) history of hypersensitivity to any RAS inhibitor; and (12) history of noncompliance with medical regimens.

The theoretical sample size necessary for obtaining statistically significant differences was calculated based on the standard deviation of the inclusion/exclusion criteria analytical parameters. Given the homogeneity of the subjects and the specificity of inclusion/exclusion criteria that made it difficult to find patients matching them, sample size was established at the lower limit of the interval obtained through the equation.

2.2. Blood Pressure, Blood, and Urine Analysis. SBP, DBP, mean BP (MBP), and heart rate over day, night, and 24 h were measured by 24 h ABPM (Diasys Integra II; Novacor, Paris, France). Office BP was recorded following the European guidelines [9].

Serum electrolytes (sodium and potassium) were analyzed by selective ion electrodes; serum urea, creatinine, lipidic profile, glycemic profile, and urine albumin and creatinine levels were determined by kinetic, colorimetric, or immunoturbidimetric assays, in the Roche Cobas® 6000 analyzer, following the manufacturer's instructions.

2.3. Urine Collection. First morning urine void was collected, centrifuged, and stored at −80°C until proteomic analysis.

2.4. Quantitative Liquid Chromatography Tandem Mass Spectrometry (LC-MSn) Analysis. Four biological replicates from each condition (control, basal, and treated) were processed. Each replicate was a pool of three or four different patients as appropriate.

2.4.1. Sample Preparation. Samples (14–28 ml) were thawed and centrifuged (4000*g*, 4°C, 20 min), filtered (Steriflip PVDF 0.22 μm pore, Millipore, Watford, UK), and concentrated using Amicon® centrifugal filters (Amicon Ultra 15 ml, Millipore) up to about 250 μl final volume. Samples were evaporated in a SpeedVac (Thermo Electron, Waltham, MA, USA) to a final volume of about 50 μl and albumin/IgG depleted using the PROTIA Proteoprep Immunoaffinity kit (Sigma-Aldrich, St Louis, MO, USA).

Each sample was immunodepleted separately. Pools of 3-4 different patients were prepared for further processing combining volumes of eluate containing equimolar amounts of protein (26.7 μg each). A total of 12 pools were prepared (4 controls, 4 diabetic basal, and 4 diabetic treated).

2.4.2. Protein Digestion and Peptide Labeling. Pooled immunodepleted samples (80 μg of protein) were digested as previously described. Each tryptic peptide mixture was labeled with the corresponding tandem mass tags (TMT) (Thermo Fisher Scientific, Rockford, IL, USA). The TMT labeling kits used provide 6 different molecular labels. Thus, only 6 samples can be analyzed together per LC-MS experiment. So, the 12 pools available were analyzed in two independent experiments each containing 2 replicates (pools) of each class. In each experiment, the six differentially TMT-labeled samples were combined in a low-bind 1.5 mL Eppendorf tube, evaporated, and desalted using a C18 SPE cartridge (3 mL, 15 mg, Agilent Technologies, Waldbronn, Germany). The SPE eluates were evaporated and resuspended in 200 μl of 30% ACN (0.1% formic acid).

2.4.3. Sample Fractionation by Strong Cation Exchange Chromatography. SCX fractionation of the TMT-labelled peptide mixtures was performed on an Agilent 1100 HPLC system (Agilent Technologies) using a Polysulfoethyl A™, 50 × 2.1 mm, 5 μm, and 200 Å column at a flow rate of 200 μl/min. A linear NH_4Cl gradient from 0 to 25% B in 38 min and then to 100% B in 20 min was used (buffer A: 30% ACN, 0.1% formic acid; buffer B: 30% ACN, 0.1% formic acid, 0.5 M NH_4Cl). Six fractions were collected from minute 10 to 52.

2.4.4. LC-MSn Analysis. One-fifth of each collected SCX fraction was analyzed by LC-MSn using an Agilent 1200 nano pump (Agilent Technologies) connected to a LTQ-Orbitrap XL instrument (Thermo Fisher Scientific) equipped with a nanoESI source (Proxeon, Odense, Denmark). Separations

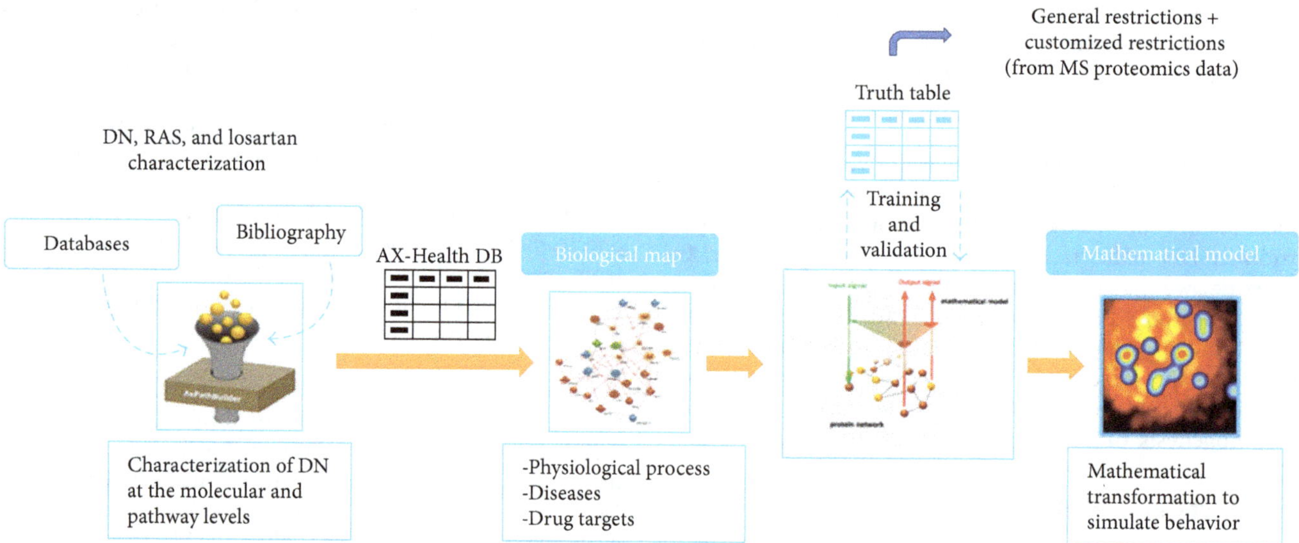

FIGURE 1: Mathematical model generation process. It includes the creation of a Biological Effector Database (BED), the construction of a biological map, and, finally, the achievement of the mathematical model.

were carried out using a C18 preconcentration cartridge (Agilent Technologies) connected to a 15 cm-long 100 μm i.d. C18 column (Nikkyo Technos Co., Japan). Separations were done at 0.4 μl/min using a linear ACN gradient from 0 to 40% in 120 min (solvent A: 0.1% formic acid, solvent B: ACN 0.1% formic acid). The spectrometric analysis was performed in an automatic data-dependent mode. A full scan followed by 1 HCD and 1 CID MS/MS scans for the 5 most abundant signals was acquired (dynamic exclusion: 1, time window: 30 s).

2.4.5. Database Search. Thermo RAW files were processed using the EasierMgf software. Database search was done using Proteome Discoverer v1.4 (Thermo-Instruments) with a 1% false discovery rate (FDR) and the UniProt 2014-10 database restricted to *Homo sapiens*. Search parameters were parent tolerance, 20 ppm; fragment tolerance, 0.8 Da; enzyme, trypsin; missed cleavages, 1; fixed modifications, TMTsixplex (N-terminal, K), carbamidomethyl (C); and variable modifications, oxidation (M).

2.5. Bioinformatic Analysis of Proteomic Data. Based on artificial intelligence and pattern recognition techniques, Therapeutic Performance Mapping System (TPMS, Anaxomics Biotech) [10, 11] creates mathematical models that integrate all the available biological, pharmacological, and medical knowledge to simulate human physiology in silico. TPMS technology includes two different and complementary strategies to solve mathematical models:

(i) Artificial neural networks (ANNs): this strategy is able to identify relationships among regions of the network (generalization). These provide a predictive value that infers the probability of the existence of a specific relationship between two or more sets of proteins (in this case, each protein and DN), based on a validation of the predictive capacity of the model towards what is described in databases.

(ii) Sampling methods: this second strategy allows to trace back observed effects to molecules and is normally applied once a key region of the map has been identified (using an ANN or as suggested by experimental work). Once a response is identified to a specific stimulus (e.g., a drug target, as identified with an ANN), it is possible to analyze mechanisms of action using the sampling methods strategy.

Mathematical models are able to suggest mechanistic hypotheses that are consistent with actual biological processes. Finally, the comparative analysis of healthy and DN mathematical models revealed functional properties and mechanistic insights specific of the pathological state of interest.

The process comprises four steps (Figure 1): (1) collection of scientific knowledge based on hand-curated databases that relate biological processes to their molecular effectors (BED) (including a specific DN, type 2 diabetes, and RAS pathway characterizations); (2) preparation of a human biological network focused on DN based on data retrieved from both public and private external databases such as KEGG, BioGRID, IntAct, REACTOME, and MINT; (3) subsequent generation of mathematical model, whereby the biological map is transformed into a mathematical model capable of both reproducing existing knowledge and predicting new data. To do this, the mathematical models were previously trained using a collection of known input-output physiological signals (e.g., a drug indication relationship), these being obtained from the literature mining and a compendium of databases that accumulate biological and clinical data [12–17], namely:

(i) Model inputs: for example, information about drugs provided by DrugBank [18], since they inhibit or activate one or more nodes of the model (their targets) triggering a perturbation through the system,

(ii) Model outputs: for example, experimental microarray data (upregulated or downregulated proteins, after the treatment). The collection of known input-output physiological signals generates a list of physiological rules or principles found to apply to all humans, or to particular pathophysiological conditions, that act as mathematical restrictions. These sets of rules are collected to form a *Truth Table*, a collection of mathematical restrictions that include the available biological knowledge on the constructed networks, together with knowledge derived from DrugBank, and the statistically significant differentially expressed proteins from transcriptomic data. Furthermore, models able to simulate the physiological behavior of diabetic patients suffering DN were generated including the differentially expressed proteins extracted from the different group comparison,

and (4) extraction of biological and clinical conclusions. To extract conclusions, the pairs of mathematical models of interest were compared with the aim of identifying the key proteins involved in the pathophysiology of the DN and in the efficacy of losartan:

(i) Identification of the key proteins and mechanism of action associated with DN pathophysiology:

(a) Model of diabetic patient suffering DN versus healthy model

(ii) Identification of the key proteins and mechanism of action associated with losartan effect:

(a) Model of diabetic patients suffering DN and treated with losartan versus model of diabetic patients suffering DN

(b) Model of diabetic patients suffering DN and treated with losartan versus model of diabetic patients

Sampling methods were used to describe with high capability all plausible relationships between nodes of the mathematical models. As the number of restrictions is always smaller than the number of parameters required by the algorithm, any process modeled by TPMS considers a population of different solutions, currently set around 10^6–10^9 since this interval is estimated to faithfully portray nature. Subsequently, TPMS traces the most probable pathways (in biological and mathematical terms) among all the possible pathways leading from the stimulus to the response through the biological network.

Mathematical models should be able to weigh the relative value of each protein ratio (node). In the mathematical algorithm, each parameter corresponds to the relative weight of a link connecting nodes (genes/proteins) in a graph (protein map). Using the sampling methods, we generated populations of solutions that comply with the biological restrictions of the Truth Table. This approach allows tracing back the biological effects on molecules or triggering effectors by analyzing the different populations of solutions. Thus, the population of solutions accounts for the variety of physiological responses that may occur in human populations. The mathematical model is challenged with the stimulus and the response, and we traced the most probable path (in biological and mathematical terms) that leads from the stimulus to the response through the biological network. Thus, it identifies the most probable MoA that achieves a physiological response when the system is stimulated. For the analysis, we used those solutions that comply with the general knowledge collated in the Truth Table (high accuracy values). That is, only MoAs that are plausible from the standpoint of currently accepted scientific understandings and the restrictions applied were considered in the analysis.

2.6. Urinary Neprilysin and VCAM-1 ELISA. Their abundance was tested in urinary samples from patients and controls using a specific enzyme-linked immunosorbent assay (ELISA). Urine neprilysin (MyBioSource, San Diego, California, USA) and human vascular cell adhesion molecule-1 (VCAM-1) ELISA (Sigma-Aldrich, St. Louis, Missouri, USA) were performed following the manufacturer's instructions.

2.7. Presentation of Data and Statistical Analyses. Patient clinical data: quantitative data are presented as the mean ± standard deviation (SD). Statistical comparisons were performed by *t*-test (unpaired or paired as appropriate using SPSS 17.0).

Proteomic data analysis: DanteR [19] was used for relative quantification. Only unique peptides were considered for the analysis. Tandem mass tag (TMT) reporter intensity data were normalized using the Loess method followed by adjustment with central tendency. ANOVA was performed and adjusted by false discovery rate (FDR) correction. Two different comparisons were carried out: (1) basal and treated versus control and (2) treated versus basal. Differential proteins were selected using an adjusted p value cutoff of 0.05 and a ratio < 0.7 (down) or >1.3 (up).

Bioinformatic analysis: mathematical models allowed the identification of key proteins associated with DN pathology and treatment efficacy; p-values used to select these key proteins were ≤ 0.005 and ≤ 0.05, respectively.

3. Results

3.1. Patients. Clinical and demographic characteristics of the study population are shown in Table 1. All patients included in the study were over 60 years old. Control and DN basal groups were balanced regarding baseline characteristics except for albuminuria levels. None of the patients had diabetic retinopathy. The 9 DN patients were treated with losartan during three months. After this period, there were no differences in terms of albuminuria, HbA1c, eGFR, cholesterol, and triglycerides levels. Figure 2 shows albumin/creatinine ratio in the three groups studied. Losartan treatment in DN patients maintained office BP

Table 1: Clinical and demographic characteristics of the study population.

	Controls	DN basal	DN treated	Statistics (student t-test)
N (gender)	12 (males)	9 (males)		N/A
Nonsmokers/smokers/ex-smokers	4/2/6	0/5/4		N/A
Age (years)	69.6 ± 9.6	71.0 ± 7.0		0.714
BMI	28.1 ± 5.2	27.0 ± 2.3		0.572
Time of type 2 DM (years)	13.8 ± 7.9	12.2 ± 4.5		0.591
HbA1c (%) (mmol/mol)	6.8 ± 0.8 (51 ± 9.0)	7.0 ± 0.7 (53 ± 7.6)	7.0 ± 0.7 (52.4 ± 7.4)	0.467
Cholesterol total (mmol/l)	4.1 ± 0.7	4.2 ± 0.8	4.3 ± 0.6	0.773
Cholesterol LDL (mmol/l)	2.1 ± 0.6	2.1 ± 0.6	2.3 ± 0.5	0.884
Triglycerides (mmol/L)	1.1 ± 0.4	1.3 ± 0.4	1.7 ± 0.8	0.196
eGFR (CKD-EPI) (ml/min/1.73 m^2)	80.4 ± 10.9	89.1 ± 16.8	85.4 ± 19.0	0.1662
Urine albumin/creatinine (mg/mmol)	0.68 ± 1.0	13.6 ± 12.2	12.5 ± 4.8	$p < 0.0001$
ABPM				
24 h SBP (mmHg)	119.4 ± 11.8	121.4 ± 11.4	n.d.	0.869
24 h DBP (mmHg)	70.8 ± 5.0	69.2 ± 7.5	n.d.	0.509
Antidiabetic drugs				
Insulin (N)	1	1		N/A
Metformin (N)	8	9		N/A
Sulfonylureas (N)	6	1		N/A
Other oral drugs (N)	2	1		N/A

Data are expressed as the mean ± SD; the statistics column refers to the comparison between control patients and DN patients before losartan treatment (basal). All comparisons between basal and treated DN patients were nonsignificant. ABPM: ambulatory blood pressure monitoring; BMI: body mass index; DM: diabetes mellitus; DN: diabetic nephropathy; DBP: diastolic blood pressure; eGFR: estimated glomerular filtration rate; HbA1c: glycated hemoglobin; n.d.: not determined; SD: standard deviation; SBP: systolic blood pressure; N/A: not applicable.

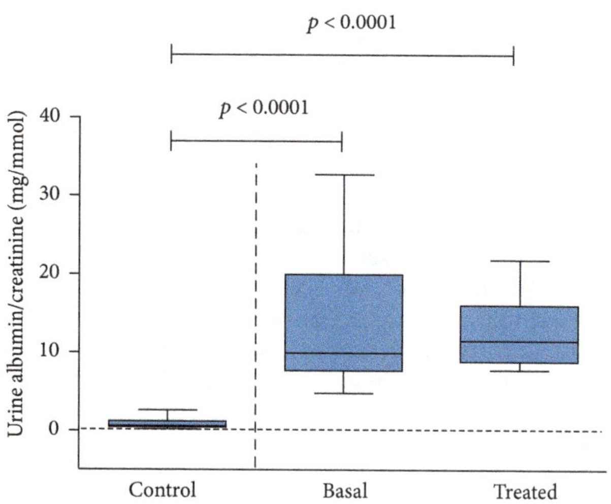

Figure 2: Box-and-whisker plots of urine albumin/creatinine ratios in mg/mmol in the three studied groups. Each value was calculated from three successive measurements. N control = 11, N basal = 9, and N treated = 9; statistical test: Student's t-test.

(SBP 144.0 ± 17.7 versus 140.0 ± 24.8 mmHg; DBP 73.6 ± 6.6 versus 75.3 ± 6.8 mmHg, basal versus treatment, resp.). Antidiabetic drugs are specified in Table 1. Ten patients from the control group and 4 from the DN group took statins. Five patients from the control group and 4 from the DN group took antiplatelet agents, being aspirin the most used.

3.2. Protein Identification and Relative Quantification. 10780 spectra corresponding to 2520 nonredundant peptides were identified through database search (1% FDR). For quantitative analysis, only peptides identified as unique (i.e., peptide sequences belonging to one single protein in the database) were considered. Overall, a total of 688 proteins could be quantified from 2191 nonredundant unique peptides. The mass spectrometry proteomic data have been deposited to the ProteomeXchange consortium via the PRIDE [20] partner repository with the dataset identifier PXD009303. This information is also available in the Supplementary data (available here).

3.3. Proteomic Data Processing and Enrichment Analysis of Differentially Abundant Proteins. We identified 166 differentially abundant proteins in basal versus control comparison, 27 between treated and basal cohorts, and 182 in treated versus control comparison (Table 2). Detailed information is provided in the supplementary data. We predicted 138 and 13 proteins as direct effectors of DN and RAS efficacy, respectively, according to its molecular characterization in the Biological Effector Database (BED) [21]. Furthermore, we found 14 differential proteins common to the three evaluated cohorts considering both upregulated and downregulated proteins. One of them, osteopontin, a bone matrix protein and proinflammatory cytokine, was also predicted as a direct effector of DN according to its BED molecular characterization (Figure 3).

Table 2: Summary of differentially abundant proteins identified for each evaluated cohort comparison that are also direct effectors of DN according to its molecular characterization in the Biological Effector Database (BED).

	Number of differentially expressed proteins			Number of DN effectors		
	Total	Upregulated proteins	Downregulated proteins	Total	Upregulated proteins	Downregulated proteins
Basal versus control	166	23	143	3	0	3
Treated versus basal	27	14	13	2	1	1
Treated versus control	182	26	156	3	3	0

DN: diabetic nephropathy.

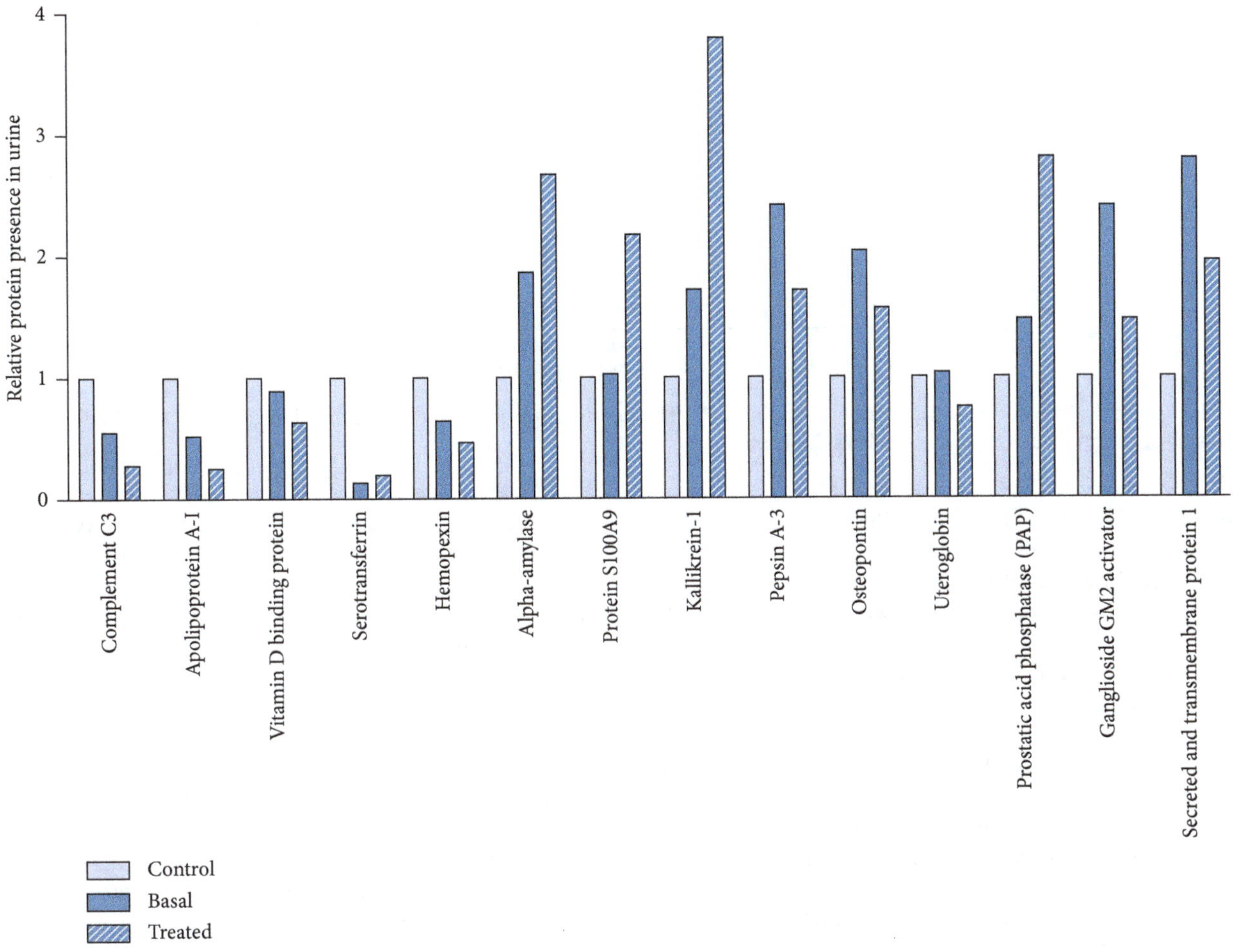

Figure 3: Differentially abundant proteins among the three cohorts. Data presented as a relative change from the control cohort.

The enrichment analysis of the differential proteins between basal and control cohorts revealed 344 enriched pathways, 263 between treated and basal cohorts, and 352 between treated and control cohorts. Interestingly, some of them are related to DN and RAS according to an artificial neural network (ANN) [22] analysis. This analysis identifies associations among different regions of the network, such as potential relationships between the enriched protein sets and DN and RAS. Specifically, the vasoactive hormone pathway is enriched in the treated versus basal cohorts' comparison. The inflammation associated with DN is an enriched pathway in the comparisons between treated versus basal and basal versus control cohorts.

3.4. Clustering Analysis. Results of hierarchical clustering, according to mathematical models, are represented in Figure 4 as a dendrogram to show distances in terms of protein expression between groups.

3.5. Key Proteins Involved in DN and RAS Efficacy. Comparative analyses among the generated mathematical models predicted 80 proteins with an important role in DN (key proteins) (supplementary data): (1) 14 of them are measurable in urine; (2) 20 have been previously considered effectors of DN; (3) 2 have also been identified as differentially abundant proteins from the cohort comparisons of proteomic data; and (4) 45 of the key proteins are directly linked to some of the

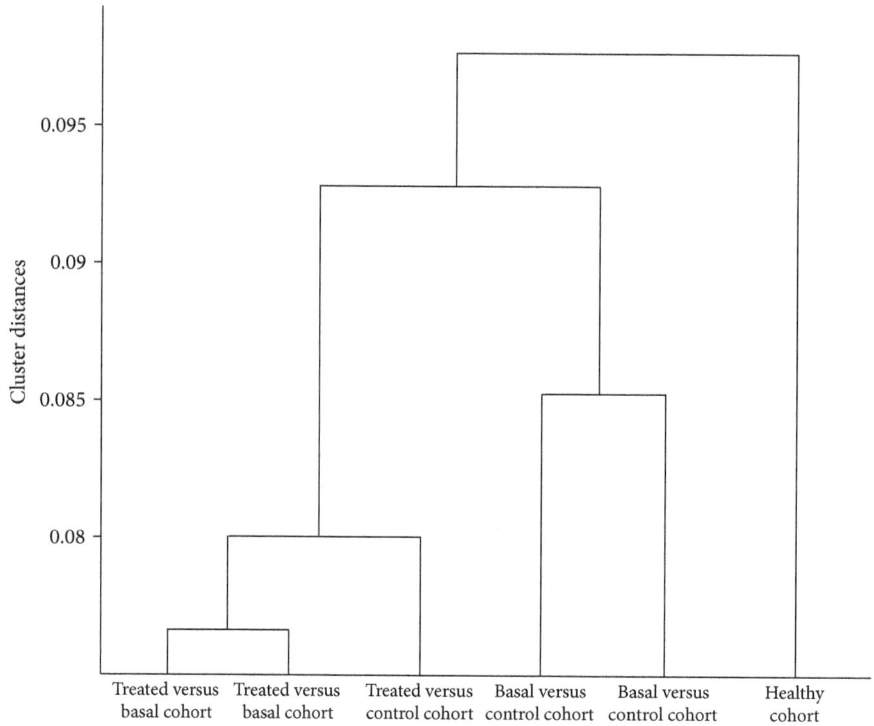

FIGURE 4: Hierarchical clustering of the mathematical models. The dendrogram was build using the Hausdorff distance between the set of mechanisms of action defined by the models in duplicate.

differentially present proteins identified from the cohort comparisons of proteomic data.

Regarding losartan effect, comparative analysis from mathematical models predicted 15 key proteins (supplementary data): (1) 7 are measurable in urine; (2) none are RAS efficacy key proteins according to the molecular characterization in our BED; (3) 4 have been also identified in the differential presence analysis of proteomic data; and (4) 9 are directly linked to one or several of the differentially present proteins identified from the cohort comparisons of proteomic data.

An effector protein is defined as an essential protein in the disease pathology according to its molecular characterization in BED and published literature, whereas a key protein is predicted through the analysis of mathematical models. Key proteins can also be effector proteins or new potential candidates (in the disease pathology or in the treatment efficacy), the role of which has not been described before. In this work, we detected 5 DN effector proteins differentially abundant among the three cohorts: osteopontin, neprilysin, fibronectin, kininogen-1, and VCAM-1 (Table 3(a)). Neprilysin and VCAM-1, however, are the only ones that are also DN disease key proteins. Additionally, we predicted 4 losartan effect key proteins differentially abundant among the three cohorts: neprilysin, VCAM-1, kininogen-1, and alpha-2-macroglobulin. Only alpha-2-macroglobulin is not a losartan effector protein (Table 3(b)).

Finally, we predicted 7 key proteins in both DN pathophysiology and losartan effect (Table 4). VCAM-1 and neprilysin stand out from the others because they are differentially abundant in the urine proteome.

3.6. Urinary Neprilysin and VCAM-1 ELISA. We were only able to detect VCAM-1 in one of the urine samples among the three cohorts through ELISA analysis. Regarding neprilysin, urine levels were higher in DN losartan-treated patients than in the untreated patients ($p = 0.0255$) (Figure 5), reinforcing the results obtained in the proteomic analysis.

4. Discussion

Albuminuria is not specific for DN and is highly variable [23]. In order to identify alternative biomarkers, we performed urinary proteomic analysis in diabetic and incipient DN patients, the latter before and after losartan treatment. Several publications support that profiling of the urinary proteome can be useful to diagnose DN and identify novel biomarkers [6, 7, 24, 25]. In our study, patients' selection criteria were strict, avoiding confounder factors such obesity, uncontrolled BP, or dyslipidemia, which are commonly associated comorbidities that also induce albuminuria. Therefore, differences in urinary proteome would correspond to the disease itself and not to associated secondary problems.

In contrast to other proteomic studies, our results were further analyzed by bioinformatic tools including mathematical models and several databases in order to reach more specific and distilled information. Thus, we predicted 5 proteins known to be involved in DN pathophysiology and 4 associated with losartan treatment. Two of them, VCAM-1 and neprilysin, are effector proteins of both disease and treatment efficacy, making them the most relevant proteins at this early stage of the disease. Levels of VCAM-1, a candidate biomarker of renal pathology [26], correlate with

TABLE 3: (a) DN effector proteins differentially abundant in the cohort comparisons and (b) losartan treatment key proteins differentially abundant in the cohort comparisons.

(a)

Protein name	Basal* versus control	Treated* versus basal	Treated* versus control
Osteopontin	Downregulated	Upregulated	Downregulated
Neprilysin	—	Downregulated	—
Fibronectin	Downregulated	—	Downregulated
Kininogen-1	—	—	Downregulated
VCAM-1	Downregulated	—	—

(b)

Protein name	Basal* versus control	Treated* versus basal	Treated* versus control
Neprilysin	—	Downregulated	—
VCAM-1	Downregulated	—	—
Kininogen-1	—	—	Downregulated
Alpha-2-M	—	—	Upregulated

*Cohort used as reference group. VCAM-1: vascular cell adhesion protein 1; Alpha-2-M: alpha-2-macroglobulin; —: no changes observed.

TABLE 4: Summary of the key proteins in both DN pathophysiology and losartan effect. The table indicates whether (1) the protein is a DN effector and for positive instances the process with which the protein is associated, (2) the protein is also differentially abundant from the cohort comparison ($d = 0$) or it is directly linked to one of them ($d = 1$), and (3) if the protein is easily measurable in urine according to bibliography review.

Protein	DN effector		Presence in proteomic data			Urine presence
	Yes/no	Process	$d = 0$	Comparison	$d = 1$	Yes/no
Neprilysin	Yes	Vasoactive hormones	Yes	Treated versus basal	Yes	Yes
Kallikrein	No		No	NA	Yes	Yes
Angiopoietin-2	Yes	Activation of angiogenesis	No	NA	No	Yes
Signal transducer and activator of transcription1-alpha/beta	Yes	JAK/STAT pathway alterations	No	NA	No	No
MAD homolog 7	Yes	Inflammation	No	NA	Yes	Yes
VCAM-1	Yes	Inflammation	Yes	Basal versus control	No	Yes
NADPH oxidase	No		No	NA	Yes	No

DN: diabetic nephropathy; N/A: not applicable; MAD homolog 7: mothers against decapentaplegic homolog 7; VCAM-1: vascular cell adhesion protein 1; NADPH oxidase: nicotinamide adenine dinucleotide phosphate hydrogen oxidase; JAK/STAT: Janus kinase/signal transducer and activator of transcription.

albuminuria in diabetic hypertensive patients [27] and with the number of infiltrating immune cells [28]. Its expression is increased in the kidneys from DN patients [29], probably because Ang II upregulates VCAM-1 [30]. In accordance with these results, we observed that VCAM-1 urine levels were increased in basal albuminuric DN patients compared to diabetic controls without renal damage, supporting its role in this process. In fact, there are preclinical studies describing the blockade of adhesion molecules as a potential therapeutic target [31].

Urine proteome also showed changes in neprilysin abundance that were also confirmed by ELISA. Neprilysin is a metalloprotease that inactivates several peptides including natriuretic peptides, bradykinin, and endothelins. It is particularly abundant in the kidney where it is bound to plasma membrane, but it is also present in a soluble form in urine and blood. The urine form appears to reflect the activity of the enzyme in the kidney [32, 33]. Our proteomic results indicate an increase of urinary neprilysin after losartan treatment in DN patients showing persistent albuminuria. To our knowledge, this is the first study that observes changes in urine neprilysin after losartan treatment in incipient DN patients. The increase of Ang II, by losartan, may favor the activity and/or expression of neprilysin through the alternative RAS activation towards the formation of Ang (1–7), without neglecting the contribution of angiotensin-converting enzyme 2 (ACE2). Indeed, the selective neprilysin inhibitor SCH39370 abolished the formation of Ang (1–7) [34].

Several studies demonstrate a potential role of neprilysin in renal damage [35]. A DN animal model showed greater attenuation of albuminuria when treated with a neprilysin inhibitor compared to a RAS blocker [36]. Vasodilatation is associated with natriuretic peptides and may result in reductions of intraglomerular pressure and proteinuria [37, 38].

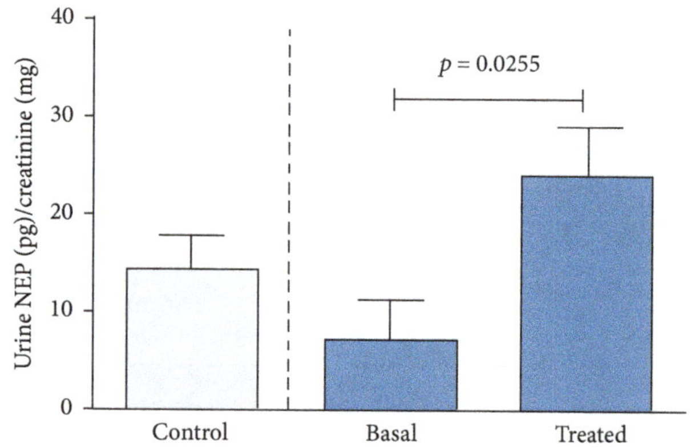

Figure 5: Quantification of urinary neprilysin (NEP) by ELISA showed an increased presence of this protein in losartan-treated patients compared to basal cohort. N control = 11, N basal = 9, and N treated = 9; statistical test: Student's t-test.

Neprilysin inhibition could increase these effects and can also impair breakdown of Ang II. Beneficial effects of neprilysin inhibition are enhanced when combined with a RAS inhibitor, which has led to the development of dual inhibition. Additionally, there is an ongoing clinical trial testing the nephroprotection effects of this double inhibition [35, 39].

Neprilysin metabolizes Ang I to Ang (1–7) and inactivates bradykinin, whereas angiotensin I-converting enzyme (ACE) catalyzes the conversion of Ang I to Ang II and it is able to inactivate bradykinin. Accordingly, changes in RAS are accompanied by changes in kallikrein-kinin system, seeming necessary to control both systems in the treatment and monitoring of DN [40]. Our results also show differences regarding kallikrein-kinin system proteins such as urine kininogen-1 and kallikrein-1. These proteins should be studied in a larger cohort to confirm their role in this disease and in RAS system pathway.

Proteomic results also show differences in extracellular matrix proteins such as fibronectin and osteopontin. Osteopontin is a glycoprotein that blocks apoptosis of macrophages and T-cells as well as fibroblasts and endothelial cells exposed to harmful stimuli. It has been suggested to have a role in albuminuria and mesangial expansion in DN [41]. There are contradictory results regarding urine osteopontin as a DN progression biomarker [42, 43]. Our results show increased levels of osteopontin in DN patients compared to diabetic controls. These results are in accordance to previous studies that demonstrated that increased Ang II stimulates the production of osteopontin in the glomerulus in DN [44]. Nevertheless, DN patients treated with losartan show lower osteopontin than basal without changes in albumin excretion. This may be explained because Ang II mediates osteopontin synthesis [45, 46] and blockade of AT1 receptors could prevent its effects.

Fibronectin is another extracellular matrix glycoprotein important in fibrosis. Our results show increased levels of fibronectin in DN patients compared to diabetic controls. Murine diabetic models develop nephropathy and increase glomerular expression and accumulation of type IV collagen and fibronectin [47–50]. Furthermore, AT1 receptor blocking by losartan did not influence urinary fibronectin [51, 52]. Our results confirm that high urinary fibronectin in DN patients is not affected by losartan treatment, suggesting an AT1 receptor-independent pathway.

Progression of DN includes inflammation of glomeruli and tubulointerstitial regions accompanied by expression of adhesion molecules and chemokines, resulting in macrophage infiltration into renal tissues [53]. Vasoactive hormones are known to be key mediators of renal injury [54]. Our urine proteomic results show proteins related to inflammation and vasoactive pathways, such as osteopontin, VCAM, neprylisin, and kininogen, that are differentially expressed in the cohorts studied. Although our patients are in an initial stage of the disease, the enrichment results already show alterations of these pathways, suggesting an early involvement in incipient DN.

In our DN patients, factors associated with albuminuria are closely controlled and this could explain partially the lack of clinic response to losartan treatment. Although activation of RAS is related to albuminuria, there are other critical factors associated with its development that probably will be more relevant in non-obese DN patients with good blood pressure, lipid, and glycemic control. There are also other reasons that could explain the lack of therapeutic responses to RAS inhibition including incomplete inhibition of RAS, lack of effects on structural hallmarks of DN, and reversibility of established renal lesions on these patients [55, 56]. Evidences suggested that microalbuminuria may not be the ideal marker of DN progression [57, 58]. Moreover, our proteomic approach pointed out some possible candidates involved in DN and losartan treatment since differences were statistically significant among the three studied groups. A validation study, on a greater cohort and during a longer period, would be necessary.

In conclusion, our results point to neprilysin and VCAM-1 as possible candidates involved in incipient DN pathology and RAS inhibition treatment in elderly males. If ongoing clinical trials with double inhibition of RAS and neprilysin are satisfactory, they could help in the clinical management of the disease. Moreover, urine detection of these proteins could serve as potential new tools as DN progression biomarkers.

Consent

It was obtained from all participants.

Conflicts of Interest

The authors declare that they have no conflict of interest.

Authors' Contributions

Patricia Fernández-Llama and Mark A. Knepper did the research idea and study design; Sílvia Ferrer, Carlos Brotons, and Francesca Calero did the patient selection; Beatriz Bardají-de-Quixano, Montserrat Carrascal, Joaquin Abian, and Elena Guillén-Gómez did the proteomic and laboratory analysis; José M. Mas did the mathematical models/statistics; Patricia Fernández-Llama, Beatriz Bardají-de-Quixano, José M. Mas, Montserrat Carrascal, Joaquin Abian, Elena Guillén-Gómez, and Mark A. Knepper did the data interpretation; Patricia Fernández-Llama, José A. Ballarin, and Mark A. Knepper did the supervision; Elena Guillén-Gómez and Beatriz Bardají-de-Quixano contributed equally to this work.

Acknowledgments

The authors thank all patients who agreed to participate. The authors thank Olga Sancho for her valuable technical assistance. The research group belongs to a Consolidated Research Group (AGAUR 2009/SGR-1116) and to REDINREN (Spanish Renal Network for Research, RETICS, Instituto de Investigación Carlos III). Funding was granted by Fondo de Investigación Sanitaria, Ministerio de Sanidad (PI10/01261) to Patricia Fernández-Llama) and ISCIII RETIC REDINREN FEDER Funds (RD12/0021/0033). The proteomics laboratory CSIC/UAB is a member of Proteored, PRB2-ISCIII and is supported by grant PT13/0001, of the PE I+D+i 2013-2016, funded by ISCIII and FEDER.

Supplementary Materials

Supplementary Tables: the excel file includes (1) peptides identified by urine proteomics with intensities and identification scores: all peptides and protein groups (tab "All_data") and unambiguous peptides pointing to a single protein that were used for statistical analysis (tab "Unique"); (2) differentially expressed proteins identified for each evaluated cohort comparison and which are direct effectors of DN, as well as the DN motives associated; (3) DN (tab "Key proteins DN") and losartan (tab "Key proteins losartan") key protein data containing the following columns: activation (sign of activation); DN effector (indicates whether it is a DN effector and the associated motive); presence in cohort comparisons in our proteomic data (the protein is also differentially abundant from the cohort comparison ($d = 0$) or it is directly linked to one of them ($d = 1$); urine presence (if the protein is easily measurable in urine according to bibliography review). Data added as an additional file through Manuscript Tracking System. *(Supplementary Materials)*

References

[1] J. Floege, R. J. Johnson, and J. Feehally, *Comprehensive Clinical Nephrology*, Saunders/Elsevier, St. Louis, MO, USA, 2010.

[2] G. Remuzzi, A. Schieppati, and P. Ruggenenti, "Nephropathy in patients with type 2 diabetes," *The New England Journal of Medicine*, vol. 346, no. 15, pp. 1145–1151, 2002.

[3] N. M. Bhensdadia, K. J. Hunt, M. F. Lopes-Virella et al., "Urine haptoglobin levels predict early renal functional decline in patients with type 2 diabetes," *Kidney International*, vol. 83, no. 6, pp. 1136–1143, 2013.

[4] M. L. Merchant, B. A. Perkins, G. M. Boratyn et al., "Urinary peptidome may predict renal function decline in type 1 diabetes and microalbuminuria," *Journal of the American Society of Nephrology*, vol. 20, no. 9, pp. 2065–2074, 2009.

[5] P. Zürbig, G. Jerums, P. Hovind et al., "Urinary proteomics for early diagnosis in diabetic nephropathy," *Diabetes*, vol. 61, no. 12, pp. 3304–3313, 2012.

[6] P. V. Rao, X. Lu, M. Standley et al., "Proteomic identification of urinary biomarkers of diabetic nephropathy," *Diabetes Care*, vol. 30, no. 3, pp. 629–637, 2007.

[7] J. A. D. van, J. W. Scholey, and A. Konvalinka, "Insights into diabetic kidney disease using urinary proteomics and bioinformatics," *Journal of the American Society of Nephrology*, vol. 28, no. 4, pp. 1050–1061, 2017.

[8] G. Mancia, R. Fagard, K. Narkiewicz et al., "2013 ESH/ESC guidelines for the management of arterial hypertension: the task force for the management of arterial hypertension of the European Society of Hypertension (ESH) and of the European Society of Cardiology (ESC)," *Journal of Hypertension*, vol. 31, no. 7, pp. 1281–1357, 2013.

[9] G. Mancia, G. de Backer, A. Dominiczak et al., "2007 guidelines for the management of arterial hypertension: the task force for the management of arterial hypertension of the European society of hypertension (ESH) and of the European society of cardiology (ESC)," *Journal of Hypertension*, vol. 25, no. 6, pp. 1105–1187, 2007.

[10] A. F. M. Altelaar, J. Munoz, and A. J. R. Heck, "Next-generation proteomics: towards an integrative view of proteome dynamics," *Nature Reviews Genetics*, vol. 14, no. 1, pp. 35–48, 2013.

[11] P. Navarro, M. Trevisan-Herraz, E. Bonzon-Kulichenko et al., "General statistical framework for quantitative proteomics by stable isotope labeling," *Journal of Proteome Research*, vol. 13, no. 3, pp. 1234–1247, 2014.

[12] M. Kanehisa, S. Goto, M. Hattori et al., "From genomics to chemical genomics: new developments in KEGG," *Nucleic Acids Research*, vol. 34, no. 90001, pp. D354–D357, 2006.

[13] D. Croft, A. F. Mundo, R. Haw et al., "The reactome pathway knowledgebase," *Nucleic Acids Research*, vol. 42, no. D1, pp. D472–D477, 2014.

[14] S. Kerrien, B. Aranda, L. Breuza et al., "The IntAct molecular interaction database in 2012," *Nucleic Acids Research*, vol. 40, no. D1, pp. D841–D846, 2012.

[15] R. Oughtred, A. Chatr-aryamontri, B. J. Breitkreutz et al., "Use of the BioGRID database for analysis of yeast protein and genetic interactions," *Cold Spring Harbor Protocols*, vol. 2016, no. 1, 2016.

[16] L. Licata, L. Briganti, D. Peluso et al., "MINT, the molecular interaction database: 2012 update," *Nucleic Acids Research*, vol. 40, no. D1, pp. D857–D861, 2012.

[17] D. S. Wishart, C. Knox, A. C. Guo et al., "DrugBank: a comprehensive resource for in silico drug discovery and exploration," *Nucleic Acids Research*, vol. 34, no. 90001, pp. D668–D672, 2006.

[18] A. Pujol, R. Mosca, J. Farrés, and P. Aloy, "Unveiling the role of network and systems biology in drug discovery," *Trends in Pharmacological Sciences*, vol. 31, no. 3, pp. 115–123, 2010.

[19] T. Taverner, Y. V. Karpievitch, A. D. Polpitiya et al., "DanteR: an extensible R-based tool for quantitative analysis of -omics data," *Bioinformatics*, vol. 28, no. 18, pp. 2404–2406, 2012.

[20] J. A. Vizcaíno, A. Csordas, N. del-Toro et al., "2016 update of the PRIDE database and its related tools," *Nucleic Acids Research*, vol. 44, no. D1, pp. D447–D456, 2016.

[21] M. Gómez-Serrano, E. Camafeita, E. García-Santos et al., "Proteome-wide alterations on adipose tissue from obese patients as age-, diabetes- and gender-specific hallmarks," *Scientific Reports*, vol. 6, no. 1, article 25756, 2016.

[22] C. M. Bishop, *Pattern Recognition and Machine Learning*, Springer, New York, NY, USA, 2006.

[23] R. J. Macisaac and G. Jerums, "Diabetic kidney disease with and without albuminuria," *Current Opinion in Nephrology and Hypertension*, vol. 20, no. 3, pp. 246–257, 2011.

[24] K. Rossing, H. Mischak, M. Dakna et al., "Urinary proteomics in diabetes and CKD," *Journal of the American Society of Nephrology*, vol. 19, no. 7, pp. 1283–1290, 2008.

[25] A. Alkhalaf, P. Zürbig, S. J. L. Bakker et al., "Multicentric validation of proteomic biomarkers in urine specific for diabetic nephropathy," *PLoS One*, vol. 5, no. 10, article e13421, 2010.

[26] S. Singh, T. Wu, C. Xie et al., "Urine VCAM-1 as a marker of renal pathology activity index in lupus nephritis," *Arthritis Research & Therapy*, vol. 14, no. 4, article R164, 2012.

[27] A. F. Rubio-Guerra, H. Vargas-Robles, J. J. Lozano Nuevo, and B. A. Escalante-Acosta, "Correlation between circulating adhesion molecule levels and albuminuria in type-2 diabetic hypertensive patients," *Kidney & Blood Pressure Research*, vol. 32, no. 2, pp. 106–109, 2009.

[28] A. F. Rubio-Guerra, L. J. Cabrera-Miranda, H. Vargas-Robles, A. Maceda-Serrano, J. J. Lozano-Nuevo, and B. A. Escalante-Acosta, "Correlation between levels of circulating adipokines and adiponectin/resistin index with carotid intima-media thickness in hypertensive type 2 diabetic patients," *Cardiology*, vol. 125, no. 3, pp. 150–153, 2013.

[29] D. Seron, J. S. Cameron, and D. O. Haskard, "Expression of VCAM-1 in the normal and diseased kidney," *Nephrology Dialysis Transplantation*, vol. 6, no. 12, pp. 917–922, 1991.

[30] O. Soehnlein, A. Schmeisser, I. Cicha et al., "ACE inhibition lowers angiotensin-II-induced monocyte adhesion to HUVEC by reduction of p65 translocation and AT1 expression," *Journal of Vascular Research*, vol. 42, no. 5, pp. 399–407, 2005.

[31] B. Fernandez-Fernandez, A. Ortiz, C. Gomez-Guerrero, and J. Egido, "Therapeutic approaches to diabetic nephropathy—beyond the RAS," *Nature Reviews Nephrology*, vol. 10, no. 6, pp. 325–346, 2014.

[32] R. Aviv, K. Gurbanov, A. Hoffman, S. Blumberg, and J. Winaver, "Urinary neutral endopeptidase 24.11 activity: modulation by chronic salt loading," *Kidney International*, vol. 47, no. 3, pp. 855–860, 1995.

[33] O. Domenig, A. Manzel, N. Grobe et al., "8D.05: the role of neprilysin in angiotensin 1-7 formation in the kidney," *Journal of Hypertension*, vol. 33, Supplement 1, pp. e114–e115, 2015.

[34] B. M. Westwood and M. C. Chappell, "Divergent pathways for the angiotensin-(1–12) metabolism in the rat circulation and kidney," *Peptides*, vol. 35, no. 2, pp. 190–195, 2012.

[35] P. Judge, R. Haynes, M. J. Landray, and C. Baigent, "Neprilysin inhibition in chronic kidney disease," *Nephrology Dialysis Transplantation*, vol. 30, no. 5, pp. 738–743, 2015.

[36] B. J. Davis, C. I. Johnston, L. M. Burrell et al., "Renoprotective effects of vasopeptidase inhibition in an experimental model of diabetic nephropathy," *Diabetologia*, vol. 46, no. 7, pp. 961–971, 2003.

[37] Z. Cao, L. M. Burrell, I. Tikkanen, F. Bonnet, M. E. Cooper, and R. E. Gilbert, "Vasopeptidase inhibition attenuates the progression of renal injury in subtotal nephrectomized rats," *Kidney International*, vol. 60, no. 2, pp. 715–721, 2001.

[38] M. W. Taal, V. D. Nenov, W. Wong et al., "Vasopeptidase inhibition affords greater renoprotection than angiotensin-converting enzyme inhibition alone," *Journal of the American Society of Nephrology*, vol. 12, no. 10, pp. 2051–2059, 2001.

[39] UK HARP-III Collaborative Group, "Randomized multicentre pilot study of sacubitril/valsartan versus irbesartan in patients with chronic kidney disease: United Kingdom Heart and Renal Protection (HARP)- III—rationale, trial design and baseline data," *Nephrology Dialysis Transplantation*, vol. 32, no. 12, pp. 2043–2051, 2016.

[40] J. B. Su, "Different cross-talk sites between the renin–angiotensin and the kallikrein–kinin systems," *Journal of the Renin-Angiotensin-Aldosterone System*, vol. 15, no. 4, pp. 319–328, 2014.

[41] S. B. Nicholas, J. Liu, J. Kim et al., "Critical role for osteopontin in diabetic nephropathy," *Kidney International*, vol. 77, no. 7, pp. 588–600, 2010.

[42] H. Yamaguchi, M. Igarashi, A. Hirata et al., "Progression of diabetic nephropathy enhances the plasma osteopontin level in type 2 diabetic patients," *Endocrine Journal*, vol. 51, no. 5, pp. 499–504, 2004.

[43] A. L. Al-Malki, "Assessment of urinary osteopontin in association with podocyte for early predication of nephropathy in diabetic patients," *Disease Markers*, vol. 2014, Article ID 493736, 5 pages, 2014.

[44] J. Lorenzen, R. Shah, A. Biser et al., "The role of osteopontin in the development of albuminuria," *Journal of the American Society of Nephrology*, vol. 19, no. 5, pp. 884–890, 2008.

[45] Z. Xie, D. R. Pimental, S. Lohan et al., "Regulation of angiotensin II-stimulated osteopontin expression in cardiac microvascular endothelial cells: role of p42/44 mitogen-activated protein kinase and reactive oxygen species," *Journal of Cellular Physiology*, vol. 188, no. 1, pp. 132–138, 2001.

[46] C. M. Giachelli, R. Pichler, D. Lombardi et al., "Osteopontin expression in angiotensin II-induced tubulointerstitial nephritis," *Kidney International*, vol. 45, no. 2, pp. 515–524, 1994.

[47] J. van den Born, A. A. van Kraats, M. A. H. Bakker et al., "Selective proteinuria in diabetic nephropathy in the rat is associated with a relative decrease in glomerular basement membrane heparan sulphate," *Diabetologia*, vol. 38, no. 2, pp. 161–172, 1995.

[48] I. S. Park, H. Kiyomoto, S. L. Abboud, and H. E. Abboud, "Expression of transforming growth factor-β and type IV collagen in early streptozotocin-induced diabetes," *Diabetes*, vol. 46, no. 3, pp. 473–480, 1997.

[49] D. Koya, M. Haneda, H. Nakagawa et al., "Amelioration of accelerated diabetic mesangial expansion by treatment with a PKC β inhibitor in diabetic db/db mice, a rodent model for type 2 diabetes," *The FASEB Journal*, vol. 14, no. 3, pp. 439–447, 2000.

[50] F. N. Ziyadeh, B. B. Hoffman, D. C. Han et al., "Long-term prevention of renal insufficiency, excess matrix gene

expression, and glomerular mesangial matrix expansion by treatment with monoclonal antitransforming growth factor-β antibody in *db/db* diabetic mice," *Proceedings of the National Academy of Sciences of the United States of America*, vol. 97, no. 14, pp. 8015–8020, 2000.

[51] D. Yavuz, N. Aksoy, Y. Taga, and S. Akalin, "P-385: effects of enalapril and losartan on urinary fibronectin excretion in hypertensive type 2 diabetic patients," *American Journal of Hypertension*, vol. 15, no. S3, article 170A, 2002.

[52] V. Woo, L. S. Ni, D. Hak et al., "Effects of losartan on urinary secretion of extracellular matrix and their modulators in type 2 diabetes mellitus patients with microalbuminuria," *Clinical and Investigative Medicine*, vol. 29, no. 6, pp. 365–372, 2006.

[53] J. F. Navarro-González, C. Mora-Fernández, M. M. de Fuentes, and J. García-Pérez, "Inflammatory molecules and pathways in the pathogenesis of diabetic nephropathy," *Nature Reviews Nephrology*, vol. 7, no. 6, pp. 327–340, 2011.

[54] S. S. Roscioni, H. J. L. Heerspink, and D. de Zeeuw, "The effect of RAAS blockade on the progression of diabetic nephropathy," *Nature Reviews Nephrology*, vol. 10, no. 2, pp. 77–87, 2014.

[55] S. Anderson and R. Komers, "Inhibition of the renin–angiotensin system: is more better?," *Kidney International*, vol. 75, no. 1, pp. 12–14, 2009.

[56] C. Zoja, D. Corna, E. Gagliardini et al., "Adding a statin to a combination of ACE inhibitor and ARB normalizes proteinuria in experimental diabetes, which translates into full renoprotection," *American Journal of Physiology-Renal Physiology*, vol. 299, no. 5, pp. F1203–F1211, 2010.

[57] H. H. Parving, B. Oxenbøll, P. A. Svendsen, J. S. Christiansen, and A. R. Andersen, "Early detection of patients at risk of developing diabetic nephropathy. A longitudinal study of urinary albumin excretion," *Acta Endocrinologica*, vol. 100, no. 4, pp. 550–555, 1982.

[58] C. E. Mogensen, "Microalbuminuria predicts clinical proteinuria and early mortality in maturity-onset diabetes," *The New England Journal of Medicine*, vol. 310, no. 6, pp. 356–360, 1984.

16

Glycyrrhizic Acid Prevents Diabetic Nephropathy by Activating AMPK/SIRT1/PGC-1α Signaling in db/db Mice

Shaozhang Hou,[1,2] Ting Zhang,[1,2] Yuan Li,[3] Fengying Guo,[1,2] and Xiu Jin[4]

[1]*Department of Pathology, School of Basic Medical Sciences, Ningxia Medical University, Yinchuan 750004, China*
[2]*Institute of Basic Medical Sciences, Ningxia Medical University, Yinchuan 750004, China*
[3]*Department of Nursing, Ningxia Medical University, Yinchuan 750004, China*
[4]*Affiliated Hospital of Jining Medical College, Jining 272000, China*

Correspondence should be addressed to Shaozhang Hou; szhou8@163.com

Academic Editor: Steven F. Abcouwer

Diabetic nephropathy (DN) is a major cause of end-stage renal disease (ESRD). Glycyrrhizic acid (GA) is an effective inhibitor of reactive oxygen species (ROS) production. We investigated the role of GA in the progression of renal injury in DN. Albumin (Alb)/creatinine (crea) levels were significantly lower, and renal histopathology was attenuated in the diabetic db/db mice that were treated with GA (15 mg/kg via intraperitoneal injection) once per day for eight weeks. These changes were associated with significantly lower levels of α-smooth muscle actin (α-SMA) and transforming growth factor β1 (TGF-β1) expression. Additionally, diabetic db/db mice displayed more terminal deoxynucleotidyl transferase-mediated nick-end labeling- (TUNEL-) positive nuclei and diabetes-induced ROS production in the kidneys, and these effects were attenuated by the treatment with GA, which activated adenosine monophosphate-activated protein kinase (AMPK)/silent information regulator 1 (SIRT1)/peroxisome proliferator-activated receptor-γ coactivator-1α (PGC-1α) signaling in the kidneys. In summary, in diabetic db/db mice, the effect of GA on DN involved, in part, the inhibition of ROS and the activation of AMPK/SIRT1/PGC-1α signaling in the kidneys. GA, therefore, shows therapeutic potential for preventing and treating DN.

1. Introduction

Diabetic nephropathy (DN) is a major cause of end-stage renal disease (ESRD) and one of the most severe microvascular complications of both type 1 and type 2 diabetes [1–4]. In diabetic patients, the pathogenesis and progression of chronic kidney disease (CKD) involve numerous factors, such as hyperglycemia-induced oxidative stress and inflammation. Hemodynamic changes and disorders of glucose metabolism can be caused by genetic factors, hyperglycemia, or changes in cytokine levels and can result in the development of DN [2, 5, 6]. Although chronic exposure to elevated glucose levels is a major cause of kidney disease, the mechanisms that lead to the development and progression of kidney injury in these patients remain unclear [7, 8]. It is therefore important to explore new approaches aimed at preventing and treating DN.

Glycyrrhizic acid (GA) is a triterpenoid saponin glycoside that is known as the most efficacious component of the licorice plant [9, 10]. Previous studies have shown that GA exhibits antiulcerative, expectorant, antiviral, anti-inflammatory, antidiabetic, anticancer, neuroprotective, and immune-enhancing properties [11, 12]. Additionally, GA has been shown to alleviate benzopyrene-induced lung injury [13], to exert a therapeutic effect on asthma by regulating immune functions [14], and to prevent renal ischemia-reperfusion injury in rabbits [15]. Furthermore, it is widely accepted that the effects of GA are mediated by both SIRT1 and AMPK [16]. However, the role that GA plays in the kidneys of type 2 diabetic animals has not been explored.

In this study, we investigated the protective effect exerted by GA against oxidative stress and found that GA activates AMPK/SIRT1/PGC-1α signaling in diabetic db/db mice. These results increase our understanding of the mechanisms underlying DN. Furthermore, these data suggest targets for the search for a potential therapy for DN.

2. Materials and Methods

2.1. Materials. GA was obtained from Tokyo Chemical Industry Co. (TCI, Tokyo, Japan). A reactive oxygen species assay kit was purchased from Beyotime (Jiangsu, China). AMPKα, p-AMPKα, SIRT1, PGC-1α, TGF-β1, and α-SMA antibodies were purchased from Abcam. β-actin was purchased from Bios (Beijing, China).

2.2. Animals and Grouping. Male db/db (BKS.Cg-m+ $Lepr^{db}$/+ $Lepr^{db}$/Jcl) and db/m (BKS.Cg-m +/+Lepr db/Jcl) mice were purchased from Mode Animal Research Center of Nanjing University. The mice were maintained in a specific pathogen-free colony in the Laboratory Animal Center of Ningxia Medical University (Yinchuan, China) in facilities with controlled temperature and humidity, and 12 : 12 hour light and dark cycle. The body weight and fasting blood glucose level were monitored weekly. The study was conducted in accordance with the "Guide for the Care and Use of Laboratory Animals" and approved by the Institutional Animal Care and Use Committee of Ningxia Medical University.

Eight-week-old male mice were divided into the following five different groups, which received either 0.9% sodium chloride (NaCl) or GA: db (db/db mice treated with NaCl, $n = 10$), db + g (db/db mice treated with GA, $n = 10$), m (db/m mice treated with NaCl, $n = 10$), m + g (db/m mice treated with GA, $n = 10$), and n (normal group, C57BL/6 mice treated with NaCl, $n = 10$. C57BL/6 mice is a common inbred strain of laboratory mouse). The groups administered with GA received a dose of 15 mg/kg via an intraperitoneal (i.p.) injection once per day for eight weeks starting when the mice were eight weeks old. The db, m, and n group mice were administered (i.p.) with 0.9% sodium chloride at the same time points. The mice were euthanized to remove the kidneys. The kidneys were rapidly fixed in normal-buffered 4% paraformaldehyde for immunohistochemical analyses, and all experiments were performed using renal cortex samples. Blood was collected from the left ventricle, and plasma was stored at −80°C.

2.3. Histological Analysis. Paraformaldehyde-fixed and paraffin-embedded renal tissues were sectioned (4 μm thickness) and stained with hematoxylin and eosin (HE) and periodic acid-Schiff (PAS). For the electron microscopic studies, tissue sections were dehydrated through an ascending series of ethanol (to 100%) and then washed in dry acetone and embedded in epoxy resin. After the sections were fixed, dehydrated, embedded, and sliced, they were stained with uranyl acetate. Ultrathin sections were counterstained with lead citrate and then examined using transmission electron microscopy (H7650).

2.4. Immunohistochemistry Assay. The protein levels of AMPKα, p-AMPKα, SIRT1, PGC-1α, TGF-β1, and α-SMA (1 : 200, Abcam, USA) were determined in each group by incubating the samples in primary antibodies overnight followed by incubation with secondary antibodies and IHC detection reagent (ZSGB-BIO, Beijing, China) at 37°C for 45 min. The results were detected using DAB (ZSGB-BIO, Beijing, China), and hematoxylin staining was used to label the nuclei. The cells were observed and photographed using an optical microscope (BX61). The number of positively stained cells was counted in five microscopic fields at 400x.

2.5. Western Blot Analysis. Protein was isolated from tissues, and the concentration of proteins in each sample was determined to ensure that the sample volumes were consistent. Equal amounts (50 μg) of protein extracts were subjected to 10%–15% sodium dodecyl sulfate-polyacrylamide gel electrophoresis (SDS-PAGE) and then transferred to polyvinylidene fluoride membranes (Millipore). The membranes were incubated overnight at 4°C with the following primary antibodies: anti-AMPKα (1 : 1000), anti-p-AMPKα (1 : 1000), anti-SIRT1 (1 : 1000), anti-PGC-1α (1 : 1000), anti-TGF-β1 (1 : 2000), anti-α-SMA (1 : 2000), and anti-β-actin (1 : 3000). The membranes were then incubated with horseradish peroxidase-conjugated secondary antibodies for 60 min at room temperature. Imaging was performed using a Bio-Rad imaging system with chemiluminescence detection reagents. The densitometry of the bands was assessed using Image-Pro Plus 6.0 software.

2.6. ROS Detection. Frozen renal cortex sections were cultured and incubated in the dark with 10 μm/L of dihydroethidium (DHE) for 30 min at 37°C. Intracellular ROS production was assessed using an Olympus FluoView1000 confocal laser scanning microscope (using Ex/Em $\lambda = 480$ nm/535 nm for DHE).

2.7. TUNEL Staining. Terminal deoxynucleotidyl transferase-mediated dUTP nick-end labeling (TUNEL) staining was used to detect apoptosis. Apoptotic cells were examined using a TdT DNA fragmentation detection kit (Roche, Mannheim, Germany) according to the manufacturer's protocol. The percentage of apoptotic cells was calculated as the ratio of the number of TUNEL-positive cells to the total number of cells.

2.8. Statistical Analysis. All quantitative data are expressed as mean ± SD. Differences between the two experimental conditions were assessed using Tukey's test. The statistical significance of these differences was analyzed using one-way ANOVA, and a value of $p < 0.05$ was considered statistically significant.

3. Results

3.1. Effect of GA on the Onset of DN in db/db Mice. Blood glucose levels, body weight, and food intake were significantly higher in db/db mice than in the other groups. Treatment with GA did not significantly alter blood glucose levels, body weight, or food intake in db/db mice. Alb/crea levels were significantly higher in the db group than in the other groups, and treatment with GA for 8 weeks significantly decreased Alb/crea levels in the db + g group but not in the db group (Figure 1).

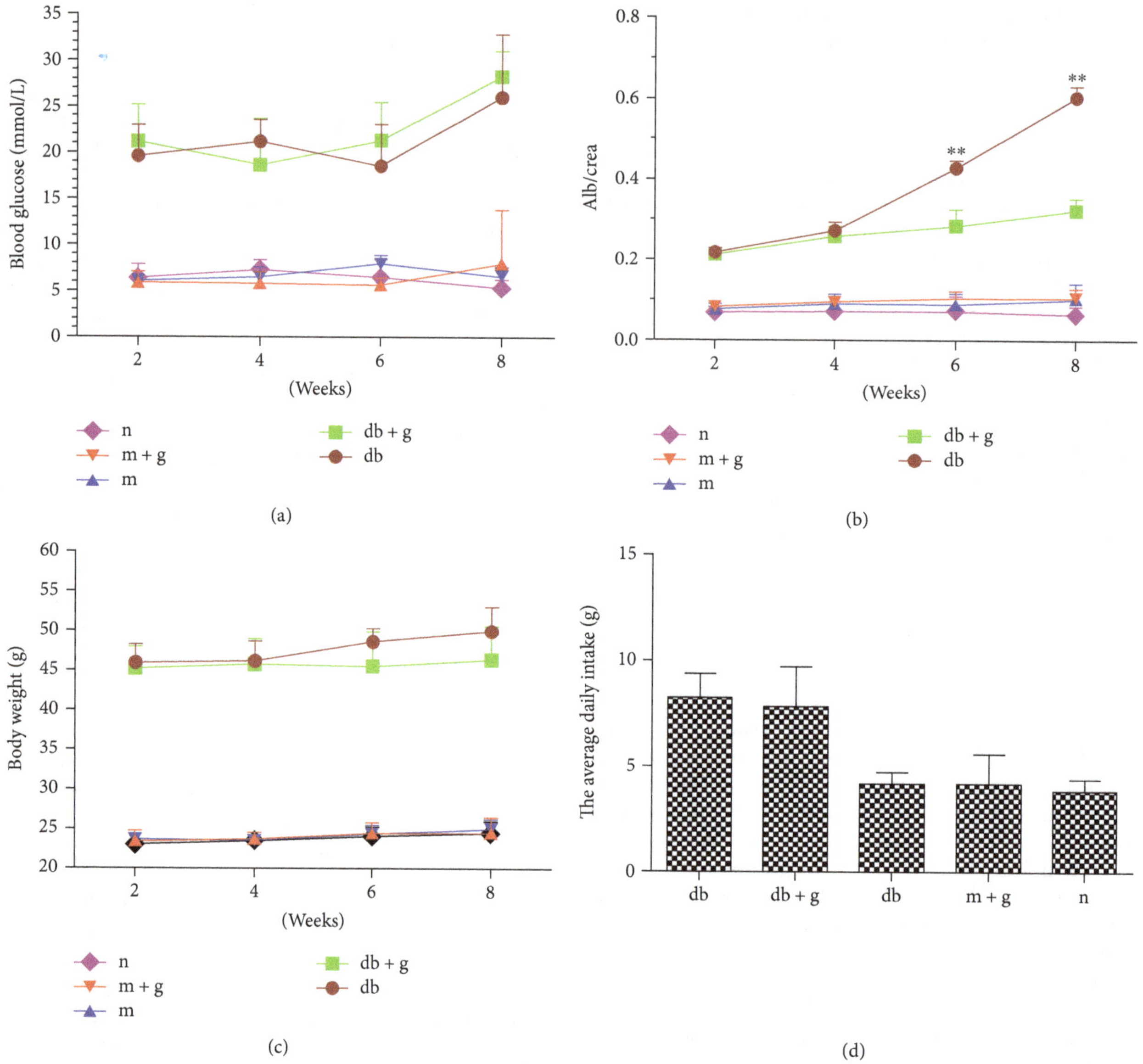

FIGURE 1: Effect of GA on the onset of DN in db/db mice. Treatment with GA did not significantly alter blood glucose levels (a), body weight (c), or food intake (d) in db/db mice. Alb/crea levels were significantly lower in the db + g group than in the db group ($^{**}p < 0.05$ versus db + g).

3.2. Histopathological Findings in db/db Mice Treated with GA. Mesangial expansion is a characteristic finding in diabetic glomerulopathy (Figure 2). HE staining revealed that the glomerular structure was normal, and there was no clear difference in proliferation in glomerular mesangial cells between the db and normal control group mice. Mesangial expansion, glomerular hypertrophy, and mesangial matrix gathering were clearly observed in the db/db mice, and these symptoms were substantially ameliorated by treatment with GA. The mesangial area was determined using PAS staining and found to be higher in the db/db mice than in the db/m and wild-type mice. Electron microscopy revealed the capillary ultrastructure of the glomerulus. Electron micrographs confirmed that in the db/db mice, mesangial volume was higher, glomeruli were irregularly thickened, and the basement membranes exhibited splitting. Treatment with GA produced clear changes. For example, basement membrane thickness was significantly decreased. Masson staining was used to dye collagen fibers blue, and the db/db group mice exhibited heavier renal fibrosis than that observed in the db + g group mice. We found that collagen fibers had significantly accumulated in the db/db group. Consistent with the changes observed in the glomerulus, treatment with GA markedly reduced the increase in collagen deposition that was observed in the renal interstitium in the db/db mice (assayed using Masson staining as shown in Figures 2(b) and 2(c)). These results indicate that treatment with GA may attenuate diabetic renal interstitial fibrosis *in vivo*.

3.3. GA Reduces Apoptosis in Renal Cells in db/db Mice. To assess cellular apoptosis in diabetic kidneys, renal tissue sections were submitted to a TUNEL assay. In 8-week-old mice, there were more apoptotic cells in the diabetic db/db mice than in the db/m mice. There were fewer apoptotic cells

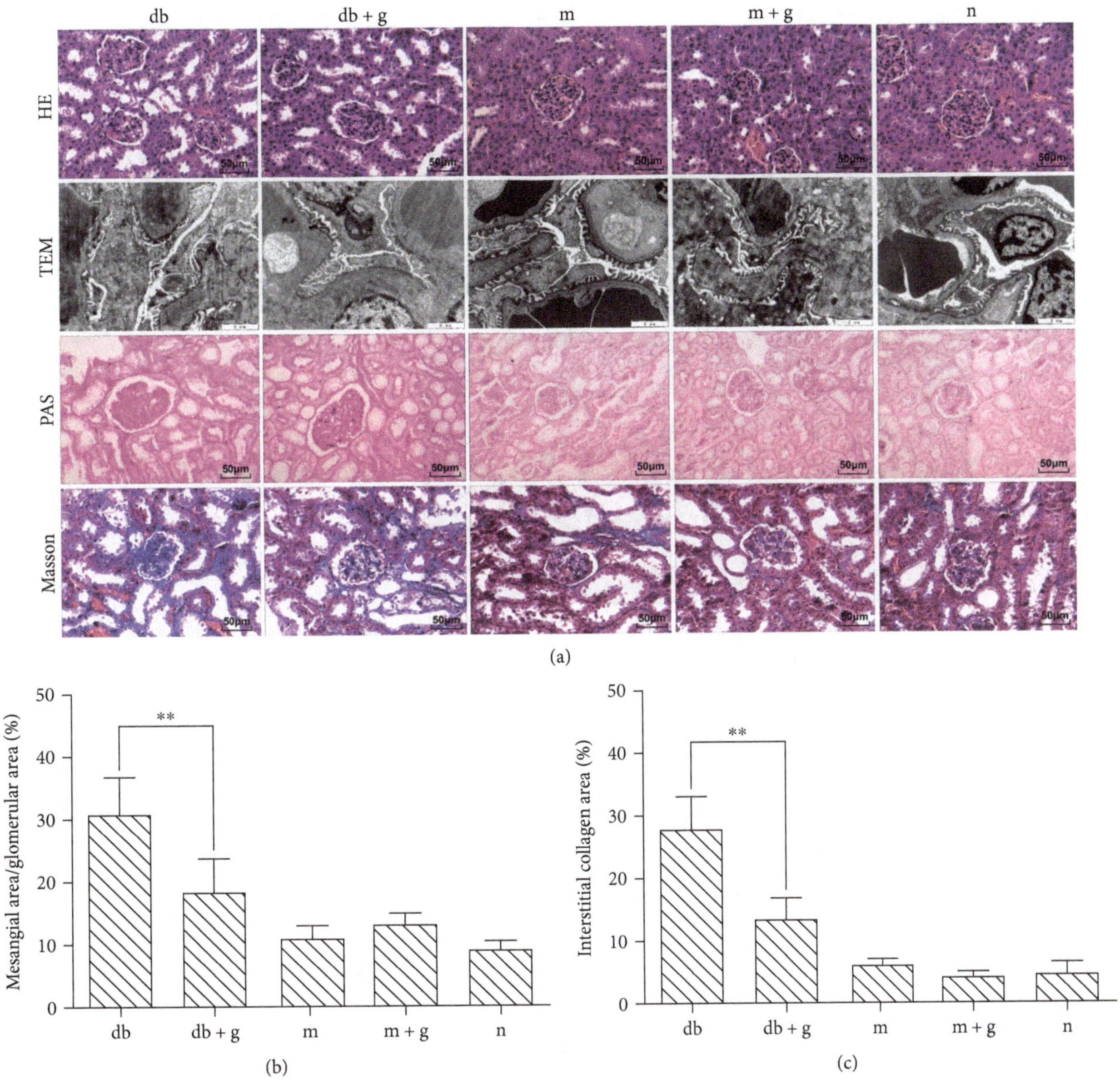

FIGURE 2: Effect of GA on kidney pathology in db/db mice. Representative sections obtained from the kidneys of mice (8 weeks old) in each group were stained with (a) HE ×400, electron microscopy (TEM) ×2000, and PAS ×400, Masson staining (blue) ×400. (b) Quantitative estimates of the mesangial fractional area (%). (c) Quantitative assessment of the interstitial collagen area (%). Values are shown as means ± SD. $^{**}p < 0.01$.

in the db/db mice treated with GA than in the corresponding db group (Figure 3). These data demonstrate that treatment with GA attenuates diabetes-induced apoptosis in type 2 diabetic kidneys.

3.4. Effect of GA on the Expression of α-SMA and TGF-β1 in db/db Mice. α-SMA and TGF-β1 have been shown to stimulate proliferation in mesangial cells and increase the synthesis of extracellular matrix (ECM), and both have been identified as key mediators of glomerular and tubulointerstitial pathologies in chronic renal diseases. Immunohistochemical and western blot analyses showed that DN increased α-SMA and TGF-β1 expression (Figure 4), and both were expressed at significantly lower levels in the db + g and db control groups ($p < 0.05$).

3.5. Effects of GA on Diabetes-Induced ROS Production in the Kidneys of db/db Mice. ROS production was measured using a DHE probe that detects superoxide. As shown in Figure 5(a), DN significantly enhanced the production of ROS in db/db mice, and pretreatment with GA prevented this DN-induced increase in ROS ($p < 0.05$). Thus, the levels of ROS were the same in the normal group, the m group, and the m + g group ($p > 0.05$). In this study, the DN-induced production of ROS was augmented in the db group but decreased in the db + g group. These data indicate that

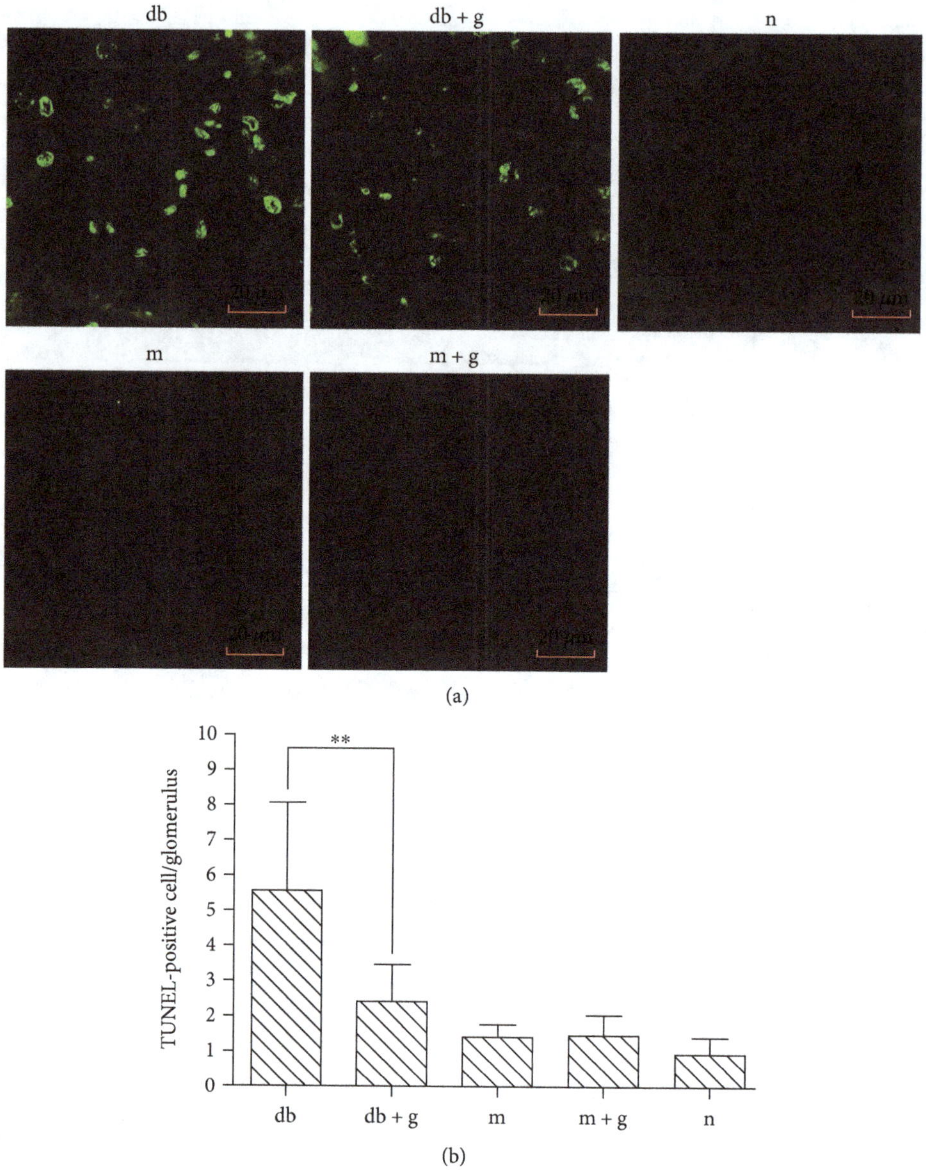

FIGURE 3: Effect of GA on apoptosis of cells in the renal cortex of db/db mice. Representative micrographs of TUNEL staining in the renal cortex (a). The same data are shown as a graph (b). The graph shows the number of TUNEL-positive cells that were detected in the glomerulus. Original magnification, ×400. $^{**}p < 0.001$ compared with the control group.

the administration of GA either impaired the generation of ROS or increased the capacity of the cell to perform endogenous ROS scavenging/antioxidant activities.

3.6. Effect of GA on p-AMPKα, SIRT1, and PGC-1α Expression in db/db Mice. In this study, we used immunohistochemistry and western blot analyses to assess the effect of GA on p-AMPKα, SIRT1, and PGC-1α protein expression levels (Figure 6). GA administration caused the expression of p-AMPKα, SIRT1, and PGC-1α to be higher in the db + g group than in the db group ($p < 0.05$). These results indicate that AMPK/SIRT1/PGC-1α signaling is induced in the kidneys of db/db mice and that GA effectively prevents DN by activating AMPK/SIRT1/PGC-1α signaling in db/db mice.

4. Discussion

In this study, we provide new information regarding the role of GA as a treatment for DN. GA has been reported to perform a variety of biological and pharmacological activities, but the mechanism by which GA alleviates DN is not fully understood and requires further study [1]. Data presented in our previous studies demonstrate that GA exerts a protective effect against DN in high-glucose-stimulated HBZY-1 cells and db/db mice [17]. In this study, we further explored the molecular mechanisms underlying the protective effects that GA exerts against DN-induced oxidative stress damage.

Pharmacologically targeting transcriptional networks to regulate or modulate gene expression programs that favor energy expenditure is an attractive option for studies aimed

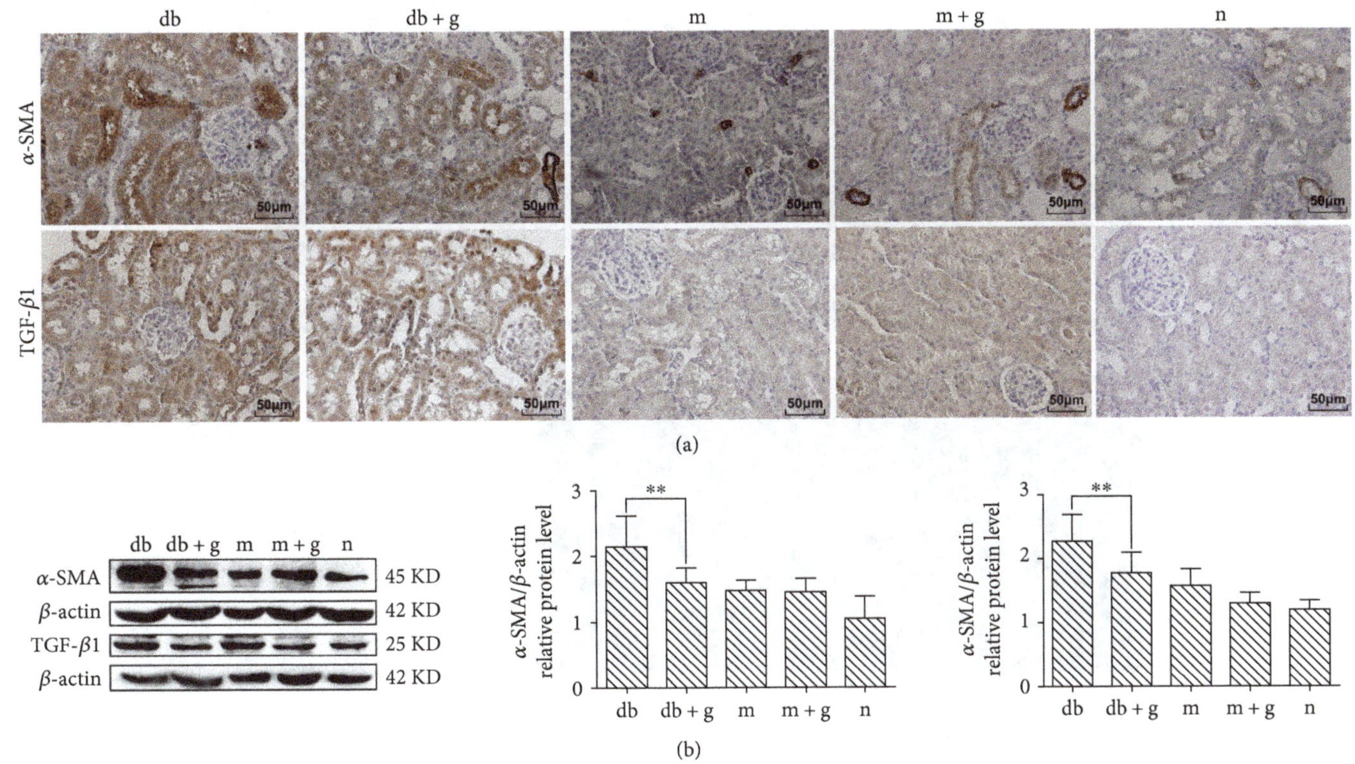

Figure 4: Effect of GA on the expression of α-SMA and TGF-β1 in the renal cortex of db/db mice. (a) Immunohistochemistry was used to detect the expression of α-SMA and TGF-β1. Original magnification: ×400. (b) Western blot assays were used to detect α-SMA and TGF-β1 in mice treated with GA. The proportion of cells with positive protein expression is shown. Histograms indicate the mean ± SD ($^{**}p < 0.05$). β-actin was detected to confirm equal loading. The gray graph indicates the relative level of protein expression in each group.

at combating metabolic diseases, particularly those that lead to diabetic complications [18]. Because AMPK, SIRT1, and PGC-1α are involved in catabolism, mitochondrial activation, angiogenesis, and enhanced cell survival, they are important targets of interest [19–22].

However, the effects of GA on the kidneys of animal models of type 2 diabetes are not well understood. We therefore chose db/db mice as a model of type 2 DM. In this study, db/m mice were used as the control group. The experimental groups were treated with 15 mg/kg of GA, and the results showed that GA had no obvious effect on the blood glucose levels, body weight, and food intake in db/db mice. In contrast, Wang et al. [23] found that GA decreased blood glucose levels. This difference is potentially due to differences in the animal models and treatment methods used in these studies. In the Wang et al. study, male BALB/cA mice were used to build a model of diabetic nephropathy, and GA was administered to diabetic mice by mixing it with a powder diet. This disparity requires further investigation. However, GA clearly reduced Alb/crea levels in the mice in this study, and we therefore speculated that GA may alleviate renal injury caused by DN in the kidneys of db/db mice. HE and PAS staining and electron microscopy showed that after treatment with GA, the kidney damage observed in the db/db mice was significantly reduced, and the glomerular structure tended to be normal, consistent with the results reported in previous studies. In this study, we show that in db/db mice, DN is associated with an increase in the accumulation of renal lipids, apoptotic renal cell injury, and oxidative stress, all of which are related to the inactivation of AMPK/SIRT1/PGC-1α signaling. DN was ameliorated by treatment with GA, which activates AMPK/SIRT1/PGC-1α signaling.

In recent years, studies of pathological cases have shown that renal cells can express renal tissue fibrosis and that the transdifferentiation of muscle fibroblasts in the renal tissue may indirectly react to the degree of renal tissue fibrosis [24]. α-SMA is expressed in muscle fibroblasts, and mature renal cells are located only in the middle of the vessel wall. Presumably, GA inhibits α-SMA expression and thereby plays a role in slowing renal fibrosis. In addition, early diabetic glomerular and tubular hypertrophy play important roles in this process [25]. In our experiments, TGF-β1 protein levels were significantly higher in db/db mice than in mice in the other groups. This finding suggests that the cell hypertrophy observed in the db group was related to the high expression level of TGF-β1, which can block ECM degradation [26, 27]. Matrix metalloproteinases (MMPs) are enzymes that play key roles in substrate degradation. TGF-β1 inhibits the synthesis of MMP and the activation of fibrinolytic enzymes [28]. Additionally, it stimulates cell receptors and the ECM to trigger cells and induce interactions between the cells and the matrix, further exacerbating the accumulation of the ECM [29, 30]. In the present study, we verified these results in mice. In the experimental db/db group, α-SMA and TGF-β1 was present at higher levels than those observed in the normal group, and their expression

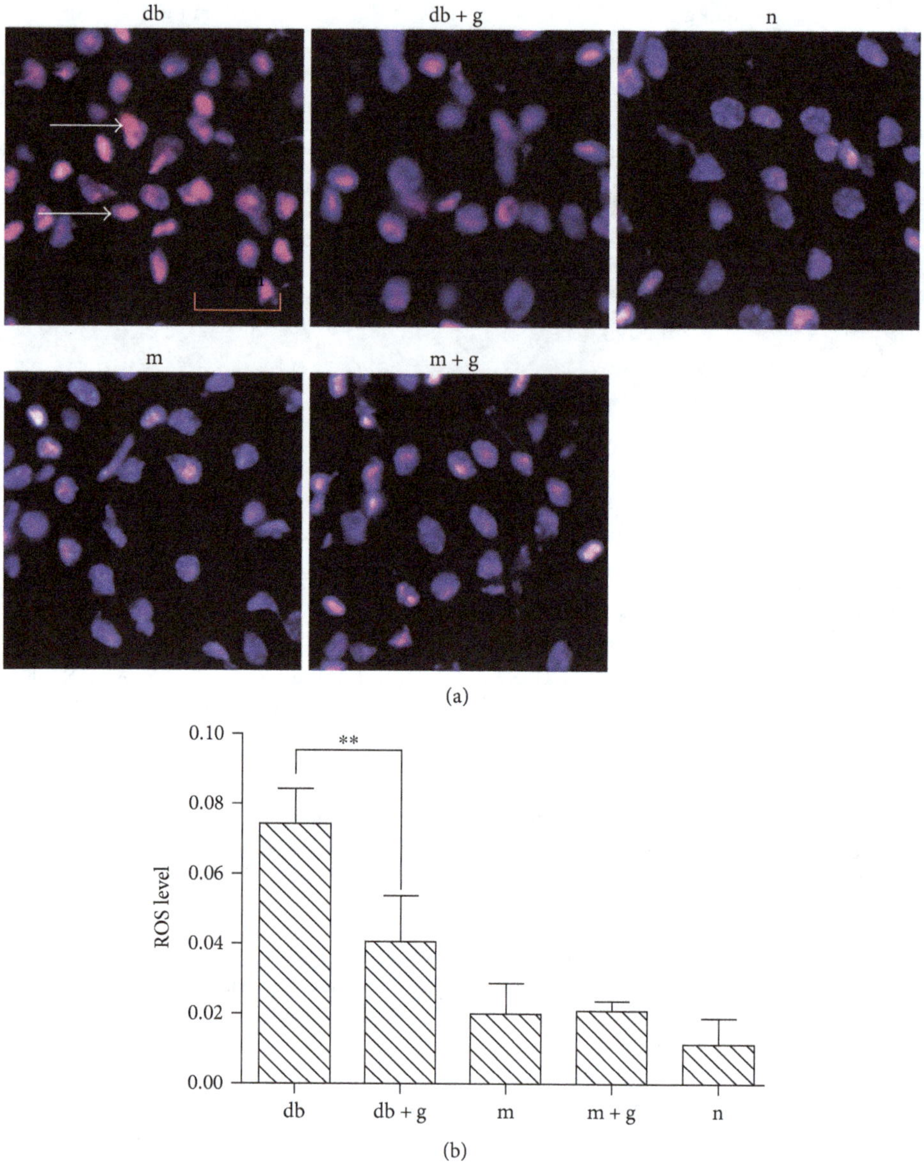

FIGURE 5: Effect of GA on ROS levels in the kidneys of db/db mice. The bar graph demonstrates the increases in ROS production observed in the renal cortex of db/db mice and the antioxidant effect of GA. The lower panels are representatives of the original recorded data. The data were collected from 3 independent experiments and are presented as means ± SD. $^{**}p < 0.05$ compared with the control. One-way ANOVA followed by Tukey's test.

was decreased after the addition of GA. Therefore, a method designed to prevent the expression of α-SMA and TGF-β1 might produce a protective effect against DN.

ROS can be generated during glucose metabolism in the mitochondria (via the electron transport chain (ETC) activity) and the plasma membrane (via NADPH oxidase (NADPHox)). But ROS are mainly produced by the mitochondria, during both physiological and pathological conditions [31]. The main antioxidant enzymes responsible for ROS removal are superoxide dismutase (SOD), glutathione reductase, glutathione peroxidase, and catalase. Evidence suggests that ROS are present in both db/db mice [32]. The importance of elevated ROS levels to the pathogenesis of microvascular complications in diabetes is well documented [33, 34]. Our results show that high glucose levels promote the generation of ROS and increase MDA and decrease SOD levels [17]. We further confirmed that high glucose levels induce ROS production, promote lipid peroxidation, and decrease antioxidant capacity. However, in the db + g group, ROS levels were decreased, and we observed that GA played an antioxidant role in these mice. A previous study showed that oxidative stress leads to lipid peroxidation as a result of the formation of harmful products by MDA [35]. In addition, the activities of antioxidant defense enzymes, which cause cellular damage, were decreased [36]. Finally, GA has been reported to play an antioxidant role in ameliorating carbon tetrachloride-induced liver injury [37].

It has been reported that AMPK/SIRT1/PGC-1α signaling is an important energy-sensing signaling pathway. It is important to note that AMPK and SIRT1 regulate each other

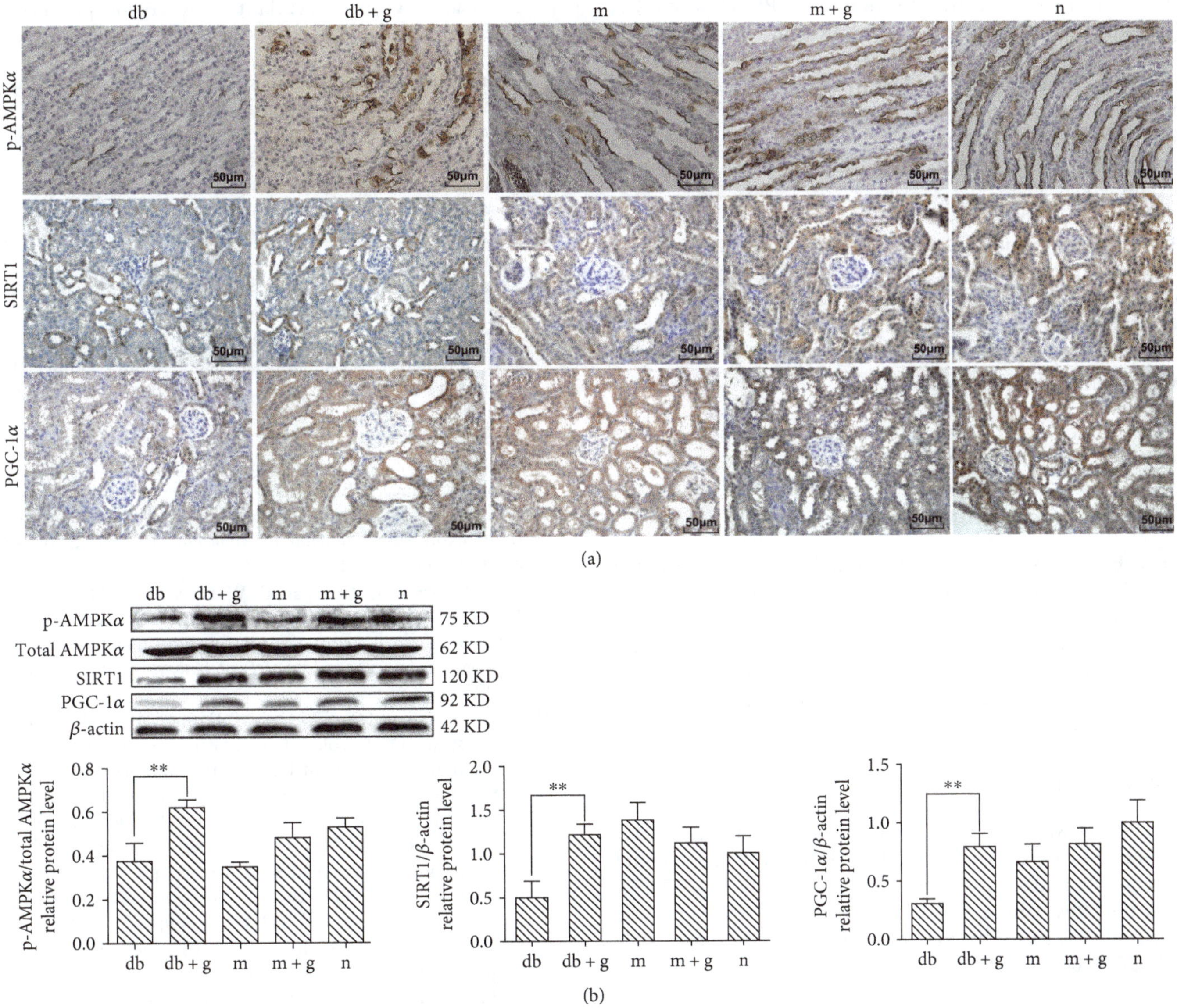

FIGURE 6: Effect of GA on p-AMPKα, SIRT1, and PGC-1α expression in the kidneys of db/db mice. (a) Immunohistochemistry was used to detect p-AMPKα, SIRT1, and PGC-1α in mice treated with GA. Original magnification: ×400. (b) Western blot analysis was used to detect specific proteins, and the proportion of cells with positive protein expression was determined. Histogram values represent the mean ± SD (**$p < 0.05$). β-actin was detected to confirm equal loading. The gray graphs show the relative protein levels in each group.

and share many common target molecules, including PGC-1α. Moreover, AMPK and SIRT1 are clinically relevant in metabolic syndrome and type 2 diabetes because their effects on target molecules lead to mitochondrial dysfunction and oxidative damage [38]. SIRT1 also responds to changes in the availability of nutrients via a forkhead-dependent pathway [39] and PGC-1α [40]. A high level of expression of PGC-1α can increase ATP levels and reduce the production of ROS. Previous studies have shown that overexpressed PGC-1α effectively suppressed ROS production and apoptosis caused by oxidative stress [41]. Thus, evidence has shown that activating AMPK and SIRT1 induces the concurrent deacetylation and phosphorylation of their target molecules and decreases susceptibility to diabetes-associated disorders. The present study suggests that the GA-mediated activation of AMPK, SIRT1, and PGC-1α may prevent both the accumulation of renal lipids and cell injury. This in vivo data demonstrates that the diabetes-induced suppression of AMPK/SIRT1/PGC-1α signaling is activated by GA. These results suggest that AMPK and SIRT1 activate each other and jointly regulate their downstream effector PGC-1α in mesangial cells [42, 43]. High glucose levels can prevent mesangial cells from transitioning from G1 to S phase, reduce the proportion of cells in G1 phase, increase the proportion of cells in S phase, and promote DNA synthesis and cell proliferation [44]. Consistent with our results, several recent studies have demonstrated that adiponectin [45] or AICAR [46] protect renal podocytes and decrease albuminuria in diabetic animals by decreasing oxidative stress and apoptosis via a mechanism involving the activation of AMPK. However, GA prevents DN by directly scavenging ROS and blocks glucose-lipid metabolism via AMPK/SIRT1-independent mechanisms [47]. The discrepancy between our results and those reported in previous studies regarding AMPK/SIRT1 signaling might reflect differences in the dose of GA that was administered and the part of the renal tissue that was examined.

Our data support the conclusion that the effect of GA on DN is associated, in part, with the inhibition of ROS and the activation of AMPK/SIRT1/PGC-1α signaling in the kidneys of diabetic db/db mice. GA therefore shows potential as a therapeutic target for preventing and treating DN.

Conflicts of Interest

The authors declare that there are no competing interests regarding the publication of this paper.

Authors' Contributions

Shaozhang Hou, Ting Zhang, and Yuan Li contributed equally as co-first authors of this work. Shaozhang Hou and Yuan Li designed the research; Ting Zhang and Xiu Jin performed the research; Ting Zhang contributed new reagents and analytic tools; Yuan Li and Fengying Guo analyzed the data; and Ting Zhang and Shaozhang Hou wrote the paper.

Acknowledgments

This study was supported by the National Natural Science Foundation of China (year 2012, 81160106), the Natural Science Foundation of Ningxia (year 2017, NZ17053), and the West China Top Class Discipline Project in Basic Medical Sciences, Ningxia Medical University (year 2017, 201-30181601).

References

[1] C. Mora-Fernández, V. Domínguez-Pimentel, M. M. de Fuentes, J. L. Górriz, A. Martínez-Castelao, and J. F. Navarro-González, "Diabetic kidney disease: from physiology to therapeutics," *The Journal of Physiology*, vol. 592, no. 18, pp. 3997–4012, 2014.

[2] L. L. Kong, H. Wu, W. P. Cui et al., "Advances in murine models of diabetic nephropathy," *Journal of Diabetes Research*, vol. 2013, Article ID 797548, 10 pages, 2013.

[3] L. Xu, B. Zhou, H. Li et al., "Serum levels of progranulin are closely associated with microvascular complication in type 2 diabetes," *Disease Markers*, vol. 2015, Article ID 357279, 9 pages, 2015.

[4] D. Schlöndorff, "Choosing the right mouse model for diabetic nephropathy," *Kidney International*, vol. 77, no. 9, pp. 749-750, 2010.

[5] M. Mauer, M. L. Caramori, P. Fioretto, and B. Najafian, "Glomerular structural-functional relationship models of diabetic nephropathy are robust in type 1 diabetic patients," *Nephrology, Dialysis, Transplantation*, vol. 30, no. 6, pp. 918–923, 2015.

[6] M. Kitada, Y. Ogura, T. Suzuki et al., "A very-low-protein diet ameliorates advanced diabetic nephropathy through autophagy induction by suppression of the mTORC1 pathway in Wistar fatty rats, an animal model of type 2 diabetes and obesity," *Diabetologia*, vol. 59, no. 6, pp. 1307–1317, 2016.

[7] R. Pothuraju, R. K. Sharma, J. Chagalamarri, S. Jangra, and P. Kumar Kavadi, "A systematic review of Gymnema sylvestre in obesity and diabetes management," *Journal of the Science of Food and Agriculture*, vol. 94, no. 5, pp. 834–840, 2014.

[8] C. Lo, M. Jun, S. V. Badve et al., "Glucose-lowering agents for treating pre-existing and new-onset diabetes in kidney transplant recipients," *The Cochrane Database of Systematic Reviews*, vol. 2, article CD009966, 2017.

[9] H. Zhao, M. Zhao, Y. Wang, F. Li, and Z. Zhang, "Glycyrrhizic acid attenuates sepsis-induced acute kidney injury by inhibiting NF-κB signaling pathway," *Evidence-Based Complementary and Alternative Medicine*, vol. 2016, Article ID 8219287, 11 pages, 2016.

[10] Y. Yao, L. Wang, P. Jin et al., "Methane alleviates carbon tetrachloride induced liver injury in mice: anti-inflammatory action demonstrated by increased PI3K/Akt/GSK-3β-mediated IL-10 expression," *Journal of Molecular Histology*, vol. 48, no. 4, pp. 301–310, 2017.

[11] J. M. Hendricks, C. Hoffman, D. W. Pascual, and M. E. Hardy, "18β-glycyrrhetinic acid delivered orally induces isolated lymphoid follicle maturation at the intestinal mucosa and attenuates rotavirus shedding," *PLoS One*, vol. 7, no. 11, article e49491, 2012.

[12] B. Schröfelbauer, J. Raffetseder, M. Hauner, A. Wolkerstorfer, W. Ernst, and O. H. Szolar, "Glycyrrhizin, the main active compound in liquorice, attenuates pro-inflammatory responses by interfering with membrane-dependent receptor signalling," *The Biochemical Journal*, vol. 421, no. 3, pp. 473–482, 2009.

[13] W. Qamar, R. Khan, A. Q. Khan et al., "Alleviation of lung injury by glycyrrhizic acid in benzo(a)pyrene exposed rats: probable role of soluble epoxide hydrolase and thioredoxin reductase," *Toxicology*, vol. 291, no. 1–3, pp. 25–31, 2012.

[14] M. U. Rehman, M. Tahir, A. Q. Khan et al., "Chrysin suppresses renal carcinogenesis via amelioration of hyperproliferation, oxidative stress and inflammation: plausible role of NF-κB," *Toxicology Letters*, vol. 216, no. 2-3, pp. 146–158, 2013.

[15] S. Subramanian, M. W. Bowyer, J. C. Egan, and T. J. Knolmayer, "Attenuation of renal ischemia-reperfusion injury with selectin inhibition in a rabbit model," *The American Journal of Surgery*, vol. 178, no. 6, pp. 573–576, 1999.

[16] H. Pang, T. Huang, J. Song, D. Li, Y. Zhao, and X. Ma, "Inhibiting HMGB1 with glycyrrhizic acid protects brain injury after DAI via its anti-inflammatory effect," *Mediators of Inflammation*, vol. 2016, Article ID 4569521, 9 pages, 2016.

[17] S. Hou, F. Zheng, Y. Li, L. Gao, and J. Zhang, "The protective effect of glycyrrhizic acid on renal tubular epithelial cell injury induced by high glucose," *International Journal of Molecular Sciences*, vol. 15, no. 9, pp. 15026–15043, 2014.

[18] W. Xin, X. Zhao, L. Liu et al., "Acetyl-CoA carboxylase 2 suppression rescues human proximal tubular cells from palmitic acid induced lipotoxicity via autophagy," *Biochemical and Biophysical Research Communications*, vol. 463, no. 3, pp. 364–369, 2015.

[19] N. Xia, S. Strand, F. Schlufter et al., "Role of SIRT1 and FOXO factors in eNOS transcriptional activation by resveratrol," *Nitric Oxide*, vol. 32, pp. 29–35, 2013.

[20] F. Yeung, J. E. Hoberg, C. S. Ramsey et al., "Modulation of NF-κB-dependent transcription and cell survival by the SIRT1 deacetylase," *The EMBO Journal*, vol. 23, no. 12, pp. 2369–2380, 2004.

[21] J. T. Rodgers, W. Lerin, W. Haas, S. P. Gygi, B. M. Spiegelman, and P. Puigserver, "Nutrient control of glucose homeostasis through a complex of PGC-1α and SIRT1," *Nature*, vol. 434, no. 7029, pp. 113–118, 2005.

[22] M. Lagouge, C. Argmann, Z. Gerhart-Hines et al., "Resveratrol improves mitochondrial function and protects against metabolic disease by activating SIRT1 and PGC-1α," *Cell*, vol. 127, no. 6, pp. 1109–1122, 2006.

[23] Z. H. Wang, C. H. Hsieh, W. H. Liu, and M. C. Yin, "Glycyrrhizic acid attenuated glycative stress in kidney of diabetic mice through enhancing glyoxalase pathway," *Molecular Nutrition & Food Research*, vol. 58, no. 7, pp. 1426–1435, 2014.

[24] A. Hartner, C. Menendez-Castro, N. Cordasic et al., "Tubulointerstitial de novo expression of the α8 integrin chain in a rodent model of renal fibrosis—a potential target for anti-fibrotic therapy?," *PLoS One*, vol. 7, no. 11, article e48362, 2012.

[25] A. Sila, Z. Ghlissi, Z. Kamoun et al., "Astaxanthin from shrimp by-products ameliorates nephropathy in diabetic rats," *European Journal of Nutrition*, vol. 54, no. 2, pp. 301–307, 2014.

[26] A. I. Serban, L. Stanca, O. I. Geicu, M. C. Munteanu, and A. Dinischiotu, "RAGE and TGF-β1 cross-talk regulate extracellular matrix turnover and cytokine synthesis in AGEs exposed fibroblast cells," *PLoS One*, vol. 11, no. 3, article e0152376, 2016.

[27] M. Pliszka, B. Oleszczak, and L. Szablewski, "Leptin at gender-specific concentrations does not affect glucose transport, expression of glucose transporters and leptin receptors in human lymphocytes," *Endocrine*, vol. 49, no. 1, pp. 97–105, 2015.

[28] X. Q. Chen, S. H. Wu, Y. Y. Luo et al., "Lipoxin A4 attenuates bronchopulmonary dysplasia via upregulation of Let-7c and downregulation of TGF-β1 signaling pathway," *Inflammation*, 2017.

[29] S. V. McLennan, D. J. Kelly, A. J. Cox et al., "Decreased matrix degradation in diabetic nephropathy: effects of ACE inhibition on the expression and activities of matrix metalloproteinases," *Diabetologia*, vol. 45, no. 2, pp. 268–275, 2002.

[30] X. Xie, W. Xia, X. Fei et al., "Relaxin inhibits high glucose-induced matrix accumulation in human Mesangial cells by interfering with TGF-β1 production and Mesangial cells phenotypic transition," *Biological and Pharmaceutical Bulletin*, vol. 38, no. 10, pp. 1464–1469, 2015.

[31] S. Di Meo, T. T. Reed, P. Venditti, and V. M. Victor, "Role of ROS and RNS sources in physiological and pathological conditions," *Oxidative Medicine and Cellular Longevity*, vol. 2016, Article ID 1245049, 44 pages, 2016.

[32] J. M. Forbes, M. T. Coughlan, and M. E. Cooper, "Oxidative stress as a major culprit in kidney disease in diabetes," *Diabetes*, vol. 57, no. 6, pp. 1446–1454, 2008.

[33] D. K. Singh, P. Winocour, and K. Farrington, "Oxidative stress in early diabetic nephropathy: fueling the fire," *Nature Reviews Endocrinology*, vol. 7, no. 3, pp. 176–184, 2011.

[34] A. Houldsworth, A. Hodgkinson, S. Shaw, A. Millward, and A. G. Demaine, "Polymorphic differences in the SOD-2 gene may affect the pathogenesis of nephropathy in patients with diabetes and diabetic complications," *Gene*, vol. 569, no. 1, pp. 41–45, 2015.

[35] L. F. C. França, A. C. C. G. Vasconcelos, F. R. P. da Silva et al., "Periodontitis changes renal structures by oxidative stress and lipid peroxidation," *Journal of Clinical Periodontology*, vol. 44, no. 6, pp. 568–576, 2017.

[36] A. Karadeniz, N. Simsek, E. Karakus et al., "Royal jelly modulates oxidative stress and apoptosis in liver and kidneys of rats treated with cisplatin," *Oxidative Medicine and Cellular Longevity*, vol. 2011, Article ID 981793, 10 pages, 2011.

[37] N. Oumi, K. A. Taniguchi, A. M. Kanai, M. Yasunaga, T. Nakanishi, and K. Sato, "A crucial role of bone morphogenetic protein signaling in the wound healing response in acute liver injury induced by carbon tetrachloride," *International Journal of Hepatology*, vol. 2012, Article ID 476820, 10 pages, 2012.

[38] C. W. Park, Y. Zhang, X. Zhang et al., "PPARα agonist fenofibrate improves diabetic nephropathy in db/db mice," *Kidney International*, vol. 69, no. 9, pp. 1511–1517, 2006.

[39] S. Nemoto, M. M. Fergusson, and T. Finkel, "Nutrient availability regulates SIRT1 through a forkhead-dependent pathway," *Science*, vol. 306, no. 5704, pp. 2105–2108, 2004.

[40] S. Nemoto, M. M. Fergusson, and T. Finkel, "SIRT1 functionally interacts with the metabolic regulator and transcriptional coactivator PGC-1α," *The Journal of Biological Chemistry*, vol. 280, no. 16, pp. 16456–16460, 2005.

[41] J. X. Ye, S. S. Wang, M. Ge, and D. J. Wang, "Suppression of endothelial PGC-1α is associated with hypoxia-induced endothelial dysfunction and provides a new therapeutic target in pulmonary arterial hypertension," *American Journal of Physiology - Lung Cellular and Molecular Physiology*, vol. 310, no. 11, pp. L1233–L1242, 2016.

[42] N. B. Ruderman, X. J. Xu, L. Nelson et al., "AMPK and SIRT1: a long-standing partnership?," *American Journal of Physiology - Endocrinology and Metabolism*, vol. 298, no. 4, pp. E751–E760, 2010.

[43] T. Okayasu, A. Tomizawa, K. Suzuki, K. Manaka, and Y. Hattori, "PPARα activators upregulate eNOS activity and inhibit cytokine-induced NF-κB activation through AMP-activated protein kinase activation," *Life Sciences*, vol. 82, no. 15-16, pp. 884–891, 2008.

[44] C. G. Mao, Z. Z. Tao, Z. Chen, C. Chen, S. M. Chen, and L. J. Wan, "Indole-3-carbinol inhibits nasopharyngeal carcinoma cell growth in vivo and in vitro through inhibition of the PI3K/Akt pathway," *Experimental and Therapeutic Medicine*, vol. 8, no. 1, pp. 207–212, 2014.

[45] K. Sharma, S. Ramachandrarao, G. Qiu et al., "Adiponectin regulates albuminuria and podocyte function in mice," *The Journal of Clinical Investigation*, vol. 118, no. 5, pp. 1645–1656, 2008.

[46] A. A. Eid, B. M. Ford, K. Block et al., "AMP-activated protein kinase (AMPK) negatively regulates Nox4-dependent activation of p53 and epithelial cell apoptosis in diabetes," *The Journal of Biological Chemistry*, vol. 285, no. 48, pp. 37503–37512, 2010.

[47] M. Kitada, S. Kume, N. Imaizumi, and D. Koya, "Resveratrol improves oxidative stress and protects against diabetic nephropathy through normalization of Mn-SOD dysfunction in AMPK/SIRT1-independent pathway," *Diabetes*, vol. 60, no. 2, pp. 634–643, 2011.

17

Therapeutic Effects of Tangshen Formula on Diabetic Nephropathy in *db/db* Mice Using Cytokine Antibody Array

Xue Mei Fan,[1] Chun Lian Huang,[1] Yi Ming Wang,[1] Ning Li,[2] Qiong Lin Liang,[1] and Guo An Luo[1,3]

[1]*Beijing Key Laboratory of Bioorganic Phosphorus Chemistry & Chemical Biology (Ministry of Education), Department of Chemistry, Tsinghua University, Beijing, China*
[2]*School of Pharmacy, China Pharmaceutical University, Nanjing, China*
[3]*State Key Laboratory for Quality Research in Chinese Medicines, Macau University of Science and Technology, Macau, China*

Correspondence should be addressed to Guo An Luo; luoga@tsinghua.edu.cn

Academic Editor: Munmun Chattopadhyay

Objective. Cytokines are essential promoters in the pathogenesis of diabetic nephropathy (DN) in type 2 diabetes. The following study investigates the adjustment mechanism of *Tangshen* formula (TSF) on cytokine expressions in *db/db* mice (DN animal model). *Materials and Methods. Db/db* mice were randomly divided into three groups. The treated groups were orally administered with TSF and losartan for 12 weeks. Biochemical and histological examinations were determined at 8 and 12 weeks posttreatment, while the cytokine antibody array analysis was applied to analyze the expression of 144 cytokines in kidney tissues at the end of the 12th week posttreatment. *Results.* TSF significantly reduced urinary albumin excretion and the levels of blood glucose, cholesterol, triglyceride, creatinine, and urea nitrogen. Furthermore, a significant decrease in glomerulus and mesangial area, as well as the downregulation of 24 cytokines and upregulated expressions of 5 cytokines, was found in the TSF-treated mice. *Conclusions.* The present study reveals that TSF could ameliorate the metabolic anomalies and renal injury in db/db mice. One of the important mechanisms for treatment of DN using the treatment of TSF is the control of the JAK/STAT signaling pathway via regulation of IL-2, IL-6, IL-13, Il-15, and IFN-γ expression.

1. Introduction

Diabetic nephropathy (DN) is one of the major microvascular complications in type 1 and type 2 diabetes and the leading cause of end-stage renal disease worldwide [1, 2]. Kidney inflammation has been reported to play an essential role in the development and progression of DN [3]. Many inflammatory cytokines are involved in the pathogenesis of DN, including cell adhesion molecules (CAMs), monocyte chemotactic protein-1 (MCP-1), tumor necrosis factor-α (TNF-α), interleukin-1 (IL-1), interleukin-6 (IL-6), interleukin-18 (IL-18), transforming growth factor-β (TGF-β), adiponectin, leptin, and resistin which are believed to be essential for DN because of cellular injury and progressive fibrosis [4]. In such circumstances, the multidetection of cytokines could be used to identify therapeutic mechanisms.

Tangshen formula (TSF), a traditional Chinese medicine composed of *Radix Astragali*, *Radix Rehmanniae*, *Radix Notoginseng*, *Radix et Rhizoma Rhei*, *Fructus Aurantii*, *Fructus Corni*, and *Ramulus Euonymi*, has been used to treat DN in clinic [5–7]. A recent clinical trial has proved the efficacy and safety of TSF in decreasing proteinuria and improving eGFR in patients with diabetic kidney disease and macroalbuminuria [5]. Previous studies have also shown that TSF is very important in regulating and ameliorating the metabolism of phospholipids [8] and purine-pyrimidine [9]. To date, there have been few reports about TSF regulating cytokine expression in patients with DN; thus, further investigations of the molecular mechanisms of TSF are needed. The purpose of this study was to evaluate the effects of TSF against DN and to explore the molecular mechanisms of multiple cytokine expressions underlying the renal-protective activity in *db/db* mice.

In addition, antihypertensive drugs such as angiotensin II-converting enzyme inhibitors (ACEI) or angiotensin II receptor blockers (ARBs) are commonly used to treat proteinuria in clinic. Losartan, angiotensin II receptor antagonists which are commonly used to treat high blood pressure, conferred significant renal benefits in patients with type 2 diabetes and nephropathy [10]. Thus, losartan was used as the positive control in this study.

2. Materials and Methods

2.1. Chemicals. Losartan potassium tablets (Lot: 110674, MSD, USA); *Tangshen* formula was provided by China-Japan Friendship Hospital (Lot: 0606320, Jiangyin Tianjiang Pharmaceutical, China); Albumin (Mouse) Elisa Kit (KA0489, Abnova, USA); RayBio®2 × Cell Lysis Buffer (Lot: 121,580, RayBiotech, USA); Biotechnologies BCA Protein Assay Kit (Lot: 201556AX, Aidlab, China); RayBio Mouse Cytokine Antibody Array G-Series 2000 (RayBiotech, USA).

2.2. Preparation of Tangshen Formula. TSF powder (prepared and standardized in Jiangyin Tianjiang Pharmaceutical, Jiangsu, China) was provided by China-Japan Friendship Hospital. Seven natural herbs, *Radix Astragali* (35.3%), *Radix Rehmanniae* (14.4%), *Radix Notoginseng* (3.5%), *Radix et Rhizoma Rhei* (7.1%), *Fructus Aurantii* (11.5%), *Fructus Corni* (10.6%), and *Ramulus Euonymi* (17.6%), were well mixed and soaked in distilled water for 30 minutes, boiled in 10 volumes of water (*v/w*) for 1 h, and extracted twice. The extract was filtrated and condensed to the final concentration of 1 g/mL and processed into powder by spray drying [11]. In our previous research, TSF had been subjected to high-performance liquid chromatography (HPLC) analysis; a Shimadzu diode array detector (DAD) was set at 280 nm to detect the constituents of TSF. Finally, fifty-nine compounds in *Tangshen* formula were identified, including flavonoids and flavonoid glycosides, iridoid glycosides, anthraquinone, and triterpenoid saponins [12].

2.3. Animals and Treatment Allocations. Obese diabetic mice lacking leptin receptor (*db/db*) carry a mutation in the leptin receptor gene and are well-established spontaneous models of obesity-induced type 2 diabetes. 19-week-old *db/db* male mice (C57BL/KsJ) weighing 40–60 g and *db/m* normal mice weighing 20–30 g were purchased from Vital River Laboratory Animal Technology Co. Ltd. (Beijing, China). All the animals were housed in an environment with temperature of 22 ± 1°C, relative humidity of 50 ± 1%, and a light/dark cycle of 12/12 hr. All animal studies (including the mouse euthanasia procedure) were done in compliance with the regulations and guidelines of Tsinghua University institutional animal care and were conducted according to the AAALAC and the IACUC guidelines (approval number: 12-LGA9; approval date: July 2012).

After acclimating to the laboratory for 1 week, biochemical indexes of blood taken from ocular venous plexus and urinary albumin in both *db/db* mice and *db/m* mice were measured, and the kidneys were collected from each mouse. Then the remaining mice were randomly divided into four groups (16 mice/group): (a) control group (*db/m* mice orally administrated with pure water); (b) model group (*db/db* mice orally administrated with pure water); (c) losartan group (*db/db* mice orally administrated with losartan, 6.50 mg/kg/day); (d) TSF group (*db/db* mice orally administrated with TSF, 2.08 g/kg/day). The treatment lasted for 12 weeks.

At 0, 8, and 12 weeks posttreatment, the mice were euthanized and the following experiments were performed: (1) blood was collected from ocular venous plexus and centrifuged at 4°C, 4000 rpm for 15 min, and the supernatant was further analyzed for biochemical indexes; (2) renal tissues were collected and immediately washed with cold phosphate-buffered saline (PBS); the left kidney was formaldehyde fixed for histological examination, while the right kidney was snap-frozen and stored in liquid nitrogen for cytokines detection.

Twenty-four-hour urine collections were obtained from the volume in each mouse after they were placed in metabolic cages the day before collecting blood samples; next, the urine was centrifuged at 4°C, 3000 rpm, for 15 min, and then the supernatant was taken to test the urinary albumin.

2.4. Blood and Urine Chemistry. The levels of blood glucose, cholesterol, triglyceride, blood urea nitrogen, and creatinine were measured by the Laboratory Medicine, Peking University Hospital. Urinary albumin was strictly measured by Albumin (Mouse) Elisa Kit according to manufacturer's instructions. The urinary albumin excretion was expressed by the total amount excreted in 24 h.

2.5. Histological Examination. Formaldehyde-fixed kidney tissues were embedded in paraffin. Sections of 4 μm thickness were cut and stained with hematoxylin and eosin (HE) and periodic acid–Schiff base (PAS). The pathological changes were observed under light microscope. PAS staining photographs were obtained and quantitatively analyzed with SPI analysis software for morphology. About 10 glomeruli from each slide were randomly selected and checked by a computed image analyzer. The mean glomerular area, mesangial area, and the mesangial area to glomerular area ratio were calculated. The percent of the mesangial area in the glomerular area in preparations stained with PAS was used as a glomerular sclerotic index. Differences in the areas and ratios mentioned above between different groups were analyzed by Student's *t*-test.

2.6. Detection of Renal Cytokines by Cytokine Antibody Array. Right kidneys from the model group in expt. week 0 and the right kidneys from model, TSF, and losartan groups in expt. week 12 then were ground under liquid nitrogen with a prechilled mortar and pestle and homogenized and treated with lysis buffer (50 mmol/L Tris, pH 7.4, 150 mmol/L NaCl, 1% Triton X-100, 1% sodium deoxycholate, 0.1% SDS,

Table 1: Blood and urine chemistry values in *db/db* mouse groups, 8 weeks posttreatment. ($n = 8$, means ± SEM).

Index	Control group	Model group	Losartan group	TSF group
Glucose ($mmol \cdot L^{-1}$)	6.01 ± 0.24	26.53 ± 5.57*	15.60 ± 4.73#	13.80 ± 3.95#
Triglycerides ($mmol \cdot L^{-1}$)	0.70 ± 0.02	0.96 ± 0.10*	0.69 ± 0.05#	0.73 ± 0.04#
Cholesterol ($mmol \cdot L^{-1}$)	2.34 ± 0.09	4.77 ± 0.46*	3.80 ± 0.56	3.66 ± 0.31#
Creatinine ($\mu mol \cdot L^{-1}$)	35.23 ± 5.48	42.67 ± 5.49*	44.20 ± 7.00	35.67 ± 2.93#
Blood urea nitrogen ($mmol \cdot L^{-1}$)	6.64 ± 0.36	9.38 ± 0.32*	7.94 ± 0.31#	7.40 ± 0.58#
Urinary albumin (μg/24 h)	28.6 ± 2.60	288.00 ± 21.91*	267.00 ± 17.96	273.00 ± 18.78

*$P < 0.05$ compared with the control group. #$P < 0.05$ compared with the model group.

Table 2: Blood and urine chemistry values in *db/db* mouse groups, 12 weeks posttreatment. ($n = 8$, means ± SEM).

Index	Control group	Model group	Losartan group	TSF group
Glucose ($mmol \cdot L^{-1}$)	7.08 ± 0.64	34.00 ± 3.48*	14.72 ± 2.77#	14.91 ± 2.94#
Triglycerides ($mmol \cdot L^{-1}$)	0.64 ± 0.03	1.13 ± 0.04*	0.96 ± 0.07#	0.95 ± 0.05#
Cholesterol ($mmol \cdot L^{-1}$)	2.51 ± 0.11	4.63 ± 0.27*	4.26 ± 0.26	4.07 ± 0.15#
Creatinine ($\mu mol \cdot L^{-1}$)	35.50 ± 2.56	44.86 ± 3.07*	30.86 ± 4.13#	32.22 ± 4.14#
Blood urea nitrogen ($mmol \cdot L^{-1}$)	6.05 ± 0.39	7.28 ± 0.33*	6.36 ± 0.58#	6.05 ± 0.39#
Urinary albumin (μg/24 h)	32.80 ± 2.37	314.00 ± 19.65*	225.00 ± 12.73#	240.00 ± 12.00#

*$P < 0.05$ compared with the control group. #$P < 0.05$ compared with the model group.

sodium orthovanadate, sodium fluoride, EDTA, etc.). The total protein concentration was analyzed using BCA protein assay kit according to the manufacturer's instructions. Each extract was diluted to the same protein concentration (1 $\mu g/\mu L$) before the cytokine antibody array analysis was performed.

Renal cytokine levels of mice were analyzed using Mouse Cytokine Antibody Array G-Series 2000 from RayBiotech, containing 144 different anti-cytokine antibodies, as well as positive and negative controls (http://www.raybiotech.com/files/manual/Antibody-Array/AAM-CYT-G2000.pdf). The assays were strictly performed according to the manufacturer's instructions. The glass slides were scanned with CapitalBio LuxScan 10 K-A Microarray Scanner using Cy3 channel. Fluorescence (intensities of obtained spots) was recorded to determine the changes in detected cytokine expressions.

2.7. Microarray Data Extraction and Analysis. The cytokine expression data were imported into the mouse cytokine semiquantitative analysis software (S02-AAM-CYT-G2000) for correction and normalization. The Matlab software (version 5.0) was used for further cluster analysis. The pathway analysis was performed on DAVID and Kyoto Encyclopedia of Genes and Genomes (KEGG) pathways.

2.8. Statistical Analysis. Values are expressed as means ± SEM, with n denoting the number of animals. Significance was evaluated using one-way ANOVA. Comparisons between two groups were performed using Student's t-test. $P < 0.05$ was considered statistically significant, while $P < 0.01$ was considered highly statistically significant.

3. Results

3.1. TSF Treatment Inhibits Blood Glucose Increase and Regulates the Disorder of Glycolipid Metabolism in db/db Mice. The levels of blood glucose, triglyceride, and cholesterol were measured to reveal the adjustment of TSF on the glycolipid metabolism in *db/db* mice (Tables 1 and 2). Briefly, the levels of blood glucose, triglyceride, and cholesterol in model group were significantly elevated compared to those of the control group. After 8 and 12 weeks of treatment, TSF administration groups showed a tendency to decrease the abnormal levels of glucose, triglyceride, and cholesterol. Nevertheless, no significant differences in cholesterol levels were observed in the in losartan-treated group compared to the model group. To sum up, these results indicated that TSF might effectively control the blood glucose and regulate glycolipid metabolism disorder.

3.2. TSF Treatment Attenuates Renal Dysfunctions

3.2.1. TSF Treatment Alleviates the Renal Dysfunctions in db/db Mice. The levels of urinary albumin excretion, blood creatinine, and urea nitrogen were detected to evaluate the diabetic renal dysfunction. As shown in Table 2, the levels of blood creatinine, urea nitrogen, and urinary albumin were significantly higher in the model group compared to the control group, while they were efficiently reduced in mice treated with TSF and losartan. This data suggested that TSF alleviates the renal dysfunctions in *db/db* mice.

3.2.2. TSF Treatment Decreases Kidney Tissue Damage in db/db Mice. The HE staining results of kidney tissues are shown in Figure 1. After 12 weeks, *db/m* kidney tissues had

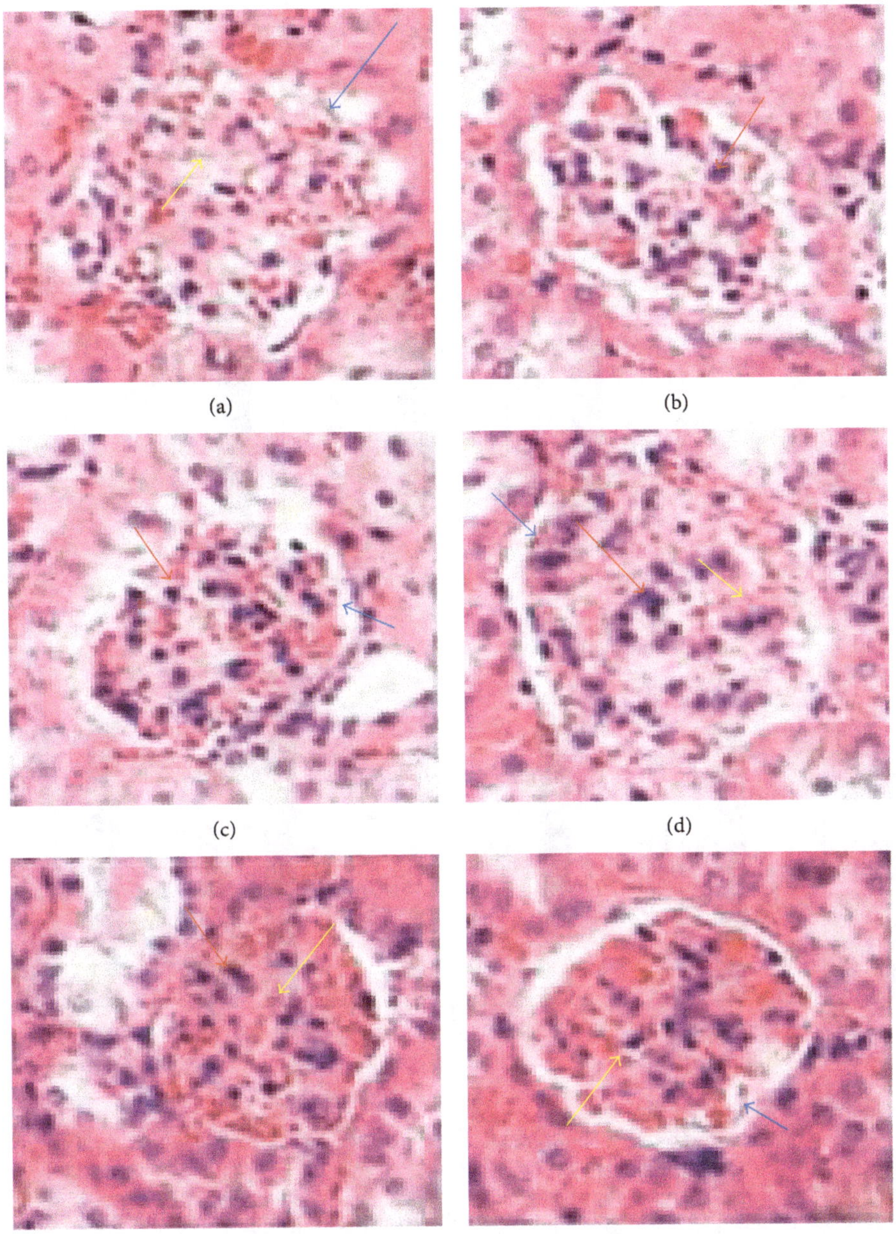

(a) (b) (c) (d) (e) (f)

FIGURE 1: Renal pathological changes after 12-week treatment (HE × 400). (a) Model group (expt. week 0). (b) Control group (expt. week 0). (c) Control group (expt. week 12). (d) Model group (expt. week 12). (e) Losartan group (expt. week 12). (f) TSF group (expt. week 12). The red arrow indicates mesangial cells, the yellow arrow indicates endothelial cells, and the blue indicates basement membrane.

intact glomerular morphology, clean cut, regular arrangement, and normal tubular structure. Contrary, increased glomerular volume, endothelial and mesangial cell proliferation, narrow capsular space, and blurred tubular structure were observed in the model group. In TSF group, mesangial expansion and glomerular volume were markedly ameliorated and the tubular structure was clear compared with the mouse model group of the same age. Similar improvement was observed in the losartan group.

According to the quantitative analysis results of PAS staining, glomerular fibrotic areas were significantly increased in *db/db* mice compared to the control group (Figure 2). After 12-week treatment with TSF, there was a significant decrease in the glomerular surface area, as well as in mesangial matrix and relative mesangial matrix area compared to model mice; while no significant differences were observed between the treated groups (Figure 2(g)).

3.2.3. TSF Treatment Improves the Abnormal Expression of Cytokines in Kidney Tissue of db/db Mice. We further examined the therapeutic effect of TSF on 144 cytokine expression in plasma of *db/db* mice using cytokine antibody array. After the semiquantitative soft analysis of the mouse cytokines, a strict significant t-test resulted in a final set of 29 differentially expressed cytokines, including 24 cytokines that were downregulated and 5 that were upregulated in *db/db* mice

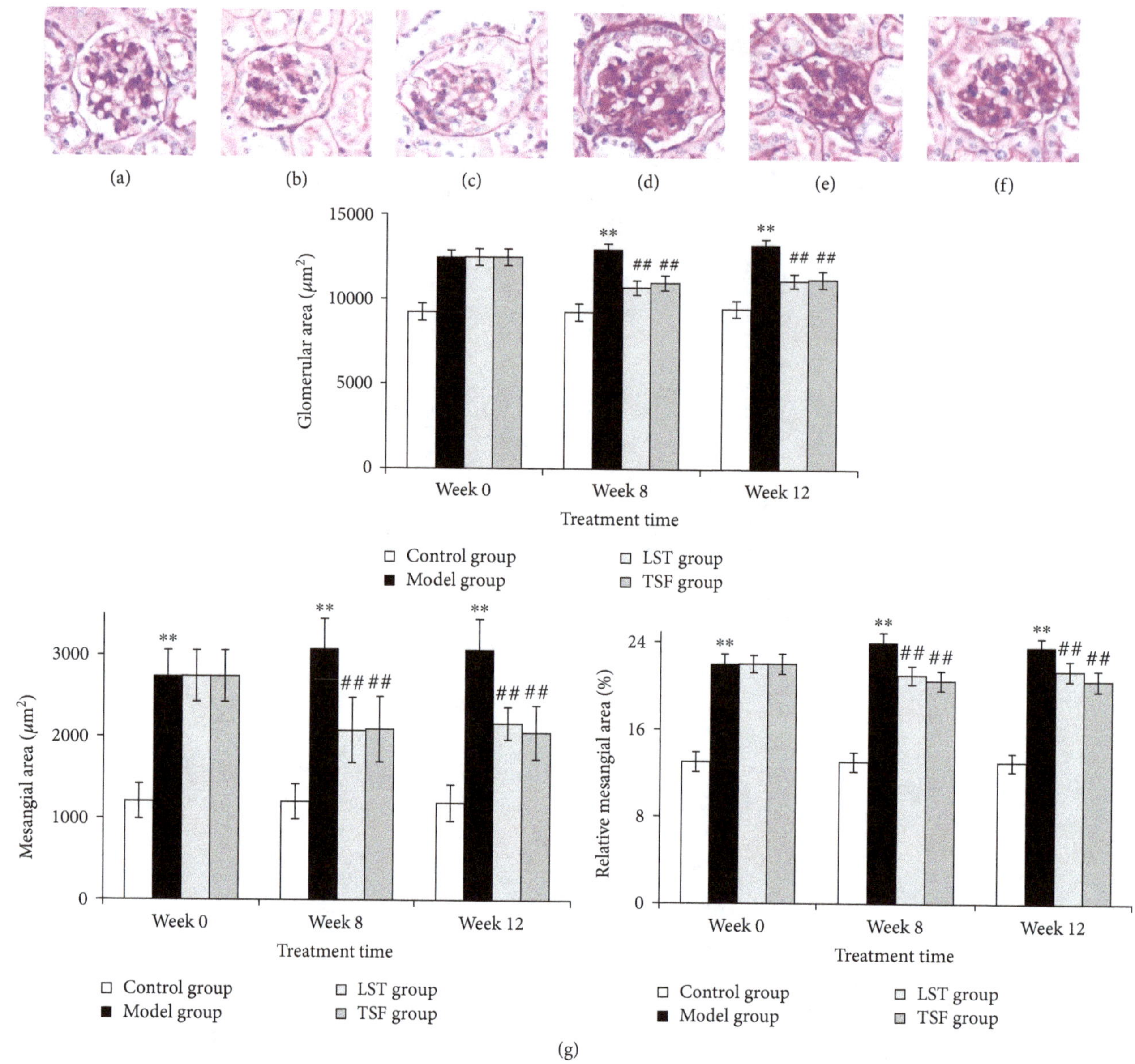

Figure 2: Renal pathological changes after 12-week treatment (PAS × 400). (a) Model group (expt. week 0); (b) control group (expt. week 0); (c) control group (expt. week 12); (d) model group (expt. week 12); (e) LST (losartan) group (expt. week 12); (f) TSF group (expt. week 12); (g) change of glomerular area, mesangial area, and the percentage of mesangial area. $^{**}P < 0.01$ compared with control group in the same time point; $^{\#\#}P < 0.01$ compared with the model group at the same time point.

after TSF treatment. 29 cytokines and the changes in their expression are shown in Table 3.

Cluster analysis was applied to observe the overall expression changes of cytokines among model, TSF and losartan groups. Before cluster analysis, the data of expt. week 12 was normalized with the data of expt. week 0's *db*/*db* mice as a reference. Then cluster result of microarray data was generated by Matlab 5.0 (Figure 3). The TSF and losartan groups could get together for a class and all are well separated separated with the model group. The results also showed that changed cytokines of the TSF group were farther away from the model group than from losartan group, indicating that TSF has a unique and effective molecular regulatory mechanism in the treatment of DN.

3.2.4. Regulated JAK/STAT Signaling Pathway Regulated via Improved the Related Cytokine Abnormal Expression May Be Mechanisms by TSF Treatment DN in db/db Mice. To gain insights into the biological roles of the differentially expressed cytokines adjusted by TSF, the pathway enrichment analysis was performed on DAVID software (KEGG pathway analysis). The significant pathways ($P < 0.001$) were cytokine-cytokine receptor interaction, JAK/STAT signaling pathway, adipocytokine signaling pathway, Toll-like receptor signaling pathway, and cell adhesion molecules (CAMs). Cytokine-cytokine receptor interaction and JAK/STAT signaling pathway were the most significant channels. In the cytokine-cytokine receptor interaction, the cytokines with altered expression were widely distributed. In the JAK/STAT

Table 3: The relative expression changes of 29 cytokines.

Number	Cytokines	Model group (expt. week 12)/model group (expt. week 0)	LST group (expt. week 12)/model group (expt. week 0)	TSF group (expt. week 12)/model group (expt. week 0)
1	VEGF	0.94	0.97	0.75
2	VEGF R2	0.90	1.48	0.64
3	IGFBP-3	1.13	1.05	0.96
4	SCF	0.95	1.00	0.67
5	IL-2	1.52	1.47	1.01
6	IL-4	3.72	3.73	2.02
7	IL-6	1.61	1.26	1.32
8	IL-13	1.19	1.14	0.96
9	IL-15	1.05	0.82	0.83
10	FAS ligand	0.99	0.78	0.65
11	ICAM-1	0.54	0.69	0.42
12	VCAM-1	0.35	0.42	0.24
13	PF4	0.93	0.67	0.56
14	TIMP-1	0.99	1.05	0.73
15	IFN-gamma	1.76	1.70	1.51
16	Decorin	2.02	1.88	1.56
17	TNF-alpha	1.50	1.26	1.27
18	IL-3	0.76	0.68	0.51
19	IL-7	1.37	1.18	1.01
20	IL-10	0.74	0.63	0.59
21	IL-17	0.74	0.65	0.54
22	MCP-1	0.64	0.59	0.41
23	M-CSF	0.70	0.64	0.53
24	CD36	0.74	0.63	0.49
25	EGF	0.59	0.36	0.75
26	IGFBP-2	0.74	0.65	0.98
27	IGF-II	0.64	0.59	0.86
28	MMP-2	0.70	0.64	0.95
29	E-cadherin	1.05	1.01	1.23

signaling pathway, the distribution of differentially expressed cytokines was more concentrated. Moreover, JAK/STAT pathway might be closely related to the pathogenesis of DN [13, 14]. Therefore, we made a further investigation of these 5 differentially expressed cytokines (Table 4) in JAK/STAT signaling pathway related to DN. Figure 4 showed the main role of these cytokines and related JAK/STAT signaling pathway in physiology and pathology.

4. Discussion

DN is one of the major microvascular complications in type 2 diabetes and a leading cause of end-stage renal disease. Using traditional Chinese medicine for DN has shown good results and has become increasingly recognized worldwide. In the present study, we verified the efficacy of TSF and discussed its action mechanisms on animal models of DN.

The determination of biochemical indexes indicated that TSF could effectively control the deterioration of DN. The levels of blood glucose, blood triglyceride, and cholesterol significantly decreased following TSF treatment; these beneficial effects can be achieved via TSF regulating action on the glycolipid metabolism. Urinary albumin, blood urea nitrogen, and blood creatinine are commonly used to characterize the renal dysfunction in clinical diagnosis. As shown in Tables 1 and 2, the urinary albumin, blood urea nitrogen, and blood creatinine levels were all reduced with TSF treatment, suggesting that TSF could effectively reduce kidney damage caused by DN. In pathological analysis, treatment with TSF resulted in a significant reduction in formation of glomerular sclerotic lesions and fibrosis that were marked in the model group. These observations suggested that the intake of TSF could slow down the progressive deterioration in pathological aspects of DN in *db*/*db* mice.

Above-mentioned results showed that TSF therapy could indeed slow down the disease progression of DN. On this basis, the molecular mechanism of TSF was further explored by cytokine antibody array. The results of protein microarray analysis revealed that the occurrence and development of DN were regulated by a variety of cytokines and growth factors.

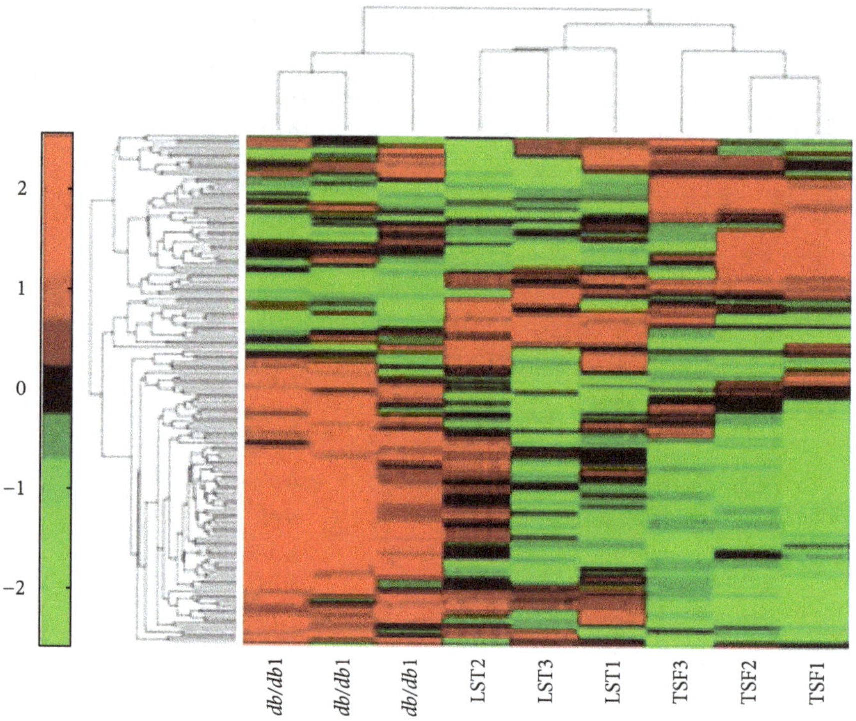

FIGURE 3: Cluster analysis result of protein microarray data. Model group, LST (losartan) group, and TSF group have 3 samples which represent biologically independent duplicates. Red indicates increased expression; green indicates reduced expression.

TABLE 4: Semiquantitative results of 5 differentially expressed cytokines in the JAK/STAT signaling pathway (means ± SEM; 3 individuals).

Cytokines	Fluorescence intensity value (IU)			
	Expt. week 0 Model group	Expt. week 12 Model group	Expt. week 12 Losartan group	Expt. week 12 TSF group
IL-2	3840 ± 83	5846 ± 202	5626 ± 94	4628 ± 116*
IL-6	1226 ± 42	1970 ± 68	1544 ± 55*	1622 ± 55*
IL-13	1020 ± 37	1210 ± 29	1161 ± 42	974 ± 23*
IL-15	2163 ± 71	2771 ± 104	2156 ± 101*	2196 ± 116*
IFN-γ	1630 ± 55	2861 ± 25	2768 ± 89	2461 ± 103*

*$P < 0.05$ compared with the model group in expt. week 12.

In this study, the expression of 29 cytokines (in total 144 proteins) significantly changed compared with the model group after TSF intervention, including IL-2, IL-6, IL-13, IL-15, and IFN-γ enriched to JAK/STAT signaling pathway. JAK/STAT pathway, an essential intracellular mechanism of cytokines and growth factors, is frequently associated with gene expression and cellular activation, proliferation, and differentiation in DN [13, 14]. In this animal experiment, the genomics of renal tissue was carried out in parallel. And the results have provided evidence for the involvement of JAK/STAT/SOCS pathway in the mechanism of Tangshen formula-treated diabetic nephropathy at the gene expression level [12]. Growth factor and inflammatory factor signaling pathways mediated by JAK/STAT are considered to be very important in diabetic nephropathy [15]. When experimental time was prolonged, the IL-2, IL-6, IL-13, and IL-15 expressions and IFN-γ were abnormally increased in the model group. However, decreased levels of these five cytokines implied that JAK/STAT pathway was inhibited following the TSE treatment. This means that TSF may affect the downstream function by regulating the expression of the five cytokines.

IL-2 has a very complex role in the development and control of inflammatory disease [16]. Accordingly, major IL-2 dysfunctions in both humans and mice are associated with the development of autoimmunity as well as immunodeficiencies [17, 18]. This finding highlights that the balance between the IL-2 pro- and anti-inflammatory effects is critical for an appropriate mounting and resolution of immune responses. However, there are no previous studies that have revealed the functionality of IL-2 in kidney tissue diagnosis of DN. In our study, renal expression of IL-2 was decreased in TSF-treated *db*/*db* mice compared with the model group.

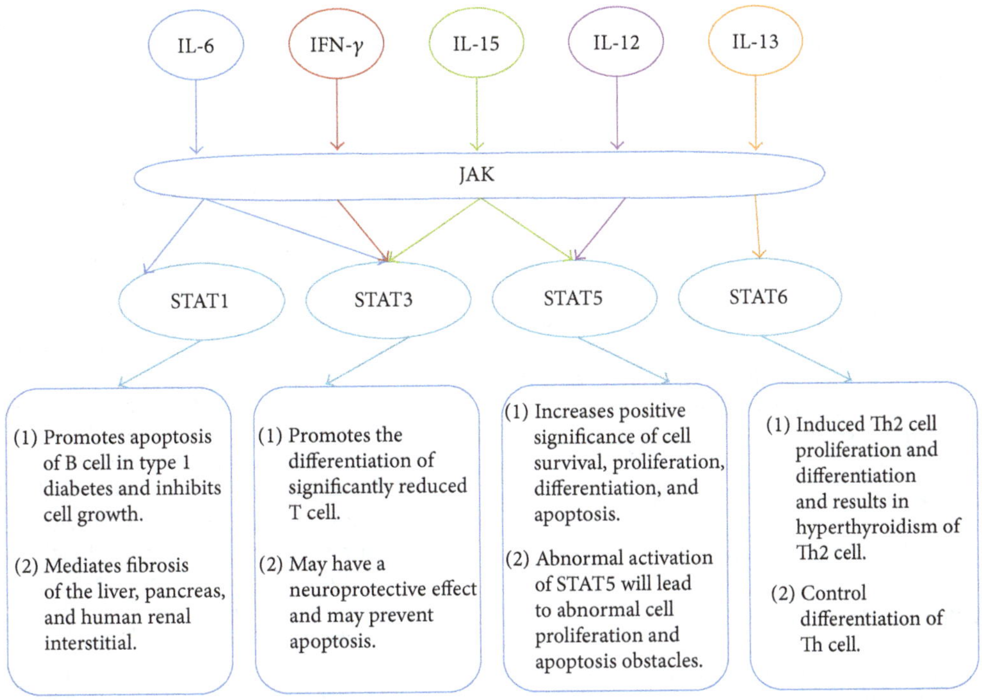

FIGURE 4: The main physiological and pathological role of IL-2, IL-6, IL-13, IL-15, and IFN-γ.

This suggested that TSF could adjust the renal level of IL-2 to an appropriate standard to improve renal immunity in *db/db* mice, eventually reducing the kidney damage.

IL-6 is a well-known pleiotropic cytokine which is the classic upstream activator of the JAK/STAT3. It has been shown that inhibition of the JAK/STAT3 pathway reduced infiltration of interstitial inflammatory cells and production of chemokines in the adriamycin-induced nephropathy model [19]. IL-6 levels and polymorphisms were also associated with the risk of DN [20]. It was reported that IL-6 was associated with reduced glomerular filtration rate (GFR) in type 2 diabetic patients [21]. Choudhary and Ahlawat have also confirmed that the elevated levels of IL-6 are independently associated with urinary albumin excretion [22]. *Lu Huang Shen Hua* capsule, a traditional Chinese medicine, could reduce urine albumin excretion, lower serum IL-6, and TNF-α levels by controlling FBG, thus having an important role in kidney protection and DNA prevention and treatment [23]. In the present study, decreased levels of IL-6 in renal and lower albuminuria were observed in TSF group compared with the model group. Therefore, we believe that TSF could attenuate the albuminuria by indirectly decreasing the IL-6 expression in renal.

IL-13 triggers a number of signaling pathways, and different effects of IL-13 are mediated through discrete mechanisms. IL-13 that activates JAK3/STAT6 signaling, including the kidney [24], has been identified as the principle signaling pathway involved in IL-13-induced responses [25]. The previous study has suggested that IL-13 overexpression in the rat could lead to podocyte injury with downregulation of nephrin, podocin, and dystroglycan, and a concurrent upregulation of B7-1 in the glomeruli, inducing a minimal change-like nephropathy that is characterized by increased proteinuria, hypoalbuminemia, hypercholesterolemia, and fusion of podocyte foot processes [26]. IL-13 has a pathogenic role in altered glomerular permeability by influencing intracellular trafficking of proteins and promoting proteolysis at the basolateral surface of glomerular visceral epithelial cells [27]. TSF treatment can significantly reduce the levels of kidney IL-13 in renal and the urine albumin excretion; therefore, we speculate that TSF may protect the renal function by regulating the IL-13 renal levels in *db/db* mice.

IL-15 is an autocrine survival factor for tubular epithelial cells, both in humans and mice that has a vital role in renal physiology [28, 29]. Increased or decreased expression of IL-15 characterizes several renal pathologies that are harmful to renal cell survival and kidney functions [30]. On the other hand, the synthesis of increased IL-15 has been linked with autoimmune diseases, such as diabetes mellitus type 1 and 2 [31]. Indeed, we found that IL-15 level in renal mouse model was significantly increased compared with the TSF-treated mice, suggesting that increased expression of IL-15 may enhance proinflammatory actions leading to the renal fibrosis. TSF could reduce the levels of IL-15 in kidney, thus ameliorating the inflammation in *db/db* mice. This finding was consistent with the supposition that although high IL-15 level enhances proinflammatory actions, extremely low IL-15 level markedly and selectively suppresses proinflammatory actions [32].

IFN-γ induces gene transcription via activation of the JAK/STAT pathway [33]. Inflammation modulates angiotensinogen (AGT) production in tissues via inflammatory cytokines. Previous studies have shown that IFN-γ increases AGT expression in hepatocytes via activating the STAT1 pathway [34], while Satou et al. have reported that IFN-γ radically regulates AGT expression in the kidney via STAT3 activity modulated by STAT1-SOCS1 axis [35]. In the present study, IFN-γ expression in the kidney of the TSF group was significantly attenuated, indicating that TSF could reduce AGT production by reducing the expression of IFN-γ and thus ameliorate the development of hypertension. However, the exact way of how the TSF regulates the expression of IFN-γ needs to be further investigated.

5. Conclusions

This study demonstrated that TSF has the ability to ameliorate impaired metabolic status of blood glucose and lipid, to improve renal function, and to slow down the renal fibrosis by regulating the JAK/STAT pathway. The next stage is to make further analysis of differentially expressed cytokines.

Conflicts of Interest

The authors declare that they have no conflicts of interest.

Authors' Contributions

Guo An Luo, Yi Ming Wang, and Qiong Lin Liang conceived and designed the experiments. Xue Mei Fan and Ning Li performed the experiments and analyzed the data. Xue Mei Fan and Chun Lian Huang wrote the paper.

Acknowledgments

This work was supported by the State Key Program of National Natural Science of China (Grant no. 81130066) and the Major National Science and Technology Project (2017ZX09301032). The authors are thankful to Professor Li Ping of China-Japan Friendship Hospital for providing them the Tangshen formula used for these studies.

References

[1] A. A. Lopes, "End-stage renal disease due to diabetes in racial/ethnic minorities and disadvantaged populations," *Ethnicity & Disease*, vol. 19, pp. 47–51, 2009.

[2] Y. M. Sun, Y. Su, J. Li, and L. F. Wang, "Recent advances in understanding the biochemical and molecular mechanism of diabetic nephropathy," *Biochemical and Biophysical Research Communications*, vol. 433, no. 4, pp. 359–361, 2013.

[3] J. Wada and H. Makino, "Inflammation and the pathogenesis of diabetic nephropathy," *Clinical Science*, vol. 124, no. 3, pp. 139–152, 2013.

[4] A. A. Elmarakby and J. C. Sullivan, "Relationship between oxidative stress and inflammatory cytokines in diabetic nephropathy," *Cardiovascular Therapeutics*, vol. 30, no. 1, pp. 49–59, 2012.

[5] P. Li, Y. P. Chen, J. P. Liu et al., "Efficacy and safety of Tangshen formula on patients with type 2 diabetic kidney disease: a multicenter double-blinded randomized placebo-controlled trial," *PLoS One*, vol. 10, no. 5, article e0126027, 2015.

[6] Q. Li, H. M. Zhang, Y. T. Fei, J. M. Xing, H. Luo, and J. P. Liu, "Treatment of diabetic nephropathy by integrative medicine: a multi-center prospective cohort study," *Chinese Journal of Integrated Traditional and Western Medicine*, vol. 32, no. 3, pp. 317–321, 2012.

[7] L. Ma and J. Hu, "Clinical observation of treatment of 36 cases of nephrosis diabetes by Western medicine and self-made Tangshen recipe," *Beijing Journal of Traditional Chinese Medicine*, vol. 24, pp. 263–265, 2005.

[8] M. Huang, C. Zhu, Q. L. Liang et al., "Effect of Tangshen formula on phospholipids metabolism in diabetic nephropathy patients," *Acta Pharmaceutica Sinica*, vol. 46, no. 7, pp. 780–786, 2011.

[9] J. F. Xia, Q. L. Liang, H. F. Zhong, Y. M. Wang, P. Li, and G. A. Luo, "Effect of Tangshen formula on the purine and pyrimidine metabolism of patients with diabetic nephropathy," *Chinese Traditional Patent Medicine*, vol. 33, pp. 13–17, 2011.

[10] B. M. Brenner, M. E. Cooper, D. de Zeeuw et al., "Effects of losartan on renal and cardiovascular outcomes in patients with type 2 diabetes and nephropathy," *The New England Journal of Medicine*, vol. 345, no. 12, pp. 861–869, 2001.

[11] H. J. Zhang, P. Li, F. J. Burczynski et al., "Attenuation of diabetic nephropathy in Otsuka long-evans Tokushima fatty (OLETF) rats with a combination of Chinese herbs (Tangshen formula)," *Evidence-Based Complementary and Alternative Medicine*, vol. 2011, Article ID 613737, 8 pages, 2011.

[12] Hu. JJ, X. M. Fan, X. S. Meng, Y. M. Wang, Q. L. Liang, and G. A. Luo, "Evidence for the involvement of JAK/STAT/SOCS pathway in the mechanism of Tangshen formula-treated diabetic nephropathy," *Planta Medica*, vol. 80, no. 08/09, pp. 614–621, 2014.

[13] A. K. Banes, S. Shaw, J. Jenkins et al., "Angiotensin II blockade prevents hyperglycemia-induced activation of JAK and STAT proteins in diabetic rat kidney glomeruli," *American Journal of Physiology-Renal Physiology*, vol. 286, pp. 653–659, 2004.

[14] M. B. Marrero, A. K. Banes-Berceli, D. M. Stern, and D. C. Eaton, "Role of the JAK/STAT signaling pathway in diabetic nephropathy," *American Journal of Physiology Renal Physiology*, vol. 290, pp. 762–768, 2006.

[15] A. K. Banes, S. Shaw, J. Jenkins et al., "Angiotensin II blockade prevents hyperglycemia-induced activation of JAK and STAT proteins in diabetic rat kidney glomeruli," *American Journal of Physiology Renal Physiology*, vol. 286, no. 4, pp. 653F–6659, 2004.

[16] R. Y. Lan, C. Selmi, and M. E. Gershwin, "The regulatory, inflammatory, and T cell programming roles of interleukin-2 (IL-2)," *Journal of Autoimmunity*, vol. 31, no. 1, pp. 7–12, 2008.

[17] C. A. Aoki, C. M. Roifman, Z. X. Lian et al., "IL-2 receptor alpha deficiency and features of primary biliary cirrhosis," *Journal of Autoimmunity*, vol. 27, no. 1, pp. 50–53, 2006.

[18] T. Kanai, J. Jenks, and K. C. Nadeau, "The STAT5b pathway defect and autoimmunity," *Frontiers in Immunology*, vol. 3, p. 234, 2012.

[19] R. Li, N. S. Yang, L. L. Zhang et al., "Inhibition of Jak/STAT signaling ameliorates mice experimental nephrotic syndrome," *American Journal of Nephrology*, vol. 27, no. 6, pp. 580–589, 2007.

[20] U. Dhamodharan, V. Viswanathan, E. Krishnamoorthy, R. Rajaram, and V. Aravindhan, "Genetic association of *IL-6*, *TNF-α* and *SDF-1* polymorphisms with serum cytokine levels in diabetic foot ulcer," *Gene*, vol. 565, no. 1, pp. 62–67, 2015.

[21] D. P. K. Ng, S. Nurbaya, S. H. J. Ye, and A. S. Krolewski, "An IL-6 haplotype on human chromosome 7p21 confers risk for

impaired renal function in type 2 diabetic patients," *Kidney International*, vol. 74, no. 4, pp. 521–527, 2008.

[22] N. Choudhary and R. S. Ahlawat, "Interleukin-6 and C-reactive protein in pathogenesis of diabetic nephropathy: new evidence linking inflammation, glycemic control, and microalbuminuria," *Iranian Journal of Kidney Diseases*, vol. 2, no. 2, pp. 72–79, 2008.

[23] X. Guan and X. Du, "Effect of Lu Huang Shen Hua capsule on levels of interleukin-6 and tumor necrosis factor-α in rats with diabetic nephropathy tumor necrosis factor-α in rats with diabetic nephropathy," *Journal of Anhui Traditional Chinese Medical College*, vol. 27, no. 5, pp. 39–41, 2008.

[24] M. Z. Zhang, X. Wang, Y. Wang et al., "IL-4/IL-13–mediated polarization of renal macrophages/dendritic cells to an M2a phenotype is essential for recovery from acute kidney injury," *Kidney International*, vol. 91, no. 2, pp. 375–386, 2017.

[25] J. E. de Vries, "The role of IL-13 and its receptor in allergy and inflammatory responses," *The Journal of Allergy and Clinical Immunity*, vol. 102, no. 2, pp. 165–169, 1998.

[26] K. W. Lai, C. L. Wei, L. K. Tan et al., "Overexpression of interleukin-13 induces minimal-change-like nephropathy in rats," *Journal of the American Society of Nephrology*, vol. 18, no. 5, pp. 1476–1485, 2007.

[27] J. G. Van Den Berg, J. Aten, C. Annink, J. H. Ravesloot, E. Weber, and J. J. Weening, "Interleukin-4 and-13 promote basolateral secretion of H^+ and cathepsin L by glomerular epithelial cells," *American Journal of Physiology Renal Physiology*, vol. 282, no. 1, pp. F26–F33, 2002.

[28] M. Shinozaki, J. Hirahashi, T. Lebedeva et al., "IL-15, a survival factor for kidney epithelial cells, counteracts apoptosis and inflammation during nephritis," *The Journal of Clinical Investigation*, vol. 109, no. 7, pp. 951–960, 2002.

[29] H. Eini, N. Tejman-Yarden, E. C. Lewis, C. Chaimovitz, M. Zlotnik, and A. Douvdevani, "Association between renal injury and reduced interleukin-15 and interleukin-15 receptor levels in acute kidney injury," *Journal of Interferon & Cytokine Research*, vol. 30, no. 1, pp. 1–8, 2010.

[30] J. Giron-Michel, S. Azzi, K. Khawam et al., "Interleukin-15 plays a central role in human kidney physiology and cancer through the γc signaling pathway," *PLoS One*, vol. 7, no. 2, article e31624, 2012.

[31] P. M. Duarte, V. R. Santos, F. A. dos Santos, S. de Lima Pereira, D. B. R. Rodrigues, and M. H. Napimoga, "Role of smoking and type 2 diabetes in the immunobalance of advanced chronic periodontitis," *Journal of Periodontology*, vol. 82, no. 3, pp. 429–438, 2011.

[32] D. G. Alleva, S. B. Kaser, M. A. Monroy, M. J. Fenton, and D. I. Beller, "IL-15 functions as a potent autocrine regulator of macrophage proinflammatory cytokine production: evidence for differential receptor subunit utilization associated with stimulation or inhibition," *The Journal of Immunology*, vol. 159, no. 6, pp. 2941–2951, 1997.

[33] B. Saha, S. Jyothi Prasanna, B. Chandrasekar, and D. Nandi, "Gene modulation and immunoregulatory roles of interferonγ," *Cytokine*, vol. 50, no. 1, pp. 1–14, 2010.

[34] S. Jain, M. Shah, Y. Li, G. Vinukonda, P. B. Sehgal, and A. Kumar, "Upregulation of human angiotensinogen (AGT) gene transcription by interferon–gamma: involvement of the STAT1-binding motif in the AGT promoter," *Biochimica et Biophysica Acta (BBA) - Gene Structure and Expression*, vol. 1759, no. 7, pp. 340–347, 1759.

[35] R. Satou, K. Miyata, R. A. Gonzalez-Villalobos, J. R. Ingelfinger, L. G. Navar, and H. Kobori, "Interferon-γ biphasically regulates angiotensinogen expression via a JAK-STAT pathway and suppressor of cytokine signaling 1 (SOCS1) in renal proximal tubular cells," *The FASEB Journal*, vol. 26, no. 5, pp. 1821–1830, 2012.

18

The *CNDP1* $(CTG)_5$ Polymorphism Is Associated with Biopsy-Proven Diabetic Nephropathy, Time on Hemodialysis, and Diabetes Duration

Thomas Albrecht,[1] Shiqi Zhang,[1,2] Jana D. Braun,[1] Li Xia,[1,2] Angelica Rodriquez,[1] Jiedong Qiu,[1] Verena Peters,[3] Claus P. Schmitt,[3] Jacob van den Born,[4] Stephan J. L. Bakker,[4] Alexander Lammert,[1] Hannes Köppel,[1] Peter Schnuelle,[1] Bernhard K. Krämer,[1] Benito A. Yard,[1] and Sibylle J. Hauske[1]

[1]*Fifth Medical Department (Nephrology/Endocrinology/Rheumatology), University Medical Center Mannheim, University of Heidelberg, Mannheim, Germany*
[2]*Department of Endocrinology, The First Affiliated Hospital of Anhui Medical University, Hefei, China*
[3]*Centre for Pediatric and Adolescent Medicine, University of Heidelberg, Heidelberg, Germany*
[4]*Nephrology, University Medical Center Groningen, University of Groningen, Groningen, Netherlands*

Correspondence should be addressed to Thomas Albrecht; t.albrecht@stud.uni-heidelberg.de

Academic Editor: Feng Wang

Considering that the homozygous *CNDP1* $(CTG)_5$ genotype affords protection against diabetic nephropathy (DN) in female patients with type 2 diabetes, this study assessed if this association remains gender-specific when applying clinical inclusion criteria (CIC-DN) or biopsy proof (BP-DN). Additionally, it assessed if the prevalence of the protective genotype changes with diabetes duration and time on hemodialysis and if this occurs in association with serum carnosinase (CN-1) activity. Whereas the distribution of the $(CTG)_5$ homozygous genotype in the no-DN and CIC-DN patients was comparable, a lower frequency was found in the BP-DN patients, particularly in females. We observed a significant trend towards high frequencies of the $(CTG)_5$ homozygous genotype with increased time on dialysis. This was also observed for diabetes duration but only reached significance when both $(CTG)_5$ homo- and heterozygous patients were included. CN-1 activity negatively correlated with time on hemodialysis and was lower in $(CTG)_5$ homozygous patients. The latter remained significant in female subjects after gender stratification. We confirm the association between the *CNDP1* genotype and DN to be likely gender-specific. Although our data also suggest that $(CTG)_5$ homozygous patients may have a survival advantage on dialysis and in diabetes, this hypothesis needs to be confirmed in a prospective cohort study.

1. Introduction

Diabetic nephropathy (DN) occurs in approximately 40% of patients with type 1 and type 2 diabetes [1] and is the leading cause of end-stage renal disease (ESRD) [2]. Compelling evidence has shown that susceptibility to DN is genetically determined [3, 4]. Amongst the reported linkage studies, there seems to be consistency in the linkage between human chromosome 18q22.3-q23 and DN [4–7]; linkage to the DN trait on chromosomes 7q21.3, 10p15.3, and 14q23.1 has also been reported [7]. Linkage with 18q22.3 was observed in populations of different ethnicities, for example, American Indians [8], Afro-Americans [9], and Caucasians [5].

Janssen et al. initially postulated that the *CNDP1* gene on chromosome 18q22.3-q23, encoding serum carnosinase (CN-1), is a susceptibility gene for DN in type 2 diabetes mellitus (T2DM) patients [10]. It was found that T2DM patients homozygous for the *CNDP1* $(CTG)_5$ allele are less frequently affected by DN compared to T2DM patients with other *CNDP1* genotypes [10]. The prevalence of the $(CTG)_5$ allele strongly varies with different ethnicities. While homozygosity for the $(CTG)_5$ allele is more frequent in the European population (38.6% in healthy controls and 29.3% in diabetic patients with ESRD) [11], this genotype seems to be much more rare in the Asian population with a high prevalence of DN [12, 13]. It has also been reported that the association between the *CNDP1* genotype and DN is sex-specific and independent of susceptibility to T2DM [14].

Since most patients with T2DM are not formally evaluated with a renal biopsy, the diagnosis of DN is based on clinical criteria, for example, persistent macroalbuminuria on at least 2 independent occasions (albumin excretion rate > 300 mg/d or >200 mg/l or ACR (albumin/creatinine ratio) > 300 mg/g). Yet, biopsy-based retrospective evaluations of the prevalence of nondiabetic renal disease (NDRD) in T2DM patients revealed a high percentage of patients having NDRD without evidence of concurrent DN [15, 16]. Although the predictive value of clinical criteria for DN in T2DM patients can be improved by the presence of proliferative retinopathy [17, 18], genetic studies that use clinical inclusion criteria (CIC) for group allocation still bear the risk of wrongly assigning patients to the DN group. In the present study, we assessed if the association between *CNDP1* and DN is still observed when applying CIC or biopsy-proven diabetic nephropathy (BP-DN) and, if so, whether this is only observed in female T2DM patients. Since also an association between the *CNDP1* $(CTG)_5$ homozygous genotype and cardiovascular mortality has been reported to be sex-specific [19], we also assessed if the prevalence of this genotype changes with diabetes duration and time on dialysis. Since T2DM patients on dialysis have a high mortality risk, it would be expected that the proportion of *CNDP1* $(CTG)_5$ homozygous patients would decrease with time on dialysis, particularly in females.

2. Materials and Methods

2.1. Patients. Patients were recruited between 2011 and 2014 from the Fifth Medical Clinic and Dialysis Unit at the University Medical Centre Mannheim and different nephrology practices in proximity (Centre for Renal Disease, Weinheim, Lindenfels, Viernheim; Nephrocare Ludwigshafen GmbH; KfH Nierenzentrum, Ludwigshafen; Nephrology Practice Frankenthal, Bad Dürkheim, Lampertheim). After screening of clinical records ($n = 384$) and patients with a biopsy-proven renal diagnosis ($n = 52$), a total of 436 patients were deemed to be eligible for this study. Due to the retrospective nature of this study, indications for renal biopsies were not uniform and the histological evaluation was undertaken by different pathologists. Out of the 436 initially selected patients, 66 were excluded because of incomplete clinical data or missing informed consent. The remaining patients ($n = 370$) were allocated to 5 different groups, that is, 130 T2DM patients without DN (no-DN), 108 T2DM patients with CIC-DN, 30 T2DM patients with BP-DN, 80 patients with CIC nondiabetic renal disease (CIC-NDRD), and 22 patients with biopsy-proven nondiabetic renal disease (BP-NDRD) (Figure 1). Patients without renal biopsy material were allocated on the basis of clinical criteria as specified below, whereas patients with renal biopsy material were allocated either to the BP-DN or to the BP-NDRD group. The ethnicity distributions in the no-DN and BP-DN groups were broadly comparable (no-DN: 75% from Germany, 12.5% from Turkey; BP-DN: 70% from Germany, 17% from Turkey).

Inclusion criteria for clinical diagnosis of DN were as follows: persistent macroalbuminuria on at least 2 independent occasions (albumin excretion rate > 300 mg/d or >200 mg/l or ACR (albumin/creatinine ratio) > 300 mg/g) in combination with the diagnosis of diabetic retinopathy (DR) (all severity degrees were allowed). This combination was obligatory to reduce the possibility that cases with proteinuria due to renal disease other than DN (NDRD) were included [20]. Anuric patients with a history of macroalbuminuria were included. Exclusion criteria were urinary tract infection or fever at the time of urine investigation, documented renal disease other than DN, and a history of kidney transplantation.

T2DM patients without DN (=control group) fulfilled the following criteria: diabetes duration of at least 15 years accompanied by normoalbuminuria on at least two independent occasions (albumin excretion rate < 30 mg/d or <20 mg/l or ACR< 30 mg/g). Since approximately 80% of the diabetic patients in this group were on ACE inhibitors or AT_1 blockers, false-negative results based on albuminuria could not be excluded. However, to minimize the possibility of DN patients in the control group, only the normoalbuminuric patients with no or mild nonproliferate DR were included since the presence of nephropathy without significant DR is rare [18, 21, 22]. Diabetes mellitus was defined by a documented history of diabetes or a fasting blood glucose of ≥7.0 mmol/l (126 mg/dl), a casual plasma glucose level of ≥11.1 mmol/l (200 mg/dl), or a HbA1c level of ≥6.5%.

Nondiabetic patients with ESRD were included in the CIC-NDRD group ($n = 80$) after screening of patient records and medications along with laboratory testing for plasma glucose or HbA1c levels to exclude diabetes.

Out of the whole cohort, 175 patients were on hemodialysis including 90 diabetic patients and 85 NDRD patients. Patients were dialyzed using a blood flow rate of 200–300 ml/min and a dialysate flow rate of approximately 500 ml/min.

Estimated GFR was calculated based on the MDRD formula [23]. Serum was used to measure CN-1 activity and concentration. Genotyping was performed on EDTA blood. All samples were stored at −20°C until use. The study protocol was approved by the local ethics committee, and all patients gave written informed consent prior to the study enrollment (no. 0193/2001).

2.2. Genotyping. Genomic DNA was isolated from whole blood using the Genomic DNA isolation kit (Promega, Mannheim, Germany) according to the manufacturer's instruction and stored at −20°C until use. A 167-base pair fragment spanning the $(CTG)_n$ polymorphism of *CNDP1* was amplified by standard PCR methods using a fluorescence

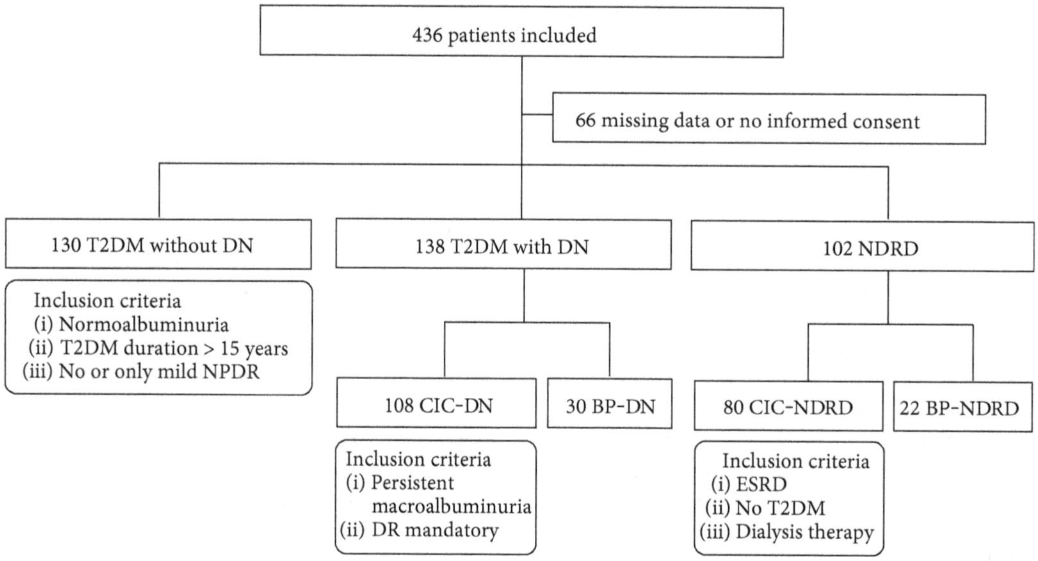

Figure 1: Flow diagram for patient recruitment and group allocation. DN: diabetic nephropathy, NDRD: nondiabetic renal disease, NPDR: nonproliferative diabetic retinopathy, CIC: clinical inclusion criteria, BP: biopsy-proven, DR: diabetic retinopathy, ESRD: end-stage renal disease.

labeled forward primer (5′FAM-AGGCAGCTGTGTGAGG TAAC-3′) and an unlabeled reverse primer (5′-GGGTGAG GAGAACATGCC-3′), respectively. Genotyping was performed by means of fragment analysis on an ABI 310 sequencing platform (ABI PRISM DNA analyzer 3100).

2.3. CN-1 Activity Assay. CN-1 activity was assayed based on the method described by Teufel et al. [24].

2.4. Statistical Analysis. Quantitative data are depicted as median with corresponding 25th and 75th percentiles (interquartile range) or, when appropriate, as mean ± SEM. Student's *t*-test was carried out for comparison of continuous variables. Qualitative data were analyzed using the χ^2 test. For pairwise comparisons, frequency tables were partitioned into respective 2×2 subtables. The significance level was corrected using the Bonferroni method based on the number of planned comparisons. Univariate and multivariate logistic regression analyses were performed to examine predictors of biopsy-proven diabetic nephropathy. Variables with a P value of <0.25 in the univariate analysis were included into a full-model multivariate analysis. To compare frequencies among groups, which have an ordering, the χ^2 test for trend (Cochran-Armitage test for trend) was carried out. Time on hemodialysis was logarithmically transformed before the correlation analysis because of its skewed distribution. The significance level α was defined as 0.05. Statistical analyses were performed with GraphPad Prism 6.0 (GraphPad Software, Inc., La Jolla, California) and Microsoft Excel/XLSTAT 19.01 (Addinsoft, New York, USA).

3. Results

3.1. Patient Characteristics. Demographic and clinical characteristics of all studied individuals are presented in Table 1. Significantly more male patients (64%) were recruited in the CIC-DN group (males: $n = 69$, females: $n = 39$) as compared to the no-DN group (50%) (males: $n = 65$, females: $n = 65$). Gender distribution in the other groups resembled the CIC-DN group (CIC-NDRD: 61% males, BP-DN: 70% males and BP-NDRD: 64% males). BP-NDRD patients were diagnosed with hypertensive nephrosclerosis, IgA nephropathy, lupus nephritis, or other categories of glomerulonephritis (e.g., granulomatosis with polyangiitis and minimal change GN). Irrespective of subgroup analyses, the distribution of the most prevalent ethnicities was comparable in the no-DN and BP-DN groups as determined by means of χ^2 test. Also, the frequency of $(CTG)_5$ homozygosity did not differ between the two major ethnicities, German and Turkish.

It should be noted that in the group of BP-DN, DM duration was shorter (time from DM diagnosis: 14 (9–20) years versus 21.0 (15–29) years, BP-DN versus CIC-DN) with more severe hyperglycemia and albuminuria (HbA1c: 7.6 (6.7–8.8) % versus 7.3 (6.8–8.2) %, albuminuria: 2070 (337–3290) mg/l versus 644 (327–2110) mg/l, BP-DN versus CIC-DN).

3.2. Association of the CNDP1 $(CTG)_5$ Homozygous Genotype with Diabetic Nephropathy. If diagnosis of DN was based on CIC alone, the frequency of the homozygous $(CTG)_5$ genotype did not significantly differ between the no-DN and CIC-DN groups (Figure 2(a), 36% versus 38%). The frequency of the protective genotype dropped to 17% when biopsy-proven DN was considered only (36% versus 17%; no-DN versus BP-DN, $P < 0.05$, NS after Bonferroni correction) (Figure 2(a)).

To confirm the previous findings of the sex-specific association between DN and the homozygous $(CTG)_5$ genotype, patients were stratified according to gender. In male patients, neither CIC-DN nor BP-DN was associated with $(CTG)_5$ homozygosity when compared to no-DN (no-DN: 34%, CIC-DN: 42%, BP-DN: 24%) (Figure 2(b)). Although the

Table 1: Demographic and clinical data of all patients.

	No-DN	CIC-DN	BP-DN	CIC-NDRD	BP-NDRD
N	130	108	30	80	22
Demographic characteristics					
Male sex—*n* (%)	65 (50)	69 (64)	21 (70)	49 (61)	14 (64)
Age—year	71 (63–75)	71 (62–76)	61 (57–69)	61 (48–74)	61 (55–78)
Clinical characteristics					
Body mass index—kg/m^2	31.1 (28–35)	29.8 (27–35)	29.9 (25–35)	24.5 (21–27)	27 (24–32)
Hypertension					
Number of AHM	3 (2–3)	3 (2–4)	3 (2–5)	3 (1.5–4)	2 (2–4)
Blood pressure—mmHg					
Systolic	129 (120–140)	135 (120–156)	140 (130–150)	135 (120–145)	140 (128–153)
Diastolic	70 (66–80)	70 (60–80)	75 (70–80)	70 (60–80)	70 (64–80)
Diabetes mellitus					
Time from diagnosis—year	16 (13–20)	21 (15–29)	14 (9–20)	—	—
HbA1c—%	7.0 (6.4–8.1)	7.3 (6.8–8.2)	7.6 (6.7–8.8)	5.6 (5.4–5.7)	5.6 (5.1–6.2)
Kidney function					
Creatinine—mg/dl	0.9 (0.8–1.1)	6.3 (3.7–8.8)	5.7 (3.0–7.3)	9.7 (7.5–11.5)	3.4 (1.7–5.0)
eGFR—ml/min	73 (61–87)	9 (6–16)	10 (6–20)	5 (4–8)	15 (8–37)
Hemodialysis—*n* (%)	0 (0)	83 (75)	18 (60)	85 (100)	8 (36)
HD duration—months*	0 (0–0)	26 (1–69)	3 (0–30)	56 (28–100)	0 (0–0.3)
Albuminuria—mg/l	9 (5–16)	644 (327–2110)	2070 (337–3290)	470 (261–1587)	556 (189–1308)
Retinopathy (DR)—n (%)					
No DR	107 (82)	1 (0)	6 (20)	—	—
NPDR	23 (18)	68 (63)	11 (37)	—	—
Proliferative DR	—	17 (16)	4 (13)	—	—
Maculopathy	—	8 (7)	3 (10)	—	—
Laser therapy	—	13 (12)	3 (10)	—	—
Polyneuropathy—*n* (%)	54 (42)	56 (52)	17 (57)	—	—
History—n (%)					
Coronary heart disease	42 (32)	74 (69)	11 (37)	24 (30)	6 (22)
Cardiovascular event	20 (15)	42 (39)	7 (23)	14 (18)	5 (23)
Arterial occlusive disease	24 (18)	56 (52)	11 (37)	17 (21)	3 (14)
Stroke	19 (15)	28 (26)	6 (20)	8 (10)	2 (9)
Statin	86 (66)	79 (73)	19 (63)	28 (35)	10 (45)
Homozygous CTG$_5$—*n* (%)	47 (36)	41 (38)	5 (17)	32 (40)	7 (32)

*Patients on hemodialysis only. Categorical data are represented as numbers (%) and continuous data as median with corresponding 25th and 75th percentiles (IQR). AHM: antihypertensive medication; eGFR: estimated glomerular filtration rate; HD: hemodialysis; DR: diabetic retinopathy; NPDR: nonproliferative diabetic retinopathy.

homozygous (CTG)$_5$ genotype was less frequent in both the female CIC-DN and the female BP-DN groups as compared to the no-DN group, this difference was only significant for BP-DN (38% versus 0%, no-DN versus BP-DN, $P < 0.05$, significant after Bonferroni correction) (Figure 2(c)).

To confirm that (CTG)$_5$ homozygosity is an independent, negative predictor for biopsy-proven diabetic nephropathy, multivariate logistic regression analysis was performed (Table 2). Seven diabetes-associated factors were selected as independent variables (age, BMI, diabetes duration, HbA1c, male sex, systolic blood pressure, and (CTG)$_5$ homozygosity). All variables except BMI showed a P value below 0.25 in univariate analysis and were consequently included in the multivariate model. The Hosmer-Lemeshow test demonstrated an excellent goodness of fit ($\chi^2 = 3949$, $P = 0.862$) of the resulting multivariate model. The area under the receiver operating characteristic curve (ROC-AUC) further indicated adequate discrimination (AUC = 0.797).

The (CTG)$_5$ homozygous genotype was significantly associated with biopsy-proven nephropathy in both univariate (OR = 0.353, $P = 0.047$) and multivariate analyses (OR = 0.307, $P = 0.046$) and, as such, identified as an independent protective factor. Interestingly, significance was reached despite the markedly lower number of cases ($n = 30$) generally

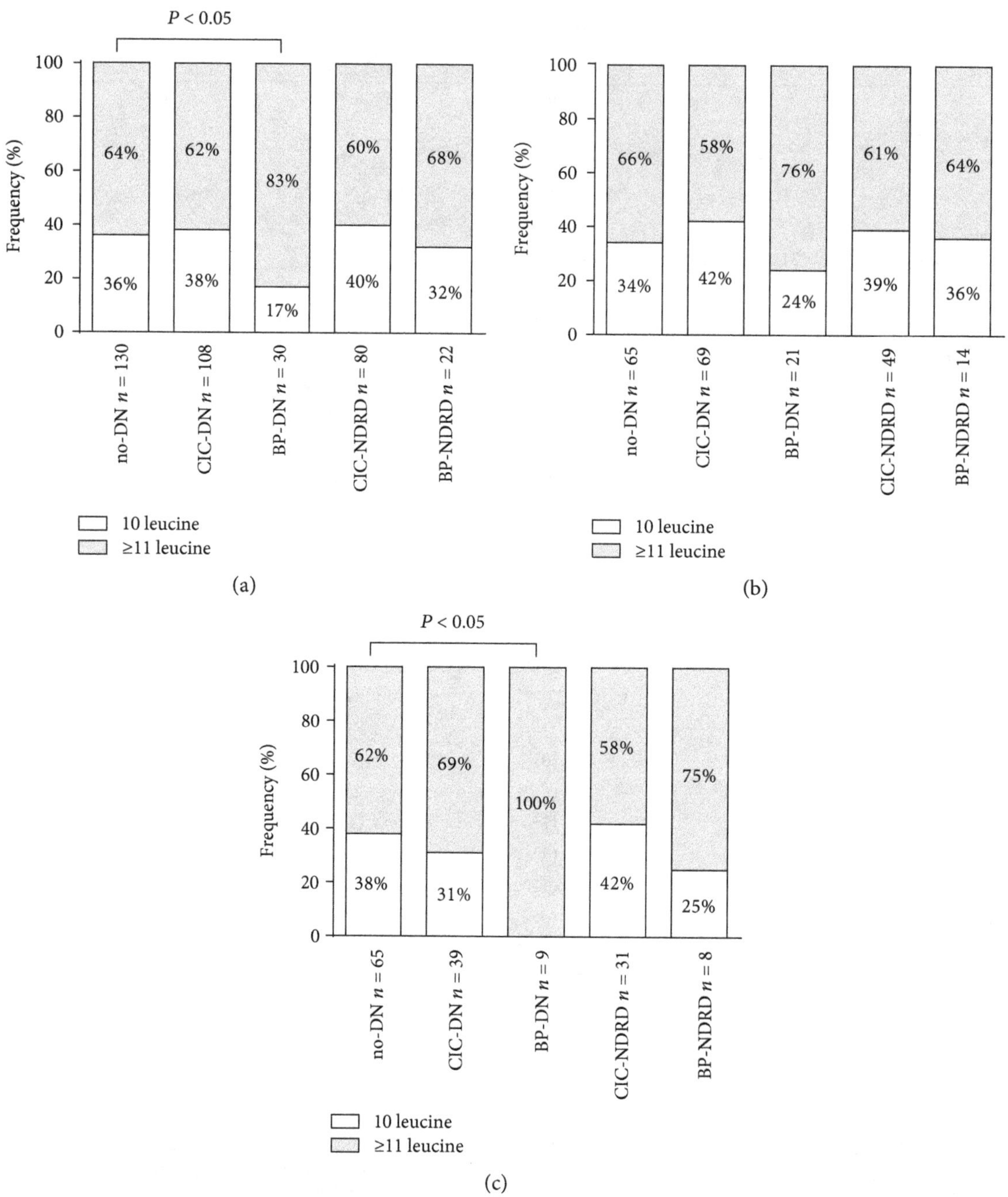

FIGURE 2: *CNDP1* $(CTG)_n$ genotype distribution in T2DM patients. Genotype distribution is depicted as homozygosity for the $(CTG)_5$ allele (10 leucine) versus all other genotypes (≥11 leucine). Planned comparisons were carried out between T2DM patients without DN and with either CIC- or BP-defined nephropathy. (a) No significant difference in genotype distribution was observed between T2DM patients with DN and without DN when applying CIC. The frequency of patients homozygous for the $(CTG)_5$ allele decreased when BP-DN was considered. However, this difference did not hold after Bonferroni correction. ((b) and (c)) Gender stratification ((b) male patients, (c) female patients) showed no significant difference in the frequency of homozygosity for the *CNDP1* $(CTG)_5$ allele between T2DM with and without DN when applying CIC. When DN was confirmed through biopsy, however, the frequency of *CNDP1* $(CTG)_5$ homozygosity significantly decreased in female T2DM patients, which remained significant after Bonferroni adjustment.

believed to be necessary for obtaining sufficient power (i.e., $n = 10$/independent variable). In the multivariate model, systolic blood pressure (OR = 1.024, $P = 0.045$) was positively and age (OR = 0.931, $P = 0.007$) and diabetes duration (OR = 0.895, $P = 0.025$) were negatively associated with biopsy-proven nephropathy, respectively.

3.3. CNDP1 Genotype Distribution over Time on Hemodialysis and Diabetes Duration. The *CNDP1* genotype distribution (*CNDP1* $(CTG)_5$ homozygous—versus all other *CNDP1* genotypes) was tested in 175 patients on hemodialysis, including 90 patients with DN according to CIC and/or BP-DN and 85 CIC-NDRD patients. Patients were stratified

Table 2: Summary of logistic regression analysis of variables predicting biopsy-proven diabetic nephropathy (male and female, $n = 160$).

	Univariate analysis			Multivariate analysis		
	OR	95% CI	P value	OR	95% CI	P value
Age (years)	0.920	0.881–0.961	<0.001	0.931	0.883–0.980	0.007
BMI (kg/m^2)	0.980	0.922–1.041	0.513	—	—	—
Diabetes duration (years)	0.886	0.813–0.966	0.006	0.895	0.812–0.986	0.025
HbA1c (%)	1.308	1.020–1.678	0.034	1.169	0.844–1.619	0.348
Male sex	2.333	0.994–5.477	0.052	1.957	0.748–5.124	0.171
SBP (mmHg)	1.021	1.000–1.042	0.052	1.024	1.001–1.047	0.045
CTG$_5$ homozygosity	0.353	0.127–0.984	0.047	0.307	0.096–0.980	0.046

Area under the ROC curve (AUC) = 0.797, $P = 0.862$ for Hosmer-Lemeshow test. BMI: body mass index; SBP: systolic blood pressure.

on the basis of hemodialysis duration, that is, time on dialysis: <30 months ($n = 60$), between 30 and 100 months ($n = 76$) and >100 months ($n = 39$). To assess the frequencies over time on hemodialysis and diabetes duration, the χ^2 test for trend was carried out.

The frequency of the (CTG)$_5$ homozygous genotype significantly increased with time on hemodialysis (<30 months: 33%, 30–100 months: 40%, >100 months: 49%, $P < 0.05$) (Figure 3(a)), while gender distribution was approximately equal in the groups. The association of the (CTG)$_5$ homozygous genotype with time on hemodialysis was not significant in the subgroup analyses after gender stratification (contingency tables not shown).

Although the frequency of the homozygous *CNDP1* (CTG)$_5$ genotype uniformly increased with diabetes duration, this trend did not reach statistical significance (<10 years: 27%, 10–15 years: 34%, 16–20 years: 37%, >20 years: 42%, $P = 0.17$) (Figure 3(b)). However, if patients with a heterozygous *CNDP1* (CTG)$_5$ genotype were included (i.e., patients with at least one (CTG)$_5$ allele), there was a clear, significant trend towards high frequencies with increasing diabetes duration (<10 years: 64%, 10–15 years: 75%, 16–20 years: 87%, >20 years: 90%, $P < 0.01$) (Figure 3(c)).

3.4. CN-1 Activities in Hemodialysis Patients. Because serum carnosinase (CN-1) activity correlates with *CNDP1* (CTG)$_n$ genotypes, that is, CN-1 activity is in general lower in individuals with less CTG copies, we also cross-sectionally assessed if serum CN-1 activity changes with time on dialysis. In line with the increased frequency of the homozygous *CNDP1* (CTG)$_5$ genotype in the groups of patients with a long history of hemodialysis, a significant negative correlation between serum CN-1 activity and log-transformed hemodialysis duration was found in all patients ($r = -0.33$; $P < 0.0001$, Figure 4(a)), T2DM patients only ($r = -0.034$, $P = 0.0006$, Figure 4(b)), and nondiabetic hemodialysis patients ($r = -0,031$, $P = 0.004$, Figure 4(c)).

To delineate if the *CNDP1* genotype is relevant for CN-1 activities in hemodialysis patients, patients on hemodialysis were stratified on the basis of homozygosity for the (CTG)$_5$ allele. Out of 174 subjects, the 65 patients carrying the homozygous *CNDP1* (CTG)$_5$ genotype showed a significantly lower serum CN-1 activity compared to patients with other genotypes (Figure 5(a), $P < 0.01$). This remained significant in female (Figure 5(c), $P < 0.05$), but not in male (Figure 5(b), $P = 0.07$) patients after gender stratification.

4. Discussion

This study examined whether the protection against DN afforded by the homozygous *CNDP1* (CTG)$_5$ genotype is still observed when applying clinical inclusion criteria or biopsy findings only and if the prevalence of the protective genotype changes in situations of increased cardiovascular mortality. Our results demonstrate that the frequency of the homozygous *CNDP1* (CTG)$_5$ genotype in the group of patients with biopsy-proven DN is significantly lower as compared to the groups of patients with no DN or with other biopsy-proven nephropathies. Our study also indicates that the frequency of homozygous *CNDP1* (CTG)$_5$ genotype tends to be higher in patients with a longer duration of hemodialysis, particularly in female patients. An analogous increase was detected for patients carrying at least one (CTG)$_5$ allele stratified for diabetes duration.

CIC for group allocations in DN studies bears the risk of wrongly assigning patients to the DN group as up to 20–50% of diabetic patients with albuminuria develop NDRD without concurrent DN [25, 26]. Although the presence of diabetic retinopathy (DR) is helpful for the prediction of DN [27] and thus improves the validity of group allocation, still DR may be absent in up to 50% of DN patients [28, 29]. Controversial studies reporting on genetic susceptibility loci for DN, including those for the *CNDP1* (CTG)$_n$ polymorphism, might partly underlie this problem.

The use of large cohorts from different consortia and subsequent meta-analysis of data obtained from genome-wide association studies (GWAS) may partly overcome this problem as the proportion of wrongly allocated patients might be outnumbered by the large number of studied patients. The GWAS approach has been successfully utilized in newer studies confirming susceptibility loci for declining glomerular filtration rate (eGFR) or albuminuria [30–32]. The *CNDP1* locus, a postulated DN susceptibility locus found by positional cloning [5] and case control studies [10], has

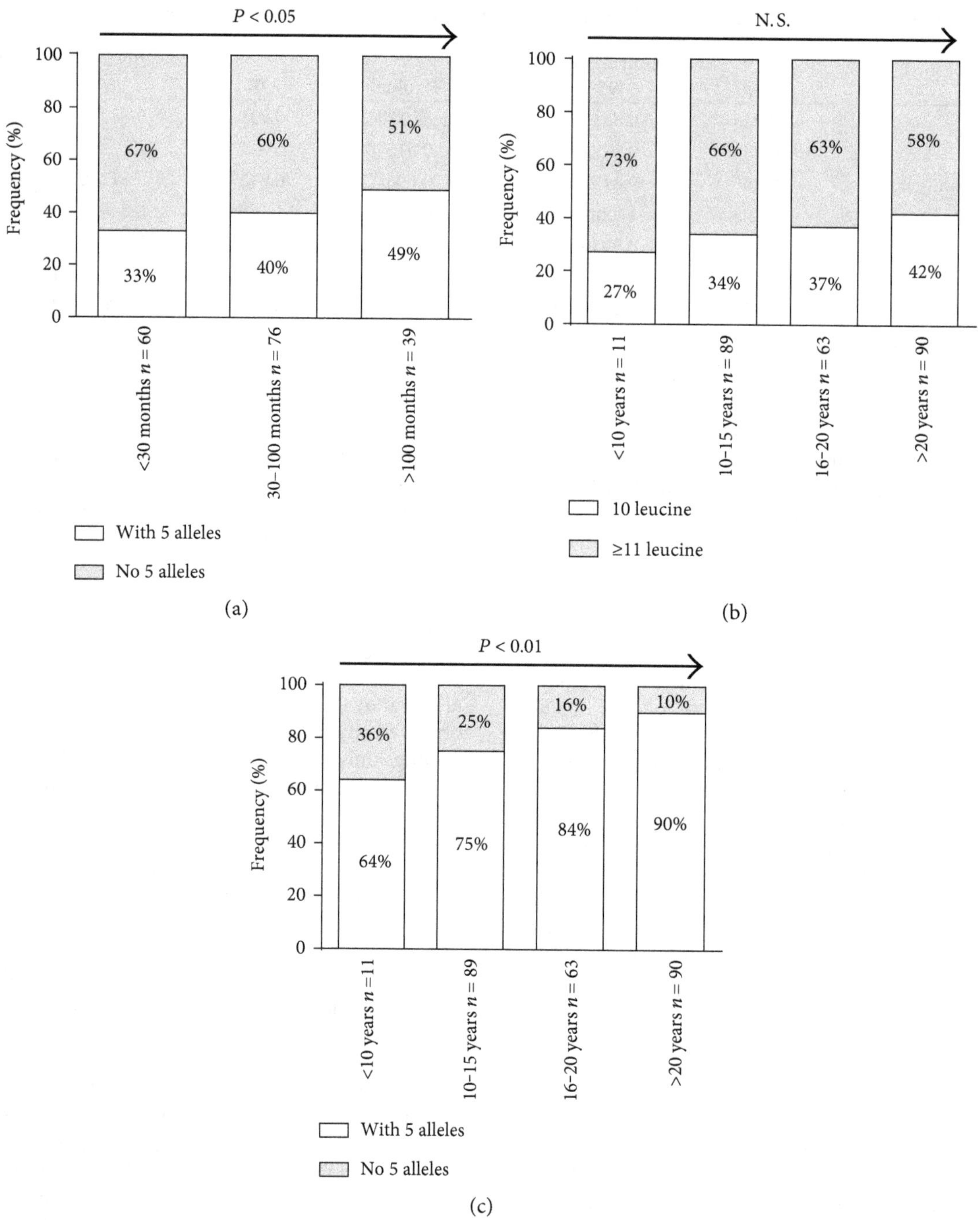

FIGURE 3: The *CNDP1* $(CTG)_5$ genotype distribution is changed with time on dialysis and diabetes duration. To assess if the frequencies change over time, the χ^2 test for trend (Cochran-Armitage test for trend) was carried out. (a) The frequency of the homozygous *CNDP1* $(CTG)_5$ genotype (10 leucine) significantly increased with time on hemodialysis. ((b) and (c)) Although the observed frequency of the homozygous (b) *CNDP1* $(CTG)_5$ genotype uniformly increased with diabetes duration, this trend did not reach statistical significance. Yet, if patients with a heterozygous (c) *CNDP1* $(CTG)_5$ genotype (one 5 allele) were included as well, a significant trend towards high frequencies with increasing diabetes duration was found. N.S.: not significant.

never been reported to be linked to DN in a GWAS approach, despite the fact that other genetic studies [11, 14, 33, 34] including a meta-analysis on 4546 DN, 7994 diabetes mellitus (DM), and 1826 healthy subjects [35] have confirmed an association between the *CNDP1* $(CTG)_n$ polymorphism and DN in T2DM patients. Significance further increased in these studies if more stringent CIC for DN, for example, the presence of proliferative DR and a longer duration of T2DM, were considered [11].

In our study, the association between the protective homozygous *CNDP1* $(CTG)_5$ genotype and DN was restricted to biopsy-proven DN and only significant in female patients using the χ^2 test. Multivariate logistic regression subsequently identified $(CTG)_5$ homozygosity as an independent protective

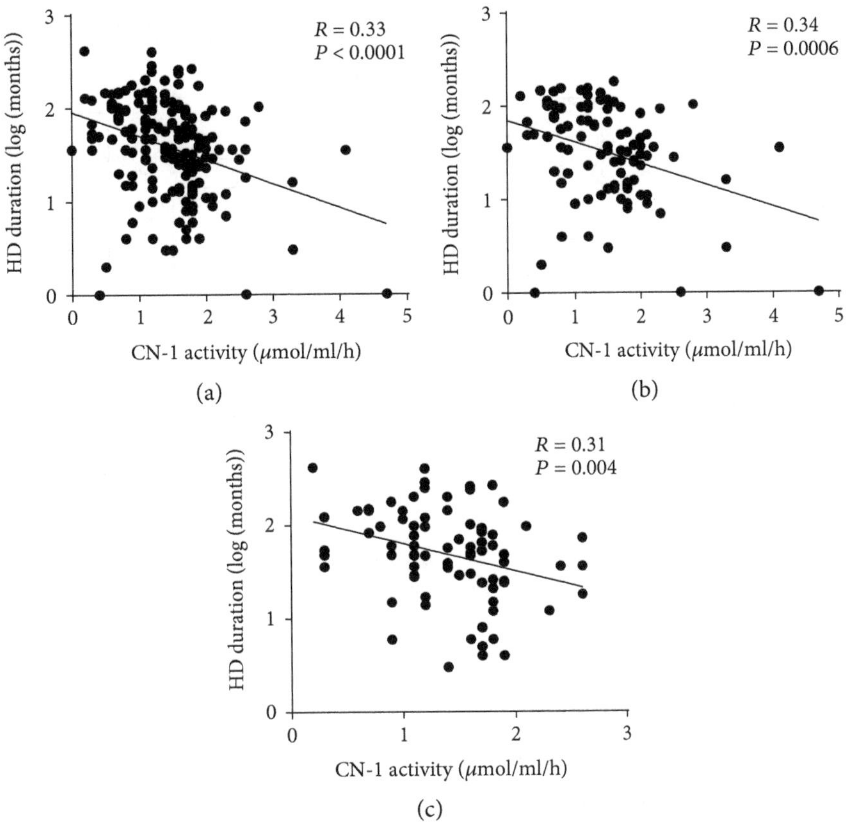

Figure 4: CN-1 activities decrease with time on dialysis. (a) Serum CN-1 activity was assessed in 175 hemodialysis patients and plotted against the log-transformed duration since hemodialysis was initiated. A significant correlation between serum CN-1 activity and log-transformed hemodialysis duration was found in all patients. ((b) and (c)) After stratification in T2DM (b) and other causes of renal failure (c), the correlation remained significant. HD: hemodialysis.

factor for biopsy-proven DN with an odds ratio of approximately 0.3. The negative association of age and diabetes duration with biopsy-proven DN in this analysis may be explained by the fact that in older diabetic patients, a renal biopsy is often waived due to the lack of consequence.

The frequencies of the homozygous *CNDP1* $(CTG)_5$ genotype in the no-DN and BP-NDRD groups were comparable, suggesting that this genotype does not afford protection against NDRD. Nonetheless, it would be prudent to be cautious with this assumption as other studies have suggested that this genotype also affords protection against other chronic kidney diseases (CKD), for example, glomerulonephritis but not tubulointerstitial nephritis [36]. In this light, the paradox between CIC-DN and BP-DN might be due to the fact that patients with NDRD were falsely included in the CIC-DN group, underscoring that clinical criteria do not provide a sufficient certainty for the diagnosis of DN in T2DM patients. It is important to note that patients in the BP-DN group had a shorter DM duration and displayed more severe hyperglycemia and albuminuria as compared to the CIC-DN group. Because of this relatively atypical DN course, these patients required a biopsy to clarify the actual underlying renal disease. Whether the change in *CNDP1* genotype distribution between CIC-DN and BP-DN underlies the severity of disease per se is unknown so far and cannot be excluded.

Our data are in agreement with a previous publication showing that the association of *CNDP1* and DN is most likely sex-specific [14]. Although also in males of the BP-DN group the frequency of the $(CTG)_5$ homozygous genotype was lower as compared to the no-DN group, it was only significantly decreased in female BP-DN patients. The sex-specific protection of *CNDP1* is generally explained by higher serum CN-1 activities in females [14].

In keeping with the recently published prospective study that the *CNDP1* genotype may impart a cardiovascular mortality risk in female, but not in male T2DM patients [19], we investigated whether genotype distribution changes with time on dialysis or diabetes duration. Since both of the latter variables are associated with an increased (cardiovascular) mortality risk, it would be expected based on the above study that the frequency of the homozygous *CNDP1* $(CTG)_5$ genotype would decrease rather than increase in patients with a long history of hemodialysis. By contrast, our data show that the frequency of the homozygous *CNDP1* $(CTG)_5$ genotype was significantly increased in patients with a long history of hemodialysis. This difference remained in both males and females although it was not statistically significant, which is likely explained by the small sample size of the subgroup analysis. Similar findings were also observed with respect to a longstanding diabetes duration when all patients carrying at least one $(CTG)_5$ allele were included.

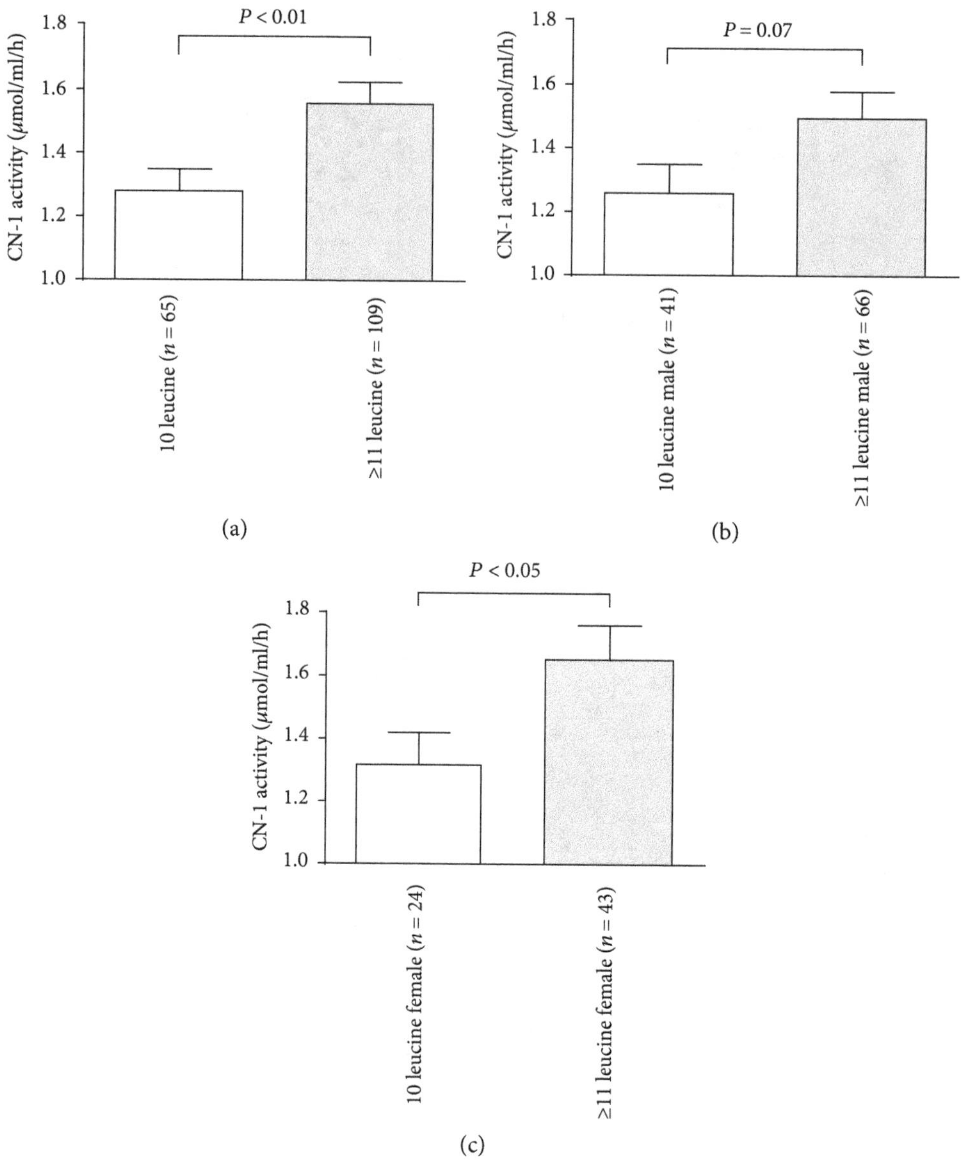

FIGURE 5: CN-1 activity correlates with *CNDP1* genotype in hemodialysis patients. (a) CN-1 activity in $(CTG)_5$ homozygous hemodialysis patients is significantly lower than that in patients carrying other genotypes. ((b) and (c)) After gender stratification differences in CN-1 activity between the $(CTG)_5$ homozygous, all other genotypes remained but only reached statistical significance in females (c).

Although our findings suggest that in patients on hemodialysis and in diabetic patients the *CNDP1* $(CTG)_5$ genotype may not impart an additional mortality risk, it should be underscored that the small group sizes and the cross-sectional design of this study impede drawing firm conclusions, in particular since a considerable number of hemodialysis patients were not diabetic. Nonetheless, these findings suggest that in patients on hemodialysis and in diabetes, the *CNDP1* $(CTG)_5$ genotype may not impart an additional mortality risk.

Serum CN-1 concentrations and activities are in part determined by $(CTG)_n$ polymorphism [10, 37]. Since this repeat is located in the hydrophobic part of the CN-1 signal peptide and is essential for the translocation of CN-1 protein during secretion, it is believed that the shorter $(CTG)_5$ variant is less efficiently secreted [37]. In line with an increased frequency of the homozygous *CNDP1* $(CTG)_5$ genotype in patients with a long history of hemodialysis, CN-1 activities were reduced. This reduction is not due to the loss of protein through hemofiltration since serum CN-1 concentrations even increase proportionally to the amount of ultrafiltrate [38].

As discussed above, we acknowledge the relatively small sample size as a major limitation of our study, accounting for a limited statistical power regarding major questions addressed. In addition, in contrast to a prospective study design, no systematic biopsy strategy with uniform indications and assigned nephropathologists could be implemented. Other studies, however, demonstrated that the histological classification of DN based on glomerulopathy shows a satisfying interobserver reproducibility [39]. We also acknowledge uncertainties regarding the procedure of patient allocation leading to limited group selectivity. This holds true especially for the diabetic control group without DN, which is based only on clinical criteria instead of a histological diagnosis. As 80% of these patients were on ACE inhibitor or AT_1-blocking drugs, albuminuria alone was not a reliable parameter. Despite the extension of the criteria by diabetes duration of >15 years and exclusion of patients which manifest retinopathy, accidental assignment of patients with DN to this group is not improbable.

In our eyes, the fact that this study still resulted in significant results in the light of these conceptual drawbacks supports a particular strong association of our findings. Our study supports the hypothesis that protection against DN is indeed afforded by the *CNDP1* $(CTG)_5$ genotype and that this association mainly applies to female T2DM patients. The restriction of this finding to the BP-DN group may be attributed to false allocation of patients with other proteinuric diseases to the CIC-DN group. In fact, 20–50% of diabetic patients with proteinuria display NDRD without concurrent DN [25, 26]. Our investigation also suggests that $(CTG)_5$ homozygous hemodialysis patients and patients with diabetes carrying at least one $(CTG)_5$ allele might have a survival benefit as compared to other genotypes. These findings warrant further conformational studies, ideally with a prospective longitudinal design.

Conflicts of Interest

The authors declare that they have no conflicts of interest.

Authors' Contributions

Thomas Albrecht and Shiqi Zhang are equally contributing authors.

Acknowledgments

This work was supported by the Deutsche Forschungsgemeinschaft (DFG) SA 2143/1-1 to Sibylle J. Hauske and Graduiertenkolleg (GRK) 1874/1 to Benito A. Yard and Sibylle J. Hauske. The authors would like to thank all involved Dialysis Units and Diabetic Centers for supporting the recruitment of patients. The authors would also like to thank Annette Breedijk (University Medical Center Mannheim) for her invaluable technical assistance and David Papke (Harvard Medical School, Boston, USA) for proofreading this manuscript.

References

[1] C. H. Hasslacher, E. Ritz, P. Wahl, and C. Michael, "Similar risks of nephropathy in patients with type I or type II diabetes mellitus," *Nephrology, Dialysis, Transplantation*, vol. 4, no. 10, pp. 859–863, 1989.

[2] J. William, D. Hogan, and D. Batlle, "Predicting the development of diabetic nephropathy and its progression," *Advances in Chronic Kidney Disease*, vol. 12, no. 2, pp. 202–211, 2005.

[3] E. R. Seaquist, F. C. Goetz, S. Rich, and J. Barbosa, "Familial clustering of diabetic kidney disease. Evidence for genetic susceptibility to diabetic nephropathy," *The New England Journal of Medicine*, vol. 320, no. 18, pp. 1161–1165, 1989.

[4] B. I. Freedman, D. W. Bowden, M. M. Sale, C. D. Langefeld, and S. S. Rich, "Genetic susceptibility contributes to renal and cardiovascular complications of type 2 diabetes mellitus," *Hypertension*, vol. 48, no. 1, pp. 8–13, 2006.

[5] I. Vardarli, L. J. Baier, R. L. Hanson et al., "Gene for susceptibility to diabetic nephropathy in type 2 diabetes maps to 18q22.3-23," *Kidney International*, vol. 62, no. 6, pp. 2176–2183, 2002.

[6] D. W. Bowden, C. J. Colicigno, C. D. Langefeld et al., "A genome scan for diabetic nephropathy in African Americans," *Kidney International*, vol. 66, no. 4, pp. 1517–1526, 2004.

[7] S. K. Iyengar, H. E. Abboud, K. A. Goddard et al., "Genome-wide scans for diabetic nephropathy and albuminuria in multiethnic populations: the family investigation of nephropathy and diabetes (FIND)," *Diabetes*, vol. 56, no. 6, pp. 1577–1585, 2007.

[8] H. A. Chakkera, R. L. Hanson, S. Kobes et al., "Association of variants in the carnosine peptidase 1 gene (CNDP1) with diabetic nephropathy in American Indians," *Molecular Genetics and Metabolism*, vol. 103, no. 2, pp. 185–190, 2011.

[9] C. W. McDonough, P. J. Hicks, L. Lu, C. D. Langefeld, B. I. Freedman, and D. W. Bowden, "The influence of carnosinase gene polymorphisms on diabetic nephropathy risk in African-Americans," *Human Genetics*, vol. 126, no. 2, pp. 265–275, 2009.

[10] B. Janssen, D. Hohenadel, P. Brinkkoetter et al., "Carnosine as a protective factor in diabetic nephropathy: association with a leucine repeat of the carnosinase gene CNDP1," *Diabetes*, vol. 54, no. 8, pp. 2320–2327, 2005.

[11] B. I. Freedman, P. J. Hicks, M. M. Sale et al., "A leucine repeat in the carnosinase gene CNDP1 is associated with diabetic end-stage renal disease in European Americans," *Nephrology, Dialysis, Transplantation*, vol. 22, no. 4, pp. 1131–1135, 2007.

[12] P. Y. Poon, C. C. Szeto, B. C. Kwan, K. M. Chow, and P. K. Li, "Relationship between carnosinase gene CNDP1 leucine repeat polymorphism and the clinical outcome of Chinese PD patients," *Clinical Nephrology*, vol. 74, no. 5, pp. 343–345, 2010.

[13] A. L. Mooyaart, I. G. van Valkengoed, P. C. Shaw et al., "Lower frequency of the 5/5 homozygous CNDP1 genotype in South Asian Surinamese," *Diabetes Research and Clinical Practice*, vol. 85, no. 3, pp. 272–278, 2009.

[14] A. L. Mooyaart, A. Zutinic, S. J. Bakker et al., "Association between CNDP1 genotype and diabetic nephropathy is sex specific," *Diabetes*, vol. 59, no. 6, pp. 1555–1559, 2010.

[15] T. T. Pham, J. J. Sim, D. A. Kujubu, I. L. Liu, and V. A. Kumar, "Prevalence of nondiabetic renal disease in diabetic patients," *American Journal of Nephrology*, vol. 27, no. 3, pp. 322–328, 2007.

[16] S. Olsen and C. E. Mogensen, "How often is NIDDM complicated with non-diabetic renal disease? An analysis of renal biopsies and the literature," *Diabetologia*, vol. 39, no. 12, pp. 1638–1645, 1996.

[17] R. Klein, B. E. Klein, and S. E. Moss, "Epidemiology of proliferative diabetic retinopathy," *Diabetes Care*, vol. 15, no. 12, pp. 1875–1891, 1992.

[18] A. Chandy, B. Pawar, M. John, and R. Isaac, "Association between diabetic nephropathy and other diabetic

microvascular and macrovascular complications," *Saudi Journal of Kidney Diseases and Transplantation*, vol. 19, no. 6, pp. 924–928, 2008.

[19] A. Alkhalaf, G. W. Landman, K. J. van Hateren et al., "Sex specific association between carnosinase gene CNDP1 and cardiovascular mortality in patients with type 2 diabetes (ZODIAC-22)," *Journal of Nephrology*, vol. 28, no. 2, pp. 201–207, 2015.

[20] H. H. Parving, M. A. Gall, P. Skøtt et al., "Prevalence and causes of albuminuria in non-insulin-dependent diabetic patients," *Kidney International*, vol. 41, no. 4, pp. 758–762, 1992.

[21] M. Kanauchi, T. Kawano, H. Uyama, H. Shiiki, and K. Dohi, "Discordance between retinopathy and nephropathy in type 2 diabetes," *Nephron*, vol. 80, no. 2, pp. 171–174, 1998.

[22] R. A. Pedro, S. A. Ramon, B. B. Marc, F. B. Juan, and M. M. Isabel, "Prevalence and relationship between diabetic retinopathy and nephropathy, and its risk factors in the north-east of Spain, a population-based study," *Ophthalmic Epidemiology*, vol. 17, no. 4, pp. 251–265, 2010.

[23] A. S. Levey, J. P. Bosch, J. B. Lewis, T. Greene, N. Rogers, and D. Roth, "A more accurate method to estimate glomerular filtration rate from serum creatinine: a new prediction equation. Modification of Diet in Renal Disease Study Group," *Annals of Internal Medicine*, vol. 130, no. 6, pp. 461–470, 1999.

[24] M. Teufel, V. Saudek, J. P. Ledig et al., "Sequence identification and characterization of human carnosinase and a closely related non-specific dipeptidase," *The Journal of Biological Chemistry*, vol. 278, no. 8, pp. 6521–6531, 2003.

[25] T. Soleymanian, G. Hamid, M. Arefi et al., "Non-diabetic renal disease with or without diabetic nephropathy in type 2 diabetes: clinical predictors and outcome," *Renal Failure*, vol. 37, no. 4, pp. 572–575, 2015.

[26] S. S. Soni, S. Gowrishankar, A. G. Kishan, and A. Raman, "Non diabetic renal disease in type 2 diabetes mellitus," *Nephrology (Carlton, Vic.)*, vol. 11, no. 6, pp. 533–537, 2006.

[27] F. He, X. Xia, X. F. Wu, X. Q. Yu, and F. X. Huang, "Diabetic retinopathy in predicting diabetic nephropathy in patients with type 2 diabetes and renal disease: a meta-analysis," *Diabetologia*, vol. 56, no. 3, pp. 457–466, 2013.

[28] G. Wolf, N. Müller, A. Mandecka, and U. A. Müller, "Association of diabetic retinopathy and renal function in patients with types 1 and 2 diabetes mellitus," *Clinical Nephrology*, vol. 68, no. 2, pp. 81–86, 2007.

[29] J. Prakash, M. Lodha, S. K. Singh, R. Vohra, and R. Raja, "Diabetic retinopathy is a poor predictor of type of nephropathy in proteinuric type 2 diabetic patients," *The Journal of the Association of Physicians of India*, vol. 55, no. 55, pp. 412–416, 2007.

[30] A. Teumer, A. Tin, R. Sorice et al., "Genome-wide association studies identify genetic loci associated with albuminuria in diabetes," *Diabetes*, vol. 65, no. 3, pp. 803–817, 2016.

[31] C. A. Böger, M. H. Chen, A. Tin et al., "CUBN is a gene locus for albuminuria," *Journal of the American Society of Nephrology*, vol. 22, no. 3, pp. 555–570, 2011.

[32] C. Pattaro, A. Teumer, M. Gorski et al., "Genetic associations at 53 loci highlight cell types and biological pathways relevant for kidney function," *Nature Communications*, vol. 7, Article ID 10023, 2016.

[33] A. Alkhalaf, S. J. Bakker, H. J. Bilo et al., "A polymorphism in the gene encoding carnosinase (CNDP1) as a predictor of mortality and progression from nephropathy to end-stage renal disease in type 1 diabetes mellitus," *Diabetologia*, vol. 53, no. 12, pp. 2562–2568, 2010.

[34] T. S. Ahluwalia, E. Lindholm, and L. C. Groop, "Common variants in CNDP1 and CNDP2, and risk of nephropathy in type 2 diabetes," *Diabetologia*, vol. 54, no. 9, pp. 2295–2302, 2011.

[35] J. M. Zhu, B. Wang, J. Li et al., "D18S880 microsatellite polymorphism of carnosinase gene and diabetic nephropathy: a meta-analysis," *Genetic Testing and Molecular Biomarkers*, vol. 17, no. 4, pp. 289–294, 2013.

[36] K. Kiliś-Pstrusińska, D. Zwolińska, W. Grzeszczak, and S. Group, "Is carnosinase 1 gene (CNDP1) polymorphism associated with chronic kidney disease progression in children and young adults? Results of a family-based study," *Archives of Medical Research*, vol. 41, no. 5, pp. 356–362, 2010.

[37] E. Riedl, H. Koeppel, P. Brinkkoetter et al., "A CTG polymorphism in the CNDP1 gene determines the secretion of serum carnosinase in Cos-7 transfected cells," *Diabetes*, vol. 56, no. 9, pp. 2410–2413, 2007.

[38] S. Zhang, H. A. Lindner, S. Kabtni et al., "Monoclonal antibody RYSK173 recognizes the dinuclear Zn center of serum carnosinase 1 (CN-1): possible consequences of Zn binding for CN-1 recognition by RYSK173," *PLoS One*, vol. 11, no. 1, article e0146831, 2016.

[39] T. W. Tervaert, A. L. Mooyaart, K. Amann et al., "Pathologic classification of diabetic nephropathy," *Journal of the American Society of Nephrology*, vol. 21, no. 4, pp. 556–563, 2010.

19

Assessment of Vitamin D-Binding Protein and Early Prediction of Nephropathy in Type 2 Saudi Diabetic Patients

Manal S. Fawzy[1,2] **and Baraah T. Abu AlSel**[3]

[1]*Department of Biochemistry, Faculty of Medicine, Northern Border University, Arar, Saudi Arabia*
[2]*Department of Medical Biochemistry, Faculty of Medicine, Suez Canal University, Ismailia, Egypt*
[3]*Department of Microbiology, Faculty of Medicine, Northern Border University, Arar, Saudi Arabia*

Correspondence should be addressed to Manal S. Fawzy; manal2_khashana@ymail.com

Academic Editor: Suat Simsek

Early detection of diabetic nephropathy (DN) represents a great challenge in an attempt to reduce the burden of chronic kidney diseases in diabetic patients. This study aimed to investigate the potential early prediction role of urinary vitamin D-binding protein (uVDBP) for the diagnosis of DN and to examine the possible correlation to serum VDBP, high-sensitivity C-reactive protein (hs-CRP), and insulin resistance in these patients. Serum and urine samples were obtained from 40 healthy volunteers and 120 patients with type 2 diabetes divided into 3 groups: normoalbuminuria, microalbuminuria, and macroalbuminuria (urinary albumin excretion rate < 30, 30–300, and >300 μg/mg, resp.); $n = 40$/group. Serum and urinary VDBP levels were quantified by ELISA. Insulin resistance has been assessed by homeostasis model assessment index (HOMAI). Correction for urine creatinine concentration was applied for urinary quantitative measurements. uVDBP levels were significantly elevated in micro- and macroalbuminuria patient groups compared with those of the normoalbuminuria patient group and controls (820.4 ± 402.8 and 1458.1 ± 210.0 compared with 193.1 ± 141.0 and 127.7 ± 21.9 ng/mg, resp.) ($P < 0.001$). There was significant correlation between serum and urinary levels of VDBP in total patient group. Receiver operating characteristic analysis of uVDBP levels showed optimum cut-off value of 216.0 ng/mg corresponding to 98.8% sensitivity and 80.0% specificity and an area under the curve of 0.973 to discriminate the normoalbuminuria from the microalbuminuria groups. In multivariate analysis, ordination plot showed obvious demarcation between the study groups caused by the higher levels of uVDBP and albumin/creatinine ratio among other variables. The study findings suggested a possible clinical application of uVDPB as an early and a good marker for the detection of early renal disease in type 2 DM Saudi patients. Large-scale validation studies are warranted to confirm the results before including uVDBP with the available list of other conventional biomarkers.

1. Introduction

Diabetes mellitus (DM) is one of the most growing chronic diseases worldwide, and its incidence has been speculated to rise up to 500 million by 2030 [1]. Recently, Saudi Arabia has been enlisted in the top ten countries with high diabetes prevalence (23.9%) due to the major socioeconomic changes that have occurred and associated with major changes in the person's lifestyle [2]. Diabetic nephropathy (DN) is a progressive kidney disease caused by glomerular as well as tubular structural and functional alterations which is induced by glucose homeostasis disturbance [3]. It occurs in approximately 30% of diabetic patients, and it is one of the main causes of end-stage renal disease (ESRD) [4]. Over the past few decades, major advances were achieved in its diagnosis and treatment, albeit it is still representing one of the late complications which associated with increased risk for cardiovascular morbidity and mortality [3]. Measuring of urine albumin levels (albumin-to-creatinine ratio) has been used conventionally to detect DN severity [5–9]. Even though persistent microalbuminuria (30–300 μg/mg) or macroalbuminuria (levels > 300 μg/mg) [10] was considered as the best available, noninvasive marker and predictor for DN risk and its progression to ESRD [3], certain studies have shown it to have inadequate specificity and sensitivity [11–13] and it does not cover all patients with renal impairment [14]. In addition, microalbuminuria was detected in other patients with kidney impairment as in cases of hypertension and glomerular basement membrane dysfunction [15]. Thus, additional studies for novel noninvasive risk markers in body fluids are required, and feasible measures for the diagnosis of DN prior to advanced renal dysfunction are considered to be of clinical importance with a public health implication [16, 17].

Vitamin D-binding protein (VDBP) (primary accession number P02774; http://www.uniprot.org/uniprot/P02774), also known as gc-globulin, is a 58 kDa glycoprotein which serves as the main carrier protein for circulating vitamin D and its metabolites, supporting the bioavailability of active 1,25-dihydroxyvitamin D (1,25(OH)$_2$D) and its precursor 25-hydroxyvitamin D (25OHD) [18, 19]. The vital role by which VDBP plays for maintaining the serum levels of the bioactive vitamin D is important for the function of a wide variety of tissues which show development of a number of diseases associated with changes in VDBP activity [20].

In addition to the transport function, VDBP is the parent molecule of VDBP-maf (macrophage-activating factor). This latter molecule is the deglycosylated product form of VDBP and has been reported to be a potent anti-angiogenic and antitumorigenic molecule [21]. Moreover, VDBP is important in the actin-scavenger system, participating in the immune responses and the inflammatory processes [20]. Studies concerning the actions of VDBP in the kidney have received increased attention and have reported that VDBP is vital for 1,25(OH)2D biosynthesis within renal proximal tubules, in which it binds 25OHD and the complex is actively recovered from the glomerular filtrate through megalin-mediated receptor endocytosis [22, 23]. Clinically, it has been demonstrated that exaggerated excretion of urinary VDBP is associated with tubular dysfunction [24]. Therefore, it was hypothesized that the loss of urinary VDBP is likely to be elevated in diabetic patients and particularly accentuated in those patients with DN [25].

In addition, it has been demonstrated that the presence of vitamin D deficiency or insufficiency in patients with diabetes is independently associated with the development of DN. Moreover, exaggerated urinary excretion of VDBP was observed in patients with type 1 diabetes, which contributed mechanistically to vitamin D deficiency in this disease [24, 26–28].

Therefore, a further possibility for the potential elevation of urinary VDBP levels identified in some studies may be associated with the relatively lower serum level and vitamin D levels. Hence, further studies are required to clarify the role of VDBP in the pathogenesis of DN in particularly type 2. This study was designed to evaluate the urinary vitamin D-binding protein in patients with type 2 DM presented with different degrees of DN and to examine the possible correlation to the available clinico-laboratory parameters to explore its validity as an early, specific, and sensitive biomarker for nephropathy and its severity in Saudi diabetic patients in the northern area of the KSA. This is a preliminary step in an attempt to early implement the preventive measurements and control the occurrence of renal failure in these patients.

2. Subjects and Methods

2.1. Participants. One hundred and twenty diabetic patients (DM type 2) and 40 age- and sex-matched apparently healthy controls have been enrolled in the current preliminary case-control study. Early morning serum and urine samples have been obtained on the same day from all participants. Patients who were attending the Prince Hospital Outpatient Diabetic Clinics, Northern Borders Area, Saudi Arabia, were divided into 3 patient groups: (1) normoalbuminuria group (urinary albumin excretion rate $< 30\,\mu$g/mg), (2) microalbuminuria group (at least two of three consecutive urine samples with albumin excretion rate 30–300 μg/mg), and (3) macroalbuminuria group (albumin excretion rate $> 300\,\mu$g/mg) [10], ($n = 40$ per group). Patients with active urinary tract infection, renal disease other than diabetic nephropathy (diagnosed by renal biopsy according to recommended protocols adopted from international standards for diagnosis of nondiabetic renal disease) [29], neoplastic disorders, severe liver disease, active or chronic infection or inflammatory disorders, hematological diseases, pregnancy or a recent history of acute myocardial infarction, stroke, or occlusive peripheral vascular disease have been excluded. Patients' medical data have been reviewed from their medical records. In addition, blood pressure, body weight, and body mass index have been measured. The control subjects were randomly selected from the general population. They had no signs or clinical symptoms of chronic diseases or cancer, and they did not take any regular medication. The study was conducted in accordance with the ethical standards of the institutional and national research committee and with the Helsinki Declaration and its later amendments or comparable ethical standards. It was approved by the Medical and Bioethics Local Committee of Northern Borders University. All participants provided written informed consent to participate in the study after being informed with its purpose.

2.2. Biochemical Analysis. Venous blood samples (8 ml) were withdrawn after an overnight fast (10–12 h); 7 ml was collected on a plain tube for serum separation after centrifugation at 2500 rpm × 15 minutes, then stored frozen at 80°C until the time of laboratory analysis. The remaining 1 ml from the blood sample was placed in EDTA tube for glycated hemoglobin (HbA1c) determination (Cobas Integra, Roche Diagnostics, USA).

Routine laboratory measurements including blood urea nitrogen (BUN), serum creatinine, fasting blood sugar (FBS), and lipid profile (total cholesterol (TC), high-density lipoprotein cholesterol (HDL-c), and triacylglycerol (TG)) were done using commercially available kits on Cobas Integra 400 plus Biochemical analyzer (Roche Diagnostics).

Table 1: Clinical and demographic characteristics of the study groups.

Variables	Control group ($n = 40$)	Diabetic groups Normal albuminuria ($n = 40$)	Microalbuminuria ($n = 40$)	Macroalbuminuria ($n = 40$)	P values
Age (years)	47.6 ± 13.6	50.6 ± 7.8	50.4 ± 12.0	45.9 ± 6.5	0.127
Gender, n (%)					
Females	32 (80.0)	35 (87.5)	33 (82.5)	34 (85.0)	0.821
Males	8 (20.0)	5 (12.5)	7 (17.5)	6 (15.0)	
Weight (kg)	74.9 ± 14.3	80.1 ± 15.1	77.2 ± 11.7	80.4 ± 18.5	0.315
Height (cm)	166.1 ± 5.2	156.4 ± 7.9^{a}	158.3 ± 9.5^{a}	154.5 ± 4.4^{ab}	**<0.001**
BMI (kg/m^2)	27.2 ± 5.5	32.8 ± 6.2^{a}	30.8 ± 4.1	33.7 ± 7.5^{a}	**<0.001**
Obesity, n (%)	12 (30.0)	30 (75.0)	18 (45.0)	25 (62.5)	**<0.001**
Hypertension, n (%)	14 (35.0)	11 (27.5)	9 (22.5)	10 (25.0)	0.625
Smoking, n (%)	7 (17.5)	2 (5.0)	3 (7.5)	3 (7.5)	0.227
FH of DM	11 (27.5)	17 (42.5)	24 (60.0)	28 (70.0)	**0.001**
DM duration (years)	—	5.5 ± 2.5	6.1 ± 2.7	6.8 ± 2.1	0.063
Insulin therapy, n (%)	—	17 (42.5)	19 (47.5)	20 (50.0)	0.791
DR, n (%)	—	14 (35.0)	16 (40.0)	19 (47.5)	0.519
CKD, n (%)					
Stage 1	—	34 (85.0)	34 (85.0)	30 (75.0)	**0.013**
Stage 2	—	6 (15.0)	6 (15.0)	10 (25.0)	

Data are expressed as mean ± SD or n (%). DM: diabetes mellitus; BMI: body mass index; FH: family history; DR: diabetic retinopathy; CKD: chronic kidney disease. Chi square test was used for qualitative variables. One-way ANOVA for quantitative variables followed by Tukey HSD post hoc test for multiple comparisons. [a]Compared to the control group; [b]compared to microalbuminuria. Bold values indicate significance at $P < 0.05$.

Low-density lipoprotein cholesterol (LDL-c) concentration was calculated by the Friedewald equation [30].

A clean-catch midstream urine samples (nearly 20 ml) were collected into a sterile plastic tube and then centrifuged for 10 minutes at 3000 rpm, 4°C, to remove cell debris and particulate matter. The supernatant was stored at −80°C for further analysis. Repeated freeze-thaw cycles were avoided. Spot urinary albumin and creatinine concentrations were measured (Siemens Healthcare Diagnostics Inc., USA) and expressed as the urinary albumin (μg)/creatinine (mg) ratio (UACR). Glomerular filtration rate was estimated (eGFR) using the four variable Modification of Diet in Renal Disease GFR formulas (age, sex, race, and serum creatinine) which are as follows: $\text{eGFR} = 186 \times (\text{serum creatinine}^{-1.154}) \times (\text{age}^{-0.203}) \times (0.742 \text{ if female})$ [31]. Quantitative estimation of serum hypersensitive C-reactive protein (hs-CRP) was done by means of particle enhanced immunonephelometry using BN system (Dade Behring, USA).

Hormonal assay for insulin was measured by Electrochemiluminescence Immunoassay (Cobas, Roche Diagnostics, USA). Insulin resistance was assessed using HOMA model (homeostasis model assessment index) = fasting insulin (μU/ml) × fasting glucose (mmol/l)/22.5 [32].

Serum and urinary VDPB were measured in duplicate using a Human Vitamin DBP Quantikine ELISA kit (DVDBP0; R&D Systems, Minneapolis, MN, USA). The assay was performed according to the instructions recommended by the manufacturer. The standard curve was created using the lyophilized human VDBP standard preparation supplied with the assay. Following the colorimetric reaction, the optical density (OD) readings were converted to concentrations in ng/ml based on quantification of the OD at 450 nm. The levels of uVDBP were normalized according to urine Cr concentrations (to avoid the influence of urine volume) and presented as uVDBP : Cr ratio (ng/mg of Cr) [33]. The intra-assay coefficient of variations of the urinary and serum VDBP were 6.2 and 5.5%, respectively.

2.3. Statistical Analysis. Statistical analysis was performed using SPSS, version 22 (Statistical Package for the Social Sciences, SPSS Inc., Chicago, Illinois, USA). Normally distributed continuous values were expressed as means ± SD and compared using analysis of variance (ANOVA) test followed by Tukey HSD post hoc test for multiple comparisons, whereas nonnormally distributed values were expressed as median with interquartile range (IQR) and compared by the Kruskal Wallis test followed by Tukey HSD multiple comparison test. Categorical variables were presented as percentage and compared by chi square test. Moreover, Pearson's correlation coefficient was used to test correlations between serum and urinary VDBP and other variables. Linear regression analysis was applied to allow us to estimate the association between a given independent variable and the outcome holding all other variables constant and to provide a way of adjusting for potentially confounding variables that have been included in the model. Receiver operating characteristics (ROC) analysis was used to calculate the area under the curve (AUC) for uVDBP and to find the best cut-off values to identify diabetic nephropathy. The results with

Table 2: Laboratory parameters of the study groups.

Variables	Control group ($n = 40$)	Diabetic groups Normal albuminuria ($n = 40$)	Microalbuminuria ($n = 40$)	Macroalbuminuria ($n = 40$)	P values
Lipid profile					
Total cholesterol (mmol/l)	4.8 ± 1.5	4.8 ± 0.7	4.6 ± 0.9	5.1 ± 1.4	0.289
HDL-c (mmol/l)	1.2 ± 0.4	1.2 ± 0.3	1.1 ± 0.4	0.9 ± 1.0	0.196
LDL-c (mmol/l)	6.9 ± 24.5	3.3 ± 0.6	3.4 ± 1.1	1.12 ± 0.4	0.417
Total triglyceride (mmol/l)	1.3 ± 0.8	1.7 ± 0.8	1.4 ± 0.5	2.7 ± 0.9 [b c]	**<0.001**
Diabetic assessment					
FBS (mmol/l)	5.5 ± 5.9	7.9 ± 5.3	12.1 ± 16.7[a]	11.8 ± 4.1[a,b]	**0.004**
HbA1c (%)	4.7 ± 0.4	7.2 ± 0.7[a]	7.5 ± 1.4[a]	9.4 ± 0.8[a,b,c]	**<0.001**
Fasting insulin (mIU/l)	9.6 ± 5.0	25.3 ± 10.4[a]	32.3 ± 14.4[a,b]	37.8 ± 16.8[a,b]	**<0.001**
HOMA-IR index	0.15 ± 0.25	0.8 ± 1.2[a]	0.4 ± 0.3[b]	0.7 ± 0.4[a]	**<0.001**
Total protein (gm/l)	74.2 ± 10.4	73.9 ± 3.2	70.7 ± 4.2	71.9 ± 5.5	0.052
Serum albumin (gm/l)	47.7 ± 7.7	35.0 ± 3.3[a]	34.1 ± 2.4[a]	34.4 ± 2.5[a]	**<0.001**
Renal function tests					
Serum urea (mmol/l)	3.5 ± 1.1	4.6 ± 1.0[a]	4.5 ± 0.9[a]	4.5 ± 1.4[a]	**<0.001**
Serum creatinine (μmol/l)	57.7 ± 12.5	56.2 ± 16.0	59.1 ± 9.8	69.2 ± 16.6[a,b,c]	**<0.001**
Albumin/creatinine ratio (μg/mg)	16.7 ± 8.7	10.5 ± 7.8	77.5 ± 65.5	803.5 ± 355[a,b,c]	**<0.001**
eGFR (ml/min/1.73 m^2)	102.4 ± 17.6	111.2 ± 36.6	107.9 ± 17.2	113.3 ± 22.9	0.232
Inflammatory markers					
hs-CRP (mg/l)	0.12 ± 0.08	0.17 ± 0.05[a]	0.17 ± 0.04[a]	0.15 ± 0.02[a,b,c]	**<0.001**
VDBP analyses					
sVDBP (μg/ml)	210.3 ± 33.8	202.4 ± 43.9	248.4 ± 36.5[a,b]	299.2 ± 50.6[a,b,c]	**<0.001**
uVDBP/uCr (ng/mg)	127.7 ± 21.9	193.1 ± 141.0	820.4 ± 402.8[a,b]	1458.1 ± 210[a,b,c]	**<0.001**

Data are expressed as mean ± SD. HDL: high-density lipoprotein cholesterol; LDL: low-density lipoprotein cholesterol; FBS: fasting blood sugar; HBA1c: hemoglobin A1c; HOMA: homeostasis model assessment; eGFR: estimated glomerular filtration rate; hs-CRP: high sensitivity C-reactive protein. [a]Compared to control group. [b]Compared to diabetic normal albuminuria group. [c]Compared to diabetic microalbuminuria group. Bold values indicate significance at $P < 0.05$.

$P < 0.05$ were considered statistically significant. Finally, for clustering the study participants according to clinico-laboratory variable interaction, PC-ORD version 6.0 was employed to run the multivariate analysis. Bray-Curtis ordination and two-way hierarchical cluster analysis were run to identify the combination of variables that could discriminate between the patient and control groups. Data profile was first examined. No outliers were detected, and no transformation was required. Ordination was run to visualize data of participants along the axis according to their resemblance. Sorensen coefficient, Euclidean residual distance, and variance-regression endpoint selection method were adjusted to calculate scores for factors by weighted averaging. In cluster analysis, flexible beta linkage method at −0.75 and Sorensen distance measure were selected [34].

3. Results

3.1. Baseline Characteristics of the Study Groups. Clinical and biochemical data for the diabetic patients categorized according to the level of albuminuria compared to the control group are shown in Tables 1 and 2, respectively. Patients and controls were matched with age and gender. No significant differences were observed with regard to history of smoking or presence of hypertension. However, diabetic patients showed a higher body mass index and a higher frequency of positive family history for diabetes. There was a significant increase of serum TG in the macroalbuminuria group compared to other groups ($P < 0.001$). For insulin resistance expressed as HOMA model, it was significantly higher in the diabetic groups versus the control group ($P < 0.001$) as expected.

3.2. Serum and Urinary VDBP Profiles. Mean urinary VDPB levels were significantly different among the study groups ($P < 0.001$) with increasing levels with the degree of albuminuria (Table 2 and Figure 1). uVDBP levels were significantly elevated in the micro- and macroalbuminuria patient groups compared to the normoalbuminuria diabetic group and normal controls (820.4 ± 402.8 and 1458.1 ± 210.0 compared with 193.1 ± 141.0 and 127.7 ± 21.9 ng/mg, resp.) ($P < 0.001$). In addition, the serum VDBP levels were also significantly elevated in the patient subgroups: normo-, micro-, and macroalbuminuria compared to controls (Table 2). There was a significant positive correlation

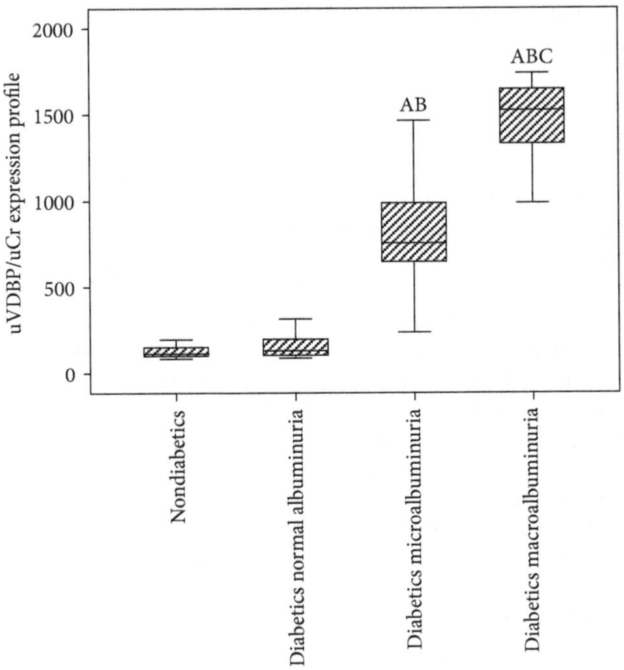

FIGURE 1: Urinary vitamin D-binding protein levels among the study groups. uVDBP, urinary vitamin D-binding protein; uCr, urinary creatinine. [A]Compared to the control group. [B]Compared to the diabetic normal albuminuria group. [C]Compared to the diabetic microalbuminuria group. Kruskal-Wallis test and Tukey HSD multiple comparison test were applied.

between serum and uVDBP levels in the whole patient group, albeit this significance was not evident when patients were stratified according to the levels of albuminuria (Table 3, Figure 2).

Receiver operating characteristic analysis of urinary VDBP levels showed optimum cut-off value of 216.0 ng/mg corresponding to 98.8% sensitivity and 80.0% specificity and an area under the curve of 0.973 to discriminate the normoalbuminuria from microalbuminuria groups (Figure 3).

Pearson's correlation between uVDBP levels and the different clinico-laboratory parameters showed its significant correlation with family history of diabetes, HbA1c %, LDL-c, total serum protein levels, and urinary albumin/creatinine ratio ($r = 0.309$, 0.584, −0.244, −0.202, and 0.775, resp.) in the total patient group (Table 3).

Univariate logistic regression analysis was executed to identify which of the predictors (independent variables) are significantly contributing to DN (Table 4). Percent accuracy classification of the model was 94.2%. Serum VDBP and uVDBP levels showed the only statistically significant independent predictors to microalbuminuria (Table 4). While the odds ratios were statistically significant, the values were near 1 (i.e., the magnitudes of the effect were 1.028- and 1.01-fold increase for sVDBP and uVDBP levels, resp.). A larger study is needed to generate a more precise estimate of effect and confirm these associations.

TABLE 3: Correlation of uVDBP with the clinical and biochemical features in diabetic nephropathy patients.

Variables	*r*	*P*
Clinical features		
Age	−0.088	0.338
Gender	0.009	0.921
BMI	0.115	0.210
FH of DM	0.309	**0.001**
DM duration	0.079	0.394
DR	0.099	0.281
CKD	−0.093	0.311
Diabetic assessment		
FBS	0.018	0.849
HbA1c	0.584	**<0.001**
Fasting insulin	−0.155	0.091
HOMA-IR index	−0.099	0.281
Lipid profile		
Total cholesterol	0.091	0.324
HDL-c	−0.052	0.575
LDL-c	−0.244	**0.007**
Total triglyceride	0.018	0.849
Total serum protein	−0.202	**0.027**
Renal function tests		
Serum urea	0.097	0.294
Serum creatinine	0.010	0.912
Albumin/creatinine ratio	0.775	**<0.001**
eGFR	0.047	0.611
Inflammatory markers		
hs-CRP	−0.167	0.089
Vitamin D-binding protein analysis		
sVDBP	0.665	**<0.001**

BMI: body mass index; FH of DM: family history of diabetes mellitus; DR: diabetic retinopathy; CKD: chronic kidney; FBS: fasting blood sugar; HOMA: homeostasis model assessment, HDL: high-density lipoprotein cholesterol; LDL: low-density lipoprotein cholesterol; eGFR: estimated glomerular filtration rate; hs-CRP: high-sensitivity C-reactive protein; sVDBP: serum vitamin D-binding protein. Bold values indicate significance at $P < 0.05$.

3.3. Multivariate Analysis. Ordination plot showed obvious demarcation between the study groups. In axis 1, uVDBP/uCr, sVDBP, and HbA1c were the most effective classifier in the negative direction explaining 96.7%, 55.6%, and 53.9% of axis variability. Whereas, axis 2 was mostly affected by platelet count, hemoglobin, and albuminuria/creatinine ratio with R^2 of 44.8%, 20.3, and 19.3%, respectively. Two-way cluster analysis also demonstrated clustering of patients and controls into separate groups (Figure 4).

4. Discussion

The identification of novel biomarkers of the early stages of DN is mandatory in an attempt to reduce the burden of chronic kidney diseases in diabetic patients [3]. To evaluate whether uVDBP levels could be a novel noninvasive

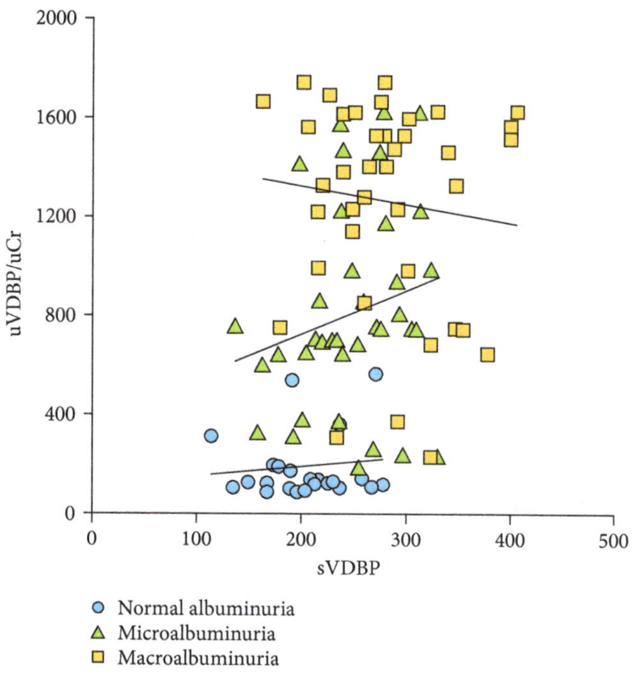

FIGURE 2: Correlation between urinary VDBP/Cr and serum VDBP levels in patient subgroups.

biomarker for DN in a sample of Saudi population, the current study results demonstrated that the uVDBP levels were highly elevated in Saudi patients with DN and were correlated significantly with the severity (degree of albuminuria) of DN. Interestingly, the human *VDBP* gene is a member of a multigene cluster [35] residing on chromosome 4 and coding for related albumin proteins (i.e., albumin, alpha-fetoprotein, and afamin) which have structural and functional similarities [36]. In the normal kidney, VDBP as a 25-(OH) vitamin D3/VDBP complex is reabsorbed by megalin-mediated endocytosis and catabolized by epithelial cells of the proximal tubules contributing to the reduction of its urinary excretion levels [37]. Clinically, it has been found that excessive excretion of uVDBP could indicate tubular dysfunction [38–40] which was considered as one of the early hallmarks of DN [41]. In line with our findings, Rao et al. [42] and Nauta et al. [43] reported elevated uVDBP levels among other DN proteomic markers in patients with diabetes compared to nondiabetics, especially when albuminuria is present. Several recent studies, in addition, support the marked increase in the uVDBP excretion in patients with normo-, micro-, and macroalbuminuria in type 1 [24, 44] as well as type 2 [25, 45, 46] diabetes, compared with that in the controls in different populations. Despite the specific mechanisms underlying the increased uVDBP excretion in patients with DN were not fully uncovered, several evidences support that the enhanced excretion of megalin/cubilin (i.e., multiligand endocytic receptors expressed in the brush border of proximal renal tubular cells and participate in the reuptake of filtered low-molecular weight proteins like albumin and VDBP from the glomerular filtrate) in the urine of patients with DN could play a role [47, 48]. Another speculated mechanism could be related to the renal injury which is associated with DN progression [25] independent of the presence of albuminuria. This speculation could be supported by the findings of Mirkovic´ et al. [49] and Chaykovska et al. [50] who found that uVDBP was increased along with the severity of renal damage independently of albuminuria in a rat model of proteinuric nephropathy that responded partially to an intensified renoprotective therapy in the former study and in contrast-induced nephropathy in the latter one. It has been postulated that the damaged tubular epithelial cells in areas of tubulointerstitial fibrosis may no longer be capable to deal with VDBP, resulting in its gross loss into the urine [49]. Additionally, it has been demonstrated that the major factors involved in the development of glomerulosclerosis and interstitial fibrosis of DN (e.g., TGF-β and angiotensin II) [51, 52] could negatively regulate the receptor-mediated endocytosis [53, 54], participating in enhanced uVDBP excretion.

In the current study, receiver operating characteristic analysis of uVDBP levels showed an area under the curve of 0.973 to discriminate the normoalbuminuria from microalbuminuria groups. Furthermore, the multivariate analysis has confirmed the role of uVDBP as a putative biomarker that could be used for clear demarcation between diabetic patients and the controls. This could support the rationale for using uVDBP as an emerging biomarker for early prediction and detection of DN as evidenced by other studies [25, 44, 45]. In addition, consistent with the results of these studies, our findings showed uVDBP positively correlated to indices of worsening glycemic control as high HbA1c % and to ACR. This latter correlation with the level of albuminuria was supported by Doorenbos et al. observation in which uVDBP excretion responded to antiproteinuric treatment in their chronic kidney disease patients [55]. Rather than family history of diabetes, LDL-c, and total protein levels, uVDBP did not show significant correlation with other clinical and laboratory features in the study population. This finding was in line with Leong et al.'s [56] results who concluded from their follow-up of 2254 Canadian individuals for ten years that apart vitamin D levels, VDBP has no demonstrable causal effect on any of the investigated cardiometabolic traits in their study.

Unexpectedly, serum VDBP levels were significantly elevated in patient subgroups relative to the controls, although the urinary loss of VDBP was enhanced. This finding could indicate increased production of serum VDBP as a compensatory mechanism as speculated by Kalousova and coworkers [57]. In addition, VDBP can interact with many functional partners (Figure 5) and have additional vital metabolic and immunological roles apart its involvement in vitamin D transport and storage [20, 58, 59]. For example, as diabetes could be considered as a chronic state of low grade inflammation [60, 61], this could contribute in part to the increasing levels of serum VDBP as a response to the proinflammatory state. Furthermore, previous reports suggested that serum VDBP level differences that are associated with common diseases could support its role either as an intermediate in several biological pathways or as an upstream player affecting vitamin D effects on common

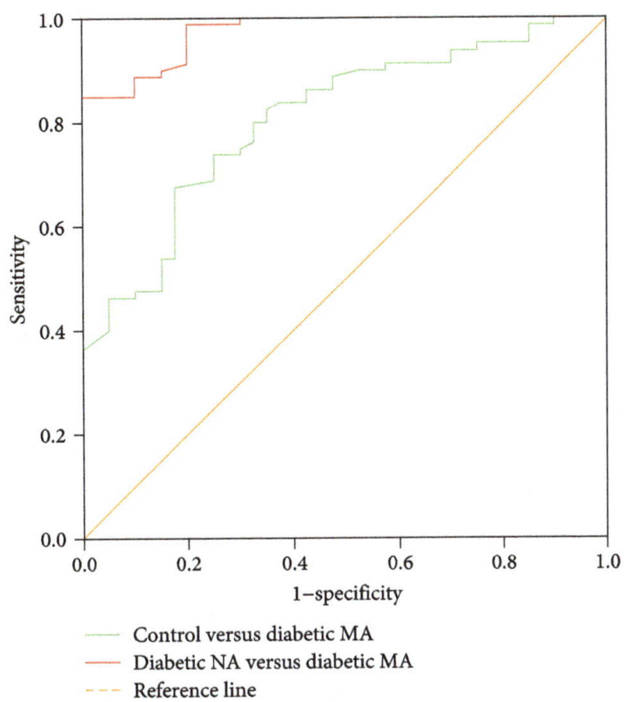

Variable	AUC ± SE	95% CI	*P* values	Cut-off value	Sensitivity	Specificity
Controls versus microalbuminuria diabetic patients	0.807 ± 0.040	0.729–0.885	<0.001	214.0 ng/mg	82.5%	65.0%
Normal albuminuria versus microalbuminuria diabetic patients	0.973 ± 0.011	0.951–0.995	<0.001	216.0 ng/mg	98.8%	80.0%

Figure 3: Diagnostic performance of uVDBP to detect patients with DN. NA: normoalbuminuria; MA: microalbuminuria; AUC: area under curve under the nonparametric assumption; 95% CI: 95% confidence interval; SE: standard error.

Table 4: Univariate logistic regression analysis.

Variables	Univariate analysis B	OR	(95% CI)	*P*
Duration of DM (year)	−0.013	0.987	(0.947–1.029)	0.544
Fasting blood sugar	0.039	1.040	(0.939–1.151)	0.453
Fasting insulin	0.012	1.012	(0.901–1.136)	0.845
sVDBP	0.027	1.028	(1.003–1.053)	**0.026**
uVDBP/uCr	0.010	1.010	(1.004–1.016)	**0.002**
Total cholesterol	−1.703	0.182	(0.030–1.100)	0.063
Serum creatinine	0.081	1.084	(0.976–1.203)	0.131

sVDBP: serum vitamin D-binding protein; uVDBP/uCr: urinary vitamin D-binding protein/urinary creatinine; B: β regression coefficient; OR: odds ratio; CI: confidence interval. Bold values indicate significance at $P < 0.05$.

diseases. This speculation was supported by analogy to other circulating steroidal hormone transporters, including sex hormone or corticosteroid binding globulins, the major effectors of steroid action independent of their function as carriers [62].

Some limitations of our study include the relatively small sample size, the cross-sectional design, and the fact that the study lack of inclusion of other types of nephropathies to which uVDBP could be assessed to confirm its specificity of this biomarker for DN. Hence, it is highly recommended that uVDBP to be validated in well-characterized larger scale cohorts with longitudinal follow-up and assessment of its response to proper DN management, as well as addressing the associations between uVDBP and the other types of nephropathy in the clinical setting. Furthermore, as it is well known, the genetic variability of VDBP could affect its circulating levels [63]; complicating the interpretation process of the serum VDBP, it is highly recommended considering its genetic variants when to interpret or associate serum VDBP levels with the disease phenotype.

5. Conclusions

Taken together, the current results suggested that uVDBP could be implicated in combination with other conventional biomarkers for the early prediction of DN in Saudi

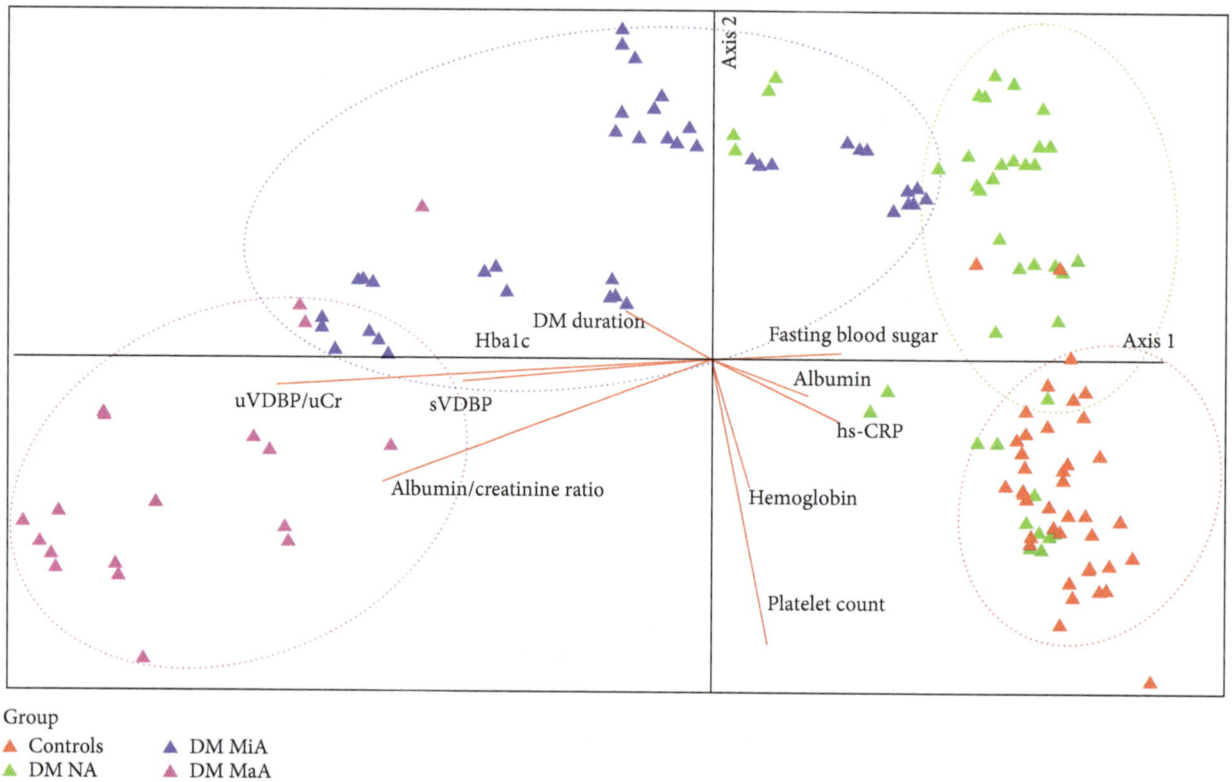

(a)

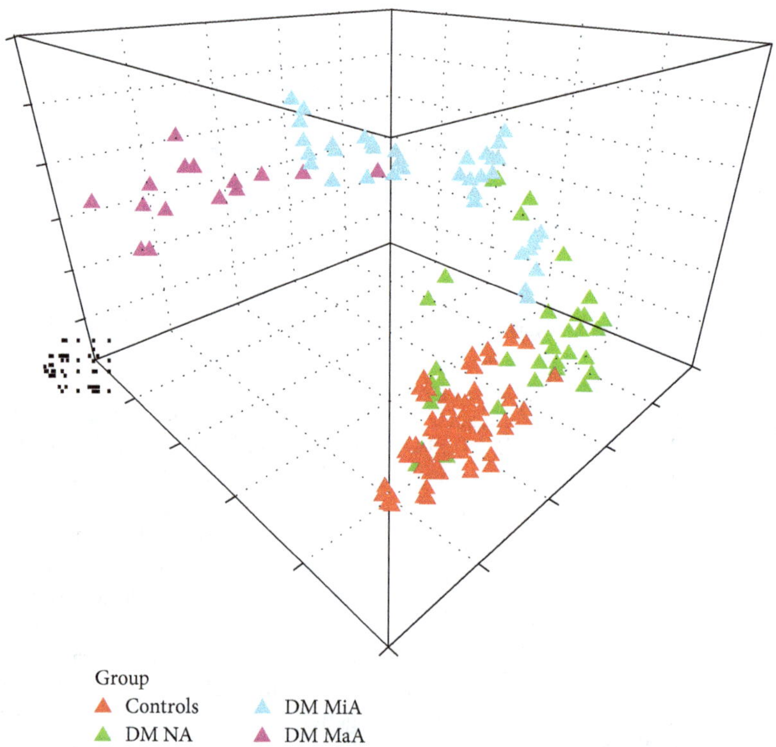

(b)

FIGURE 4: Continued.

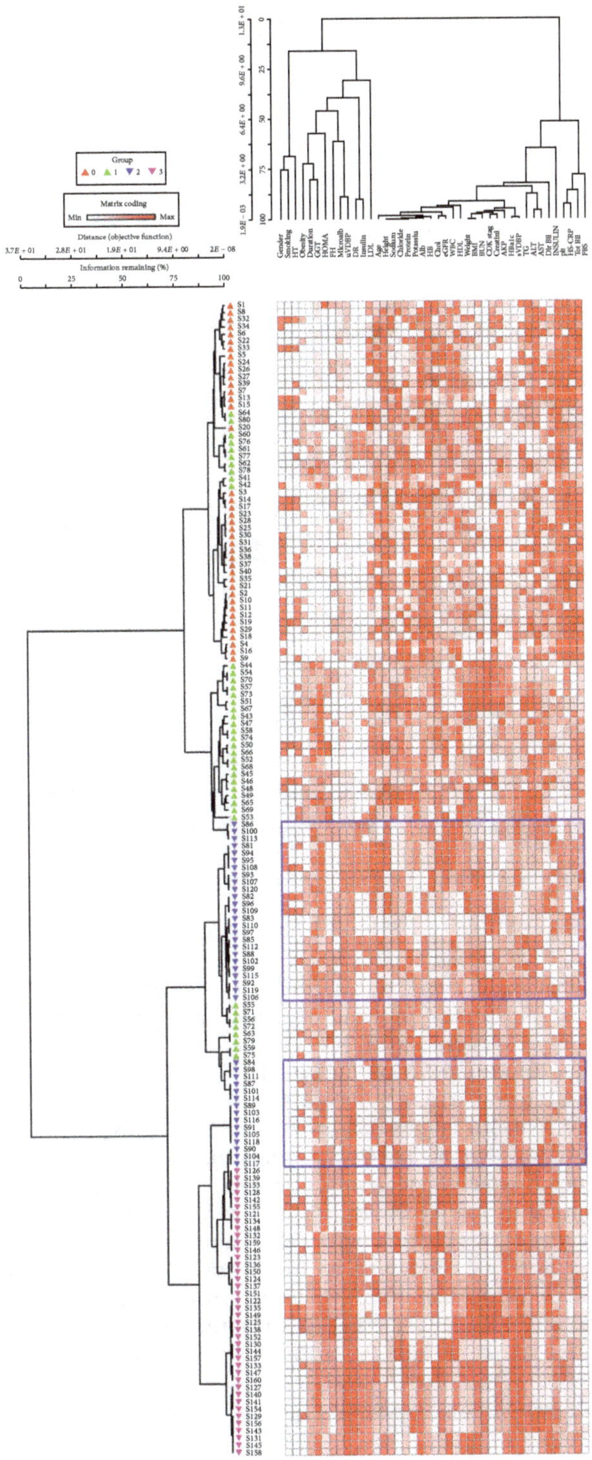

(c)

FIGURE 4: Multivariate analysis of the study participants. (a) Despite some mixing between groups, the study participants were clustered into four distinct groups: (1) one control group (red) which was mostly affected by high hemoglobin level, (2) diabetic without albuminuria (green) at the positive direction of axis 1 which was influenced by high fasting blood sugar levels, (3) diabetic microalbuminuria (blue), and (4) diabetic macroalbuminuria (pink) in the negative direction of axis 1 which was greatly affected by high level of uVDBP/Ucr, sVDBP, albumin/creatinine ratio, and HbA1c. (b) 3D ordination plot shows also separation between the controls (red) and other patient subgroups along axes 1 and 2. uVDBP was a potential factor contributing to this separation. (c) Two-way hierarchical cluster analysis shows clear cut between macroalbuminuria and the other 3 groups with 100% separation. However, the diabetic normoalbuminuria group shares some characteristics with the normal controls and microalbuminuria group.

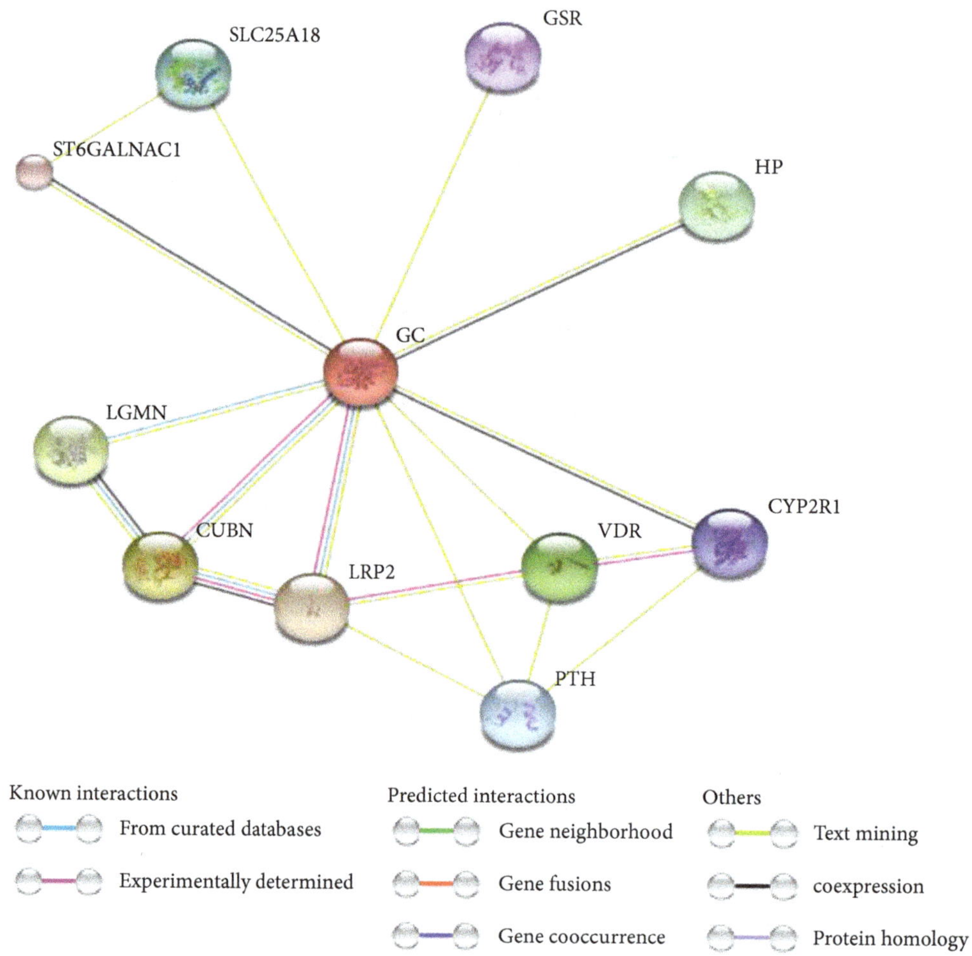

FIGURE 5: STRING analysis of vitamin D-binding protein (i.e., Gc, group-specific component protein) (accession number P02774) with its predicted functional partners. Network nodes represent proteins; each node represents all the proteins produced by a single, protein-coding gene locus. Edges represent protein-protein associations (i.e., contribute to a shared function; this does not necessarily mean they are physically binding each other). The line colors of the edges indicate the type of interaction evidence that is explained in the figure key (right side). LRP2, low-density lipoprotein receptor-related protein 2 or megalin, is a multiligand endocytic receptor that is expressed in many tissues but primarily in absorptive epithelial tissues such as the kidney; CUBN, cubilin, an intrinsic factor-cobalamin receptor cotransporter which plays a role in lipoprotein, vitamin, and iron metabolism, by facilitating their uptake. LGMN, legumain, has a strict specificity for hydrolysis of asparaginyl bonds required for normal lysosomal protein degradation in renal proximal tubules and plays a role in the regulation of cell proliferation via its role in EGFR degradation; VDR, vitamin D (1,25-dihydroxyvitamin D3), is a nuclear receptor that mediates the action of vitamin D3 by controlling the expression of hormone-sensitive genes and plays a central role in calcium homeostasis; HP, haptoglobin, captures and combines with free plasma hemoglobin to allow hepatic recycling of heme iron and to prevent kidney damage. SLC25A18, solute carrier family 25 (glutamate carrier), is member 18 which involved in glutamate transport with H^+ across the inner mitochondrial membrane; PTH, parathyroid hormone; CYP2R1, cytochrome P450, family 2, subfamily R, polypeptide 1 which has a D-25-hydroxylase activity on both forms of vitamin D: D2 and D3. GSR, glutathione reductase, maintains high levels of reduced glutathione in the cytosol. ST6GALNAC1 transfers a sialic acid, N-acetylneuraminic acid (NeuAc), in an alpha-2,6 linkage to O-linked GalNAc residues [data source: https://string-db.org, version 10.5].

population. This could improve the early diagnosis of DN and help in prevention of progress to ESRD by applying early and personalized targeted therapy after validation of the findings in larger scale studies.

Consent

Informed consent was obtained from all individual participants included in the study.

Conflicts of Interest

The authors declare that they have no any conflict of interest.

Acknowledgments

The authors would like to thank all participants who agree to join this work. This research was conducted at the Northern Borders University, Arar, KSA, and it was approved by the Deanship of the Scientific Research in NBU.

References

[1] M. E. Hellemons, J. Kerschbaum, S. J. L. Bakker et al., "Validity of biomarkers predicting onset or progression of nephropathy in patients with type 2 diabetes: a systematic review," *Diabetic Medicine*, vol. 29, no. 5, pp. 567–577, 2012.

[2] Z. Naeem, "Burden of diabetes mellitus in Saudi Arabia," *International Journal of Health Sciences*, vol. 9, no. 3, pp. V–VI, 2015.

[3] C. G. Campion, O. Sanchez-Ferras, and S. N. Batchu, "Potential role of serum and urinary biomarkers in diagnosis and prognosis of diabetic nephropathy," *Canadian Journal of Kidney Health and Disease*, vol. 4, 2017.

[4] International Diabetes Federation, *IDF Diabetes Atlas*, 2015, 7th edition, 2017, http://idf.org.

[5] A. I. Adler, R. J. Stevens, S. E. Manley, R. W. Bilous, C. A. Cull, and R. R. Holman, "Development and progression of nephropathy in type 2 diabetes: the United Kingdom Prospective Diabetes Study (UKPDS 64)," *Kidney International*, vol. 63, no. 1, pp. 225–232, 2003.

[6] D. De Zeeuw, G. Remuzzi, H. H. Parving et al., "Proteinuria, a target for renoprotection in patients with type 2 diabetic nephropathy: lessons from RENAAL," *Kidney International*, vol. 65, no. 6, pp. 2309–2320, 2004.

[7] S. Araki, M. Haneda, D. Koya et al., "Reduction in microalbuminuria as an integrated indicator for renal and cardiovascular risk reduction in patients with type 2 diabetes," *Diabetes*, vol. 56, no. 6, pp. 1727–1730, 2007.

[8] B. F. Palmer, "Proteinuria as a therapeutic target in patients with chronic kidney disease," *American Journal of Nephrology*, vol. 27, no. 3, pp. 287–293, 2007.

[9] G. Cerasola, S. Cottone, and G. Mulè, "The progressive pathway of microalbuminuria: from early marker of renal damage to strong cardiovascular risk predictor," *Journal of Hypertension*, vol. 28, no. 12, pp. 2357–2369, 2010.

[10] W.F. Keane and G. Eknoyan, "Proteinuria, albuminuria, risk, assessment, detection, elimination (PARADE): a position paper of the National Kidney Foundation," *American Journal of Kidney Diseases*, vol. 33, no. 5, pp. 1004–1010, 1999.

[11] B. P. Tabaei, A. S. Al-Kassab, L. L. Ilag, C. M. Zawacki, and W. H. Herman, "Does microalbuminuria predict diabetic nephropathy?," *Diabetes Care*, vol. 24, no. 9, pp. 1560–1566, 2001.

[12] B. A. Perkins, L. H. Ficociello, B. Roshan, J. H. Warram, and A. S. Krolewski, "In patients with type 1 diabetes and new-onset microalbuminuria the development of advanced chronic kidney disease may not require progression to proteinuria," *Kidney International*, vol. 77, no. 1, pp. 57–64, 2010.

[13] J. M. Halimi, "The emerging concept of chronic kidney disease without clinical proteinuria in diabetic patients," *Diabetes & Metabolism*, vol. 38, no. 4, pp. 291–297, 2012.

[14] N. J. Radcliffe, J. M. Seah, M. Clarke, R. J. Macisaac, G. Jerums, and E. I. Ekinci, "Clinical predictive factors in diabetic kidney disease progression," *Journal of Diabetes Investigation*, vol. 8, no. 1, pp. 6–18, 2017.

[15] A. L. Al-Malki, "Assessment of urinary osteopontin in association with podocyte for early predication of nephropathy in diabetic patients," *Disease Markers*, vol. 2014, Article ID 493736, 5 pages, 2014.

[16] T. Narita, M. Hosoba, M. Kakei, and S. Ito, "Increased urinary excretions of immunoglobulin G, ceruloplasmin, and transferrin predict development of microalbuminuria in patients with type 2 diabetes," *Diabetes Care*, vol. 29, no. 1, pp. 142–144, 2006.

[17] G. Tramonti and Y. S. Kanwar, "Review and discussion of tubular biomarkers in the diagnosis and management of diabetic nephropathy," *Endocrine*, vol. 43, no. 3, pp. 494–503, 2013.

[18] R. F. Chun, B. E. Peercy, J. S. Adams, and M. Hewison, "Vitamin D binding protein and monocyte response to 25-hydroxyvitamin D and 1,25-dihydroxyvitamin D: analysis by mathematical modeling," *PLoS One*, vol. 7, no. 1, article e30773, 2012.

[19] S. Christakos, D. V. Ajibade, P. Dhawan, A. J. Fechner, and L. J. Mady, "Vitamin D: metabolism," *Endocrinology and Metabolism Clinics of North America*, vol. 39, no. 2, pp. 243–253, 2010.

[20] F. Li, D. N. Chen, C. W. He et al., "Identification of urinary Gc-globulin as a novel biomarker for bladder cancer by two-dimensional fluorescent differential gel electrophoresis (2D-DIGE)," *Journal of Proteomics*, vol. 77, pp. 225–236, 2012.

[21] N. Yamamoto and V. R. Naraparaju, "Vitamin D_3-binding protein as a precursor for macrophage activating factor in the inflammation-primed macrophage activation cascade in rats," *Cellular Immunology*, vol. 170, no. 2, pp. 161–167, 1996.

[22] A. Nykjaer, D. Dragun, D. Walther et al., "An endocytic pathway essential for renal uptake and activation of the steroid 25-(OH) vitamin D_3," *Cell*, vol. 96, no. 4, pp. 507–515, 1999.

[23] D. Zehnder, R. Bland, M. C. Williams et al., "Extrarenal expression of 25-hydroxyvitamin D3-1α-hydroxylase," *The Journal of Clinical Endocrinology & Metabolism*, vol. 86, no. 2, pp. 888–894, 2001.

[24] K. M. Thrailkill, C. H. Jo, G. E. Cockrell, C. S. Moreau, and J. L. Fowlkes, "Enhanced excretion of vitamin D binding protein in type 1 diabetes: a role in vitamin D deficiency?," *The Journal of Clinical Endocrinology & Metabolism*, vol. 96, no. 1, pp. 142–149, 2011.

[25] X.-Q. Tian, L.-M. Zhao, J.-P. Ge, Y. Zhang, and Y.-C. Xu, "Elevated urinary level of vitamin D-binding protein as a novel biomarker for diabetic nephropathy," *Experimental and Therapeutic Medicine*, vol. 7, no. 2, pp. 411–416, 2014.

[26] B. M. Svoren, L. K. Volkening, J. R. Wood, and L. M. Laffel, "Significant vitamin D deficiency in youth with type 1 diabetes mellitus," *The Journal of Pediatrics*, vol. 154, no. 1, pp. 132–134, 2009.

[27] A. A. Tahrani, A. Ball, L. Shepherd, A. Rahim, A. F. Jones, and A. Bates, "The prevalence of vitamin D abnormalities in South Asians with type 2 diabetes mellitus in the UK," *The International Journal of Clinical Practice*, vol. 64, no. 3, pp. 351–355, 2010.

[28] D. Blanton, Z. Han, L. Bierschenk et al., "Reduced serum vitamin D–binding protein levels are associated with Type 1 diabetes," *Diabetes*, vol. 60, no. 10, pp. 2566–2570, 2011.

[29] A.A. Ghani, S. Al Waheeb, A Al Sahow, and N Hussain, "Renal biopsy in patients with type 2 diabetes mellitus: indications and nature of the lesions," *Annals of Saudi Medicine*, vol. 29, no. 6, pp. 450–453, 2009.

[30] W. T. Friedewald, R. I. Levy, and D. S. Fredrickson, "Estimation of the concentration of low-density lipoprotein cholesterol in plasma, without use of the preparative ultracentrifuge," *Clinical Chemistry*, vol. 18, no. 6, pp. 499–502, 1972.

[31] A. S. Levey, J. P. Bosch, J. B. Lewis et al., "A more accurate method to estimate glomerular filtration rate from serum creatinine: a new prediction equation," *Annals of Internal Medicine*, vol. 130, no. 6, pp. 461–470, 1999.

[32] D. R. Mattews, J. P. Hosker, A. S. Rudenski, B. A. Naylor, D. F. Treacher, and R. C. Turner, "Homeostasis model assessment: insulin resistance and β-cell function from fasting plasma glucose and insulin concentrations in man," *Diabetologia*, vol. 28, no. 7, pp. 412–419, 1985.

[33] S. Cho, Y. S. Choi, S. Y. Yim et al., "Urinary vitamin D-binding protein is elevated in patients with endometriosis," *Human Reproduction*, vol. 27, no. 2, pp. 515–522, 2012.

[34] B. McCune and M. J. Mefford, *PC-ORD. Multivariate Analysis of Ecological Data, Version 6*, MjM Software, Gleneden Beach, OR, USA, 2011.

[35] Y.-H. Song, A. K. Naumova, S. A. Liebhaber, and N. E. Cooke, "Physical and meiotic mapping of the region of human chromosome 4q11–q13 encompassing the vitamin D binding protein DBP/Gc-globulin and albumin multigene cluster," *Genome Research*, vol. 9, no. 6, pp. 581–587, 1999.

[36] A. Mozzi, D. Forni, R. Cagliani et al., "Albuminoid genes: evolving at the interface of dispensability and selection," *Genome Biology and Evolution*, vol. 6, no. 11, pp. 2983–2997, 2014.

[37] R. Mahadevappa, R. Nielsen, E. I. Christensen, and H. Birn, "Megalin in acute kidney injury—foe and friend," *American Journal of Physiology Renal Physiology*, vol. 306, no. 2, pp. F147–F154, 2014.

[38] K. Colston, N. J. Williams, and H. J. Cleeve, "Studies on vitamin D binding protein in the nephrotic syndrome," *Clinical Chemistry*, vol. 31, no. 5, pp. 718–721, 1985.

[39] A. Vilasi, P. R. Cutillas, A. D. Maher et al., "Combined proteomic and metabonomic studies in three genetic forms of the renal Fanconi syndrome," *American Journal of Physiology Renal Physiology*, vol. 293, no. 2, pp. F456–F467, 2007.

[40] M. Uchida, H. Teranishi, K. Aoshima, T. Katoh, M. Kasuya, and H. Inadera, "Elevated urinary levels of vitamin D-binding protein in the inhabitants of a cadmium polluted area, Jinzu River basin, Japan," *The Tohoku Journal of Experimental Medicine*, vol. 211, no. 3, pp. 269–274, 2007.

[41] R. E. Gilbert and M. E. Cooper, "The tubulointerstitium in progressive diabetic kidney disease: more than an aftermath of glomerular injury?," *Kidney International*, vol. 56, no. 5, pp. 1627–1637, 1999.

[42] P. V. Rao, X. Lu, M. Standley et al., "Proteomic identification of urinary biomarkers of diabetic nephropathy," *Diabetes Care*, vol. 30, no. 3, pp. 629–637, 2007.

[43] F. L. Nauta, W. E. Boertien, S. J. L. Bakker et al., "Glomerular and tubular damage markers are elevated in patients with diabetes," *Diabetes Care*, vol. 34, no. 4, pp. 975–981, 2011.

[44] H. Y. Kim, Y. Ah Lee, H. W. Jung et al., "A lack of association between vitamin D-binding protein and 25-hydroxyvitamin D concentrations in pediatric type 1 diabetes without microalbuminuria," *Annals of Pediatric Endocrinology & Metabolism*, vol. 22, no. 4, pp. 247–252, 2015.

[45] A. Shoukry, S. E. Bdeer, and R. H. El-Sokkary, "Urinary monocyte chemoattractant protein-1 and vitamin D-binding protein as biomarkers for early detection of diabetic nephropathy in type 2 diabetes mellitus," *Molecular and Cellular Biochemistry*, vol. 408, no. 1-2, pp. 25–35, 2015.

[46] S. A. Khodeir, N. M. Kotb, K. M. Okasha, K. A. Ahmed, and H. M. Nagy, "Urinary level of vitamin D-binding protein as a new biomarker for diabetic nephropathy," *Journal of the Egyptian Society Nephrology and Transplantation*, vol. 16, no. 1, pp. 32–38, 2016.

[47] J. R. Leheste, B. Rolinski, H. Vorum et al., "Megalin knockout mice as an animal model of low molecular weight proteinuria," *The American Journal of Pathology*, vol. 155, no. 4, pp. 1361–1370, 1999.

[48] K. M. Thrailkill, T. Nimmo, R. C. Bunn et al., "Microalbuminuria in type 1 diabetes is associated with enhanced excretion of the endocytic multiligand receptors megalin and cubilin," *Diabetes Care*, vol. 32, no. 7, pp. 1266–1268, 2009.

[49] K. Mirkovic′, C. R. Doorenbos, W. A. Dam et al., "Urinary vitamin D binding protein: a potential novel marker of renal interstitial inflammation and fibrosis," *PLoS One*, vol. 8, no. 2, article e55887, 2013.

[50] L. Chaykovska, F. Heunisch, G. von Einem et al., "Urinary vitamin D binding protein and KIM-1 are potent new biomarkers of major adverse renal events in patients undergoing coronary angiography," *PLoS One*, vol. 11, no. 1, article e0145723, 2016.

[51] K. B. Gomes, K. F. Rodrigues, and A. P. Fernandes, "The role of transforming growth factor-beta in diabetic nephropathy," *International Journal of Medical Genetics*, vol. 2014, Article ID 180270, 6 pages, 2014.

[52] D. J. Leehey, A. K. Singh, N. Alavi, and R. Singh, "Role of angiotensin II in diabetic nephropathy," *Kidney International*, vol. 58, Supplement 77, pp. S93–S98, 2000.

[53] M. Gekle, P. Knaus, R. Nielsen et al., "Transforming growth factor-β1 reduces megalin- and cubilin-mediated endocytosis of albumin in proximal-tubule-derived opossum kidney cells," *The Journal of Physiology*, vol. 552, no. 2, pp. 471–481, 2003.

[54] M. Hosojima, H. Sato, K. Yamamoto et al., "Regulation of megalin expression in cultured proximal tubule cells by angiotensin II type 1A receptor- and insulin-mediated signaling cross talk," *Endocrinology*, vol. 150, no. 2, pp. 871–878, 2009.

[55] C. R. C. Doorenbos, M. M. de Cuba, L. Vogt et al., "Antiproteinuric treatment reduces urinary loss of vitamin D-binding protein but does not affect vitamin D status in patients with chronic kidney disease," *The Journal of Steroid Biochemistry and Molecular Biology*, vol. 128, no. 1-2, pp. 56–61, 2012.

[56] A. Leong, W. Rehman, Z. Dastani et al., "The causal effect of vitamin D binding protein (DBP) levels on calcemic and cardiometabolic diseases: a Mendelian randomization study," *PLoS Medicine*, vol. 11, no. 10, article e1001751, 2014.

[57] M. Kalousova, S. Dusilova-Sulkova, O. Zakiyanov et al., "Vitamin D binding protein is not involved in Vitamin D deficiency in patients with chronic kidney disease," *BioMed Research International*, vol. 2015, Article ID 492365, 8 pages, 2015.

[58] J. G. Haddad, "Plasma vitamin D-binding protein (Gc-globulin): multiple tasks," *The Journal of Steroid Biochemistry and Molecular Biology*, vol. 53, no. 1–6, pp. 579–582, 1995.

[59] R. F. Chun, "New perspectives on the vitamin D binding protein," *Cell Biochemistry & Function*, vol. 30, no. 6, pp. 445–456, 2012.

[60] G. Lowe, M. Woodward, G. Hillis et al., "Circulating inflammatory markers and the risk of vascular complications and mortality in people with type 2 diabetes and cardiovascular disease or risk factors: the advance study," *Diabetes*, vol. 63, no. 3, pp. 1115–1123, 2014.

[61] A. M. Castro, L. E. Macedo-de la Concha, and C. A. Pantoja-Meléndez, "Low-grade inflammation and its relation to obesity

and chronic degenerative diseases," *Revista Médica del Hospital General de México*, vol. 80, no. 2, pp. 101–105, 2016.

[62] J. D. Caldwell and G. F. Jirikowski, "Sex hormone binding globulin and corticosteroid binding globulin as major effectors of steroid action," *Steroids*, vol. 81, pp. 13–16, 2013.

[63] M. Speeckaert, G. Huang, J. R. Delanghe, and Y. E. C. Taes, "Biological and clinical aspects of the vitamin D binding protein (Gc-globulin) and its polymorphism," *Clinica Chimica Acta*, vol. 372, no. 1-2, pp. 33–42, 2006.

20

The Involvement of Notch1-RBP-Jk/Msx2 Signaling Pathway in Aortic Calcification of Diabetic Nephropathy Rats

Caipan Gong,[1] Li Li,[1] Chunmei Qin,[2] Weihua Wu,[1] Qi Liu,[1] Ying Li,[1] Linwang Gan,[1] and Santao Ou[1]

[1]*Department of Nephrology, The Affiliated Hospital of Southwest Medical University, Luzhou, Sichuan 646000, China*
[2]*Department of Nephrology, Luzhou People's Hospital, Luzhou, Sichuan 646000, China*

Correspondence should be addressed to Santao Ou; ousantao@163.com

Academic Editor: Mark Yorek

Background. This study explored the changes in expression of vascular smooth muscle cell (VSMC) markers and osteogenic markers, as well as the involvement of Notch1-RBP-Jk/Msx2 pathway in a rat model of diabetic nephropathy (DN) with vascular calcification. *Methods.* A rat model of DN with concomitant vascular calcification was created by intraperitoneal injection of streptozotocin followed by administration of vitamin D3 and nicotine. Biochemical analysis and histological examination of aortic tissue were performed. VSMC markers and osteogenic markers as well as target molecules in Notch1-RBP-Jk/Msx2 were determined by quantitative real-time polymerase chain reaction and immunohistochemical analysis. *Results.* Serum calcium and phosphorus levels were significantly increased in model rats as compared to that in normal controls. Diabetic rats with vascular calcification exhibited mineral deposits in aortic intima-media accompanied by decreased expression of VSMC markers and increased expression of osteogenic markers. Notch1, RBP-Jk, Msx2, Jagged1, and N1-ICD were barely expressed in the aortic wall of normal rats. In contrast, these were significantly increased in the model group at all time points (8, 12, and 16 weeks), as compared to that in the normal rats. *Conclusion.* Activation of the Notch1-RBP-Jk/Msx2 signaling pathway may be involved in the development and progression of vascular calcification in DN.

1. Introduction

Vascular calcification is a key pathological process that contributes to cardiovascular complications of chronic kidney disease (CKD) and is also an independent risk factor for cardiovascular events and mortality in patients with CKD [1, 2]. Diabetic nephropathy (DN) is a leading cause of CKD and is associated with high incidence and quick progression of vascular calcification [3]. About 78% of diabetic patients with preserved kidney function were shown to exhibit varying degrees of vascular calcification in femoral, posterior tibial, and dorsalis pedis arteries [4].

Vascular calcification is a complex, irreversible biological process, which involves differentiation of vascular smooth muscle cells (VSMCs) into chondrocyte- or osteoblast-like cells (chondrogenesis or osteogenesis). It is accompanied by downregulation of contractile VSMC markers, such as alpha-smooth muscle actin (α-SMA) and smooth muscle 22 alpha (SM22α), and upregulation of various osteogenic transcription factors, such as runt-related transcription factor 2 (Runx2), Msx2, alkaline phosphatase (ALP), osteopontin (OPN), and bone morphogenetic protein 2 (BMP2) [5–8]. Several signaling pathways such as Wnt/β-catenin and Notch1-RBP-Jk are believed to be involved in the process of vascular calcification [9, 10]. However, the precise regulatory mechanism of vascular calcification process is not yet clear.

Recent studies have shown that Notch1 signaling pathway, a regulator of angiogenesis and osteogenesis, plays a role in the development of vascular calcification [6, 10, 11]. In mammals, the highly conserved Notch pathway involves four type I transmembrane receptors (Notch1–4), five classical ligands [Jagged 1, 2, and Delta-like (DLL) 1, 3, and 4], and nonclassical ligand DNER, in the regulation of a variety of biological processes, such as cell proliferation, differentiation, and apoptosis [12]. Notch pathway has been extensively studied in the field of tumor growth and targeted therapy [13]; however, its possible involvement in the pathogenesis of diabetic vascular calcification, as well as the specific underlying mechanisms, has rarely been reported.

In this study, we used a modified animal model of vascular calcification in the context of DN by administering a high-fat diet and injection of streptozotocin (STZ), followed by intragastric administration of nicotine and intramuscular injection of vitamin D3. The study explored the changes in expressions of VSMC markers, α-SMA and SM22α, and osteogenic markers, Runx2 and ALP, and further investigated the relationship between the target molecules in Notch1-RBP-Jk/Msx2 pathway and vascular calcification in aortic tissues in the rat model.

2. Methods and Materials

2.1. Animal Model. Specific pathogen-free Sprague-Dawley (SD) rats ($n = 42$, male, 4–6 weeks old; weight: 170–220 g) were obtained from the animal center at the Southwest Medical University. The experimental protocol was approved by the ethics committee of the Animal Care and Use Committee at the Southwest Medical University [Permit number, SYSK (CHUAN) 2013-065]. The rats were kept under observation for one week prior to the start of the experiment. They were then randomly divided into two groups, that is, normal controls (Nor group, $n = 18$) and DN rats with vitamin D3/nicotine-induced vascular calcification (DN + VDN group, $n = 24$).

Twenty-four SD rats were fed high-fat diet for four weeks. The high-fat diet contained 55% carbohydrate, 10% lard, 10% soybean oil, 11% protein, 2.5% cholesterol, and 11.5% fiber. Following 12 h fasting, the rats were administered a single intraperitoneal injection of streptozotocin, 35 mg/kg (STZ, Sigma Chemical Co., St. Louis, MO, USA) in citrate buffer (1%, *w*/*v*). Three days after the injection of STZ, whole-blood specimens were obtained from mouse tail-vein. Twenty-two rats with blood glucose level > 16.7 mmol/L for 3 consecutive days were deemed to have developed diabetes mellitus. DN was identified based on 24 h urinary protein excretion >30 mg and increase in urine volume by ≥50% from the baseline. Two weeks later, one rat that did not meet the criteria was excluded. After establishment of the DN model, the DN rats were administered intramuscular injection of vitamin D3 (300,000 U/kg) once daily at 9:00 Hrs and intragastric nicotine (Merck, Darmstadt, Germany) dissolved in peanut oil (25 mg/kg, 5 mL/kg) twice daily (at 9:00 and 18:00 Hrs) [14]. The Nor rats were fed standard chow for four weeks, followed by administration of an equal volume of citrate buffer (vehicle). The control rats were administered intramuscular injection of saline and an equal volume of intragastric peanut oil following the same schedule. The rats were sacrificed at 8, 12, and 16 weeks ($n = 6$ at each time point). During the experiment, food and water intake by the rats, their mental state, and blood glucose levels in tail-vein blood were monitored to avoid ketoacidosis or accidental death. The rats were administered subcutaneous insulin injection if the blood glucose level exceeded 26 mmol/L. The timeline of the experimental interventions in the study is shown in Figure 1.

The general conditions of all rats were monitored daily, including mental state, activities, and fur. Body weight was recorded every week throughout the experiment.

24 h urinary protein excretion of diabetic rats was determined at 2 weeks after diagnosis of diabetes and before sacrifice. Successful modeling of DN was confirmed if 24 h urinary protein excretion was more than 30 mg. The rats were fasted for 24 h and then placed in metabolic cages for 24-hour urine collection. Urine protein concentrations were determined by Beckman automatic biochemistry analyzer (Beckman Coulter, Fullerton, CA, USA).

2.2. Biochemical and Histological Analysis. After weighing, the rats were anesthetized by an intraperitoneal injection of 2% pentobarbital sodium (Sigma Chemical Co., St. Louis, MO, USA) at a dose of 50 mg/kg and then fixed on an operation table. The abdominal aorta was separated after exposure of the abdominal cavity. The blood was collected from the abdominal aorta and centrifuged at 5000 rpm/min for 10 min at 4°C. The supernatant was collected and labeled and then stored at −20°C until further processing. Serum creatinine (Scr), blood urea nitrogen (BUN), serum calcium (Ca), and phosphorus (P) were measured using an automatic biochemical analyzer.

After blood sample collection, the aorta was resected. The aortic lumen was rinsed with cold saline. The thoracic and abdominal aortic tissues were immersed in 4% formalin solution for at least 24 hours and treated with graded series of ethanol for dehydration and paraffin-embedded, and 4 μm thick sections were prepared. Sections were then stained with von Kossa (Shanghai GenMed, China) and counterstained with Nuclear fast red (Shanghai GenMed, China) to visualize the nuclei. The sections were mounted on glass slides, and three randomly selected fields per slice were examined under an inverted phase contrast microscope (Nikon, Japan).

The degree of vascular calcification was semiquantitatively assessed by two independent observers according to the following scale [15]: 0, no mineral content; 1, a few small dispersed concretions; 2, numerous small dispersed concretions; 3, large granular concretions; and 4, large areas occupied by fused mineral deposits. In case of disagreement, the average of the two scores was considered in the final analysis.

2.3. Molecular and Immunohistochemical Analysis. Total RNA was extracted from frozen thoracic aorta tissues of rats using an Eastep® Super kit (Shanghai ProMega, China), and total RNA sample was reverse-transcribed into complementary DNA (cDNA) using the Eastep RT Master Mix (5x) Kit (Shanghai ProMega, China). The sequences of the primers used are shown in Supplementary Table 1. DNA amplification was performed on a StepOne real-time polymerase chain reaction (PCR) system (Eppendorf, Germany) with Eastep qPCR Master Mix

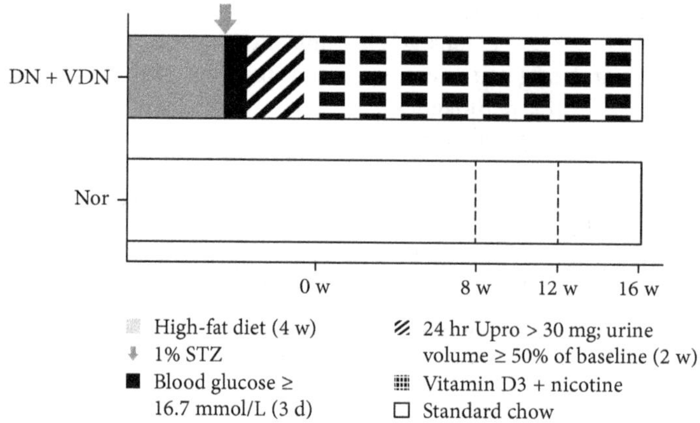

FIGURE 1: Schematic illustration of the experimental protocol. W: week; STZ: streptozotocin; Upro: urine protein. Nor group: normal controls; DN + VDN group: diabetic nephropathy rats with vitamin D3/nicotine-induced vascular calcification.

(2x) Kit (Shanghai ProMega, China) using the following thermal conditions: an initial step at 95°C for 2 minutes, followed by 40 cycles of 95°C for 15 seconds, 60°C for 1 minute, and 95°C for 15 seconds, and a final phase at 60°C for 5 minutes. The relative amount of mRNA of each sample was calculated using the $2^{-\Delta\Delta CT}$ method and corrected by reference to the expression of GAPDH (loading control).

The following primary antibodies were used for immunohistochemical analysis: monoclonal rabbit anti-rat RBP-Jk, Msx2, and N1-ICD (Shanghai Bioworld Tech Inc., China); monoclonal rabbit anti-rat Jagged1 and Runx2 (Beijing BioTech Inc., China); monoclonal rabbit anti-rat Notch1 (Wuhan Proteintech Group Inc., China); and monoclonal mouse anti-rat α-SMA (Wuhan Boster Bio-Tech., Ltd, China). Immunohistochemical staining was performed according to the manufacturer's instructions. Briefly, paraffin-embedded thoracic aortic tissues were cut into 4 μm thick sections. After antigen retrieval by heating in a microwave, the sections were incubated overnight with primary antibodies at 4°C. After rinsing with phosphate-buffered saline (PBS), the sections were incubated with anti-mouse or anti-rabbit secondary antibodies coupled to horseradish peroxidase (Zhongshan Golden Bridge Biotechnology, Beijing, China). The reaction was visualized using 3, 3′-Diaminobenzidine (DAB, Zhongshan Golden Bridge Biotechnology, China). The sections were rinsed with water and counterstained with Mayer's hematoxylin (Beijing Solarbio Biotech, China). The known positive control in the kit was used as the positive control and replacement of the primary antibody with PBS was used for the negative control. Positive immunostaining was presented as brown or yellow granules in the cytoplasm and/or nucleus. Five visual fields were randomly selected and assessed for immunoreactive areas at 200x magnification using an inverted phase-contrast microscope (Nikon, Japan). The image was analyzed by Image-Pro Plus 6.0 software (Media Cybernetics Inc., Rockville, MD, USA), with color histogram in HSI model (H: 0–30, S: 0–255, I: 0–230); optical density range was 0–6000. The cumulative optical density (IOD) and area of the selected regions were acquired by the software, and the IOD/area was calculated as mean ± standard deviation (SD) for analysis.

2.4. Statistical Analysis. All statistical analysis was performed using SPSS17.0 software (SPSS Inc., Chicago, IL, USA). Quantitative data are presented as mean ± SD. The normality of distribution of the continuous quantitative variables was assessed by the Kolmogorov-Smirnov test. Intergroup and intragroup differences were assessed using the independent sample t-test and one-way analysis of variance, respectively. Scores of von Kossa staining were analyzed by the Wilcoxon rank-sum test. $p < 0.05$ was considered statistically significant.

3. Results

3.1. The General Condition of the Rats. Compared with rats in the Nor group, the DN rats exhibited polydipsia, polyphagia, polyuria, loss of body weight, dull fur, and reduced activities at 8 weeks after establishment of the model. Rats in the DN + VDN group showed arched back and piloerection, abdominal bulge, and tail ulcers at 12 weeks, and severe depression at 16 weeks.

The body weight of normal rats gradually increased over time. On the contrary, rats in the DN + VDN group lost substantial weight with the progression of diabetes; between-group differences at 8, 12, and 16 weeks were statistically significant ($p < 0.001$, Figure 2(a), Supplementary Table 2). Rats in the DN + VDN group presented remarkable increase in blood glucose level, 24 h urine protein excretion, Scr, and serum BUN levels, as compared to that in the Nor group at 8, 12, and 16 weeks ($p < 0.01$ or $p < 0.001$; Figures 2(b)–2(e); Supplementary Table 2).

In addition, rats in the DN + VDN group exhibited elevated serum phosphorus levels at 16 weeks ($p < 0.05$), elevated serum calcium levels at 8, 12, and 16 weeks ($p < 0.05$ or $p < 0.01$), and resultant increase in calcium-phosphorus product at 8, 12, and 16 weeks ($p < 0.05$ or $p < 0.01$; Figures 2(f)–2(h); Supplementary Table 2).

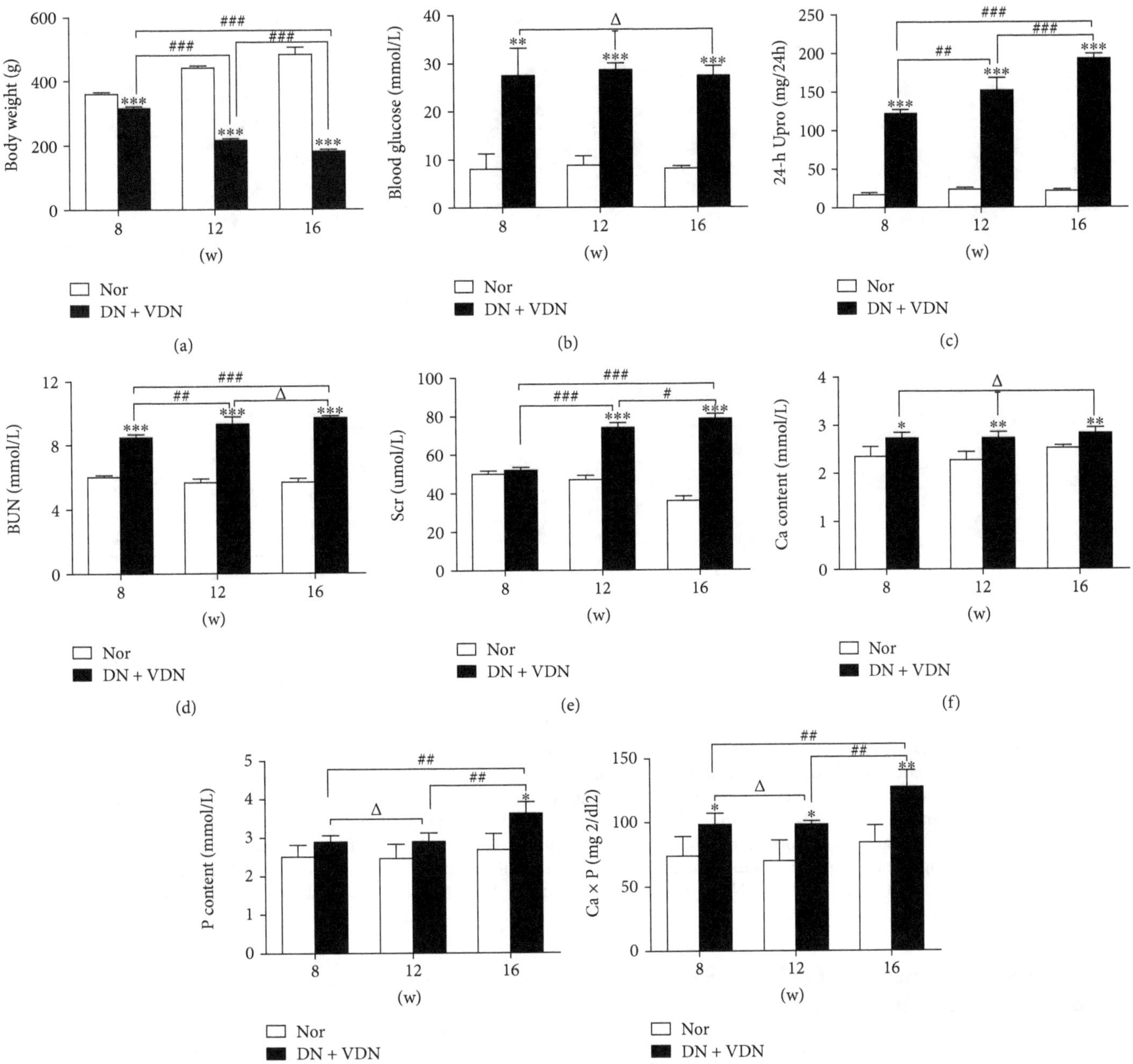

FIGURE 2: Body weight and various biochemical indicators of rats at 8, 12, and 16 weeks. (a) body weight; (b) blood glucose; (c) 24 h urine protein excretion (24 h Upro); (d) blood urea nitrogen (BUN); (e) serum creatinine (Scr); (f) serum calcium (Ca); (g) serum phosphorus (P); and (h) calcium-phosphorus product (Ca x P). Data presented as mean ± standard deviation (SD). $^{*}p < 0.05$, $^{**}p < 0.01$, and $^{***}p < 0.001$ versus Nor group; $^{\Delta}p > 0.05$, $^{\#}p < 0.05$, $^{\#\#}p < 0.01$, and $^{\#\#\#}p < 0.001$. Nor group: normal controls; DN + VDN group: diabetic nephropathy rats with vitamin D3/nicotine-induced vascular calcification.

3.2. Characteristics of Aortic Vascular Calcification in DN Rats. The absence of calcium salt deposition in aortic tissue of normal rats was revealed by von Kossa staining, irrespective of the time point (8 weeks, Figure 3(a); 16 weeks, Figure 3(b)). In contrast, rats in the DN + VDN group exhibited scattered, punctated deposition of calcium salts in the form of dark brown granules among the elastic fibers of the intima media at the end of the 8th week (Figure 3(c)); a large quantity of aggregated deposits of calcium salts was observed in vascular wall at the end of the 12th week (Figure 3(d)); finally, a wide area of confluent calcification plaque was observed at the end of the 16th week (Figure 3(e)). The distribution of scores in both groups is shown in Figure 3(f). The DN + VDN group had higher scores as compared to those of the Nor group ($p < 0.05$).

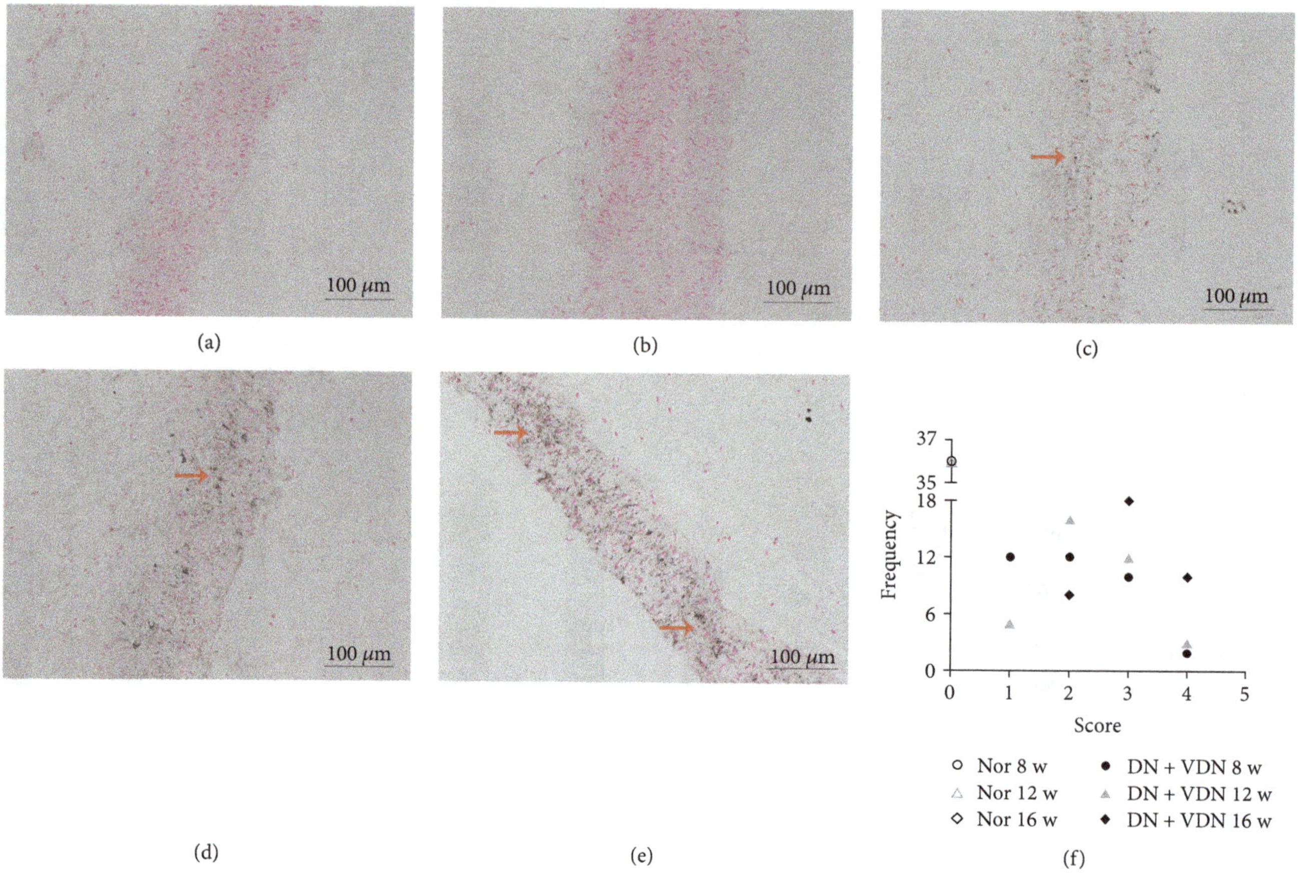

FIGURE 3: Histological analysis of aortic calcification with von Kossa staining. The von Kossa staining of aortic tissues from normal rats and DN + VDN rats. No deposition of calcium salts was observed in aortic tissues of normal rats at 8 (a) and 16 weeks (b). In contrast, rats in the DN + VDN group exhibited scattered, punctated deposition of calcium salts in the form of dark brown granules interspersed with the elastic fibers in arterial intima-media at the end of the 8th week (c); and a large quantity of aggregated deposits of calcium salts in vascular wall at the end of the 12th week (d); and finally formed a wide area of confluent calcification plaque at the end of the 16th week (e). (f) rats in the DN + VDN group had significantly higher vascular calcification scores than those of normal rats at 8, 12, and 16 weeks ($p < 0.001$). Data presented as mean ± standard deviation (SD). Nor group: normal controls; DN + VDN group: diabetic nephropathy rats with vitamin D3/nicotine-induced vascular calcification.

4. 3.3 mRNA Expressions of α-SMA, SM22α, Runx2, and ALP in Aortic Tissues

Real-time PCR showed that the mRNA expressions of α-SMA and SM22α in aortic tissue were significantly decreased at all time points (8, 12, and 16 weeks), as compared with the Nor group ($p < 0.05$, $p < 0.01$, or $p < 0.001$; Figures 4(a) and 4(b)). In contrast, the mRNA expressions of Runx2 and ALP in aortic tissues were upregulated after modeling ($p < 0.05$ and $p < 0.01$ versus Nor group; Figures 4(c) and 4(d)).

4.1. 3.4 Detection of α-SMA and Runx2 Levels by Immunohistochemical Analysis. During the experiments, α-SMA protein was extensively expressed in the aortic wall of normal rats, and there was no significant difference at any of the time points (8, 12, and 16 weeks, $p > 0.05$; Figures 5(a)–5(c)). However, the expression of α-SMA in the aortic tissue of DN + VDN group was significantly lower than that in the Nor group at the same time point ($p < 0.05$ or $p < 0.01$ versus Nor group at 8, 12, and 16 weeks; Figures 5(d)–5(g)).

In addition, Runx2 protein was weakly expressed in the wall of the aorta in normal rats (8, 12, and 16 weeks; Figures 5(h)–5(j)), whereas its expression was significantly increased in the DN + VDN group at each time point ($p < 0.05$ versus Nor group at 8, 12, and 16 weeks; Figures 5(k)–5(n)).

5. 3.5 mRNA Expression of Notch1, RBP-Jk, Msx2, and Jagged1 in Aortic Tissues

As compared with the normal rats, the mRNA expressions of Notch1, RBP-Jk, Msx2, and Jagged1 in aortic tissues were persistently increased till 12 weeks ($p < 0.01$ and $p < 0.001$ *versus* Nor group) and then substantially decreased, although these were still higher than the normal levels ($p < 0.05$, $p < 0.01$, or $p < 0.001$; Figures 6(a)–6(d)).

5.1. 3.6 Detection of Notch1, RBP-Jk, Msx2, Jagged1, and N1-ICD Levels by Immunohistochemical Analysis. Notch1, RBP-

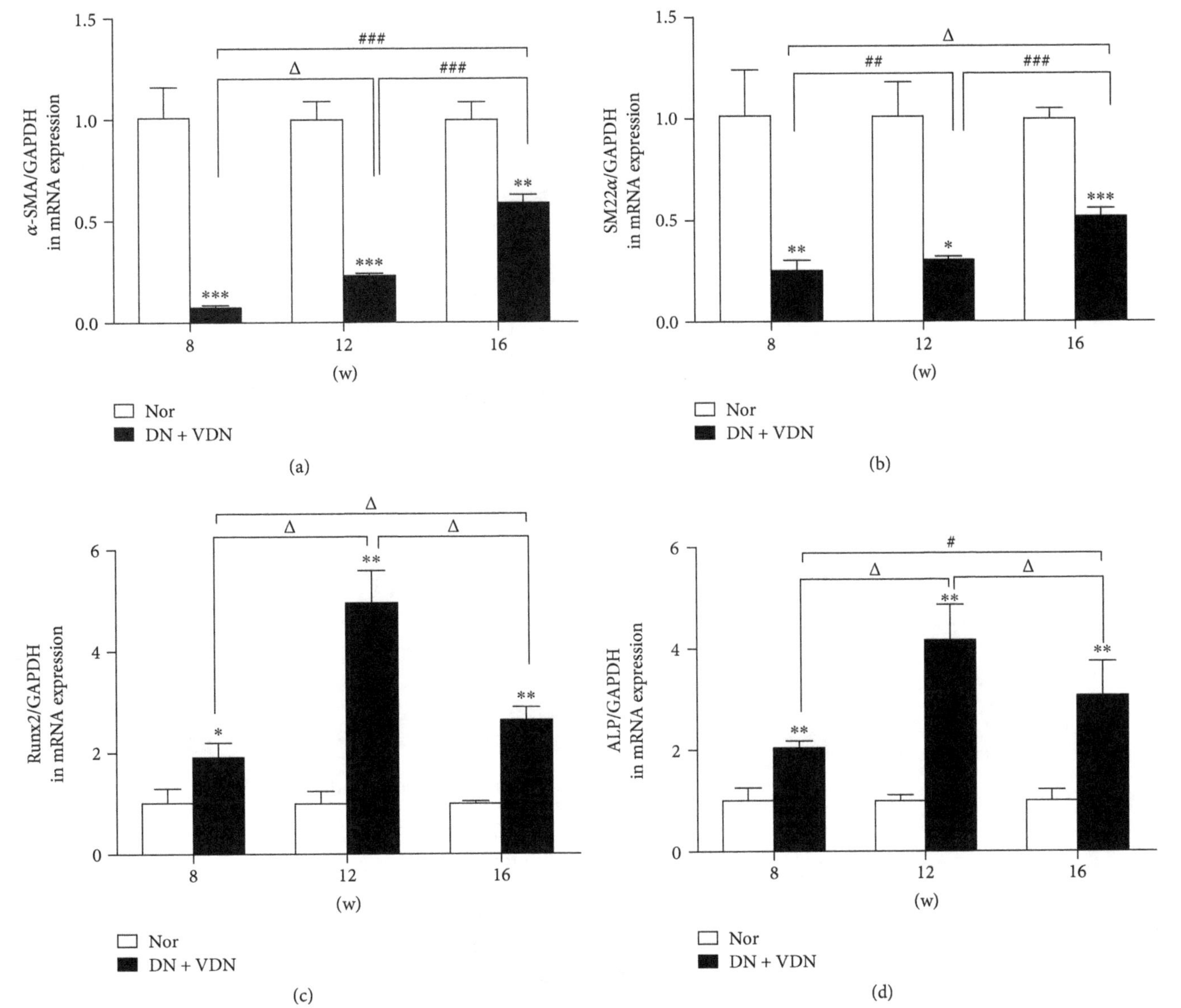

FIGURE 4: Quantitative assessment of mRNA expressions of α-SMA (a), SM22α (b), Runx2 (c), and ALP (d) in aortic tissues. Data presented as mean ± standard deviation (SD). $^{*}p < 0.05$, $^{**}p < 0.01$, and $^{***}p < 0.001$ versus Nor group; $^{\Delta}p > 0.05$, $^{\#}p < 0.05$, $^{\#\#}p < 0.01$, and $^{\#\#\#}p < 0.001$. Nor group: normal controls; DN + VDN group: diabetic nephropathy rats with vitamin D3/nicotine-induced vascular calcification.

Jk, Msx2, Jagged1, and N1-ICD were barely expressed in the aortic wall of normal rats. However, the expressions of these proteins in the DN + VDN group were significantly increased at all time points as compared to that in the normal rats (8, 12, and 16 weeks; $p < 0.05$, $p < 0.01$, or $p < 0.001$; Figure 7). The positive staining was mainly distributed in the media of the aorta.

6. 4. Discussion

Intramuscular injection of vitamin D3 and/or intragastric administration of nicotine are commonly used to establish a rat model of vascular calcification [14, 16, 17]. High dose of vitamin D induces and exacerbates oxidative stress and results in extensive vascular calcification [18]. Nicotine releases catecholamines and promotes calcium deposition in blood vessels [16]. The combination of vitamin D3 and nicotine leads to a substantial increase (approximately more than 20-fold) in calcium content of the aorta in rats [16]. This model can simulate the pathological vascular calcification observed in diabetes, end-stage renal disease, and aging-related calcification [19], with high stability and excellent reproducibility.

In this study, we used a rat model of DN with concomitant vascular calcification by intraperitoneal injection of STZ followed by administration of vitamin D3 and nicotine. The rats exhibited typical characteristics of DN, including weight loss, persistent proteinuria, robust increase in serum BUN, and creatinine. Vitamin D can increase the serum calcium level, whereas nicotine toxicity induces calcium overload and even necrosis of VSMCs [19, 20]. The released calcium and other minerals are accumulated among the elastic fibers in the arterial walls. In this study, we observed a significant increase in serum calcium levels in model rats at all

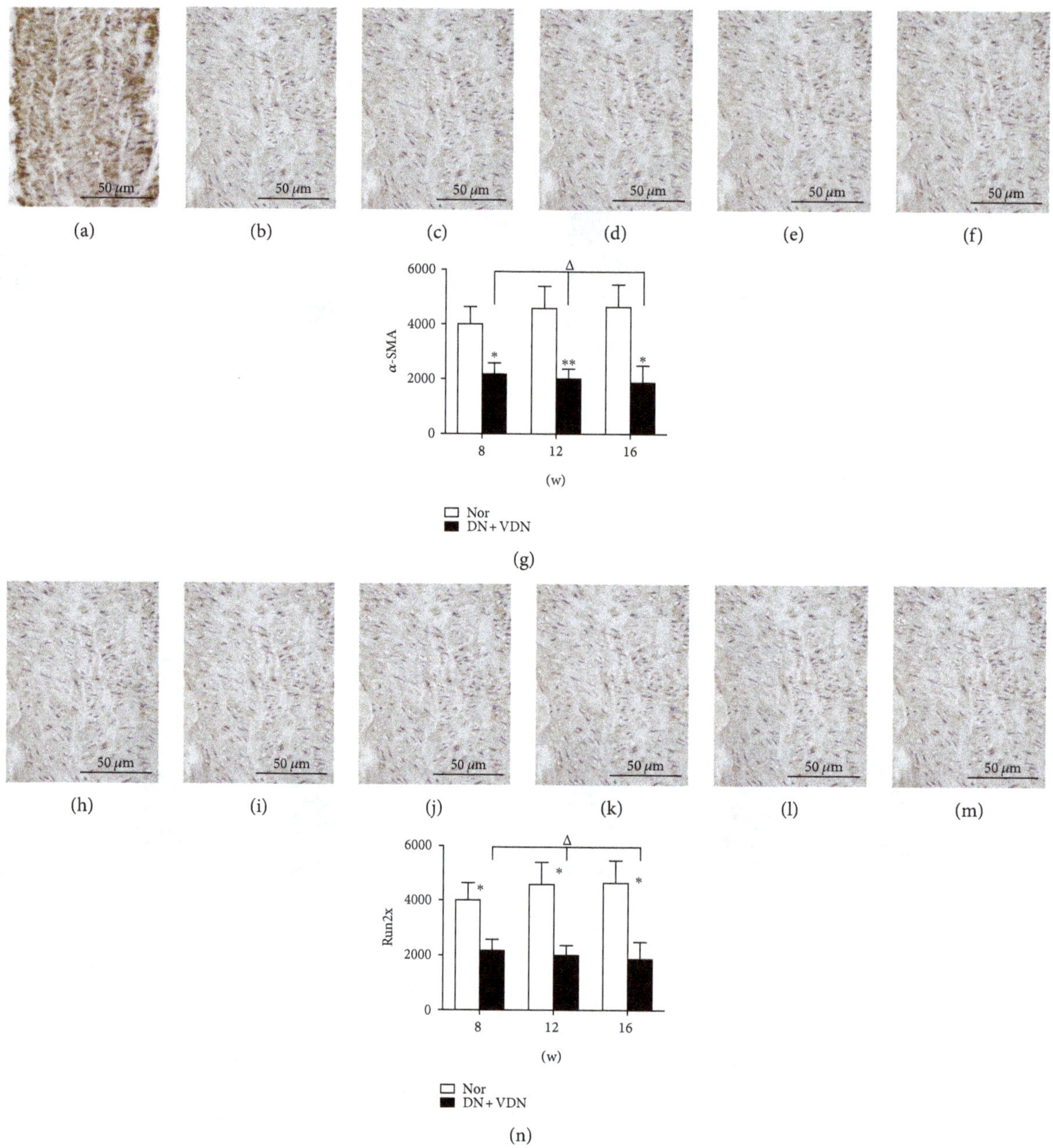

FIGURE 5: Detection of α-SMA and Runx2 levels by immunohistochemical analysis. α-SMA protein was extensively expressed in the aortic wall of normal rats at 8 weeks (a), 12 weeks (b), and 16 weeks (c), whereas the expression of α-SMA in the aortic tissue of DN + VDN group was significantly decreased at all time points, 8 weeks (d), 12 weeks (e), and 16 weeks (f). (g) Quantitative analysis of α-SMA was performed. Runx2 protein was weakly expressed in the wall of the aorta in normal rats at 8 weeks (h), 12 weeks (i), and 16 weeks (j). Its expression was significantly increased in the DN + VDN group at 8 weeks (k), 12 weeks (l), and 16 weeks (m). (n) Quantitative analysis of Runx2 was performed. Data presented as mean ± standard deviation (SD). $^{*}p < 0.05$ and $^{**}p < 0.01$ versus Nor group; $^{\Delta}p > 0.05$. Nor group: normal controls; DN + VDN group: diabetic nephropathy rats with vitamin D3/nicotine-induced vascular calcification.

time points (8, 12, and 16 weeks); however, serum phosphorus level was not significantly different until 16 weeks. These results are consistent with the fact that hyperphosphatemia usually appears in the late stages of CKD [21]. The increase in serum calcium levels as well as calcium-phosphorus products can promote calcification. Hyperphosphatemia-related vascular calcification in patients with DN, end-stage renal disease, and metabolic syndrome occurs mainly in the arterial media [22, 23]. Histological studies of model rats demonstrated deposition of calcium salts, which indicates successful establishment of a rat model of vascular calcification. The effect of vascular calcification in patients with DN is not well understood. Thus, an in-depth understanding of the pathogenesis of vascular calcification in the context of DN will be of great significance and may facilitate the search for a new therapeutic target.

Vascular calcification resulting from deposition of calcium phosphorus or hydroxyapatite in the vessel wall is a

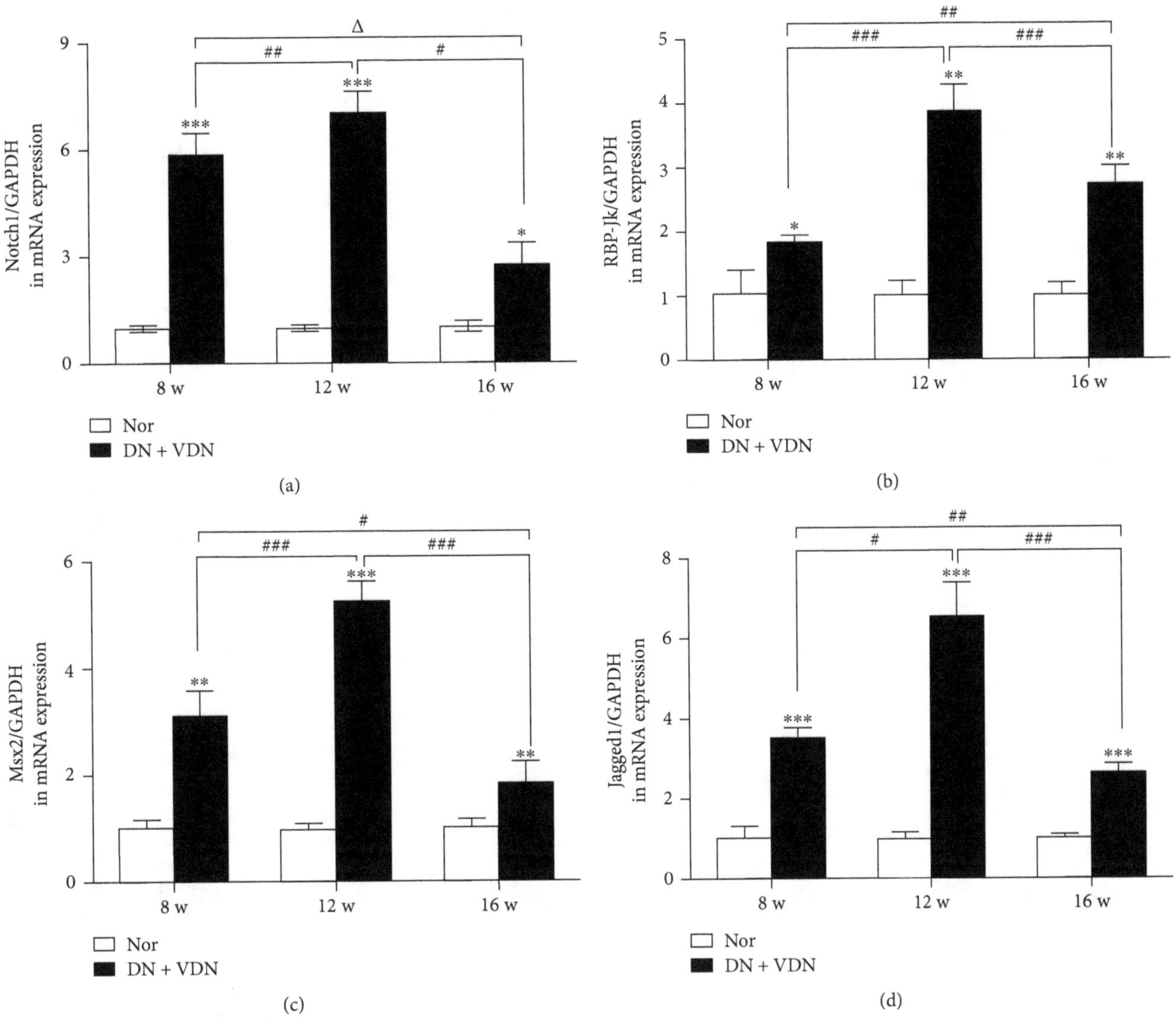

FIGURE 6: The mRNA expressions of Notch1 (a), RBP-Jk (b), Msx2 (c), and Jagged1 (d) in aortic tissues. Data presented as mean ± standard deviation (SD). $^{*}p < 0.05$, $^{**}p < 0.01$, and $^{***}p < 0.001$ versus Nor group; $^{\Delta}p > 0.05$, $^{\#}p < 0.05$, $^{\#\#}p < 0.01$, and $^{\#\#\#}p < 0.001$. Nor group: normal controls; DN + VDN group: diabetic nephropathy rats with vitamin D3/nicotine-induced vascular calcification.

complex pathological process regulated by a variety of regulatory factors and pathways. A number of studies have revealed that VSMCs play a central role in the initiation and progression of vascular calcification, during which they undergo phenotypic differentiation, for example, into osteoblast-like cells. The process is accompanied by overexpression of osteogenic markers such as Msx2, ALP, OPN, and type I collagen, which are involved in ectopic mineralization and bone formation [6, 8, 10]. In this study, real-time PCR showed a significant decrease in the mRNA expression of VSMC markers (α-SMA and SM22α) in aortic tissue of model rats; while the mRNA expressions of osteogenic markers (Runx2 and ALP) were remarkably increased, especially at 12 weeks. The expressions of these proteins were gradually restored to near normal levels over time although they were still lower (α-SMA and SM22α) or higher (Runx2 and ALP) than those in control animals, perhaps due to a compensatory mechanism of the body, which requires further investigation. These results were partially consistent with the immunohistochemical analysis, although some discrepancies between mRNA expressions of α-SMA and Runx2 and results of quantitative immunohistochemistry were observed. Further efforts are needed to explain these discrepancies. These results indicated that DN rats with vascular calcification exhibited mineral deposits in the arterial intima-media accompanied by phenotypic changes of VSMCs and activation of osteogenic factors.

Vascular calcification is associated with multiple signaling pathways, including BMP2/SMADs, receptor for advanced glycation end products (RAGE)/JAK2, Wnt/β-catenin, and Notch1 [10, 24]. Also, the involvement of Notch signaling pathway in DN has been elucidated [25, 26]. In this study, extensive arterial calcification in rats with DN was accompanied by upregulation of Notch1, RBP-Jk, Msx2, Jagged1, and N1-ICD proteins, which suggests the activation of Notch1 signaling pathway. There may be at least two possible

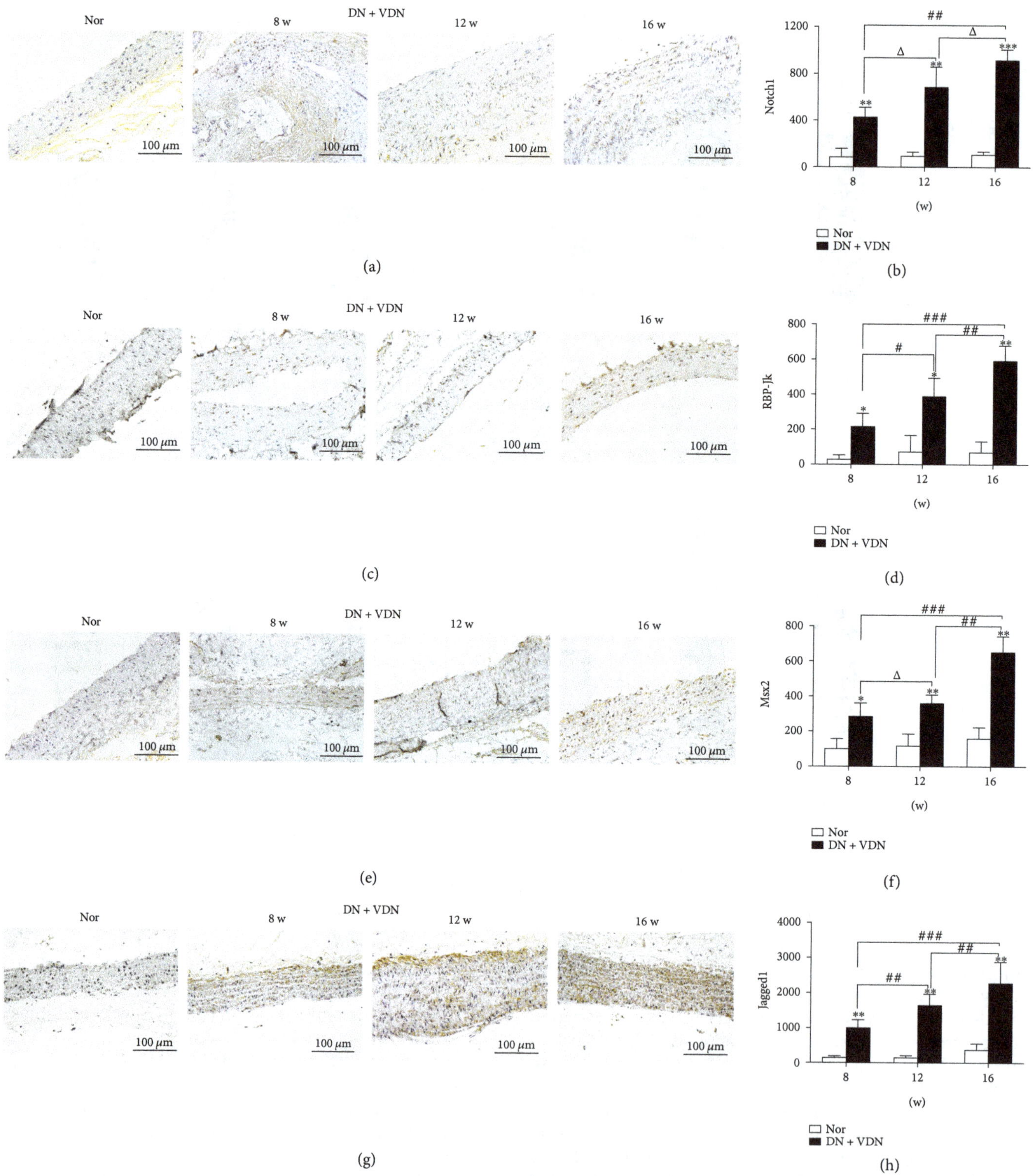

FIGURE 7: Continued.

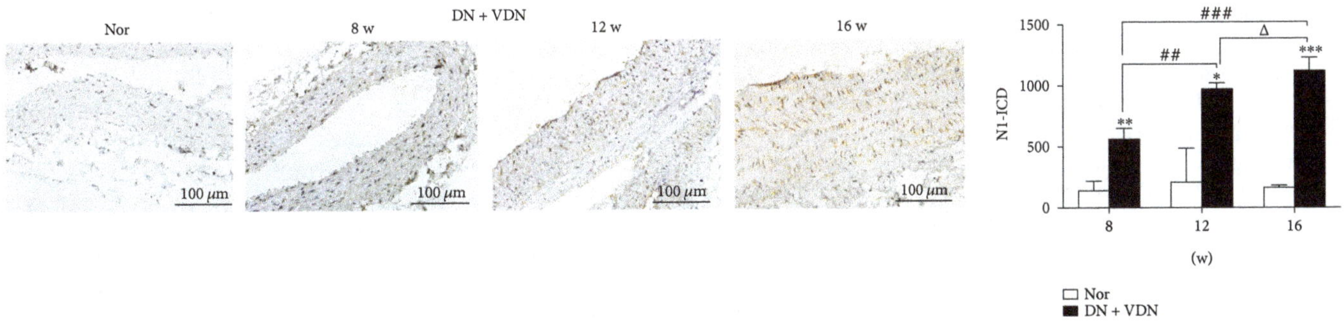

(i) (j)

FIGURE 7: Detection of Notch1, RBP-Jk, Msx2, Jagged1, and N1-ICD levels by immunohistochemical analysis. The representative images and quantitative analysis of Notch1 (a-b), RBP-Jk (c-d), Msx2 (e-f), Jagged1 (g-h), and N1-ICD (i-j) in aortic tissues. The left panel of histological images: Nor group; right panel: DN + VDN group at 8, 12 , and 16 weeks, respectively. Data presented as mean ± standard deviation (SD). $^{*}p < 0.05$, $^{**}p < 0.01$, and $^{***}p < 0.001$ versus Nor group; $^{\Delta}p > 0.05$, $^{\#}p < 0.05$, $^{\#\#}p < 0.01$, and $^{\#\#\#}p < 0.001$. Nor group: normal controls; DN + VDN group: diabetic nephropathy rats with vitamin D3/nicotine-induced vascular calcification.

mechanisms involved. Hyperglycemia can increase the expression of Notch1 protein and its downstream molecules involved in the pathogenesis of endothelial cell injury [27]. Culture of VSMCs *in vitro* with serum from diabetic patients was shown to induce an increase in calcium content of VSMCs [28]. In a study by Suga et al. [29], RAGE overexpression induced the expression of ALP and Msx2 and calcium deposition in human aortic VSMCs that were cultured with the sera of patients with diabetes; on the contrary, silencing of Msx2 effectively inhibited osteogenic differentiation of VSMCs, which indicates that activation of Notch/Msx2 signal pathway under high glucose induces osteogenic differentiation of VSMCs and contributes to aortic calcification. Secondly, in the late stage of DN, impaired renal function causes hyperphosphatemia which stimulates Notch1-RBP-Jk signaling pathway to induce the expression of target gene Msx2, resulting in osteogenic differentiation and mineralization of VSMCs [6, 11]. Interestingly, the expressions of target molecules in Notch1-RBP-Jk/Msx2 pathway might show a fluctuant increase, probably due to a synergistic or offsetting effect of various pathologic factors. For instance, hyperglycemia and hyperphosphatemia trigger the activation of Notch1-RBP-Jk/Msx2 pathway in DN to varying degrees and at different time periods, whereas the compensatory mechanism of the body may restore their levels. Therefore, further investigation is required to confirm and extend these results.

In conclusion, activation of Notch1-RBP-Jk/Msx2 signaling pathway may be involved in the development and progression of vascular calcification in DN. In subsequent research, efforts will be made to identify a novel therapeutic target, blocking of which leads to the prevention and treatment of vascular calcification in DN.

Abbreviations

ALP: Alkaline phosphatase
α-SMA: Alpha-smooth muscle actin
BMP2: Bone morphogenetic protein 2
BUN: Blood urea nitrogen
CKD: Chronic kidney disease
N1-ICD: Intracellular Notch1 domain
OPN: Osteopontin
PBS: Phosphate-buffered saline
PCR: Polymerase chain reaction
RAGE: Receptor for advanced glycation end products
Runx2: Runt-related transcription factor2
Scr: Serum creatinine
SM22α: Smooth muscle 22 alpha
STZ: Streptozotocin
VDN: Vitamin D3 and nicotine
VSMC: Vascular smooth muscle cell.

Conflicts of Interest

All authors declared there were no conflicts of interests involved.

Authors' Contributions

Caipan Gong and Li Li contributed equally to this work.

References

[1] S. Disthabanchong, "Vascular calcification in chronic kidney disease: pathogenesis and clinical implication," *World Journal of Nephrology*, vol. 1, no. 2, pp. 43–53, 2012.

[2] M. Mizobuchi, D. Towler, and E. Slatopolsky, "Vascular calcification: the killer of patients with chronic kidney disease," *Journal of the American Society of Nephrology*, vol. 20, no. 7, pp. 1453–1464, 2009.

[3] R. Pálsson and U. D. Patel, "Cardiovascular complications of diabetic kidney disease," *Advances in Chronic Kidney Disease*, vol. 21, no. 3, pp. 273–280, 2014.

[4] D. K. Singh, P. Winocour, B. Summerhayes et al., "Prevalence and progression of peripheral vascular calcification in type 2 diabetes subjects with preserved kidney function," *Diabetes Research and Clinical Practice*, vol. 97, no. 1, pp. 158–165, 2012.

[5] P. Ciceri, F. Elli, I. Brenna et al., "Lanthanum prevents high phosphate-induced vascular calcification by preserving vascular smooth muscle lineage markers," *Calcified Tissue International*, vol. 92, no. 6, pp. 521–530, 2013.

[6] T. Shimizu, T. Tanaka, T. Iso et al., "Notch signaling induces osteogenic differentiation and mineralization of vascular smooth muscle cells: role of Msx2 gene induction via Notch-RBP-Jk signaling," *Arteriosclerosis Thrombosis and Vascular Biology*, vol. 29, no. 7, pp. 1104–1111, 2009.

[7] Y. Chen, A. B. Bangash, J. Song et al., "Activation of CD137 signaling accelerates vascular calcification in vivo and vitro," *International Journal of Cardiology*, vol. 230, pp. 198–203, 2017.

[8] W. Feng, K. Zhang, Y. Liu et al., "Apocynin attenuates angiotensin II-induced vascular smooth muscle cells osteogenic switching via suppressing extracellular signal-regulated kinase 1/2," *Oncotarget*, vol. 7, no. 50, pp. 83588–83600, 2016.

[9] A. Verhulst, P. Evenepoel, and P. C. D'Haese, "Ligand trap for the activin type IIA receptor. The long-sought drug to overcome the calcification paradox in CKD?," *Kidney International*, vol. 91, no. 1, pp. 11–13, 2017.

[10] S. Zhou, F. Xin, H. Xin, W. Li, H. Qiu, and S. Guan, "Osteoprotegerin inhibits calcification of vascular smooth muscle cell via down regulation of the Notch1-RBP-Jκ/Msx2 signaling pathway," *PLoS One*, vol. 8, no. 7, article e68987, 2013.

[11] T. Shimizu, T. Tanaka, T. Iso et al., "Notch signaling pathway enhances bone morphogenetic protein 2 (BMP2) responsiveness of Msx2 gene to induce osteogenic differentiation and mineralization of vascular smooth muscle cells," *Journal of Biological Chemistry*, vol. 286, no. 21, pp. 19138–19148, 2011.

[12] J. T. Baeten and B. Lilly, "Notch signaling in vascular smooth muscle cells," *Advances in Pharmacology*, vol. 78, pp. 351–382, 2017.

[13] C. S. Nowell and F. Radtke, "Notch as a tumour suppressor," *Nature Reviews Cancer*, vol. 17, no. 3, pp. 149–159, 2017.

[14] Y. Lu, Y. Bian, Y. Wang, R. Bai, J. Wang, and C. Xiao, "Globular adiponectin reduces vascular calcification via inhibition of ER-stress-mediated smooth muscle cell apoptosis," *International Journal of Clinical & Experimental Pathology*, vol. 8, no. 3, pp. 2545–2554, 2015.

[15] K. Janda, M. Krzanowski, M. Gajda et al., "Vascular effects of advanced glycation end-products: content of immunohistochemically detected AGEs in radial artery samples as a predictor for arterial calcification and cardiovascular risk in asymptomatic patients with chronic kidney disease," *Disease Markers*, vol. 2015, Article ID 153978, 9 pages, 2015.

[16] R. Wallin, N. Wajih, G. T. Greenwood, and D. C. Sane, "Arterial calcification: a review of mechanisms, animal models, and the prospects for therapy," *Medicinal Research Reviews*, vol. 21, no. 4, pp. 274–301, 2001.

[17] Q. Wei, X. Ren, Y. Jiang, H. Jin, N. Liu, and J. Li, "Advanced glycation end products accelerate rat vascular calcification through RAGE/oxidative stress," *BMC Cardiovascular Disorders*, vol. 13, no. 1, p. 13, 2013.

[18] F. T. Tang, S. R. Chen, X. Q. Wu et al., "Hypercholesterolemia accelerates vascular calcification induced by excessive vitamin D via oxidative stress," *Calcified Tissue International*, vol. 79, no. 5, pp. 326–339, 2006.

[19] X. Ren, Q. Wei, H. Shao, Z. Sun, and N. Liu, "A rat model of diabetic artery calcification," *Journal of Endocrinological Investigation*, vol. 35, no. 5, pp. 497–503, 2012.

[20] G. M. Hass, R. E. Trueheart, C. B. Taylor, and M. Stumpe, "An experimental histologic study of hypervitaminosis D," *American Journal of Pathology*, vol. 34, no. 3, pp. 395–431, 1958.

[21] J. T. Daugirdas, G. M. Chertow, B. Larive et al., "Effects of frequent hemodialysis on measures of CKD mineral and bone disorder," *Journal of the American Society of Nephrology*, vol. 23, no. 4, pp. 727–738, 2012.

[22] G. M. London, A. P. Guerin, S. J. Marchais, F. Métivier, B. Pannier, and H. Adda, "Arterial media calcification in end-stage renal disease: impact on all-cause and cardiovascular mortality," *Nephrology Dialysis Transplantation*, vol. 18, no. 9, pp. 1731–1740, 2003.

[23] L. A. Peres and P. P. Pércio, "Mineral and bone disorder and vascular calcification in patients with chronic kidney disease," *Jornal Brasileiro de Nefrologia*, vol. 36, no. 2, pp. 201–207, 2014.

[24] M. R. Brodeur, C. Bouvet, S. Bouchard et al., "Reduction of advanced-glycation end products levels and inhibition of RAGE signaling decreases rat vascular calcification induced by diabetes," *PLoS One*, vol. 9, no. 1, article e85922, 2014.

[25] R. Bonegio and K. Susztak, "Notch signaling in diabetic nephropathy," *Experimental Cell Research*, vol. 318, no. 9, pp. 986–992, 2012.

[26] D. Kavanagh, G. J. McKay, C. C. Patterson et al., "Association analysis of Notch pathway signalling genes in diabetic nephropathy," *Diabetologia*, vol. 54, no. 2, pp. 334–338, 2011.

[27] Y. Qiu, B. Du, F. Xie et al., "Vaccarin attenuates high glucose-induced human EA•hy926 endothelial cell injury through inhibition of Notch signaling," *Molecular Medicine Reports*, vol. 13, no. 3, pp. 2143–2150, 2016.

[28] T. Tanikawa, Y. Okada, R. Tanikawa, and Y. Tanaka, "Advanced glycation end products induce calcification of vascular smooth muscle cells through RAGE/p38 MAPK," *Journal of Vascular Research*, vol. 46, no. 6, pp. 572–580, 2009.

[29] T. Suga, T. Iso, T. Shimizu et al., "Activation of receptor for advanced glycation end products induces osteogenic differentiation of vascular smooth muscle cells," *Journal of Atherosclerosis and Thrombosis*, vol. 18, no. 8, pp. 670–683, 2011.

Study on Association of Pentraxin 3 and Diabetic Nephropathy in a Rat Model

Xuehai Chen,[1] Jiao Luo,[1] Minmin Wu,[1] Zhuo Pan,[1] Yue Xie,[1] Hongwei Wang,[1] Bicheng Chen,[1,2] and Hong Zhu[3]

[1]*Department of Surgery, The First Affiliated Hospital of Wenzhou Medical University, Wenzhou, Zhejiang 325000, China*
[2]*Zhejiang Provincial Top Key Discipline in Surgery, Wenzhou Key Laboratory of Surgery, Department of Surgery, The First Affiliated Hospital of Wenzhou Medical University, Wenzhou, Zhejiang 325000, China*
[3]*Department of Endocrinology, The First Affiliated Hospital of Wenzhou Medical University, Wenzhou, Zhejiang 325000, China*

Correspondence should be addressed to Bicheng Chen; bisonch@163.com and Hong Zhu; wyyynfm@126.com

Academic Editor: Mark Yorek

Diabetic nephropathy (DN) is a serious microvascular complication of diabetes. Compared with other therapies for diabetic patients, islet transplantation can effectively prevent and reverse diabetes-induced microvascular disease, such as diabetic retinopathy and nephropathy. PTX3 is the only long pentraxin that can be detected in renal tissue. In this study, we investigated the expression of PTX3 when early DN was reversed after islet transplantation. *Methods.* Diabetes was induced in rats by injecting streptozotocin (STZ). Twelve weeks later, the diabetic rats were divided into 2 groups: the islet transplantation group (IT) and the diabetic nephropathy group (DN). Renal injury, renal function, and the expression of PTX3 in the plasma and the kidneys were assessed with urinalysis, immunohistochemical staining, and Western blot, respectively. *Results.* The expression of PTX3 in the kidney was significantly decreased in the DN group but increased in the IT group because of the reversal of DN. *Conclusions.* Our data showed that the level of PTX3 in renal tissue is closely related to renal injury in DN. This may be used to quantify the extent of renal injury in DN, provide a potential early indicator of renal tubular injury in early DN patients, and assess DN clinical progression.

1. Introduction

In recent decades, the prevalence of diabetes in Chinese adults has risen to 9.7% [1]. Diabetic nephropathy (DN), a serious microvascular complication of diabetes, remains the main cause of end-stage renal disease. The major characteristic changes of DN include glomerular mesangial expansion, glomerular basement membrane thickening, progressive renal dysfunction, and persistent proteinuria [2]. Current management of hyperglycemia around the world depends on the lifetime injection of insulin. However, lifetime insulin administration has a high cost to patients, an elevated risk of hypoglycemia caused by improper insulin use, and can cause skin hypersensitivity reactions [3]. Previous studies showed that strict blood glucose control, the administration of angiotensin II receptor blockers (ARB), lipid lowering, and so forth can delay but not reverse the progress of DN. In 1990, Tzakis et al. reported the successful transplantation of isolated islet cells into diabetic patients for the first time [4]. Islet transplantation, a new treatment in modern society, permits more effective blood sugar control and better patient economic performance. More importantly, islet transplantation can effectively prevent and reverse diabetes-induced microvascular diseases, such as diabetic retinopathy and nephropathy [5, 6]. Our previous work found that in a rat model of early diabetic nephropathy, islet transplantation could stop and reverse the progression of diabetic nephropathy [7].

Pentraxin 3 (PTX3), a member of the long pentraxin group, has a structural homology with short pentraxins such as C-reactive protein (CRP) and serum amyloid P component (SAP) [8]. However, in contrast to CRP and SAP, which are produced in the liver, PTX3 is synthesized by extrahepatic tissues and cells in response to inflammatory stimulation, such as by interleukin 6 (IL-6) [8, 9]. PTX3 is composed of eight identical protomer subunits by disulfide bonds and is a member of the highly conserved pentraxin superfamily. PTX3 is produced and released by multiple different cell types, such as endothelial cells, monocytes/macrophages, skeletal muscle, and vascular smooth muscle cells, in response to tissue injury or inflammation [10]. In prior studies, it was demonstrated that as a modulator of inflammatory processes, PTX3 was involved in angiogenesis, atherosclerotic lesions, and extracellular matrix formation [11]. It has also been reported that PTX3 can control the interaction between dendritic cell (DC) maturation and apoptotic cells and then participate in the scavenging of apoptotic cells in the body [12].

PTX3 is the only long pentraxin that can be detected in renal tissue [13]. PTX3 mRNA is expressed in normal proximal renal tubular epithelial cells [10] but is marginally present in normal human glomeruli [13]. The expression of PTX3 was increased in renal endothelial cells in an ischemia-reperfusion injury model [14] and in the glomerular mesangial and endothelial cells of patients with type I membranous glomerulonephritis or IgA nephropathy [13]. However, in renal biopsies of patients with diffuse proliferative lupus nephropathy, membranous glomerulonephritis, or focal segmental glomerulosclerosis, the expression of PTX3 in the glomeruli was almost negative [13]. Instead, in the above renal diseases, PTX3 was expressed in the renal interstitial and tubules. Only one study on the association between PTX3 and DN is currently available, which reported that the expression of PTX3 was remarkably decreased in experimental diabetic nephropathy compared with controls [15].

In this study, we evaluated the expression of PTX3 and other related renal injury parameters in the renal tissue of diabetic rats with early diabetic nephropathy. Furthermore, we investigated the expression of PTX3 when early DN was reversed after islet transplantation.

2. Materials and Methods

2.1. Animal Model and Groups. A total of 35 male Wistar rats weighting 250–300 g were purchased from the Experimental Animal Center of Wenzhou Medical University. All rats were housed with a 12 h light/dark cycle at 24°C and provided with food ad libitum for a week before the beginning of experimental procedures. All animal experiments were approved by the Wenzhou Medical University Management Committee for Medical Laboratory Animal Sciences. Twelve rats were used as islet donors, 6 rats were used as normal controls (NC group), and the others ($n = 17$) received a single intraperitoneal injection of streptozotocin (STZ) (55 mg/kg of body weight, Sigma-Aldrich, St. Louis, MO, USA) in sodium citrate buffer (pH 4.5) after fasting for 12 hours. One week after injection, blood was taken from the tail vein for 3 consecutive days to measure plasma glucose concentration with an AccuChek glucometer (Roche Diagnostics, Indianapolis, IN). When all blood plasma glucose concentrations were ≥16.67 mmol/L, the diabetic rat model was established. After 12 weeks, the early diabetic nephropathy rat model was defined on the basis of urine ACR and protein-to-creatinine ratio. The diabetic nephropathy rats were randomly divided into two groups and studied 4 weeks later: rats in the untreated group (DN group, $n = 6$) which did not receive treatment and in the islet-transplanted group (IT group, $n = 6$) where rats received an islet transplantation.

2.2. Islet Isolation and Purification. This method was described in a previous study [16]. Donor rats were anesthetized with 5% isoflurane mixed with 0.5 L/min oxygen, followed by a reduced concentration of isoflurane (2%) to maintain anesthesia. After disinfection of the abdominal skin, a U-incision was cut in the abdomen, and the pancreas was completely exposed. The entrance of the common bile duct into the duodenum was located and ligated, and 10 mL of collagenase V (2 mg/mL, dissolved in Hank's solution) was injected into the common bile duct using retrograde intubation. After complete perfusion, the expanded pancreas was carefully transferred to a sterile 50 mL centrifuge tube, to which 2 mL of precold V collagenase solution was added in advance, and then was digested for 3 min at 37 ± 0.5°C. The pancreatic tissue was transferred into a 50 mL centrifuge tube, and ingestion was terminated by adding 40 mL of Hank's solution. After gradient centrifugation, the islet cells were manually pick up under a microscope and cultured in RPMI-1640 (Gibco, Carlsbad, CA, USA) containing 10% fetal bovine serum (FBS; Gibco, Invitrogen Inc., USA) at 37°C and 5% CO_2 for 6 hours.

2.3. Preparation of Islets before Transplantation. The islet cells were randomly divided into two parts. One part was stained with fluorescein diacetate-propidium iodide (FDA-PI) to detect islet cell activity. After the other part was counted, these islets were aspirated into a 1 mL syringe connected to P50 polyethylene tubing and then transferred to the head end. Total islet equivalents (IEQ) were calculated according to the appropriate formula [17]. Approximately 1000–1200 IEQ of purified islets were obtained.

2.4. Islet Transplantation under the Kidney Capsule. This method was previously reported by Napoli et al. [18]. Recipient rats were anesthetized with isoflurane, and their left flank was shaved and disinfected with 75% alcohol and iodophor. The kidney was gently squeezed out through a small lumbar incision, and polyethylene tubing was inserted under the kidney capsule. The islets in the tubing were pushed gently, and the tubing was removed until the islets were completely transplanted under the kidney capsule.

2.5. Urine, Blood, and Tissue Sampling. At weeks 12 and 16, the 24 h urine sample was collected with a rat metabolic cage. Urine protein concentration was measured using the sulfosalicylic acid precipitation method, and the creatinine concentration was assessed with a creatinine assay kit (Bioassay Systems, Hayward, CA). Albuminuria was measured using a rat albumin-specific ELISA kit (Exocell Laboratories, Philadelphia, PA). Commercial assay kits for serum creatinine (Scr) and blood urea nitrogen (BUN) were purchased from the Nanjing Jiancheng Institute of Biotechnology

(Nanjing, China). Scr and BUN concentrations were measured according to the protocols provided by the manufacturers. The nonfasting blood glucose and body weight of members of each group were measured twice per week. At week 16, all rats were sacrificed after anesthesia with isoflurane. Select kidney tissue was fixed in 4% paraformaldehyde for histopathologic staining. The remaining tissue was stored in liquid nitrogen. After gradient alcohol dehydration and xylene transparence, the kidney tissue was incorporated into a wax block and cut into 4 μm sections.

2.6. Histopathology. Kidney tissues fixed in formaldehyde were dehydrated, embedded in paraffin, and cut into 4 μm thick sections. Sections treated with hematoxylin-eosin (HE) staining were observed with a light microscope at a high magnification.

2.7. Immunohistochemical Staining. For immunohistochemical analysis, paraffin-embedded kidney tissue sections (4 μm thick) were used. Sections were placed on glass slides, deparaffinized, and hydrated with xylene and graded alcohol. Sections were preincubated in a boiling sodium citrate buffer for antigen retrieval. Primary antibodies (1 : 200) for PTX3 (Bioworld Technology Inc., St. Louis Park, MN, USA), α-SMA (Abcam, Cambridge, MA, USA), caspase 3 (Abcam, Cambridge, MA, USA), and TGF-β1 (Abcam, Cambridge, MA, USA) were added and incubated at 4°C overnight. The tissue sections were then incubated for 1 h with HRP-conjugated anti-rabbit IgG. After DAB and hematoxylin staining, tissue sections were viewed under an optical microscope. The average optical density was calculated by Image-Pro Plus 6.0 image analysis software (Media Cybernetics, Silver Spring, MD).

2.8. Western Blot Analysis. Western blot analysis was performed to measure the protein expression of PTX3, Bax, Bcl-2, NPHS-2, and GAPDH. Kidney tissues were lysed with RIPA buffer, and protein concentrations were measured with a BCA assay kit (Beyotime Biotechnology, Jiangsu, China) according to the manufacturer's protocol. Proteins were separated with 12% sodium dodecyl sulfate-polyacrylamide gels (SDS-PAGE), then transferred to a polyvinylidene fluoride (PVDF) membrane (Millipore Corporation, Bedford, MA, USA). The membrane was blocked with 5% fat-free milk for 1 h at room temperature and then further incubated overnight at 4°C with the following primary antibodies: PTX3 (Bioworld Technology Inc., St. Louis Park, MN, USA, 1 : 1000), Bax (Cell Signaling Technology Inc., Danvers, MA, USA, 1 : 1000), Bcl-2 (Cell Signaling Technology Inc., Danvers, MA, USA 1 : 1000), NPHS-2 (Abcam, Cambridge, MA, USA), and GAPDH (Bioworld Technology Inc., St. Louis Park, MN, USA, 1 : 10,000). The membranes were then incubated with horseradish peroxidase- (HRP-) conjugated secondary antibody (goat anti-rabbit IgG; Bioworld Technology Inc., St. Louis Park, MN, USA) diluted to 1 : 10,000 at 37°C for 1 h. Protein bands were detected using Image Lab Software (Bio-Rad Laboratories Inc., Berkeley, CA, USA).

2.9. Enzyme-Linked Immunosorbent Assay (ELISA). The levels of plasma ptx3 in each groups were measured according to the manufacturer's protocol (USCN, Wuhan USCN Business Co. Ltd.). The absorbance was measured at 450 nm using a Varioskan Flash™ multimode microplate reader (Thermo Fisher Scientific, Waltham, MA, USA).

2.10. Statistical Analysis. All data were analyzed using GraphPad Prism 5 (GraphPad software, version 5, San Diego, CA, USA), and values are expressed as the mean ± standard deviation. Multiple comparisons between groups were performed with a one-way ANOVA. $p < 0.05$ was considered significant.

3. Results

3.1. Evaluation of an Early Diabetic Nephropathy Model in Rats. As shown in Figures 1(a) and 1(b), the blood glucose of the DN group injected with STZ increased rapidly and maintained levels of 25 mmol/L after 1 week. Compared with the normal group, the blood glucose of the DN group changed significantly, and body weight continued to decrease with time. Figures 1(c) and 1(d) show that the urine protein-to-creatinine ratio (6.512 ± 0.512 mg/mmol) and the urine microalbumin-to-creatinine ratio (215 ± 13.2 mg/mmol) in the DN group increased significantly compared with those of the normal group (1.159 ± 0.32 mg/mmol and 24.275 ± 3.8 mg/mmol, resp.) ($p < 0.01$; $p < 0.001$). Changes in rat blood glucose, body weight, and urine protein-to-creatinine and urine microalbumin-to-creatinine ratios demonstrate that a model of early DN was successfully established [19, 20].

3.2. Evaluation of Islet Transplantation. Figure 1 shows that the blood glucose in the IT group returned to 7.5 mmol/L, while its weight increased significantly 2 weeks following islet transplantation (IT). Compared with the DN group, the urine protein-to-creatinine and microalbumin-to-creatinine ratios of the normal group significantly decreased ($p < 0.001$). In Figure 2, the results of renal HE and islet transplantation staining show pancreatic islet cells under the renal capsule.

3.3. Evaluation of Renal Function. Figures 1(e) and 1(f) show that the SCR (49 ± 2.72 μmol/L) and the BUN (33.2 ± 10.6 mmol/L) in the DN group increased significantly compared with those of the normal group (23.94 ± 1.4 µmol/L and 5.8 ± 0.74 mmol/L, resp.) ($p < 0.001$ and $p < 0.01$, resp.). Compared with the DN group, the SCR and BUN of the IT group (23.1 ± 5.3 μmol/L and 7.38 ± 2.02 mmol/L, resp.) ($p < 0.001$ and $p < 0.01$, resp.) significantly decreased. These dates showed that the islet transplantation improved the kidney in early diabetic nephropathy rats.

3.4. Expression of PTX3 in Renal Tissue. The expression of PTX3 in the kidney was evaluated with Western blot and immunohistochemistry. In Figure 3(a), Western blot showed that PTX3 expression in the DN group was significantly lower than in the normal group ($p < 0.01$), while PTX3 expression in the IT group was significantly higher than in the DN group ($p < 0.01$). Further, PTX3 expression in the IT group was closest to that of the normal group. In Figures 3(b) and 3(c), immunohistochemistry showed that

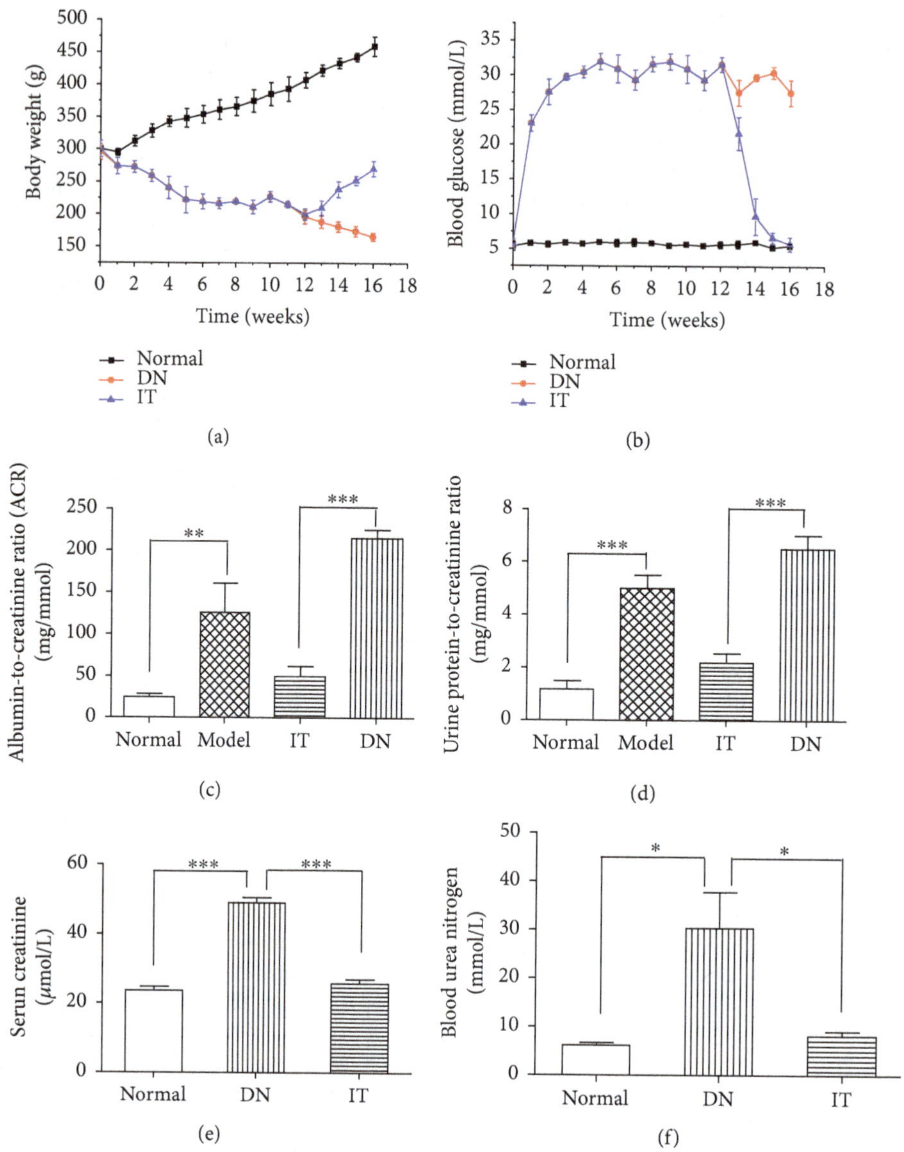

Figure 1: Changes in rat blood glucose, body weight, and urine protein-to-creatinine ratio and urine microalbumin-to-creatinine ratio. (a) Changes in body weight. (b) Rat blood glucose for each group. (c) Urine microalbumin-to-creatinine ratio. (d) Urine protein-to-creatinine ratio. (e) Serum creatinine. (f) Blood urea nitrogen. $^{*}p < 0.05$, $^{**}p < 0.01$, and $^{***}p < 0.001$.

the expression of PTX3 in the DN group was lower than that in the normal group ($p < 0.05$), while PTX3 expression in the IT group was significantly higher than that in the DN group ($p < 0.01$). PTX3 expression in the kidneys of the normal group was mainly located in renal tubular epithelial cells.

3.5. Expression of PTX3 in Plasma. The expression of plasma PTX3 was evaluated by enzyme-linked immunosorbent assay (ELISA). In Figure 3(d), mean plasma ptx3 in the DN group (9851.4 ± 808.6 pg/mL) was significantly higher compared to those in the normal group (7457.7 ± 158.5 pg/mL) and IT group (6314.6 ± 1086.4 pg/mL) ($p < 0.01$ and $p < 0.001$, resp.).

3.6. Assessment of Renal Injury. Immunohistochemistry and Western blots were used to evaluate the degree of renal injury in each group. In Figure 4(a), the Bax/Bcl-2 ratio of the DN group was higher than that of the normal and IT groups ($p < 0.01$ and $p < 0.05$, resp.). In Figure 4(b), the expression of NPHS-2 in the DN group was lower than that of the normal and IT groups ($p < 0.001$ and $p < 0.05$, resp.). In Figures 5 and 6, the expression of α-SMA, cleaved caspase-3, and TGF-β1 in the DN group was significantly higher than that in the normal and IT groups ($p < 0.01$, $p < 0.001$, and $p < 0.05$, resp.).

4. Discussion

At present, there are approximately 300 million diabetic patients in the world, a figure that will likely reach 500 million by 2030 [21]. Approximately 20–40% of diabetic patients develop diabetic nephropathy [22]. As one of the most common microvascular complications of diabetes, the prevalence of DN has had a rapid growth trend. The prevention and

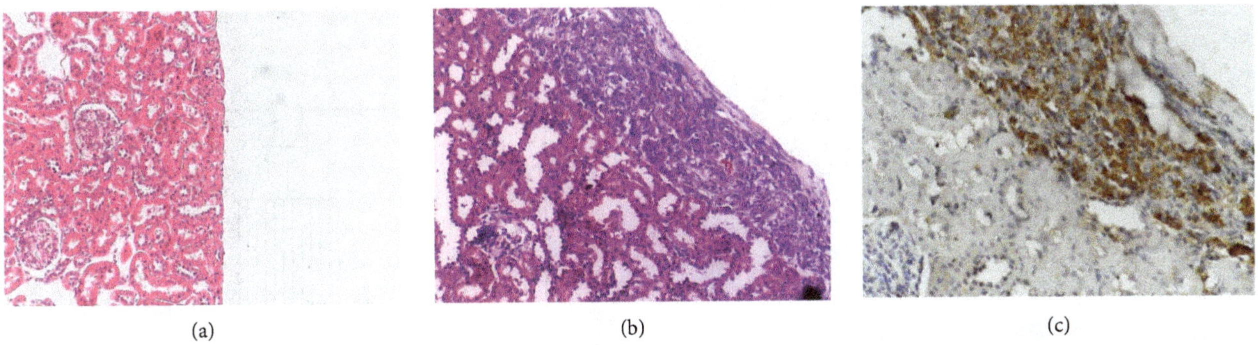

FIGURE 2: Evaluation of islet transplantation. (a) Normal renal HE staining. (b) IT group renal HE staining (200x). (c) Anti-insulin immunohistochemistry (400x).

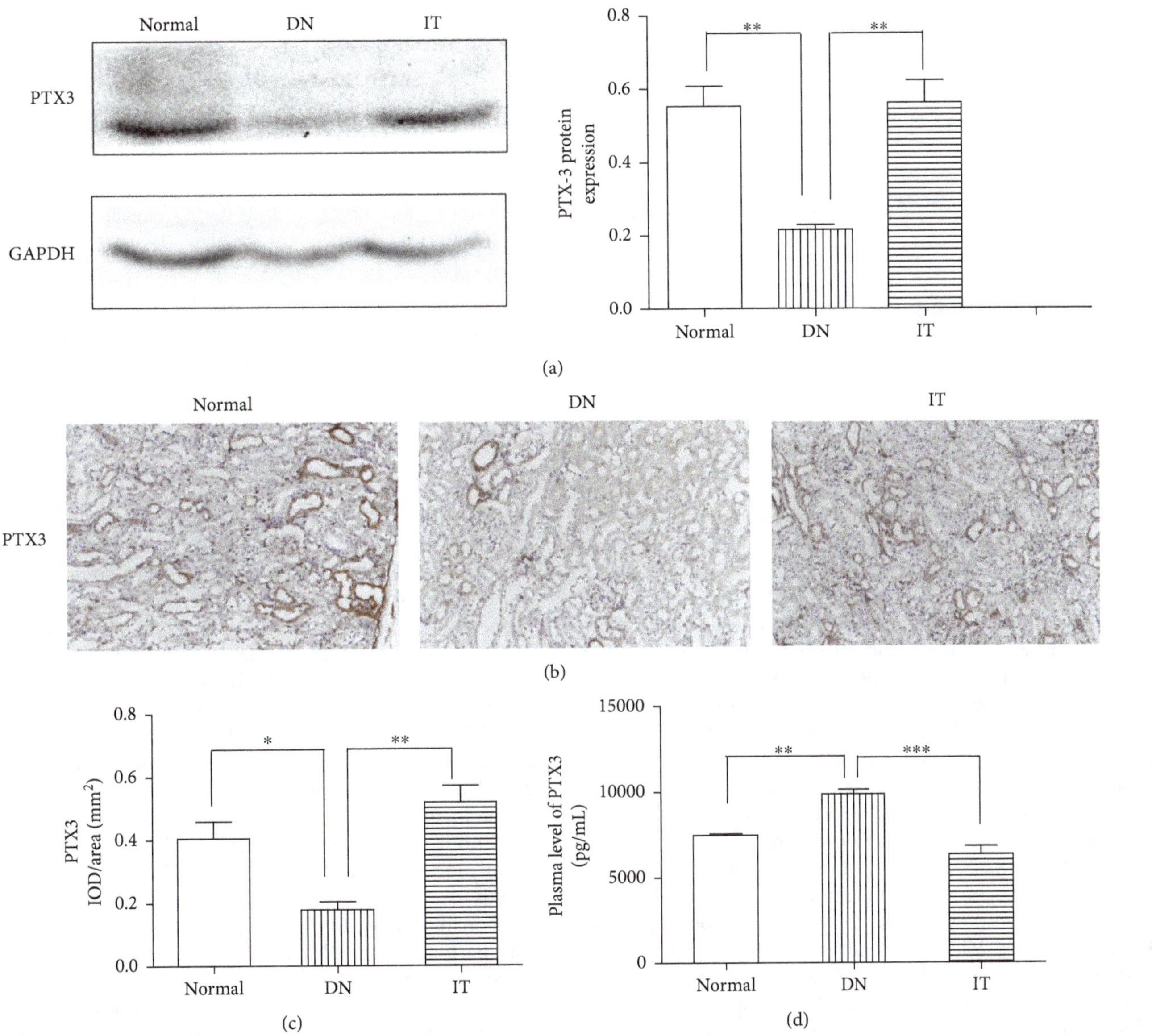

FIGURE 3: The expression of PTX3 in each group. (a) The expression of PTX3 protein as detected by Western blot. (b, c) The expression of PTX3 protein as detected by immunohistochemistry. (d) The plasma PTX3 concentration. $^{*}p < 0.05$, $^{**}p < 0.01$, and $^{***}p < 0.001$.

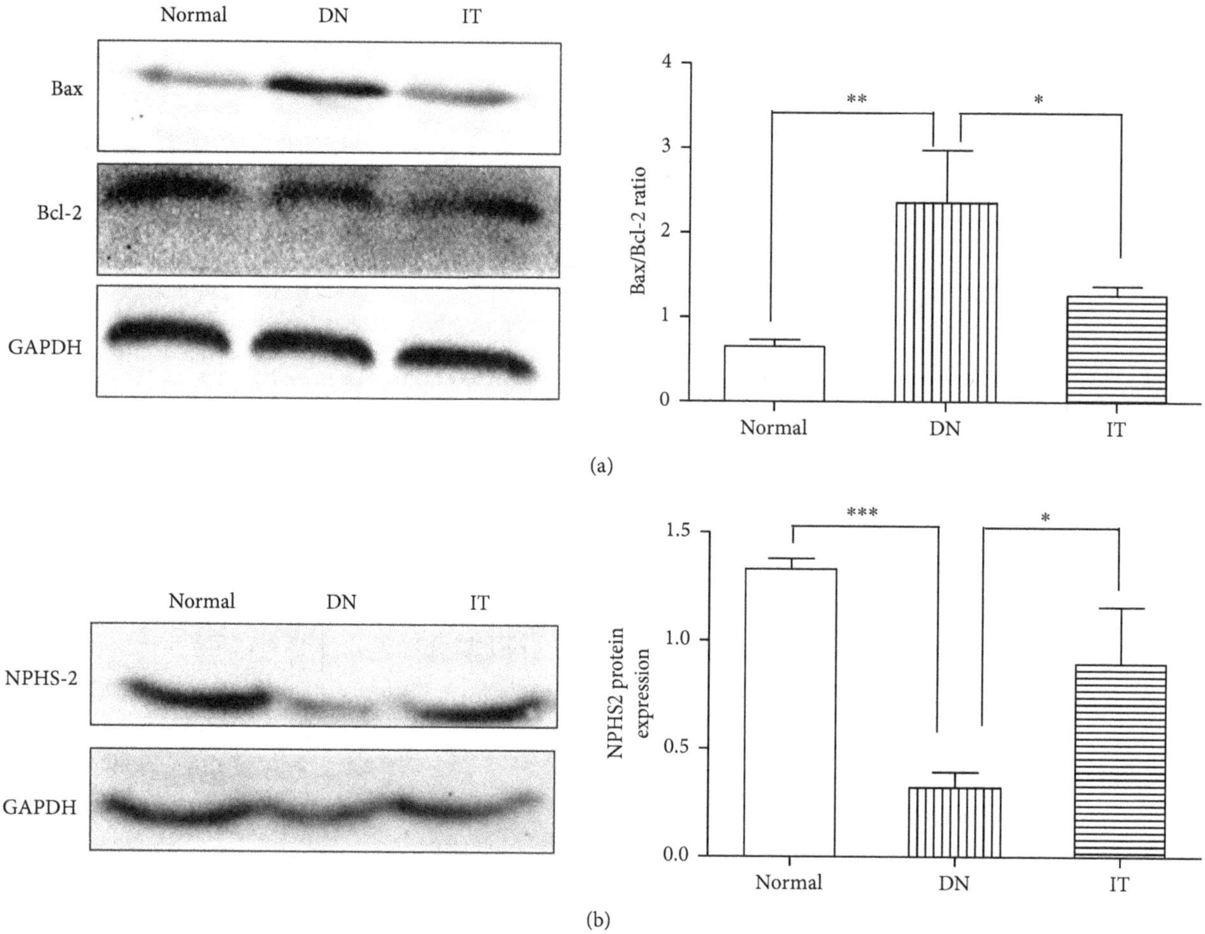

Figure 4: Western blot analysis of Bax, Bcl-2, and NPHS-2 in the renal tissues in each group. (a) Bax and Bcl-2. (b) NPHS-2. $^{*}p < 0.05$, $^{**}p < 0.01$, and $^{***}p < 0.001$.

diagnosis of renal injury in early diabetic nephropathy can help improve the life expectancy, quality of life, and economic burden of diabetic patients.

PTX3 is the first cloned long pentraxin that can be detected in renal tissue [13]. The relationship between PTX3 and various acute and chronic kidney diseases is a hot topic. The levels of plasma PTX3 in early acute ischemia-reperfusion renal injuries and chronic kidney disease are response to be increased [23, 24], and the expression of PTX3 in the renal tubular epithelial cells during ischemia-reperfusion kidney injuries and the glomerular endothelial cells in patients with IgA nephropathy [13] and type I membranous proliferative glomerulonephritis were increased. Hence, PTX3 was previously thought to have a potential pathogenic effect as a proinflammatory cytokine [25, 26]. However, in recent years, an increasing number of studies have shown that PTX3 does not cause kidney damage [27] and that an elevated plasma PTX3 concentration is likely a marker of immune inflammatory response and is a physiologic protective defense mechanism, with an anti-inflammatory and protective effect on the kidneys. Previous studies have demonstrated that PTX3 can limit inflammation, promote the repair/regeneration of damaged tissue [28], and induce and maintain immune tolerance. PTX3 binds P-selectin, which allows white blood cells to roll into the apoptotic membrane of activated microvascular endothelial cells, thereby limiting subsequent leukocyte adhesion and cross-endothelial migration. This would limit the recruitment of neutrophils and macrophages in the ischemic kidney [14], stimulating tubular repair [27]. Lech et al. [14] noted that PTX3-deficient mice had worse ischemic acute kidney injuries, which were improved following recombinant PTX3 injection. Another study [29] showed that PTX3 treatment inhibited interstitial fibrosis induced by an acute kidney injury, reduced serum creatinine levels, and decreased the expression of collagen and smooth muscle actin in mice.

In our study, the expression of PTX3 in the kidney was mainly located in renal tubular epithelial cells and was significantly decreased in our DN model. To further explore the relationship between PTX3 and DN, islet transplantation was performed in DN rats to treat diabetic nephropathy. Here, we provide the first evidence that the expression of PTX3 in the IT group was significantly greater than in the DN group and was similar to normal animals. But the expression of plasma PTX3 was though contrary to the above results. In the recent studies, the concentration of plasma PTX3 has been reported as a close and independent determinant of proteinuria, impaired kidney function, and endothelial dysfunction [24, 30]. The increased level of plasma PTX3

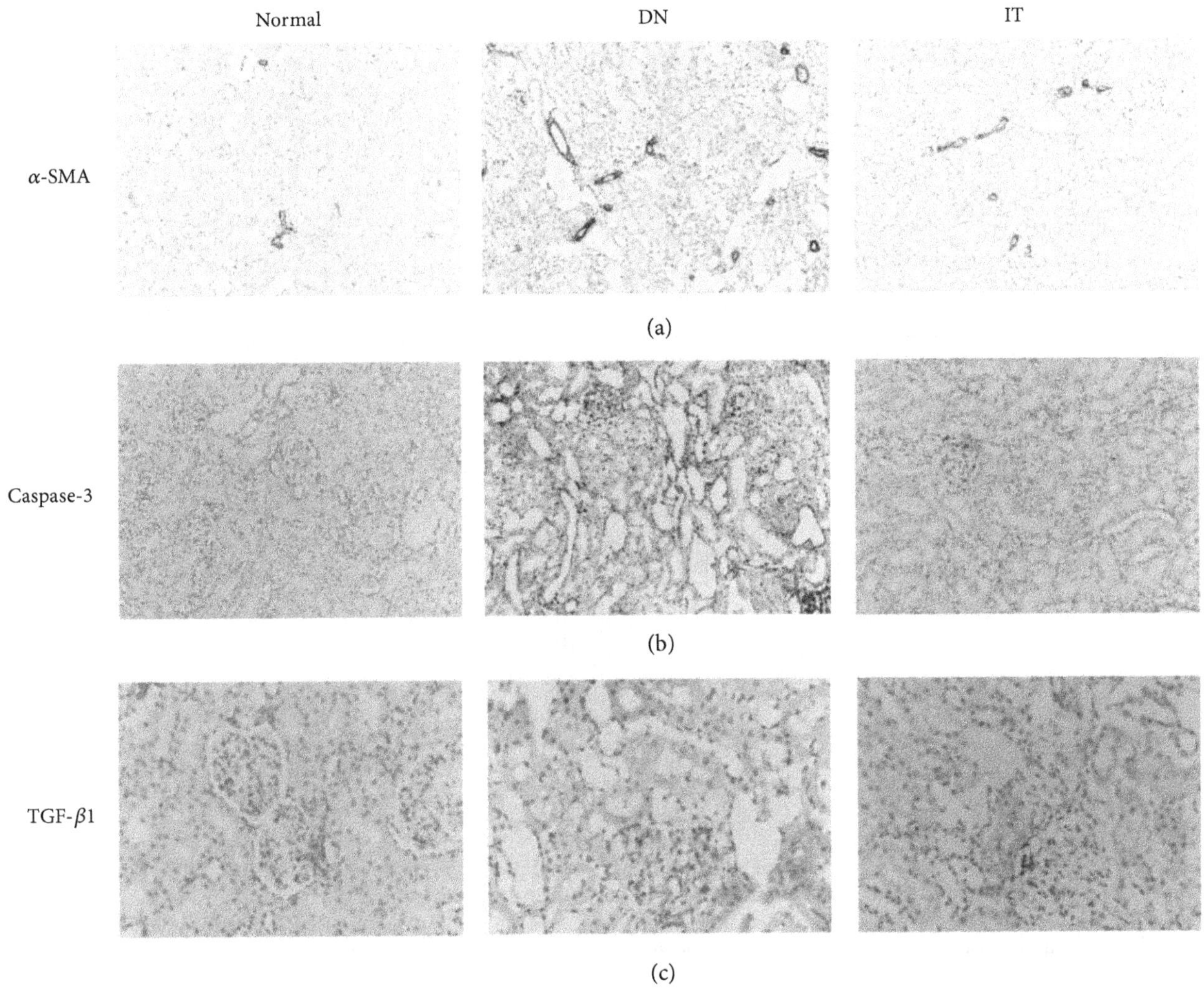

FIGURE 5: Immunohistochemistry was used to detect the expression of renal fibrogenic and interstitial fibrosis factors and apoptotic proteins. (a) α-SMA. (b) Caspase-3. (c) TGF-β1.

in the DN group showed that the kidney function is damaged and the endothelial cell is dysfunction. The results of SCR and BUN proved this conclusion in our study. However, plasma PTX3 of the rats in the IT group is lower as compared to that of the DN group, demonstrating that the renal function and the endothelial cells are restored. All of the aforementioned evidence suggests that PTX3 is involved in the development of DN. However, its mechanism of action still remains unclear.

Previous studies have found that renal tubule cell apoptosis and renal interstitial fibrosis play an important role in the development of DN beyond glomerular filtration barrier damage and glomerular sclerosis [31]. Renal tubule lesions occur earlier than glomerular lesions and are closely related to the extent and severity of renal dysfunction [31]. In hyperglycemic conditions, cell culture and animal experiments showed a significant amount of renal tubular epithelial cell apoptosis [32]. The proapoptotic protein bax and the antiapoptotic protein bcl-2, which belong to the bcl-2 family, are very important regulatory factors in the apoptotic pathway. Caspase-3, which cleaves DNA-dependent protein kinases to destroy cell structure proteins, is the most important proapoptotic protease during apoptosis [33]. The present study demonstrated that the expression of Bax/Bcl-2 in the DN group was higher than in the normal group. The immunohistochemistry staining of cleaved caspase-3 showed that there was a large amount of renal tubular epithelial cell apoptosis in the DN model. Further, the expression of Bax/Bcl-2 and cleaved caspase-3 was reversed after islet transplantation. These data suggest that the apoptosis of renal tubular epithelial cells is linked to DN. According to the expression of PTX3 in the kidney, we therefore hypothesize that renal tubular epithelial cell apoptosis and progressive loss result in the gradual decline of PTX3 synthesis and secretion. Furthermore, PTX3 is an important contributor to the development of cell apoptosis. Soluble and membranous forms of PTX3 can independently prevent and promote the autoimmune process, suggesting that PTX3 has a dual effect and that its function may be dependent on the environment, treatment structure, cytokine spectrum, and gene mutations [34]. Under infectious and inflammatory conditions, PTX3 regulates the autoimmune response, induces apoptosis, and promotes the leakage of cellular contents. By controlling the interaction between mature dendritic cells

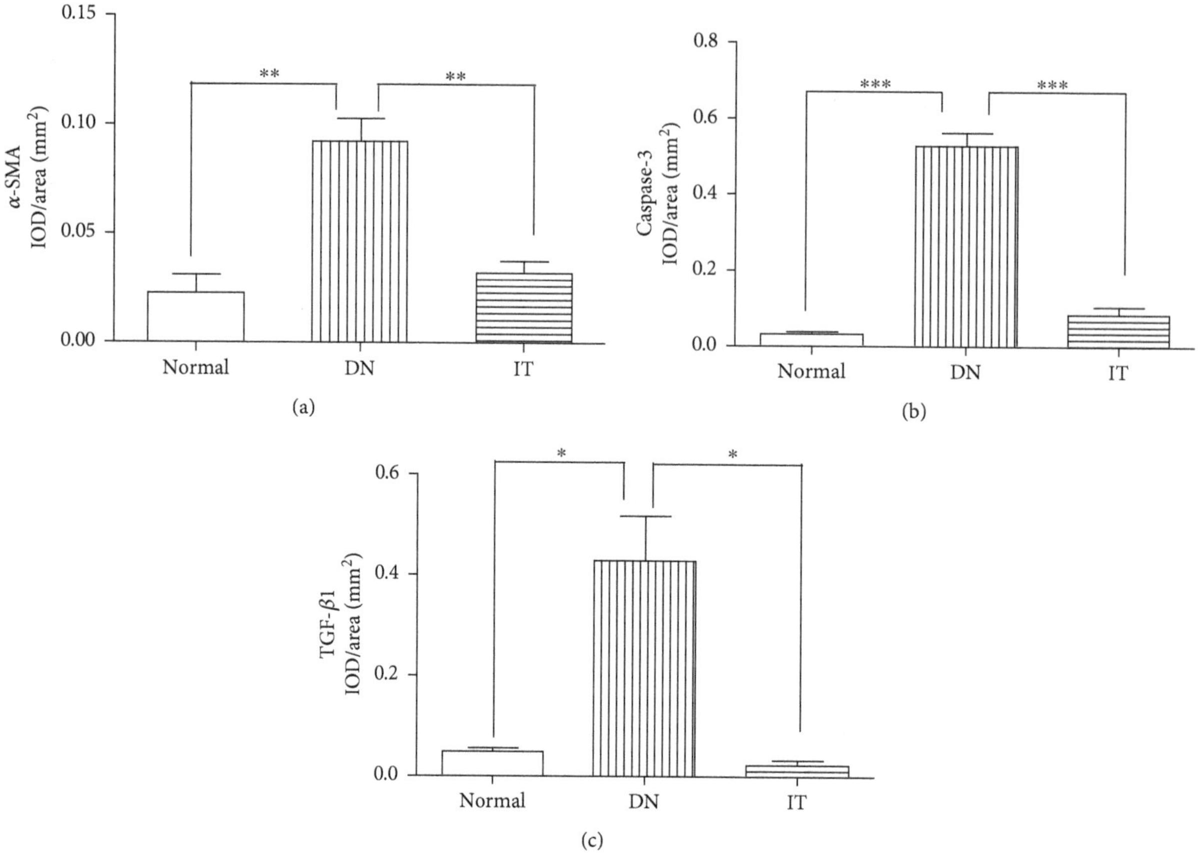

FIGURE 6: Measurement of the IOD/area of immunohistochemical staining of renal fibrogenic and interstitial fibrosis factors and apoptotic proteins. (a) Measurement of the IOD/area of α-SMA, $^{**}p < 0.05$. (b) Measurement of the IOD/area of caspase-3, $^{*}p = 0.018$ and $^{***}p < 0.001$. (c) Measurement of the IOD/area of TGF-β1, $^{*}p < 0.05$. IOD/area: integrated optical density/area. The mean of IOD/area of positive staining was used to accurately measure the degree of positive expression in immunohistochemistry samples.

and apoptotic cells, PTX3 participates in the removal of apoptotic cells [12, 35]. Under inflammatory and other conditions, PTX3 induces the activation of the classical complement pathway, specifically binding apoptotic cells and cell debris on the surface of complement component C3b/iC3b, promoting complement-mediated apoptosis and cell clearance [28]. The acceleration of cellular apoptosis in DN led to a further decrease in PTX3 expression.

We detected an elevated TGF-β1 and α-SMA expression and decreased NPHS-2 (podocin) expression in the DN group as compared with the normal and IT groups. TGF-β1 and α-SMA are the major factors in the progression of renal fibrosis in DN. NPHS-2 (podocin), a protein encoded by the NPHS-2 gene, interacts with nephrin and CD2AP, an important component of the membrane, in the same way as the glomerular filtration barrier [36]. The reduction expression of NPHS-2 may thus lead to proteinuria [37]. On the basis of these findings, we found that the level of PTX3 in renal tissue was closely related to renal injury in DN. But the mechanism how the PTX3 influence the renal injury in DN is still unclear. Maybe we will investigate the reasons in the future.

In conclusion, the present study found that the level of PTX3 in renal tissue is closely related to renal injury in DN. The expression of PTX3 in the kidney was significantly decreased in the DN group, while it was increased in the IT group because of the reversal of DN. This may be used to quantify the extent of renal injury in DN, provide a potential indicator in the early assessment of renal tubule injury in early DN patients, and assess DN clinical progression. This also could provide better advice for clinical treatment in diabetes patients to prevent the development and progress of DN.

Conflicts of Interest

All authors declare that there are no financial or nonfinancial competing interests regarding the publication of this paper.

Authors' Contributions

Xuehai Chen and Jiao Luo are co-first coauthors, and these authors contributed equally to this work.

Acknowledgments

The authors thank Professor Roland Anderson from Lund University for the language polish. This project was sponsored by the National Health and Family Planning Commission of Zhejiang Province (2013ZDA014), the

National Natural Science of China (81572087), the Natural Science Foundation of Zhejiang Province (LY17H070005, LY2H05004, and LY16H030013), and the Wenzhou Municipal Science and Bureau (Y20140672 and Y20150062).

References

[1] R. Xue, D. Gui, L. Zheng, R. Zhai, F. Wang, and N. Wang, "Mechanistic insight and management of diabetic nephropathy: recent progress and future perspective," *Journal of Diabetes Research*, vol. 2017, Article ID 1839809, 7 pages, 2017.

[2] H. Yokoyama and T. Deckert, "Central role of TGF-β in the pathogenesis of diabetic nephropathy and macrovascular complications: a hypothesis," *Diabetic Medicine*, vol. 13, no. 4, pp. 313–320, 1996.

[3] A. L. Lima, T. Illing, S. Schliemann, and P. Elsner, "Cutaneous manifestations of diabetes mellitus: a review," *American Journal of Clinical Dermatology*, vol. 18, no. 4, pp. 541–553, 2017.

[4] A. G. Tzakis, Y. Zeng, J. J. Fung et al., "Pancreatic islet transplantation after upper abdominal exeriteration and liver replacement," *The Lancet*, vol. 336, no. 8712, pp. 402–405, 1990.

[5] T. C. Lee, N. R. Barshes, C. A. O'Mahony et al., "The effect of pancreatic islet transplantation on progression of diabetic retinopathy and neuropathy," *Transplantation Proceedings*, vol. 37, no. 5, pp. 2263–2265, 2005.

[6] Health Quality Ontario, "Pancreas islet transplantation for patients with type 1 diabetes mellitus: a clinical evidence review," *Ontario Health Technology Assessment Series*, vol. 15, no. 16, pp. 1–84, 2015.

[7] Y. He, Z. Xu, M. Zhou et al., "Reversal of early diabetic nephropathy by islet transplantation under the kidney capsule in a rat model," *Journal of Diabetes Research*, vol. 2016, Article ID 4157313, 12 pages, 2016.

[8] H. Gewurz, X. H. Zhang, and T. F. Lint, "Structure and function of the pentraxins," *Current Opinion in Immunology*, vol. 7, no. 1, pp. 54–64, 1995.

[9] M. Lech, C. Rommele, and H. J. Anders, "Pentraxins in nephrology: C-reactive protein, serum amyloid P and pentraxin-3," *Nephrology, Dialysis, Transplantation*, vol. 28, no. 4, pp. 803–811, 2013.

[10] A. J. Nauta, S. de Haij, B. Bottazzi et al., "Human renal epithelial cells produce the long pentraxin PTX_3," *Kidney International*, vol. 67, no. 2, pp. 543–553, 2005.

[11] M. Presta, M. Camozzi, G. Salvatori, and M. Rusnati, "Role of the soluble pattern recognition receptor PTX3 in vascular biology," *Journal of Cellular and Molecular Medicine*, vol. 11, no. 4, pp. 723–738, 2007.

[12] P. Rovere, G. Peri, F. Fazzini et al., "The long pentraxin PTX3 binds to apoptotic cells and regulates their clearance by antigen-presenting dendritic cells," *Blood*, vol. 96, no. 13, pp. 4300–4306, 2000.

[13] B. Bussolati, G. Peri, G. Salvidio, D. Verzola, A. Mantovani, and G. Camussi, "The long pentraxin PTX3 is synthesized in IgA glomerulonephritis and activates mesangial cells," *The Journal of Immunology*, vol. 170, no. 3, pp. 1466–1472, 2003.

[14] M. Lech, C. Römmele, R. Gröbmayr et al., "Endogenous and exogenous pentraxin-3 limits postischemic acute and chronic kidney injury," *Kidney International*, vol. 83, no. 4, pp. 647–661, 2013.

[15] H. Sun, J. Tian, W. Xian, T. Xie, and X. Yang, "Pentraxin-3 attenuates renal damage in diabetic nephropathy by promoting M2 macrophage differentiation," *Inflammation*, vol. 38, no. 5, pp. 1739–1747, 2015.

[16] E. J. Zmuda, C. A. Powell, and T. Hai, "A method for murine islet isolation and subcapsular kidney transplantation," *Journal of Visualized Experiments*, no. 50, 2011.

[17] N. Lembert, J. Wesche, P. Petersen, M. Doser, H. D. Becker, and H. P. Ammon, "Areal density measurement is a convenient method for the determination of porcine islet equivalents without counting and sizing individual islets," *Cell Transplantation*, vol. 12, no. 1, pp. 33–41, 2003.

[18] R. Napoli, A. M. Davalli, M. F. Hirshman, R. Weitgasser, G. C. Weir, and E. S. Horton, "Islet transplantation under the kidney capsule fully corrects the impaired skeletal muscle glucose transport system of streptozocin diabetic rats," *Journal of Clinical Investigation*, vol. 97, no. 6, pp. 1389–1397, 1996.

[19] G. H. Tesch and T. J. Allen, "Rodent models of streptozotocin-induced diabetic nephropathy (methods in renal research)," *Nephrology*, vol. 12, no. 3, pp. 261–266, 2007.

[20] V. Usuelli and E. La Rocca, "Novel therapeutic approaches for diabetic nephropathy and retinopathy," *Pharmacological Research*, vol. 98, pp. 39–44, 2015.

[21] H. K. Yang and K. H. Yoon, "Current status of encapsulated islet transplantation," *Journal of Diabetes and its Complications*, vol. 29, no. 5, pp. 737–743, 2015.

[22] J. Chen, W. W. Zhang, K. H. Chen et al., "Urinary DcR2 is a novel biomarker for tubulointerstitial injury in patients with diabetic nephropathy," *American Journal of Physiology-Renal Physiology*, vol. 313, no. 2, pp. F273–F281, 2017.

[23] B. Sjoberg, A. R. Qureshi, B. Anderstam, A. Alvestrand, and P. Barany, "Pentraxin 3, a sensitive early marker of hemodialysis-induced inflammation," *Blood Purification*, vol. 34, no. 3-4, pp. 290–297, 2012.

[24] M. E. Suliman, M. I. Yilmaz, J. J. Carrero et al., "Novel links between the long pentraxin 3, endothelial dysfunction, and albuminuria in early and advanced chronic kidney disease," *Clinical Journal of the American Society of Nephrology*, vol. 3, no. 4, pp. 976–985, 2008.

[25] M. I. Yilmaz, J. Axelsson, A. Sonmez et al., "Effect of renin angiotensin system blockade on pentraxin 3 levels in type-2 diabetic patients with proteinuria," *Clinical Journal of the American Society of Nephrology*, vol. 4, no. 3, pp. 535–541, 2009.

[26] J. Chen, M. M. Matzuk, X. J. Zhou, and L. CY, "Endothelial pentraxin 3 contributes to murine ischemic acute kidney injury," *Kidney International*, vol. 82, no. 11, pp. 1195–1207, 2012.

[27] M. M. Speeckaert, R. Speeckaert, J. J. Carrero, R. Vanholder, and J. R. Delanghe, "Biology of human pentraxin 3 (PTX3) in acute and chronic kidney disease," *Journal of Clinical Immunology*, vol. 33, no. 5, pp. 881–890, 2013.

[28] P. Kunes, V. Lonsky, J. Mand'ak et al., "Essential PTX3 biology (not only) for cardiologists and cardiac surgeons," *Acta Medica*, vol. 50, no. 1, pp. 29–33, 2007.

[29] Y. Xiao, N. Yang, Q. Zhang, Y. Wang, S. Yang, and Z. Liu, "Pentraxin 3 inhibits acute renal injury-induced interstitial fibrosis through suppression of IL-6/Stat3 pathway," *Inflammation*, vol. 37, no. 5, pp. 1895–1901, 2014.

[30] T. Celik, M. I. Yilmaz, S. Balta et al., "The relationship between plasma whole blood viscosity and cardiovascular events in patients with chronic kidney disease," *Clinical and Applied Thrombosis/Hemostasis*, vol. 23, no. 6, pp. 663–670, 2016.

[31] R. C. Blantz and P. Singh, "Glomerular and tubular function in the diabetic kidney," *Advances in Chronic Kidney Disease*, vol. 21, no. 3, pp. 297–303, 2014.

[32] X. Q. Zhang, J. J. Dong, T. Cai, X. Shen, X. J. Zhou, and L. Liao, "High glucose induces apoptosis via upregulation of Bim expression in proximal tubule epithelial cells," *Oncotarget*, vol. 8, no. 15, pp. 24119–24129, 2017.

[33] C. A. Odonkor and S. Achilefu, "Modulation of effector caspase cleavage determines response of breast and lung tumor cell lines to chemotherapy," *Cancer Investigation*, vol. 27, no. 4, pp. 417–429, 2009.

[34] O. D. Ortega-Hernandez, N. Bassi, Y. Shoenfeld, and J. M. Anaya, "The long pentraxin 3 and its role in autoimmunity," *Seminars in Arthritis and Rheumatism*, vol. 39, no. 1, pp. 38–54, 2009.

[35] G. Deyab, I. Hokstad, J. E. Whist et al., "Anti-rheumatic treatment is not associated with reduction of pentraxin 3 in rheumatoid arthritis, psoriatic arthritis and ankylosing spondylitis," *PLoS One*, vol. 12, no. 2, article e0169830, 2017.

[36] K. Schwarz, M. Simons, J. Reiser et al., "Podocin, a raft-associated component of the glomerular slit diaphragm, interacts with CD2AP and nephrin," *Journal of Clinical Investigation*, vol. 108, no. 11, pp. 1621–1629, 2001.

[37] M. Tabatabaeifar, T. Wlodkowski, I. Simic et al., "An inducible mouse model of podocin-mutation-related nephrotic syndrome," *PLoS One*, vol. 12, no. 10, article e0186574, 2017.

Permissions

All chapters in this book were first published in JDR, by Hindawi Publishing Corporation; hereby published with permission under the Creative Commons Attribution License or equivalent. Every chapter published in this book has been scrutinized by our experts. Their significance has been extensively debated. The topics covered herein carry significant findings which will fuel the growth of the discipline. They may even be implemented as practical applications or may be referred to as a beginning point for another development.

The contributors of this book come from diverse backgrounds, making this book a truly international effort. This book will bring forth new frontiers with its revolutionizing research information and detailed analysis of the nascent developments around the world.

We would like to thank all the contributing authors for lending their expertise to make the book truly unique. They have played a crucial role in the development of this book. Without their invaluable contributions this book wouldn't have been possible. They have made vital efforts to compile up to date information on the varied aspects of this subject to make this book a valuable addition to the collection of many professionals and students.

This book was conceptualized with the vision of imparting up-to-date information and advanced data in this field. To ensure the same, a matchless editorial board was set up. Every individual on the board went through rigorous rounds of assessment to prove their worth. After which they invested a large part of their time researching and compiling the most relevant data for our readers.

The editorial board has been involved in producing this book since its inception. They have spent rigorous hours researching and exploring the diverse topics which have resulted in the successful publishing of this book. They have passed on their knowledge of decades through this book. To expedite this challenging task, the publisher supported the team at every step. A small team of assistant editors was also appointed to further simplify the editing procedure and attain best results for the readers.

Apart from the editorial board, the designing team has also invested a significant amount of their time in understanding the subject and creating the most relevant covers. They scrutinized every image to scout for the most suitable representation of the subject and create an appropriate cover for the book.

The publishing team has been an ardent support to the editorial, designing and production team. Their endless efforts to recruit the best for this project, has resulted in the accomplishment of this book. They are a veteran in the field of academics and their pool of knowledge is as vast as their experience in printing. Their expertise and guidance has proved useful at every step. Their uncompromising quality standards have made this book an exceptional effort. Their encouragement from time to time has been an inspiration for everyone.

The publisher and the editorial board hope that this book will prove to be a valuable piece of knowledge for researchers, students, practitioners and scholars across the globe.

List of Contributors

Chao Wang, Xiao-xia Hou, Hong-liang Rui, Li-jing Li, Jing Zhao, Min Yang, Li-jun Sun, Hong-rui Dong, Hong Cheng and Yi-Pu Chen
Division of Nephrology, Beijing Anzhen Hospital, Capital Medical University, Beijing 100029, China

Yang Long
Department of Endocrinology, Affiliated Hospital of Southwest Medical University, Luzhou, Sichuan 646000, China

Luping Zhou, Ting Zhang, Man Guo, Jingya Ding and Ludan Qin
Department of Endocrinology, Affiliated Hospital of Southwest Medical University, Luzhou, Sichuan 646000, China
The Graduate School of Southwest Medical University, Luzhou, Sichuan 646000, China

Wei Huang and Chenlin Gao
Department of Endocrinology, Affiliated Hospital of Southwest Medical University, Luzhou, Sichuan 646000, China
Faculty of Chinese Medicine, Macau University of Science and Technology, Avenida Wai Long, Taipa, Macau, China
State Key Laboratory of Quality Research in Chinese Medicine, Macau University of Science and Technology, Avenida Wai Long, Taipa, Macau, China

Zihao Xu
The Graduate School of Southwest Medical University, Luzhou, Sichuan 646000, China

Youhua Xu and Yan Liu
Faculty of Chinese Medicine, Macau University of Science and Technology, Avenida Wai Long, Taipa, Macau, China
State Key Laboratory of Quality Research in Chinese Medicine, Macau University of Science and Technology, Avenida Wai Long, Taipa, Macau, China

Yong Xu
Department of Endocrinology, Affiliated Hospital of Southwest Medical University, Luzhou, Sichuan 646000, China
Key Laboratory of Medical Electrophysiology of Ministry of Education, Collaborative Innovation Center for Prevention and Treatment of Cardiovascular Disease of Sichuan Province, Southwest Medical University, Luzhou, Sichuan 646000, China

Wenpeng Cui, Xu Min and Ping Luo
Department of Nephrology, The Second Hospital of Jilin University, Changchun, Jilin 130041, China

Xiaohong Xu
Department of Gynaecology and Obstetrics, The Second Hospital of Jilin University, Changchun, Jilin 130041, China

Bing Du
Department of Cardiology, The First Hospital of Jilin University, Changchun, Jilin 130031, China

Victoria L. Newton, Jonathan D. Guck and Natalie J. Gardiner
Division of Diabetes, Endocrinology and Gastroenterology, School of Medical Sciences, Faculty of Biology, Medicine and Health, University of Manchester, Oxford Road, Manchester M13 9PT, UK

Mary A. Cotter and Norman E. Cameron
School of Medical Sciences, University of Aberdeen, Aberdeen, UK

Hanyu Zhu, Guangyan Cai, Xiangmei Chen, Wenjia Geng, Xiaoli Yang, Minghui Wu and Dong Zhang
Department of Nephrology, Chinese PLA General Hospital, Chinese PLA Institute of Nephrology, State Key Laboratory of Kidney Diseases, National Clinical Research Center of Kidney Diseases, Beijing Key Laboratory of Kidney Disease, Beijing, China

Moyan Liu
Department of Nephrology, General Hospital of Jinan Military Command, Jinan, China

Hanjie Yu, Xiawei Liu, Yaogang Zhong, Jian Shu, Xinle Fu and Zheng Li
Laboratory for Functional Glycomics, College of Life Sciences, Northwest University, Xi'an, China

Liang Ma, Yongwei Jiang, Qian Liu and Yongtong Cao
Clinical Laboratory, China-Japan Friendship Hospital, Beijing, China

Meihua Yan, Tingting Zhao, Hailing Zhao, Haojun Zhang and Ping Li
Beijing Key Lab Immune-Mediated Inflammatory Diseases, Institute of Clinical Medical Science, China-Japan Friendship Hospital, Beijing, China

Xiaomu Kong
Department of Endocrinology, China-Japan Friendship Hospital, Beijing, China

Peng Liu
Graduate School of Peking Union Medical College, Chinese Academy of Medical Sciences and Peking Union Medical College, Beijing, China

Inbal Dahan and Nadia Thawho
Diabetes and Metabolism Lab, The Baruch Padeh Medical Center, Poriya, Lower Galilee, Israel

Farid Nakhoul
Diabetes and Metabolism Lab, The Baruch Padeh Medical Center, Poriya, Lower Galilee, Israel
Nephrology and Hypertension Division, The Baruch Padeh Medical Center, Poriya, Lower Galilee, Israel
The Azrieli Faculty of Medicine in Zfat in the Galilee, Bar-Ilan University, Ramat-Gan, Israel

Evgeny Farber
Nephrology and Hypertension Division, The Baruch Padeh Medical Center, Poriya, Lower Galilee, Israel

Nakhoul Nakhoul
The Azrieli Faculty of Medicine in Zfat in the Galilee, Bar-Ilan University, Ramat-Gan, Israel

Rabea Asleh and Andrew P. Levy
The Vascular Medicine Lab, Technion, Faculty of Medicine, Rappaport Institute, Haifa, Israel

Yan Chun Li
Department of Medicine, The University of Chicago, Chicago, IL 60637, USA

Ofer Ben-Izhak
Department of Pathology, Rambam Health Care Campus, Haifa, Israel
Technion, Haifa, Israel

Hailing Zhao, Meihua Yan, Tingting Zhao, Haojun Zhang, Yanzhen Liu and Ping Li
Beijing Key Lab for Immune-Mediated Inflammatory Diseases, Institute of Clinical Medical Science, China-Japan Friendship Hospital, Beijing, China

Liang Ma
Clinical Laboratory, China-Japan Friendship Hospital, Beijing, China

Yan Wang and Peng Liu
Beijing Key Lab for Immune-Mediated Inflammatory Diseases, Institute of Clinical Medical Science, China-Japan Friendship Hospital, Beijing, China
Graduate School of Peking Union Medical College, Chinese Academy of Medical Science and Peking Union Medical College, Beijing, China

Jing Sun, Yangwei Wang, Wenpeng Cui, Yan Lou, Guangdong Sun, Dongmei Zhang and Lining Miao
Department of Nephrology, Second Hospital of Jilin University, Changchun 130041, China

Luigi Rossi, Antonella Di Franco, Francesca Indrio, Rossella Lella, Luigi Laviola, Francesco Giorgino and Loreto Gesualdo
DETO, University of Bari, Bari, Italy

Maria Celeste Nicoletti, Monica Carmosino, Lisa Mastrofrancesco, Maria Svelto and Giuseppe Procino
Department of Biosciences, Biotechnologies and Biopharmaceutics, University of Bari, Bari, Italy

Haoran Dai
Department of Nephrology, Shunyi Branch, Beijing Hospital of Traditional Chinese Medicine, Station East 5, Shunyi District, Beijing 101300, China

Qingquan Liu and Baoli Liu
Department of Nephrology, Shunyi Branch, Beijing Hospital of Traditional Chinese Medicine, Station East 5, Shunyi District, Beijing 101300, China
Beijing Hospital of Traditional Chinese Medicine Affiliated to Capital Medical University, 23 Meishuguanhou Street, Dongcheng District, Beijing 100010, China

Yu Yang
Department of Endocrinology, Metabolism, and Genetics, Jiangxi Provincial Children's Hospital, Nanchang, Jiangxi, China

Hui Huang
Department of Endocrinology, Metabolism, and Genetics, Jiangxi Provincial Children's Hospital, Nanchang, Jiangxi, China
Pediatric Research Institute, Department of Pediatrics, University of Louisville, Louisville, KY, USA

Zheng Xu
Pediatric Research Institute, Department of Pediatrics, University of Louisville, Louisville, KY, USA
Department of Cardiovascular Disorders, The First Hospital of Jilin University, Changchun, China

Jun-kai Duan
Department of Cardiovascular Disorders, Jiangxi Provincial Children's Hospital, Nanchang, Jiangxi, China

Yingying Zhang, Siqi Zhao, Depei Wu, Xingmei Liu, Mingjun Shi, Yuanyuan Wang, Fan Zhang, Jing Ding, Ying Xiao and Bing Guo
Department of Pathophysiology, Guizhou Medical University, Guiyang, Guizhou 550025, China
Laboratory of Pathogenesis Research, Drug Prevention and Treatment of Major Diseases, Guizhou Medical University, Guiyang, Guizhou 550025, China

Bancha Satirapoj
Division of Nephrology, Department of Medicine, Phramongkutklao Hospital and College of Medicine, Bangkok, Thailand

Elena Guillén-Gómez
Molecular Biology Laboratory, Fundació Puigvert, Barcelona, Spain
Universitat Autònoma de Barcelona, Institut d'Investigació Biomèdica Sant Pau (IIB Sant Pau), Barcelona, Spain

Beatriz Bardají-de-Quixano
Universitat Autònoma de Barcelona, Institut d'Investigació Biomèdica Sant Pau (IIB Sant Pau), Barcelona, Spain
Renal Transplantation Unit, Nephrology Department, Fundació Puigvert, Barcelona, Spain

Sílvia Ferrer
Maragall Primary Health Care Center, Barcelona, Spain

Carlos Brotons
Universitat Autònoma de Barcelona, Institut d'Investigació Biomèdica Sant Pau (IIB Sant Pau), Barcelona, Spain
Sardenya Primary Health Care Center, Barcelona, Spain

Mark A. Knepper
Epithelial Systems Biology Laboratory, National Heart, Lung, and Blood Institute (NIH), Bethesda, MD, USA

Montserrat Carrascal and Joaquin Abian
Proteomics Laboratory CSIC/UAB, Institut d'Investigacions Biomèdiques de Barcelona (IIBB-CSIC-IDIBAPS), Barcelona, Spain

José M. Mas
Anaxomics Biotech SL, Barcelona, Spain

Francesca Calero, José A. Ballarín and Patricia Fernández-Llama
Universitat Autònoma de Barcelona, Institut d'Investigació Biomèdica Sant Pau (IIB Sant Pau), Barcelona, Spain
Hypertension Unit, Nephrology Department, Fundació Puigvert, Barcelona, Spain

Shaozhang Hou, Ting Zhang and Fengying Guo
Department of Pathology, School of Basic Medical Sciences, Ningxia Medical University, Yinchuan 750004, China
Institute of Basic Medical Sciences, Ningxia Medical University, Yinchuan 750004, China

Yuan Li
Department of Nursing, Ningxia Medical University, Yinchuan 750004, China

Xiu Jin
Affiliated Hospital of Jining Medical College, Jining 272000, China

Xue Mei Fan, Chun Lian Huang, Yi Ming Wang and Qiong Lin Liang
Beijing Key Laboratory of Bioorganic Phosphorus Chemistry & Chemical Biology (Ministry of Education), Department of Chemistry, Tsinghua University, Beijing, China

Ning Li
School of Pharmacy, China Pharmaceutical University, Nanjing, China

Guo An Luo
Beijing Key Laboratory of Bioorganic Phosphorus Chemistry & Chemical Biology (Ministry of Education), Department of Chemistry, Tsinghua University, Beijing, China
State Key Laboratory for Quality Research in Chinese Medicines, Macau University of Science and Technology, Macau, China

Thomas Albrecht, Jana D. Braun, Angelica Rodriquez, Jiedong Qiu, Alexander Lammert, Hannes Köppel, Peter Schnuelle, Bernhard K. Krämer, Benito A. Yard and Sibylle J. Hauske
Fifth Medical Department (Nephrology/Endocrinology/Rheumatology), University Medical Center Mannheim, University of Heidelberg, Mannheim, Germany

Shiqi Zhang and Li Xia
Fifth Medical Department (Nephrology/Endocrinology/Rheumatology), University Medical Center Mannheim, University of Heidelberg, Mannheim, Germany
Department of Endocrinology, The First Affiliated Hospital of Anhui Medical University, Hefei, China

Verena Peters and Claus P. Schmitt
Centre for Pediatric and Adolescent Medicine, University of Heidelberg, Heidelberg, Germany

Jacob van den Born and Stephan J. L. Bakker
Nephrology, University Medical Center Groningen, University of Groningen, Groningen, Netherlands

Manal S. Fawzy
Department of Biochemistry, Faculty of Medicine, Northern Border University, Arar, Saudi Arabia
Department of Medical Biochemistry, Faculty of Medicine, Suez Canal University, Ismailia, Egypt

Baraah T. Abu AlSel
Department of Microbiology, Faculty of Medicine, Northern Border University, Arar, Saudi Arabia

Caipan Gong, Li Li, Weihua Wu, Qi Liu, Ying Li, Linwang Gan and Santao Ou
Department of Nephrology, The Affiliated Hospital of Southwest Medical University, Luzhou, Sichuan 646000, China

Chunmei Qin
Department of Nephrology, Luzhou People's Hospital, Luzhou, Sichuan 646000, China

Xuehai Chen, Jiao Luo, Minmin Wu, Zhuo Pan, Yue Xie and Hongwei Wang
Department of Surgery, The First Affiliated Hospital of Wenzhou Medical University, Wenzhou, Zhejiang 325000, China

Bicheng Chen
Department of Surgery, The First Affiliated Hospital of Wenzhou Medical University, Wenzhou, Zhejiang 325000, China
Zhejiang Provincial Top Key Discipline in Surgery, Wenzhou Key Laboratory of Surgery, Department of Surgery, The First Affiliated Hospital of Wenzhou Medical University, Wenzhou, Zhejiang 325000, China

Hong Zhu
Department of Endocrinology, The First Affiliated Hospital of Wenzhou Medical University, Wenzhou, Zhejiang 325000, China

Index

P

R

S

T

U

V

W

www.ingramcontent.com/pod-product-compliance
Lightning Source LLC
LaVergne TN
LVHW060518210926
848485LV00005B/1103
* 9 7 8 1 6 3 9 2 7 1 1 4 6 *